GLOBAL MENTAL HEALTH
PRINCIPLES AND PRACTICE

Edited by

Vikram Patel, MRCPsych, PhD, FMedSci

Centre for Global Mental Health
London School of Hygiene and Tropical Medicine
London, United Kingdom;
Sangath, Goa, India; and
Centre for Mental Health Public Health Foundation of India
New Delhi, India

Harry Minas, MBBS, BMedSc, DPM, FRANZCP

Centre for International Mental Health
School of Population and Global Health
The University of Melbourne
Parkville, Victoria, Australia

Alex Cohen, PhD

Centre for Global Mental Health
London School of Hygiene & Tropical Medicine
London, United Kingdom

Martin J. Prince, MD, FRCPsych

Centre for Global Mental Health
London School of Hygiene & Tropical Medicine
London, United Kingdom

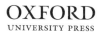

OXFORD
UNIVERSITY PRESS

OXFORD
UNIVERSITY PRESS

Oxford University Press is a department of the University of Oxford.
It furthers the University's objective of excellence in research, scholarship,
and education by publishing worldwide.

Oxford   New York
Auckland   Cape Town   Dar es Salaam   Hong Kong   Karachi
Kuala Lumpur   Madrid   Melbourne   Mexico City   Nairobi
New Delhi   Shanghai   Taipei   Toronto

With offices in
Argentina   Austria   Brazil   Chile   Czech Republic   France   Greece
Guatemala   Hungary   Italy   Japan   Poland   Portugal   Singapore
South Korea   Switzerland   Thailand   Turkey   Ukraine   Vietnam

Oxford is a registered trademark of Oxford University Press in the UK
and certain other countries.

Published in the United States of America by
Oxford University Press
198 Madison Avenue, New York, NY 10016

Library of Congress Cataloging-in-Publication Data
Global mental health : principles and practice / edited by
Vikram Patel, Harry Minas, Alex Cohen, Martin J. Prince.
     p. ; cm.
Includes bibliographical references and index.
ISBN 978–0–19–992018–1 (alk. paper)
I. Patel, Vikram, editor of compilation.   II. Minas, I. H. (I. Harry), editor of compilation.
III. Cohen, Alex, 1950–editor of compilation.   IV. Prince, Martin (Martin James), 1960– editor of
compilation.
[DNLM: 1. Mental Health Services.   2. Health Services Accessibility.   3. Mental Disorders.
4. World Health. WM 30.1]
RA790.5
362.19689—dc23
2013011540

9 8 7 6 5 4 3 2 1
Printed in the United States of America
on acid-free paper

Global
Mental Health

Contents

Contributors

Jordi Alonso, MD, PhD
Health Services Research Unit
Institut Hospital del Mar
   d'Investigacions Mèdiques
Barcelona, Spain

Jude Awuba, MPH
Office for Research on Disparities
   and Global Mental Health
National Institute of Mental Health
National Institutes of Health
Bethesda, Maryland

Margaret Barry, PhD
World Health Organization
   Collaborating Centre for Health
   Promotion Research
School of Health Sciences
National University of Ireland
Galway, Ireland

Pierre Bastin, MD
International Committee of the
   Red Cross
Geneva, Switzerland

Arvin Bhana, PhD
Department of Psychology
University of KwaZulu-Natal
Berea, South Africa

Grant Blashki, MD, FRACGP
Nossal Institute for Global Health
Melbourne School of Population
   and Global Health
The University of Melbourne
Parkville, Victoria, Australia

**José Miguel Caldas de Almeida,
   MD, PhD**
Department of Psychiatry and
   Mental Health
New University of Lisbon
   Medical School
Lisbon, Portugal

Meena Cabral de Mello, PsyD
Department of Child and Adolescent
   Health and Development
World Health Organization
Geneva, Switzerland

Claudina Cayetano, MD
Pan American Health Organization /
   World Health Organization
Panama City, Panama

Prabha S. Chandra, MD, FRCPsych
Department of Psychiatry
National Institute of Mental Health and
   Neurosciences
Bangalore, India

Somnath Chatterji
Multi-Country Studies
Health Statistics and Information Systems
World Health Organization
Geneva, Switzerland

Alex Cohen, PhD
Centre for Global Mental Health
London School of Hygiene & Tropical
   Medicine
London, United Kingdom

Pamela Y. Collins, MD, MPH
Office for Research on Disparities and
    Global Mental Health
Office of Rural Mental Health Research
National Institute of Mental Health
National Institutes of Health
Bethesda, Maryland

Mario R. Dal Poz, MD, PhD
Social Medicine Institute
University of the State of Rio de Janeiro
Rio de Janeiro, Brazil

Amy M. Daniels, PhD
Autism Speaks
New York, New York

Mary De Silva, PhD
Centre for Global Mental Health
London School of Hygiene and Tropical
    Medicine
London, United Kingdom

Julian Eaton, MRCPsych
CBM International
Lomé, Togo

Abebaw Fekadu, MRCPsych, MD, PhD
Addis Ababa University
Addis Ababa, Ethiopia

Jane Fisher, PhD
School of Public Health and Preventive
    Medicine
Monash University
Clayton, Victoria, Australia

Ana Soledade Graeff-Martins, MD, DSc
Department of Psychiatry
Universidade de São Paulo
São Paulo, Brazil

Oye Gureje, PhD, DSc
Department of Psychiatry
University of Ibadan
Ibadan, Nigeria

Hesham Hamoda, MD, MPH
Department of Psychiatry
Children's Hospital, Boston
Harvard Medical School
Boston, Massachusetts

Charlotte Hanlon, MRCPsych, PhD
Department of Psychiatry
Addis Ababa University
Addis Ababa, Ethiopia

Yanling He, MD
Department of Psychiatry
Shanghai Jiao Tong University
School of Medicine
Shanghai Mental Health Center
Shanghai, China

Helen Herrman, MD
Department of Psychiatry
Centre for Youth Mental Health
University of Melbourne
Parkville, Victoria, Australia

Mark J. D. Jordans, PhD
Department of Research and
    Development
HealthNet TPO
Amsterdam, The Netherlands

Ritsuko Kakuma, PhD
Centre for International Mental Health
School of Population and
    Global Health
The University of Melbourne
Parkville, Victoria, Australia

Ronald C. Kessler, PhD
Department of Health Care Policy
Harvard Medical School
Boston, Massachusetts

Christian Kieling, MD
Department of Psychiatry
Hospital de Clinicas de Porto
    Alegre; and
Universidade Federal do Rio
    Grande do Sul
Porto Alegre, Brazil

Laurence J. Kirmayer, MD, FRCPC
Division of Social and Transcultural
    Psychiatry
McGill University
Montreal, Quebec, Canada

Crick Lund, PhD
Alan J. Flisher Centre for Public
    Mental Health
Department of Psychiatry and
    Mental Health
University of Cape Town
Cape Town, South Africa

John Mahoney
Centre for International Mental Health
School of Population and Global Health
The University of Melbourne
Parkville, Victoria, Australia

Pallab K. Maulik, MD, PhD
George Institute for Global Health
Hyderabad, India

Rosie Mayston, PhD
Centre for Global Mental Health
Institute of Psychiatry
King's College London
London, United Kingdom

Ryan McBain
Department of Global Health and
    Population
Harvard School of Public Health
Boston, Massachusetts

Nisha Mehta, MBBS
Health Service and Population Research
    Department
King's College London, Institute of
    Psychiatry
London, United Kingdom

**Harry Minas, MBBS, BMedSc, DPM,
    FRANZCP**
Centre for International Mental Health
School of Population and Global Health
The University of Melbourne
Parkville, Victoria, Australia

Jodi Morris, PhD
Department of Psychology
University of British Columbia
Kelowna, British Columbia, Canada

**Vikram Patel, MRCPsych, PhD,
    FMedSci**
Centre for Global Mental Health
London School of Hygiene and Tropical
    Medicine
London, United Kingdom
Sangath, Goa, India; and
Centre for Mental Health Public Health
    Foundation of India
New Delhi, India

Inge Petersen, PhD
School of Psychology
University of KwaZulu-Natal
Berea, South Africa

Martin J. Prince, MD, FRCPsych
Centre for Global Mental Health
Institute of Psychiatry
King's College London
London, United Kingdom

Atif Rahman, PhD
Institute of Psychology Health and
    Society
University of Liverpool
Liverpool, United Kingdom

Luis Augusto Rohde, MD, PhD
Department of Psychiatry
Hospital de Clinicas de Porto
    Alegre; and
Universidade Federal do Rio
    Grande do Sul
Porto Alegre, Brazil

Graciela Rojas, MD
Department of Psychiatry and
    Mental Health
University of Chile
Santiago, Chile

Renato Souza, MD
Hospital das Clinicas da Faculdade
    de Medicina
Universidade de São Paulo
São Paulo, Brazil

Stephen Stansfeld, MBBS, PhD, MRCP, FRCPsych
Centre for Psychiatry
Wolfson Institute of Preventive
 Medicine; and
Barts and the London School of
 Medicine and Dentistry
Queen Mary University
 of London
London, United Kingdom

Dan J. Stein, MD, PhD
Department of Psychiatry and
 Mental Health
University of Cape Town
Cape Town, South Africa

Leslie Swartz, PhD
Department of Psychology
Stellenbosch University
Matieland, South Africa

Graham Thornicroft, MBBS, PhD, FRCPsych, FAcadMed
Centre for Global Mental
 Health
Health Service and Population Research
 Department
King's College London, Institute of
 Psychiatry
London, United Kingdom

Wietse A. Tol, PhD
Johns Hopkins Bloomberg School of
 Public Health
Baltimore, Maryland

Mark Tomlinson, PhD
Department of Psychology
Stellenbosch University
Stellenbosch, South Africa

Mark Van Ommeren, PhD
Department of Mental Health and
 Substance Abuse
World Health Organization
Geneva, Switzerland

Inka Weissbecker, PhD
International Medical Corps
Washington DC, District of Columbia

Benedict Weobong
Sangath, Goa, India; and the
London School of Hygiene and Tropical
 Medicine
London, United Kingdom

Harvey Whiteford, MBBS, MPH, DUniv, FRANZCP, FAFPM
Departments of Psychiatry and
 Population Health
University of Queensland
The Park, Queensland, Australia

Preface

Global health has been defined as "an area for study, research and practice that places a priority on improving health and achieving equity in health for all people worldwide"[1]. Global mental health is the pursuit of the same objectives in the domain of mental health. The global situation for people with mental disorders is in urgent need of substantial improvement, particularly in low-resource, post-conflict and post-disaster settings. Legislative and human rights protections are frequently lacking, and people with mental disorders experience stigma and discrimination, are frequently excluded from education, housing, employment and other benefits of citizenship, and live impoverished and marginalized lives. There are insufficient human resources and services, and those that do exist are often concentrated in urban centers. In most of the world mental health and social care services are inaccessible or of poor quality.

The emergence of the discipline of global mental health can be traced to a long and distinguished history of inter-disciplinary research and development. In recent years, several major developments have shaped and supported the growth of the discipline. These have included the demonstration of the burden and impact of mental disorders in all countries; the World Health Organization's Mental Health Gap Action Program that synthesized evidence on effective treatments for mental disorders in non-specialized health care settings; the evidence supporting the effectiveness of the delivery of these treatments by non-specialist health workers; the emergence of civil society platforms, such as the Movement for Global Mental Health; the establishment of research priorities in the field, notably the Grand Challenges in Global Mental Health, which are now backed by major new funding; and the strengthening of political commitment in many countries, and at the global level as exemplified by the WHO's global mental health action plan in May 2013, to invest in mental health.

While there is increasing acknowledgment of the importance of mental disorders for global health and development, there is a need to further develop both the scientific foundations of global mental health and the practical methods for implementing and scaling up mental health programs. This textbook is organized around these two inter-connected needs - scientific foundations and practice. The 20 chapters comprehensively review the discipline, first outlining the principles of global mental health and then considering key areas of practice. The 54 authors are drawn from 18 countries and reflect the rich contribution to the discipline by scholars and practitioners from every continent. While the discipline is global in its ambition, the textbook emphasizes the most pressing issues pertaining to low and middle income countries. Each chapter synthesizes the available evidence, illustrated with case studies where appropriate, and considers practical implications. The language and content is accessible to all with an interest in the field and does not assume specialised knowledge.

Global mental health is the discipline which seeks to address one of the most neglected global health issues of our times. It is also one of the most exciting and dynamic disciplines of global health, with the rapidly increasing involvement of researchers, practitioners, advocates, funding agencies and, most importantly, people who live with a mental disorder and their families and friends. However, it is still early in the life of this discipline. We hope this textbook will inform and inspire students and practitioners to contribute to the continued growth of global mental health, to ensure that it remains a vibrant and indispensible part of global health, and to contribute to improving the lives of people who are now among the most neglected and vulnerable throughout the world.

Vikram Patel, Harry Minas, Alex Cohen and Martin J. Prince
June 2013

PART ONE
PRINCIPLES OF GLOBAL MENTAL HEALTH

1 A Brief History of Global Mental Health

Alex Cohen, Vikram Patel, and
Harry Minas

Before the year 2001, the term *global mental health* was used to denote a measure of the overall level of stress (primarily depression and anxiety) in a given population.[1] To the best of our knowledge, David Satcher, then Surgeon General of the United States, was the first to use the phrase to denote a field within public health. His commentary, *Global Mental Health: Its Time Has Come*,[2] anticipated the publication of the World Health Organization's *World Health Report 2001*, which was devoted to mental health.[3] However, the term was not in general usage until 2007 when *The Lancet* used it to name one of the series the journal commissions "to highlight clinically important topics and areas of health and medicine often overlooked by mainstream research programmes and other medical publications."[4] Soon thereafter, the phrase began to be used widely, and, in 2010, *global mental health* was declared to be an emerging field within global health, one that aimed to improve treatments, increase access to services, and reduce human rights abuses of people experiencing mental disorders.[5]

THE ANCIENT WORLD

Despite the apparent newness of global mental health as a field, concerns about mental disorders—for example, explanatory models and approaches to treatment—have been circulating the globe for thousands of years. Although we do not know the extent to which the scholars and physicians of ancient China, India, and Greece communicated or were familiar with the teachings of the others, it is indeed striking that their theories of disease, and thus mental disorders, were similarly based on the idea that imbalances in life forces were the causes of disease; for example, the *yin* and *yang* of traditional Chinese medicine,[6] the humoral theories of disease posited in Ayurvedic medicine,[7] and the Hippocratic traditions of ancient Greece.[8] Furthermore, similar explanatory models gave rise to the development of similar, physiologically based treatments: traditional Chinese medicine offered herbal potions and acupuncture;[9] Ayurveda offered massage and Yoga;[7] and, the Hippocratic tradition offered massage, baths, balanced diet, and exercise.[10]

THE DEVELOPMENT OF INSTITUTIONAL CARE

In the world of antiquity—ancient Egypt, Greece, Rome, and the Judeo-Christian Middle East—from the time of the oldest written accounts of mental disorders (ca. twentieth century BCE)[11] to the establishment of the first general hospitals by Islamic physicians in the eighth century CE,[12] care of persons with mental disorders was the legal responsibility of families.[10] The only "institutional" care that existed took place when families brought ill members to temples, churches, or other places of religious or spiritual importance.[8,12*] For example, in ancient Greece, people worshipped at the "grave sites of…mythological and mythohistorical figures" in the belief that this would cure illnesses.[8†]

Although there are accounts from as early as the third century CE of the confinement of mentally ill people in Syrian Catholic churches, true institutional care appeared somewhat later in the Islamic world of the Middle East and North Africa. Indeed, "the special provision for the insane [was] a remarkable aspect" of the medieval Islamic medical tradition."[13] In contrast to the earlier Christian custom of utilizing exorcism to cure mental disorders,[12] Islamic physicians followed Greek medical teachings and focused on the physical causes of disease and emphasized physiological, rather than spiritual, treatments.[13]

There is general agreement that medieval Islamic hospitals were distinguished by "relaxed atmospheres," which featured fountains and gardens and treatments that included baths, bloodletting, leeches, cupping, a variety of drugs, and careful attention to diet.[13] In addition, psychosocial interventions, such as dancing, singing, and theater, were employed. At the same time, however, chaining or shackling of patients was common and, perhaps, necessary (see below).

When considering the Islamic hospitals, one must be cautious on five counts. First, there is some disagreement about when and where the first institutional care for persons with mental disorders was established. By some accounts, the first asylums were established early in the eighth century in Fez and Bagdad,[14] and perhaps as early as the seventh century.[15] However, other accounts maintain that although the first Islamic general hospital was established in Damascus in 707 CE, the earliest institutional care for mentally ill persons only took place somewhat later, in a Cairo hospital that was founded in 872 CE.[12]

Second, there is some question about the extent to which the Islamic hospitals were unique. For example, these institutions may have owed much of their development to charitable traditions in Eastern Christianity,[16] and it was certainly the case that people with mental disorders were often confined in churches as a form of treatment,[12] a practice that may have emerged from earlier, similar practices in Greece and Rome.[15]

Third, even with the establishment of hospitals, the care of persons with mental disorders remained, above all, the responsibility of their families and took place at home.[12] The Islamic hospitals "were intended primarily for the poor" who could not be maintained at home because their families were not able to afford the necessary "expensive drugs [and] medical care."

---

* In the remainder of the world, China, South Asia, sub-Saharan Africa, and South America, the care of persons with mental illness probably did not become "institutionalized" until the advent of colonial psychiatry (see below).

† Such practices were also followed in medieval Christian Europe, most famously at the Church of St. Dymphna in Geel, Belgium. Today, Islamic *dargahs*—shrines to deceased religious figures—continue to be sites where people seek spiritual cures for mental disorders.

Fourth, it is not clear whether psychiatric care and treatment took place in institutions devoted exclusively to the care and treatment of persons with mental disorders, in divisions within general hospitals, or both.[12,13,17] It is also possible that the institutional treatment of persons with mental disorders first took place within general hospitals and that, over time, the services expanded and evolved into stand-alone psychiatric facilities. Further investigations of the historical record are necessary to determine where, how, and why hospitals for persons with mental disorders came into existence.

Fifth, although it is generally believed that the Islamic hospitals provided humane care,[17] a sixteenth-century account of a facility in Constantinople described horrendous conditions in which patients were beaten, chained, and displayed for "public amusement."[18‡] However, one historian has conjectured, "The harsh conditions of the asylum should not be misconstrued....The chains and irons...were simply necessary devices to prevent harm to the insane or to others." Whether such practices were forms of abuse or benign protection remains an open question.[13]

Whatever proves to be the precise history of the development of institutional care in the centuries that saw the decline of the Roman Empire and the rise of Christianity and Islam in the Middle East, it is certainly true that by the thirteenth century, institutional care for persons with mental disorders could be found from Damascus in the east to Fez in the west.[20] This approach to the care and treatment of persons with mental disorders expanded north with the Moorish invasion of Spain in the first few decades of the eighth century.[21] Historical research suggests that institutional care for persons with mental disorders was probably established only in the fourteenth century, when Sultan Mohammed I founded a hospital in Granada that took in persons with mental disorders.[15] Moreover, such institutions were not unique to the Islamic regions of Spain. Psychiatric facilities were established in Catholic regions as well: in Valencia (1409), Saragossa (1435), Seville (1436), Toledo (1483), Valladolid (1489), Granada (1507), and Madrid (1540). Then, in 1567, this tradition was brought across the Atlantic when a psychiatric hospital was established in Mexico. This was the first institution of its kind in the Western Hemisphere, the first instance of what would later be called "colonial psychiatry," and the first truly global expansion of institutional mental health care.

However, contrary to claims that Spain was the site of the first European institutions to provide treatment and care for persons with mental disorders,[22] there is evidence that institutional care began to appear in Europe two or three centuries after the establishment of the Islamic hospitals in the Middle East and prior to those in Spain. According to one account, institutions for the treatment and care of persons with mental disorders were established in: Metz (France), Milan (Italy), and Ghent (Flanders) (twelfth century); Uppsala (Sweden), Bergamo (Italy), Elbing (Germany) London (England),§ and Florence (Italy) (fourteenth century); and Bruges, Mons, and Antwerp (Flanders) (fifteenth century).[15,23] Psychiatric institutions were not founded in Scandinavia until the eighteenth century when a "madhouse" was established in Sweden** and a Norwegian royal ordinance decreed that hospitals must set aside beds for the purpose of treating mentally ill persons.[24] The extent to which the model for these hospitals was based on a tradition of Christian charity or was a product of earlier Islamic practices in Spain—or some combination of both—remains to be determined.[25]

The Aztec, Mayan, and Incan empires of Central and South America were roughly contemporaneous to the rise and expansion of institutional care in the Middle East,

---

‡ In London at about the same time, paying to view the mad inmates of Bethlem Hospital was a popular pastime, too.[19]

§ This was Bethlem Hospital, which became the very symbol of the horrendous conditions in institutions for people with mental disorders and whose name was transformed into the term *bedlam*.

** Readers will notice the contradictory statements about when the first institutions for persons with mental disorders were established in Sweden. This points to the need for more historical research.

North Africa, and Europe. However, the relative lack of written records and the need to rely on the accounts of Spanish explorers and missionaries leaves little reliable evidence about the treatment and care of persons with mental disorders in that part of the world. There is physical evidence that trephination[††] was practiced, but we cannot be certain of its purpose. The utilization of psychotropic and hallucinogens was apparently widespread, as were religious practices, baths, bloodletting, and fasting.[26]

The lack of written records also means that we know little about the treatment of mental disorders among the peoples of sub-Saharan Africa before the onslaught of European colonialism. What we do know about traditional practices stems mostly from studies conducted since the middle of the twentieth century. Although much of this work has made claims for the effectiveness of traditional practices, there is little systematic evidence to support those conclusions and much evidence that contradicts it.[27] The relative effectiveness of traditional practices remains an important topic for future research.

About 200 years after the establishment of a mental asylum in Mexico, hospital care for mentally ill persons was initiated in Pennsylvania Hospital in Philadelphia,[28] and the first mental asylum in North America opened in 1773 in the Colony of Virginia.[29‡‡] This was followed in the first half of the nineteenth century with the establishment, first, of private and then, later, state-run psychiatric hospitals throughout the United States. In Canada, a hospital in Quebec may have started admitting mentally ill persons as early as 1714, but the establishment of psychiatric asylums in most provinces only took place in the decades following 1840.[30]

The developments in North America closely paralleled those taking place at the same time in Europe.[31] For example, although institutional care for mentally ill persons in England can be traced to the fifteenth century,[32] the great expansion of public asylums in England began in 1808 with the County Asylums Act.[31] France established a state-run system of asylums in 1838,[33] and between 1830 and 1850, Christian religious orders in Belgium opened 18 asylums.[23]

This all-too-brief account of the globalization of institutional treatment and care for persons with mental disorders might make it appear that the progression from a few Islamic hospitals that appeared beginning in the ninth century, to the many huge asylums of Europe, North America, and elsewhere in the nineteenth and twentieth centuries was a process that, once started, was inevitable.[28] However, there was a moment in the mid-nineteenth century when the future of the asylum was questioned and the merits of an alternative were considered. The debate was set off, at least in part, by overcrowding and the expense of state-run asylum systems.[32] Together, these concerns prompted a global search for solutions.

Ironically, the search focused on a system of care that had its origins in the medieval Flemish village of Geel, where, beginning in the fourteenth century, Christian pilgrims came to pray at the shrine of St. Dymphna, the patron saint of the insane.[23] During the ensuing centuries, and as increasing numbers of pilgrims came to and stayed in Geel, a system was established whereby families in the village were being paid to take in mentally ill "boarders." This became, in effect, the first program of foster care for mentally ill persons and is cited as the first example of a community mental health program.[34§§]

[††] The surgical practice of drilling a hole into the skull. It is believed that this was done to relieve a person of "evil spirits."

[‡‡] Prior to the founding of these institutions, many mentally ill persons in North America had been placed in almshouses, a strategy that was also followed in Britain and Europe.

[§§] One must be cautious about being overly idealistic about Geel. One observer has noted: "To generations of psychiatrists Geel has served as an image of the humanitarian and compassionate care of mentally ill people.... [It] has also served as an inspiration if not a model for family care programs in Europe and North America. Viewed from afar, programs take on a halo effect, while neighbors view them more realistically and with less reverence...." (Hewitt RT. Family care after a thousand years. *Am J Psychiatry* 1962;119:120–21).

As asylums became ever more overcrowded and expensive to maintain, and as the accumulation of chronic cases became more of a problem, people began to search for alternatives to institutional care, and the system in Geel became of increasing interest. In English and French medical journals of the 1850s and 1860s, one can find dozens of accounts of visits to Geel by physicians and asylum superintendents. One can also find reports of debates in London[35] and Paris[36] about whether versions of the Geel system could or should be adapted elsewhere. In the United States, a fierce debate in the late 1860s contested whether a modification of the Geel system would be implemented at the State Lunatic Hospital at Worcester, Massachusetts.[37] All of these debates ended in the same way: support for the continued expansion of hospitals won out, while explorations of an alternative were abandoned. As a result, considerations of community care for persons with mental disorders did not reemerge, for all practical purposes, until the 1950s.

The debate about the future of the asylum, and its aftermath, took place at much the same time that the European powers were colonizing great regions of Africa and Asia. With this came the spread of Western psychiatry and the establishment of mental asylums across much of the globe. A full account of colonial psychiatry is not possible here, but some brief comments are necessary. First, for example, beginning toward the end of the eighteenth century and continuing until the early twentieth century, British authorities established asylums in India,[38] Singapore,[39] South Africa,[40] and Nigeria.[41]**** Second, the establishment of these institutions meant that the essential feature of the mental health systems of Europe—the large, custodial asylum—became the dominant feature of the mental health systems of the colonies. In fact, the *idea* that asylums provided efficacious treatments extended to countries that never were colonized. For example, Japan established its first asylum in 1879,[43] and Thailand did the same 10 years later.[44] Third, the end of colonialism, mostly in the late 1950s and early 1960s, took place at the very same time that community-based mental health systems were being developed in Western Europe and North America. This left little opportunity for the development of alternatives, and psychiatric hospitals continue to dominate what exists of many mental health systems in low-income countries.[45,46]

DECLINE OF THE ASYLUM AND DEINSTITUTIONALIZATION

For most of the nineteenth century, medical superintendents of asylums had, at least in the United States and Britain, maintained that early recognition of and treatment for (i.e., institutionalization) mental illness resulted in high rates of cure. However, doubts about the "curability of insanity" began to appear in the second half of the nineteenth century and diminished earlier optimism about the efficacy of institutional care.[47] As early as 1857, *The Lancet* published commentaries that were critical of asylum care.[48] More damaging to the image of asylums was a series of essays by Pliny Earle, the superintendent of an asylum in Northampton, Massachusetts, who demonstrated that hospital statistics had conflated discharges and cures and, thus, that presented rates of cure that were greatly overestimated.[49,50] This disclosure, along with the resultant disillusionment and the introduction of psychoanalytic approaches to the treatment of non-psychotic disorders, meant that the discipline of psychiatry increasingly turned away from institutional care and, instead, emphasized office-based practice that provided services to "a more treatable, more affluent clientele."[51] Although the recognition that institutional care did not promote cures and was, in fact, associated with generally poor conditions, the numbers of people hospitalized for mental disorders continued to increase in the industrialized world throughout

---

**** In contrast, the French followed another, perhaps worse, strategy; instead of founding an asylum, the colonial authorities sent mentally ill Algerians to asylums in France where they were not only badly treated but also removed from anything familiar.[42]

the first half of the twentieth century.[29,52] For example, in Britain, the number of patients in psychiatric hospitals peaked at 148,100 in 1954,[53] and, in the United States, the number of persons in psychiatric hospitals reached 559,000 in 1955.[54]

Following World War II, institutional care, a practice that for more than 1,000 years had played an important role in the treatment of persons with mental disorders, began to be considered, at least in many of the industrialized nations of the West, as both ineffective and inhumane. This change in perspectives came about as the result of several factors:

1. increased belief in the efficacy of care that took place in the community;[55,56]
2. a growing awareness of abusive conditions in many psychiatric hospitals and that the effects of long-term institutionalization were at least as harmful as chronic mental disorder itself;[53,57]
3. the expense of caring for patients in large institutions;[53,58]
4. the discovery in 1954 of chlorpromazine, the first effective anti-psychotic medication, which offered people with chronic mental disorders the prospect of living in the community rather than in institutions;[57] and,
5. an increasing appreciation of the civil and human rights of persons with mental disorders.[55]

As a result of these factors, psychiatric hospitals in many Western industrialized countries, as well as in several countries of South America, were either downsized or closed.[52,59] These changes came to be known as *deinstitutionalization*, and community services became the principal approach to care. However, this change did not happen everywhere. The number of hospital beds has continued to increase in Japan, for example, and institutional care remains dominant in many low- and middle-income countries.[45]

There is wide acknowledgement that deinstitutionalization only partly achieved its aims. Too often, patients in hospitals were discharged without proper planning or sufficient resources to support their living in the community. As a result, many discharged patients were simply transferred to other types of institutions, such as prisons, forensic hospitals, and supportive housing.[59] In the United States, the results of deinstitutionalization have been especially mixed. Although it has resulted in the development of community services, a lack of community mental health centers and supportive services has meant that large numbers of mentally ill persons became homeless, entered the legal system and were imprisoned, or now live in adult homes that recreate the very worst aspects of the old asylums.[60,61] Thus, the neglect and abuses that had characterized the institutional care of the past were replaced all too frequently by comparative neglect in the community.[62]

COMMUNITY-BASED MENTAL HEALTH SERVICES

Although there had been, even before deinstitutionalization, a growing belief in the effectiveness of community-based mental health services (CBMHS), the great expansion of such services came about with the recognition that persons with mental disorders would no longer receive long-term hospital care but would require more than medication in order to live in the community and were in need of a range of social and rehabilitation services that would be provided "in collaboration with…local agencies."[63,64] CBMHS have been shown to be as effective, if not more so, than hospital-based services in high- and low-income countries, alike;[45,65] however, it is not necessarily true that community services are less expensive than hospital services.[66] More important than cost, the provision of services in the community is in keeping with the following:

The principle of the least restrictive [care] requires that persons are always offered treatment in settings that have the least possible effect on their personal freedom and their status and privileges in the community, including their ability to continue to work, move about and conduct their affairs.[67]

CBMHS have been in place for more than 50 years in the Western industrialized countries, and have an equally long history in some low-income countries. For example, beginning in the late 1940s, India experimented with outpatient and community care,[68,69] while at about the same time, Thomas Lambo established a day hospital in Abeokuta, Nigeria, which provided treatment for people with severe mental illnesses but also allowed them to return to a community setting each day.[70][†††] In the 1960s, a number of "psychiatric villages" were established in Tanzania for patients who could be discharged from the hospital but were not yet able to return to life in the community.[72] Throughout the world, community mental health services are now at the forefront of strategies to address the needs of persons with mental disorders.[64]

COMPARATIVE AND CULTURAL PSYCHIATRY

The current interest in the field of global mental health can be traced, at least in part, to the emergence of *comparative psychiatry*, which later came to be called *cross-cultural psychiatry*. No doubt, curiosity about mental disorders among different sociocultural groups was prompted by accounts from explorers and colonial psychiatrists. As early as the 1820s, Sir Andrew Halliday commented upon the apparent absence of insanity among Africans, slaves in the West Indies, and the peasants of Wales, the West Hebrides, and rural Ireland.[73] In 1904, Emil Kraepelin, one of the founders of modern psychiatry, visited the Dutch asylum of Buitenzorg in Java because he conjectured that cross-cultural comparisons had the potential to provide insights into the causes of mental disorders.[74] There, Kraepelin compared the expression of psychoses among Europeans and Javanese and noted, "Of the numerous forms of dementia praecox [schizophrenia] encountered among the Javanese not one of the symptoms common among Europeans was missing, but they were all much less florid, less distinctively marked."[‡‡‡] Following his visit to Java, Kraepelin wrote an essay, "Comparative Psychiatry," which established the field of cultural psychiatry. Since then, cultural psychiatry has attracted the interest of researchers from a range of disciplines, such as psychiatry, anthropology, sociology, and psychology, and has been dominated by two contrasting perspectives. The first has been the conviction that, while culture may influence some aspects of the expression of psychopathology, the core syndromes—for example, depression or schizophrenia—are the product of universal biological and psychological processes.[76] The alternative perspective is that human experience is ultimately shaped by culture and that one cannot assume the universal nature of psychiatric syndromes. These perspectives continue to be debated,[77] but the field of global mental health has arrived at something of a consensus: although there is ample evidence of differences in the expression of and responses to mental disorders, it is generally agreed that these "health conditions [affect] people in all cultures and societies, and [are] neither a figment of the 'Western' imagination nor a colonial export."[77] (See Chapter 3.)

[†††] Ironically, this "traditional" African approach to care and treatment was likened to the practices that originated in the medieval village of Geel.[71]

[‡‡‡] Unfortunately, Kraepelin then went on to speculate, using the racial theories that were common at the time,[75] that "the relative absence of delusions among the Javanese might be related to the lower stage of intellectual development attained, and the rarity of auditory hallucinations might reflect the fact that speech counts far less than it does with us and that thoughts tend to be governed more by sensory images."[74]

The origins of global mental health can also be found in the following cross-national epidemiological studies. First, the Cornell-Aro Mental Health Research Project,[78] which compared the prevalence and presentation of mental disorders in regions of Nova Scotia, Canada, and Western Nigeria, found an association between social cohesion and the prevalence of mental disorders. The project, which utilized rigorous diagnostic criteria, inspired the initiation of many other cross-national studies of the epidemiology of mental disorders.[79,80,81] In turn, this work led to the establishment of the World Health Organization (WHO) International Consortium in Psychiatric Epidemiology,[82] which went on to undertake epidemiological surveys of mental disorders in 28 countries and among a sample of more than 150,000 persons.[83] Second, the WHO International Pilot Study of Schizophrenia (IPSS),[84] a nine-country study, established that it was possible to a conduct a valid and reliable epidemiological cross-cultural study of schizophrenia. Results from the IPSS also suggested that the prognosis for schizophrenia varied according to whether the settings in which the research took place were deemed "developed" or "developing."[85] The findings of the IPSS were supported by a more rigorous, 10-country study[86] and the International Study of Schizophrenia, a long-term follow-up of cohorts in the WHO and other studies.[87] The foundations of both of these studies can be found in: a research project that examined the epidemiology of mental disorders among different ethnic groups in Taiwan[88]; the work of the WHO Expert Committee on Mental Health,[89–91] which sought to establish reliable and valid methods of diagnosing mental disorders in populations; and efforts by the U.S. National Institute of Mental Health to address the challenges of "field studies" of mental disorders.[92]

In 1972–1973, the *British Journal of Psychiatry* published what must be considered the first global mental health series (see Panel 1.1). Three papers reviewed psychiatry and

PANEL 1.1 Global Mental Health Series

- *British Journal of Psychiatry*
  1972: *Psychiatry in Latin America*[26]
  1972: *Aspects of clinical psychiatry in sub-Saharan Africa*[93]
  1973: *Psychiatry in South-East Asia*[96]
  1973: *Psychiatric problems of developing countries*[97]
  1976: *Psychiatric priorities in developing countries*[99]
- *The Lancet series on global mental health*
  2007: http://www.thelancet.com/series/global-mental-health
  2011: http://www.thelancet.com/series/global-mental-health-2011
- *PLoS Medicine: Mental health in low- and middle-income countries*
  2009–2010: http://www.ploscollections.org/article/browseIssue.action?issue=info%3Adoi%2F10.1371%2Fissue.pcol.v07.i06
- *PLoS Medicine: Putting evidence into practice: The PLoS Medicine series on global mental health practice*
  2012: http://www.plosmedicine.org/article/info%3Adoi%2F10.1371%2Fjournal.pmed.1001226
- *Harvard Review of Psychiatry: Special issue: Global mental health*
  2012: http://informahealthcare.com/toc/hrp/20/1
- *Transcultural Psychiatry: Special section: Communities and global mental health*
  2012: http://tps.sagepub.com/content/49/3-4.toc
- *International Psychiatry*: Ongoing series of country profiles http://www.rcpsych.ac.uk/publications/journals/ipinfo1.aspx
- *World Psychiatry*: Frequent papers of relevance to global mental health

the mental health challenges in Africa,[93§§§] Latin America,[26] and South-East Asia,[96] while a fourth paper, by the British psychiatrist G. M. Carstairs,[97] summarized the challenges facing developing countries, in general. What is striking about the series, and the paper by Carstairs in particular, is that the major issues in the field were identified long before the term *global mental health* was coined. These issues included: the large burden of disease imposed by mental disorders in low-income countries, the lack of necessary human resources, the pervasive consequences of stigma, and, several years before the Alma Ata Conference on Primary Health Care and decades before the concept of *task-sharing* came into common usage, Carstairs suggested:

One thing is clear: in the developing countries there is no place for "demarcation disputes" about who should do what. Even such medical prerogatives as the dispensing of drugs and injections, and the giving of ECT may have to be delegated to nurses and other auxiliaries who have been instructed in these tasks and have first practiced them under supervision.[97] (p. 275)

These reviews apparently prompted the WHO Department of Mental Health to take an increased interest in treatment services. In 1974, it convened an Expert Committee on the organization of mental health services in developing countries.[98] In its conclusions, the committee echoed Carstairs:

In the developing countries, trained mental health professionals are very scarce indeed. Clearly, if basic mental health care is to be brought within reach of the mass of the population, this will have to be done by non-specialized health workers—at all levels, from the primary health worker to the nurse or doctor—working in collaboration with, and supported by, more specialized personnel.[98] (p. 33)

Soon after this report was issued, the *British Journal of Psychiatry* followed up with the publication of a paper in which R. Giel and T. W. Harding suggested that there was a need to focus efforts on a "limited range of priority conditions"; that is, chronic mental disorders (e.g., mental retardation, addiction, and dementia), epilepsy, and functional psychoses.[99] In spite of the high prevalence of more common mental disorders such as depression and anxiety, Giel and Harding did not recommend them as priorities because of what they considered to be the inherent difficulties of identifying and treating these disorders, and their presumed responsiveness to traditional forms of treatment. Instead, Giel and Harding maintained that the most important task was to educate health workers to recognize the psychological basis of many somatic complaints with the aim of reducing the inappropriate use of medical resources.

This work prompted the WHO Department of Mental Health to add services research to its portfolio. In 1975, the Department initiated the Collaborative Study on Strategies for Extending Mental Health Care, a project whose overall goal was to examine the feasibility and effectiveness of mental health programs, mostly in primary care settings, in seven developing countries.[100] This was to be achieved through: (1) the development of cross-culturally valid psychiatric surveys; (2) training primary care health workers in the recognition and management of mental disorders; (3) the establishment of mental health programs in primary care settings; and (4) evaluation of each of these activities. However, the available reports about the projects offered scant descriptions of the seven programs and little evidence of their effectiveness, and were not followed up by later reports.[101] Nevertheless, the Collaborative Study prompted the development of primary-care mental health programs in a number of low-income countries—such as Nepal,[102] India,[103] Iran,[104]

§§§ Fifteen years later, Australian psychiatrist G. A. German updated his review.[94,95]

Nicaragua,[105] Tanzania,[106] and Botswana[107]—and the integration of mental health services into primary care became the most important policy in global mental health.[101]

EMERGENCE OF GLOBAL MENTAL HEALTH

One would think that these activities, along with the development of effective pharmacological and psychosocial interventions for a range of conditions, might have resulted in the recognition that mental disorders were a public health priority in high- and low-income countries alike (Chapter 12).[108] In fact, the key impetus for the emergence of the field of global mental health was something else entirely: the publication of the *World Development Report 1993*.[109] The report featured the initial findings of the Global Burden of Disease Study (GBD), a collaboration between the World Bank and the WHO. Prior to the GBD study, statistics about health were mostly measures of mortality. Therefore, infectious diseases were prioritized in international public health, while the morbidity from non-communicable and chronic diseases was neglected. To address this imbalance, the GBD study developed Disability-Adjusted Life Years (DALYs), a metric that combines "the loss of life from premature death…with the loss of healthy life from disability." Much to the surprise of many people, computation of the DALYs showed that even in developing economies, about 8% of the global burden of disease was due to mental health problems (see Chpter 6).[110]

In 1995, faculty in the Department of Social Medicine at Harvard Medical School produced the book *World Mental Health: Problems and Priorities in Low-Income Countries*,[110] which used the evidence from the GBD study to highlight the burden of mental disorders and the growing mental health crisis in low-income countries. In brief, the book, which was the first comprehensive work of its kind, comprised reviews that examined the major mental health issues that were confronting low-income countries, including: violence; substance abuse; dislocation; the mental health problems of women, young people, and the elderly; and the general lack of mental health services. *World Mental Health* concluded with a series of recommendations that essentially called for the expansion and improvement of services, training and research (see Table 1.1). The book was sent to policy-makers, researchers, and academics throughout the world and was remarkably influential. Not long after its publication and its launch at the United Nations, the World Federation for Mental Health (with funding from the MacArthur Foundation) was able to place a mental health advisor in the Health, Nutrition, and Population Division at the World Bank; the Nations for Mental Health Program was initiated at the WHO; the WHO established the World Mental Health Survey Consortium with the aim of developing cross-culturally valid epidemiological research instruments;[111] the U.S. Surgeon General issued two reports on mental health;[112,113] and the U.S. Institute of Medicine issued a report on neuropsychiatric disorders in the developing world.[114]

These activities, in turn, sparked a host of projects at the WHO. Perhaps the best known and most influential was the publication of the *World Health Report 2001*, the first WHO report devoted entirely to mental health.[3] The report, which was titled *Mental Health: New Understandings, New Hope*, was a comprehensive review of the burden of mental disorders and behavioral disorders, as well as public health, policy, and services approaches to mental health. The report concluded with a number of recommendations, which for the most part echoed those of the previous *World Mental Health*, but added the need to provide care in primary settings, provide education to the public, and work in the policy domain. (See Table 1.1.) Perhaps of more interest than the recommendations were the various scenarios for achieving the recommendations in settings of low, medium, and high resources. These context-dependent scenarios were suggested because of the recognition that many countries did not have the resources to take similar actions to address the recommendations. Therefore, the scenarios were provided

TABLE 1.1 Recommendations and Calls to Action

Policy	• Establish national policies, programs, and legislation (WHO).
	• Integrate the treatment of brain disorders into primary care; secondary and tertiary centers should train and oversee primary care staff, provide referral capacity and supervision (IOM).
	• Integrate mental health services into general health care (Lancet CTA).
Stigma/Public Awareness	• Educate the public (WHO).
	• Increase public and professional awareness; reduce stigma and discrimination (IOM).
Resources	• Improve and expand mental health training at all levels of medical education and for all health professionals (WMH).
	• Develop human resources (WHO).
	• Capacity building to develop leadership, training, and operational research (IOM).
	• International donors must begin to make mental health a priority and contribute substantial resources (Lancet CTA).
Prevention/ Promotion	• Make prevention of mental disorders a focus of concern (WMH).
Scale Up Services and Improve Treatment	• Upgrade quality of mental health services in Asia, Africa, and Latin America (WMH).
	• Provide treatment in primary care (WHO).
	• Use low-cost, effective interventions and follow best-practice guidelines; provide essential medications; implementation must be accompanied by ongoing research to examine applicability and sustainability (IOM).
	• Health ministries should scale up packages of interventions that provide effective treatments and protect human rights (Lancet CTA).
Research	• Expand research in five essential domains: epidemiology, effects of violence, women's mental health, mental health services, and prevention (WMH).
	• Support more research (WHO).
	• Operational research to assess cost-effectiveness of specific treatments; epidemiological research on incidence, prevalence, and burden of brain disorders (IOM).
	• Data collection and monitoring mechanisms must be strengthened (Lancet CTA).

Abbreviations:

• IOM: *Neurological, psychiatric, and developmental disorders: Meeting the challenge in the developing world*

• Lancet CTA: *Lancet Call to Action*

• WHO: *World Health Report 2001; Mental health: new understanding, new hope*

• WMH: *World mental health: Problems and priorities in low-income countries*

"to help guide developing countries in particular towards what is possible within their resource limitations."

At about the same time, the WHO Department of Mental Health and Substance Abuse initiated a number of activities, including the development of materials on the development of mental health policies and services, collation of information on the availability of mental health resources across the world, and the development of guidelines for psychosocial interventions in emergency settings (see Panel 1.2).

In December 2006, the United Nations General Assembly adopted the Convention on the Rights of Persons with Disabilities. The Convention "is the first legally binding international human rights instrument that offers comprehensive protection for persons with physical or mental impairments."[115] As important, if not more so, the Convention shifted the focus from an individual model of disability, which considered persons with disabilities as in need of interventions that enable them to better function in society, to a social model of disability that emphasized "the social determinants of disability"; in other words, the social barriers that transform impairment into disability. The Convention set out a range of rights that, in general, recognize that persons with mental and physical disabilities should be able to have "full and effective participation in society on an equal basis with others,"[116] and, thus, obligated signatories to guarantee a wide range of economic, social, and cultural rights to all persons with disabilities.

It was at about this time that two important institutions in the United Kingdom began to provide significant funding for global mental health projects. First, the U.K. Department for International Development (DFiD) funded a research consortium to review mental health policies in four countries of sub-Saharan Africa with the eventual goal of conducting "interventions to assist in the development and implementation of mental health policies in those countries."[117] Second, the Wellcome Trust, one of the world's largest funders of medical research, began to fund mental health research projects in low-income countries.

The publication of the *Lancet* series on global mental health, in September 2007, marked an important milestone in the development of the field. The series consisted of

---

PANEL 1.2 WHO Activities 2001–2006

- The **Mental Health Policy and Service Guidance package:** developed to inform the development of policies and services and to maximize the use of available resources. The package contains 14 modules (http://www.who.int/mental_health/policy/essentialpackage1/en/index.html), which address topics that range from mental health policy, to financing, to human resources and training, to information systems, to monitoring and evaluation.

- The **ATLAS project** (http://apps.who.int/globalatlas/default.asp): an ongoing effort to document mental health resources in the member states of WHO.[135] Data are collected on the following: governance, financing, mental health services, human resources, available medications, and information systems. Having these data allows for comparisons across countries and, more importantly, provides the ability to assess changes over time in individual countries. (See Chapter 9.)

- **WHO-AIMS (World Health Organization–Assessment Instrument for Mental Health Systems)** (http://www.who.int/mental_health/evidence/WHO-AIMS/en/index.html): an extension of the ATLAS project in that it collects much more detailed information about national mental health systems. Reports are now available on 42 countries (http://whqlibdoc.who.int/publications/2009/9789241547741_eng.pdf). Eventually, reports will be available on a total of 100 countries. (See Chapter 9.)

- The **Guidelines on Mental Health and Psychosocial Support in Emergency Settings:**[136] Much of the impetus for organizing the group was the all-too-often chaotic and inappropriate responses to the 2004 tsunami that devastated several countries on the rim of the Indian Ocean. The guidelines emphasize multisectoral activities that take into account the mental, physical, and social needs of the populations affected by armed conflict or natural disasters.

six papers that reviewed, with a focus on low- and middle-income countries, the burden of mental disorders,[118] mental health resources,[45] evidence on treatment and prevention,[119] an overview of extant mental health systems,[120] barriers to improvement of services,[121] and a call to scale up services for mental disorders (see Table 1.1).[122] Given that *The Lancet* is, arguably, the most prestigious public health journal in the world, the series elevated global mental health to a prominence that it had not had previously.

Less than a year later, WHO launched the mental health Gap Action Programme (mhGAP) (see Chapter 12) which had the goal of increasing the ability of countries to reduce the burden of and the treatment gap for mental, neurological, and substance abuse disorders (MNS).[123] At the core of program is the collection of "the best available scientific and epidemiological evidence about MNS conditions that have been identified as priorities"; that is, depression, schizophrenia and other psychotic disorders, suicide, epilepsy, dementia, disorders due to use of alcohol, disorders due to use of illicit drugs, and mental disorders in children. That evidence has now been collected and organized into the mhGAP Intervention Guide (see http://www.who.int/mental_health/evidence/mhGAP_intervention_guide/en/index.html), which provides guidelines for the identification, treatment, and management of the priority conditions in general health care settings. The focus on non-specialized settings was chosen because of the lack of mental health professionals in low- and middle-income countries and, therefore, the need to address the burden of MNS disorders by utilizing other health care providers—a strategy suggested almost 40 years before by a WHO expert committee.[98]

The next milestone, in 2010, was the establishment of the Grand Challenges in Global Mental Health initiative (GCGMH—http://grandchallengesgmh.nimh.nih.gov/). (See Chapter 19.) Funded by the U.S. National Institute of Mental Health (NIMH), supported by the Global Alliance for Chronic Diseases, and guided by an executive committee and scientific advisory board composed of researchers and academics from around the world, GCGMH enrolled a panel of 422 experts to participate in a "Delphi exercise," the aim of which was to identify "the major scientific thrusts that will be needed to make a significant impact on the lives of people living with neuropsychiatric disorders." Four of the five leading challenges identified in the exercise involved improving treatments and expanding access to care: (1) integrate screening and core packages of services into routine primary health care; (2) reduce the cost and improve the supply of effective medications; (3) provide effective and affordable community-based care and rehabilitation; and (4) improve the access of children to evidence-based mental health care in low- and middle-income countries.[124] The fifth leading challenge—to strengthen the mental health component in the training of all health-care personnel—was closely related and could be seen as essential to any efforts to improve and expand the availability of care. Thus, the results of GCGMH, to a great extent, mirrored the call to scale up mental health services that was expressed in the concluding paper of the 2007 *Lancet* series on global mental health.

OPPORTUNITIES AND CHALLENGES

The future of global mental health is filled with opportunities and challenges. Interest in the field has continued to grow, as is evidenced by increasing opportunities in training and expanding activities by non-governmental organizations (NGOs) (see Panels 1.3 and 1.4 at chapter end), as well as increased funding for research, capacity building, and service development in low and middle income countries (LAMICs) (see Panel 1.5 at chapter end). However, along with the opportunities there are many barriers to progress. Of these, three barriers stand out as being of paramount importance: lack of resources, "imperfections in our current state of knowledge about the nature of mental disorders and the armamentarium of effective treatments,"[77] and human rights abuses.

PANEL 1.3 Global Mental Health Courses

- *International Mental Health Leadership Program*—University of Melbourne, Australia
  http://cimh.unimelb.edu.au/learning_and_teaching/leadership_programs/international_mental_health_leadership_program
- *Leadership in Mental Health*—Sangath, Goa, India
  http://www.sangath.com/details.php?nav_id=9
- *International Master in Mental Health Policy and Services*—Universidade NOVA de Lisboa, Portugal
  http://www.globalmentalhealth.org/node/565
- *Mental Health in Complex Emergencies*—Center for International Humanitarian Cooperation, Geneva, Switzerland
  http://www.cihc.org/mhce
- *Global Mental Health: Trauma and Recovery Certificate Program*—Harvard Program in Refugee Trauma, Orvieto, Italy
  http://hprt-cambridge.org/?page_id=31
- *MSc in Global Mental Health*—London School of Hygiene and Tropical Medicine and the Institute of Psychiatry, King's College London, U.K.
  http://www.lshtm.ac.uk/study/masters/msgmh.html
- *Mental Health Leadership and Advocacy Programme for Anglophone West Africa*—University of Ibadan, Nigeria
  http://www.mhlap.org/

Lack of resources—human, financial, and technical—has consequences for nearly every aspect of global mental health. Services cannot be delivered without a sufficient number of adequately trained specialist and non-specialist health workers. Mental health systems cannot be improved, developed, or expanded without financial investments. And technical resources, such as information systems, are required for such activities as program monitoring and evaluation, ensuring adequate and consistent supplies of medication, and maintaining patient records. On the positive side, concerted efforts are now being made to address the lack of human resources through the strategy that has come to be called *task-sharing,* whereby non-specialist health workers are trained to take on the more routine aspects of interventions while the mental health specialists devote most of their time to training, supervision, and attending to the most difficult cases. As noted earlier, Carstairs recommended this strategy 40 years ago.[97] What is new is the accumulation of evidence on how this strategy can be carried out successfully. This evidence has now been synthesized in the Packages of Care series in *PLoS Medicine*[125–131] and the WHO mhGAP Intervention Guide.[132] As more evidence becomes available through services research and practical experience, the strategy of task-shifting will, no doubt, become better defined and more effective.

As successful as task-shifting might be, however, it will not make up for the financial deficiencies in the health systems of LAMICs. Indeed, the implementation of task-shifting requires investment. Therefore, financial constraints, and by extension technical constraints, will remain significant barriers into the foreseeable future. The ability of global mental health to garner these resources—from national governments, international agencies, and private organizations—might be considered another grand challenge.

Despite advances in psychopharmacology, the development of psychological and psychosocial interventions, knowledge of how environment–gene interactions contribute to risk for mental disorders, a great accumulation of epidemiological evidence, and

PANEL 1.4 International NGOs and the Development of Global Mental Health

Non-governmental organizations have played an important role in the development of global mental health.[137,138] The World Federation for Mental Health (WFMH)— an outgrowth of the earlier International Committee for Mental Hygiene[139]—was founded in 1948 amidst a wave of postwar idealism about "world citizenship," and in the belief that good mental health would promote world peace. For several decades, WFMH was virtually the only NGO that had a central focus on mental health and mental health systems. Other NGOs came into field in the 1990s, often as a result of the desire to respond to and alleviate the psychological trauma of people who have suffered humanitarian crises. In addition, there are probably thousands of local NGOs that are conducting service delivery, research, and advocacy.[140] The following are brief descriptions of a few of the international NGOs that have been prominent in global mental health.

- From the beginning, the mission of **WFMH** has been "to promote, among all people and nations, the highest possible level of mental health in its broadest biological, medical, educational and social aspects." It engages in mental health advocacy at the United Nations and the World Health Organization. Its network includes mental health organizations, members of various health professions, consumers of mental health services, and family members. In 1992, WFMH established World Mental Health Day, which is now celebrated around the world. For more information about WFMH, to go http://www.wfmh.org.[****]

- Founded in 1908, **CBM** is an international development organization that focuses on work with people with disabilities in the poorest countries of the world. The programs supported by CBM and its partners have been supporting people with mental health needs, including epilepsy, for many years. However, it was the crisis of the Asian tsunami of 2004 that prompted CMB to consider psychosocial disabilities more generally. The aims the mental health component of CBM's work are to scale up services to meet the needs of people with psychosocial disabilities in low-income countries by working with partners to provide care that is appropriate, affordable, accessible, and of high quality, and to protect the human rights and promote the social inclusion of people with psychosocial disabilities. At present, the mental health work of CBM is most active in West Africa, where 16 community-based rehabilitation projects include mental health services; several independent mental health projects are providing services; and two projects are focusing on human rights, advocacy, and awareness-raising.[††††]

- **International Medical Corps** has made sustainable, accessible mental health care a cornerstone of its relief and development programming. IMC's mental health and psychosocial programs are informed by local needs, build on community resources and structures, involve training of national counterparts, and are designed to be integrated into existing services such as health or nutrition. As of 2011, IMC had a total of 28 programs with mental health and psychosocial support components in a total of 15 countries in the Middle East and Caucasus, Asia, and sub-Saharan Africa.[‡‡‡‡]

[****] Information provided by Elena L. Berger (Director, Programs and Government Affairs, WFMH).

[††††] Information provided by Julian Eaton, Mental Health Advisor, CBM West Africa.

[‡‡‡‡] Information provided by Inka Weissbecker, Global Mental Health & Psychosocial Advisor, International Medical Corps.

- Due to its mandate to protect and assist victims of armed conflict, the **International Committee of the Red Cross** works with many populations that are facing high levels of psychological distress, and the integration of mental health services and psychosocial support into protection and assistance activities is now considered an essential component of the ICRC's multidisciplinary and comprehensive response to humanitarian crises. The neutrality, independence, and impartiality of ICRC gives it access to these populations that, all too often, cannot be reached by other organizations. The ICRC also plans to develop its capacity to support countries in post-conflict situations by integrating mental health services into primary health care.§§§§

- **HealthNet TPO** has, since 1992, worked on strengthening mental health systems in fragile states in Asia, Central Africa, and Eastern Europe. The organization follows a public mental health paradigm, integrating universal, selective, and indicated interventions in the development of systems of care that are feasible within the context of complex emergencies.[141] HealthNet TPO tries to capitalize on opportunities that arise in the context of limited human resources and inadequate infrastructures in order to build systems of care that focus on accessible, acceptable, and effective community-services. It uses operational and scientific research to develop effective, evidence-based, and context-sensitive models of care in complex emergencies,[142–145] and works on capacity-building geared towards sustainability.*****

- The **Global Initiative on Psychiatry** is an international not-for-profit organization whose mission is to promote humane, ethical, and effective mental health care throughout the world and to support a global network of individuals and organizations to develop, advocate for, and carry out necessary reforms. GIP also supports international campaigns against unethical behavior, political abuse, and other violations of human rights in the field of mental health. At present, GIP works in three dozen countries in Europe, Africa, and Asia. The organization has been awarded two prizes for its efforts: the Human Rights Award from the American Psychiatric Association and the 2000 Geneva Prize for Human Rights in Psychiatry.†††††

- **BasicNeeds** was established in 2000 to bring about lasting change in the lives of people with mental illness or epilepsy by addressing their illness, poverty, and social exclusion. Mental Health and Development, the operational model of BasicNeeds, is now being implemented in Ghana, Tanzania, Kenya, Uganda, Lao PDR, Vietnam, Sri Lanka, India, Nepal, China, and the United Kingdom. Since its inception, BasicNeeds has reached 104,234 affected individuals.‡‡‡‡‡

§§§§ Information provided by Renato Oliverira e Souza, Mental Health and Psychosocial Support Adviser, ICRC.
***** Information provided by Mark J. D. Jordans, Head of Research, HealthNet TPO.
††††† Information provided by Benedetto Saraceno, Chairman, GIP.
‡‡‡‡‡ Information provided by Chris Underhill, Founder Director, and Shoba Raja, Director, Policy and Practice, BasicNeeds.

PANEL 1.5 Opportunities

The Grand Challenges in Global Mental Health program has had at least two substantive outcomes that promise to move the field forward, far beyond previous developments. First, NIMH has funded five collaborative research "hubs" in Latin America, sub-Saharan Africa, and South Asia. Each hub links leading academic institutions in high- and low-income countries with the intention of conducting research and providing capacity-building activities. The ultimate goal of the hubs will be to expand the knowledge base for mental health interventions in low-resource settings.

Grand Challenges Canada has established Integrated Innovations in Global Mental Health, a program that has awarded about $20 million CAD to 15 projects with the goal of improving diagnosis and care of mental disorders in low-income settings.[146] A second round of funding has been announced that will provide a further $10 million CAD. Another initiative of Grand Challenges Canada may prove to be of particular importance—because it may attract younger participants with fresh ideas—Stars in Global Health,[147] which offers proof-of-concept awards initially, and much larger "transition to scale" grants to successful investigators. The full application for the Phase I grants is a two-minute video setting out the bold idea. In the current round of funding, more than 400 videos from 42 countries were submitted. Successful grants will be determined by an online vote by the general public (see http://www.grandchallenges.ca/grand-challenges/gc4-non-communicable-diseases/mentalhealth/).

The U.K. Department of International Development has continued its commitment to global mental health by funding the Programme for Improving Mental Health Care (PRIME), a six-year project in which a consortium of research institutions and ministries of health in five countries in Asia and Africa (Ethiopia, India, Nepal, South Africa, and Uganda) will collaborate to produce evidence on the implementation and scaling up of mental health programs. In addition, the European Commission has funded a WHO project to implement the mhGAP treatment guidelines in Nigeria and Ethiopia.[148] A third project, Emerging Mental Health Systems in Low- and Middle-Income Countries (EMERALD)—also funded by the European Commission—will use the knowledge gained from these two other projects and identify the key system barriers to, and possible solutions for, scaling up mental health services in low- and middle-income countries (Graham Thornicroft, personal communication).

The Wellcome Trust has also continued its support of global mental health by funding a range of research projects in a number of low-income countries. For example: (1) PREMIUM is a five-year project to develop psychological treatments for depression and alcohol use disorders that can be delivered by non-specialist health workers in India; and (2) Stepped Care Treatment of Depression in Primary Care Centers is a 3.5-year trial of an intervention that will be delivered by non-physician health workers.

The Gulbenkian Global Mental Health Platform,[149] an initiative of the Calouste Gulbenkian Foundation, in collaboration with NOVA University of Lisbon and WHO, is a new initiative whose aim is to promote a U.N. Summit on mental health. To achieve this goal, the Platform will provide support work on the social determinants of mental disorders, the interrelationships of physical and mental disorders, the development of community-based approaches to care, and protection of the human rights of people with mental disorders.

The Movement for Global Mental Health, which was launched shortly after the first global mental health series in *The Lancet*, is a network of individuals and organizations committed to the improvement of services for people with mental disorders. The Movement, which has a particular focus on low- and middle-income countries, holds biannual summits and maintains a website (http://www.globalmentalhealth. org/home) that provides links to news items, publications, activities worldwide, fund-raising opportunities, training opportunities, and other resources.

expanded knowledge of how culture shapes expressions of and responses to distress, our understanding of mental disorders and their treatment is less than desired.[77] Thus, there is an urgent need for research—in LAMIs and high-income countries, alike—that addresses the questions of etiology, treatment, and cultural variations that are raised by the "Grand Challenges" in Global Mental Health Initiative and cultural psychiatry critiques (see Chapter 3). Nevertheless, the need for more research must not be used as an excuse for delaying the response to what we know is an extensive need.[119,133] Rather, we must use the knowledge that we do possess and continue to explore improvements and alternatives to what we have, while constantly being vigilant about whether the interventions (biomedical and psychosocial) utilized provide real benefits to those in need and their families.

The issue of human rights abuses that many persons with mental disorders are subjected to constitutes the third major challenge to the future of global mental health. The human rights of people with mental disorders are abused in health and social protection institutions, in religious shrines, in sites of traditional healing practices, and in communities. The U.N. Convention on the Rights of People with Disabilities represents progress, but this international legal instrument, not ratified by all countries (and recently rejected by the U.S. Senate), must be matched with concrete actions at the level of states, professional associations, communities, and families. States must not tolerate the existence of institutions or practices that dehumanize patients. Professional associations (psychiatric, psychological, and legal) must not ignore and, thus implicitly approve of, conditions in health and social institutions that are unacceptable. Communities must not shun persons with mental disorders. Families must not relegate ill members to backrooms or cages or shackles, or abandon them to the streets. In sum, perhaps the greatest challenge to global mental health is that it must overcome what Arthur Kleinman has called "a failure of humanity,"[134] as evidenced in its willingness to consider those with mental disorders as somehow less than human and less deserving of decent care.

Despite these barriers, the opportunities provide reason to believe that the field of global mental health will, in the coming years, make contributions that will improve the lives of persons and families who live with the burden of mental disorders. To quote one of the editors of this volume:

The story of Global Mental Health is far from complete—where the field might be ten years from now may not be possible to predict accurately, but the portents are promising. If nothing else, however, the promising developments in recent years will renew the passion and commitment of the armies of advocates, from academics and practitioners to those who live with mental illness and their loved ones, to ensure that the cause of global mental health remains in the foreground of global health.[77]

1. Wells KB, Sherbourne CD. Functioning and utility for current health of patients with depression or chronic medical conditions in managed, primary care practices. *Arch Gen Psychiatry.* 1999;56:897–904.

2. Satcher D. Global mental health: its time has come. *JAMA.* 2001;285:1697.

3. WHO. *Mental health: New understanding, new hope.* Geneva: World Health Organization; 2001.

4. *The Lancet.* The Lancet Series. N.d. [cited 2012 17 November]; Available from: http://www.thelancet.com/series.

5. Patel V, Prince M. Global mental health: a new global health field comes of age. *JAMA.* 2010;303:1976–7.

6. Koran L. Psychiatry in mainland China: history and recent status. *Am J Psychiatry.* 1972;128:970.

7. Bhugra D. Psychiatry in ancient Indian texts: a review. *Hist Psychiatry.* 1992;3:167–86.

8. Simon B. Mind and madness in classical antiquity. In: Wallace ER, Gach J (eds.). *History of psychiatry and medical psychology.* New York: Springer US; 2008:175–97.

9. Liu X. Psychiatry in traditional Chinese medicine. *Br J Psychiatry.* 1981;138:429.

10. Milns RD. Squibb academic lecture: attitudes towards mental illness in antiquity. *Aust NZ J Psychiatry.* 1986;20:454–62.

11. Okasha A. Mental health in Egypt. *Israel J Psychiatry & Relat Sci.* 2005;42:116.

12. Dols MW. The origins of the Islamic hospital: myth and reality. *Bull Hist Med.* 1987;61:367–90.

13. Dols MW. Insanity and its treatment in Islamic society. *Med Hist.* 1987;31:1–14.

14. Syed EU, Hussein SA, Haidry SE. Prevalence of emotional and behavioural problems among primary school children in Karachi, Pakistan—multi-informant survey. *Indian J Pediatr.* 2009;76:623–7.

15. Mora G. Mental disturbances, unusual mental states, and their interpretation during the Middle Ages. In: Wallace ER, Gach J (eds.). *History of psychiatry and medical psychology.* New York: Springer US; 2008:199–226.

16. Horden P. Responses to possession and insanity in the early Byzantine world. *Soc Hist Med.* 1993;6:177–94.

17. Mohit A. Mental health and psychiatry in the Middle East: historical development. *East Mediterr Health J.* 2001;7:336–47.

18. Peloso PF. Hospital care of madness in the Turk sixteenth century according to the witness of G. A. Menavino from Genoa. *Hist Psychiatry.* 1998;9:35–38.

19. Andrews J, Briggs A, Porter R, Tucker P, Waddington K. *The history of Bethlem.* London: Routledge; 1997.

20. Mora G. Italy. In: Howells JG (ed.). *World history of psychiatry.* New York: Brunner/Mazel; 1975:39–89.

21. Lopez Ibor JJ. Spain and Portugal. In: Howells JG (ed.). *World history of psychiatry.* New York: Brunner/Mazel; 1975:90–118.

22. Rumbaut RD. The first psychiatric hospital of the Western world. *Am J Psychiatry.* 1972;128:1305–9.

23. Pierloot RA. Belgium. In: Howells JG (ed.). *World history of psychiatry.* New York: Brunner/Mazel; 1975:136–49.

24. Retterstol N. Scandinavia and Finland. In: Howells JG (ed.). *World history of psychiatry.* New York: Brunner/Mazel; 1975:207–37.

25. Weiner DB. The madman in the light of reason: Enlightenment psychiatry: Part I. In: Wallace ER, Gach J (eds.). *History of psychiatry and medical psychology.* New York: Springer US; 2008:255–77.

26. Leon CA. Psychiatry in Latin America. *Br J Psychiatry.* 1972;121:121–36.

27. Edgerton RB. Traditional treatment for mental illness in Africa: a review. *Cult Med Psychiatry.* 1980;4:167–89.

28. Rothman DJ. *The discovery of the asylum: social order and disorder in the new republic.* Rev. ed. New York: Aldine de Gruyter; 2002.

29. Grob GN. *The mad among us: a history of the care of America's mentally ill.* New York: Free Press; 1994.

30. Sussman S. The first asylums in Canada: a response to neglectful community care and current trends. *Can J Psychiatry.* 1998;43:260–4.

31. Shorter E. The historical development of mental health services in Europe. In: Knapp M, McDaid D, Mossialos E, Thornicroft G (eds.). *Mental health policy and practice across Europe: the future direction of mental health care*. Berkshire, England: Open University Press; 2007:15–33.

32. Scull A. *Most solitary of afflictions: madness and society in Britain, 1700–1900*. New Haven, CT: Yale University Press; 2005.

33. Goldstein J. *Console and classify: the French psychiatric profession in the nineteenth century*. Chicago: University of Chicago Press; 2001.

34. Goldstein JL, Godemont MML. The legend and lessons of Geel, Belgium: a 1500-year-old legend, a 21st-century model. *Community Ment Health J*. 2003;39:441–58.

35. Bucknill J. Valedictory address to the British Association of Medical Officers of Asylums and Hospitals for the Insane. *J Ment Sci*. 1861;7:309–18.

36. Annales Médico-Psychologiques. Discussion sur la colonisation des aliénés. *Annales Médico-Psychologiques*. 1862;8(3. Serie):650–65, 83–9.

37. Morrissey JP, Goldman HH. The ambiguous legacy: 1856–1968. In: Morrissey JP, Goldman HH, Klerman LV (eds.). *The enduring asylum: cycles of institutional reform at Worcester State Hospital*. New York: Grune & Stratton; 1980:45–95.

38. Weiss MG. The treatment of insane patients in India in the lunatic asylums of the nineteenth century. *Indian J Psychiatry*. 1983;25:312–6.

39. Ng BY, Chee KT. A brief history of psychiatry in Singapore. *Int Rev Psychiatry*. 2006;18:355–61.

40. Swartz S. "Work of mercy and necessity": British rule and psychiatric practice in the Cape Colony, 1891–1910. *Int J Ment Health*. 1999;28:72–90.

41. Sadowsky J. Psychiatry and colonial ideology in Nigeria. *Bull Hist Med*. 1997;71:94–111.

42. Bègue JM. French psychiatry in Algeria (1830–1962): from colonial to transcultural. *Hist Psychiatry*. 1996;7:533.

43. Barton WE. Mental hospitals in Japan. *Psychiatr Serv*. 1963;14:489–91.

44. Siriwanarangsan P, Liknapichitkul D, Khandelwal SK. Thailand mental health country profile. *Int Rev Psychiatry*. 2004;16:150–8.

45. Saxena S, Thornicroft G, Knapp M, Whiteford H. Resources for mental health: scarcity, inequity, and inefficiency. *Lancet*. 2007;370:878–89.

46. Mills J. Modern psychiatry in India: the British role in establishing an Asian system, 1858–1947. *Int Rev Psychiatry*. 2006;18:333–43.

47. *The Lancet*. Report of the Lancet Commission on lunatic asylums. *Lancet*. 1877;109:464–7.

48. *The Lancet*. The crime of lunacy, and how we punish it. *Lancet*. 1857;70:62–4.

49. Earle P. The curability of insanity. *Am J Insanity*. 1877;33:483–533.

50. Earle P. *The curability of insanity: a series of studies*. Philadelphia: J.B. Lippincott Co.; 1887.

51. Scull A. *Social order/mental disorder: Anglo-American psychiatry in historical perspective*. Berkeley: University of California Press; 1989.

52. Fakhoury W, Priebe S. Deinstitutionalization and reinstitutionalization: major changes in the provision of mental healthcare. *Psychiatry*. 2007;6:313–6.

53. Thornicroft G, Bebbington P. Deinstitutionalisation—from hospital closure to service development. *Br J Psychiatry*. 1989;155:739–53.

54. Goldman HH. The demography of deinstitutionalization. *New Directions for Mental Health Services*. 1983;17:31–40.

55. Grob GN. From hospital to community: mental health policy in modern America. *Psychiatric Q*. 1991;62:187–212.

56. Warner R. Deinstitutionalization: How did we get where we are? *J Social Issues*. 1989;45:17–30.

57. Greenblatt M. Deinstitutionalization and reinstitutionalization of the mentally ill. In: Robertson MJ, Greenblatt M (eds.). *Homelessness: a national perspective*. New York: Plenum Press; 1992:47–56.

58. Bachrach LL. What we know about homelessness among mentally ill persons: an analytical review and commentary. *Hosp Community Psychiatry*. 1992;43:453–64.

59. Fakhoury W, Priebe S. The process of deinstitutionalization: an international overview. *Curr Opin Psychiatry*. 2002;15:187.

60. Jencks C. *The homeless*. Cambridge, MA: Harvard University Press; 1994.

61. Levy CJ. Ingredients of a failing system: a lack of state money, a group without a voice. *New York Times*. April 28, 2002. Section 1, p. 32.

62. Scull A. Deinstitutionalization: Cycles of despair. *J Mind & Behav*. 1990;11:301–11.

63. Thornicroft G, Tansella M. *The mental health matrix: a manual to improve services.* Cambridge, UK: Cambridge University Press; 1999.

64. Thornicroft G, Alem A, Dos Santos RA, et al. WPA guidance on steps, obstacles and mistakes to avoid in the implementation of community mental health care. *World Psychiatry.* 2010;9:67–77.

65. Wiley-Exley E. Evaluations of community mental health care in low- and middle-income countries: A 10-year review of the literature. *Soc Sci Med.* 2007;64:1231–41.

66. Killaspy H. From the asylum to community care: learning from experience. *Br Med Bull.* 2006;79–80:245–58.

67. World Health Organization. *Mental health legislation and human rights.* Geneva: World Health Organization; 2003.

68. Kapur RL. The story of community mental health in India. In: Agarwal DSP, Goel D, India Directorate General of Health Services (eds.). *Mental health: An Indian perspective, 1946–2003.* New Delhi: Published for Directorate General of Health Services, Ministry of Health & Family Welfare,[by] Elsevier; 2004:92–100.

69. Menon S. Mental health in independent India: the early years. In: Agarwal DSP, Goel D, India Directorate General of Health Services (eds.). *Mental health: An Indian perspective, 1946–2003.* New Delhi: Published for Directorate General of Health Services, Ministry of Health & Family Welfare,[by] Elsevier; 2004:30–6.

70. Lambo TA. Neuro-psychiatric observations in the Western region of Nigeria. *BMJ.* 1956;2:1388–94.

71. The Lancet. The village of Aro. *Lancet.* 1964;284:513–4.

72. Swift CR. Mental health programming in a developing country: any relevance elsewhere? *Am J Orthopsychiatry.* 1972;42:517–26.

73. Halliday A. *A general view of the present state of lunatics and lunatic asylums in Great Britain and Ireland, and in some other kingdoms.* London: William Clowes; 1828.

74. Kraepelin E. Comparative psychiatry. In: Littlewood R, Dein S (eds.). *Cultural psychiatry and medical anthropology: An introduction and reader.* London: Athlone Press; 2000[1904]:38–42.

75. Shepherd M. Two faces of Emil Kraepelin. *Br J Psychiatry.* 1995;167:174–83.

76. Kirmayer LJ. Beyond the "new cross-cultural psychiatry": cultural biology, discursive psychology and the ironies of globalization. *Transcult Psychiatry.* 2006;43:126.

77. Patel V. Global mental health: from science to action. *Harv Rev Psychiatry.* 2012;20:6–12.

78. Leighton AH, Lambo TA, Hughes CC, Leighton DC, Murphy JM, Macklin DB. *Psychiatric disorder among the Yoruba: a report from the Cornell-Aro mental health research project in the Western Region, Nigeria.* Ithaca, NY: Cornell University Press; 1963.

79. Weissman MM, Bland RC, Canino GJ, et al. The cross national epidemiology of obsessive compulsive disorder. The Cross National Collaborative Group. *J Clin Psychiatry.* 1994;55:5–10.

80. Weissman MM, Bland RC, Canino GJ, et al. Cross-national epidemiology of major depression and bipolar disorder. *JAMA.* 1996;276:293–9.

81. Weissman MM, Bland RC, Canino GJ, et al. Prevalence of suicide ideation and suicide attempts in nine countries. *Psychol Med.* 1999;29:9–17.

82. Kessler RC. The World Health Organization International Consortium in Psychiatric Epidemiology (ICPE): initial work and future directions—the NAPE Lecture 1998. *Acta Psychiatr Scand.* 1999;99(1):2–9.

83. Kessler RC, Üstün TB. *The WHO World Mental Health Surveys: global perspectives on the epidemiology of mental disorders.* Cambridge, UK: Cambridge University Press; 2008:xviii, 580.

84. Sartorius N, Shapiro R, Kimura M, Barrett K. WHO international pilot study of schizophrenia. *Psychol Med.* 1972;2:422–5.

85. Sartorius N, Jablensky A, Shapiro R. Cross-cultural differences in the short-term prognosis of schizophrenic psychoses. *Schizophr Bull.* 1978;4:102–13.

86. Jablensky A, Sartorius N, Ernberg G, et al. Schizophrenia: manifestations, incidence and course in different cultures: a World Health Organization ten-country study. *Psychol Med.* 1992;20:1–97.

87. Hopper K, Harrison G, Janca A, Sartorius N. *Recovery from schizophrenia: an international perspective.* Oxford, UK: Oxford University Press; 2007.

88. Lin TY. A study of incidence of mental disorders in Chinese and other cultures. *Psychiatry.* 1953;16:313–36.

89. Reid DD. *Epidemiological methods in the study of mental disorders.* Geneva: World Health Organization; 1960.

90. Lin TY, Standley C. *The scope of epidemiology in psychiatry.* Geneva, Switzerland: World Health Organization; 1962.

91. Lin T. The epidemiological study of mental disorders by WHO. *Soc Psychiatry.* 1967;1:204–6.

92. Zubin J. *Field studies in the mental disorders: proceedings of the Work Conference on Problems in Field Studies in the Mental Disorders, February 15–19, 1959...supported by USPHS grant no. 3m-9146, National Institute of Mental Health.* New York: Grune & Stratton; 1961.

93. German GA. Aspects of clinical psychiatry in sub-Saharan Africa. *Br J Psychiatry.* 1972;121:461–79.

94. German GA. Mental health in Africa: I. The extent of mental health problems in Africa today: an update of epidemiological knowledge. *Br J Psychiatry.* 1987;151:435–9.

95. German GA. Mental health in Africa: II. The nature of mental disorder in Africa today, some clinical observations. *Br J Psychiatry.* 1987;151:440–6.

96. Neki JS. Psychiatry in South-East Asia. *Br J Psychiatry.* 1973;123:257–69.

97. Carstairs GM. Psychiatric problems of developing countries: based on the Morison lecture delivered at the Royal College of Physicians of Edinburgh, on May 25, 1972. *Br J Psychiatry.* 1973;123:271–7.

98. WHO. *Organization of mental health services in the developing countries.* Geneva: World Health Organization; 1975.

99. Giel R, Harding TW. Psychiatric priorities in developing countries. *Br J Psychiatry.* 1976;128:513–22.

100. Sartorius N, Harding TW. The WHO collaborative study on strategies for extending mental health care, I: The genesis of the study. *Am J Psychiatry.* 1983;140:1470–3.

101. Cohen A. *The effectiveness of mental health services in primary care: The view from the developing world.* Geneva, Switzerland: World Health Organization; 2001.

102. Acland S. Mental health services in primary care: the case of Nepal. In: Cohen A, Kleinman A, Saraceno B (eds.). *The world mental health casebook: social and mental health programs in low-income countries.* New York: Kluwer Academic/Plenum Press; 2002:121–52.

103. Isaac MK, Kapur RL, Chandrashekar CR, Kapur M, Pathasarathy R. Mental health delivery through rural primary care—development and evaluation of a training programme. *Indian J Psychiatry.* 1982;24:131–8.

104. Yasamy MT, Shahmohammadi D, Bagheri Yazdi SA, et al. Mental health in the Islamic Republic of Iran: achievements and areas of need. *East Mediterr Health J.* 2001;7:381–91.

105. Byng R. Primary mental health care in Nicaragua. *Soc Sci Med.* 1993;36:625–9.

106. Kempinski R. Mental health and primary health care in Tanzania. *Acta Psychiatr Scand.* 1991;83:112–21.

107. Ben-Tovim DI. Factors influencing the integration of psychiatric care into primary health care in Botswana. *Int J Ment Health.* 1984;12:107–22.

108. Cohen A, Kleinman A, Saraceno B. Introduction. In: Cohen A, Kleinman A, Saraceno B (eds.). *World mental health casebook: social and mental health programs in low-income countries.* New York: Kluwer Academic/Plenum Press; 2002:1–26.

109. World Bank. *World development report 1993: Investing in health.* New York: Oxford University Press; 1993.

110. Desjarlais R, Eisenberg L, Good B, Kleinman A. *World mental health: Problems and priorities in low-income countries.* New York: Oxford University Press; 1995.

111. Demyttenaere K, Bruffaerts R, Posada-Villa J, et al. Prevalence, severity, and unmet need for treatment of mental disorders in the World Health Organization World Mental Health Surveys. *JAMA.* 2004;291:2581–90.

112. U. S. Department of Health and Human Services. *Mental health: a report of the Surgeon General.* Rockville, MD: U.S. Department of Health and Human Services Center for Mental Health Services, National Institutes of Health, National Institute of Mental Health; 1999.

113. U.S. Department of Health and Human Services. *Mental health: culture, race, and ethnicity.* Rockville, MD: U.S. Department of Health and Human Services, Public Health Service, Office of the Surgeon General; 2001.

114. Institute of Medicine. *Neurological, psychiatric, and developmental disorders: Meeting the challenge in the developing world.* Washington, DC: National Academy Press; 2001.

115. Stuart H. United Nations convention on the rights of persons with disabilities: a roadmap for change. *Curr Opin Psychiatry.* 2012;25:365–9.

116. United Nations General Assembly. *Convention on the rights of persons with disabilities.* New York: United Nations; 2006.

117. Flisher AJ, Lund C, Funk M, et al. Mental health policy development and implementation in four African countries. *J Health Psychol.* 2007;12:505–16.

118. Prince M, Patel V, Saxena S, et al. No health without mental health. *Lancet.* 2007;370:859–77.

119. Patel V, Araya R, Chisholm D, et al. Treatment and prevention of mental disorders in low and middle income countries. *Lancet.* 2007;370:991–1005.

120. Jacob KS, Sharan P, Mirza I, et al. Mental health systems in countries: where are we now? *Lancet.* 2007;370:1061–77.

121. Saraceno B, van Ommeren M, Batniji R, et al. Barriers to improvement of mental health services in low-income and middle-income countries. *Lancet.* 2007;370:1164–74.

122. Lancet Global Mental Health Group. Scale up services for mental disorders: a call for action. *Lancet.* 2007;370:1241–52.

123. WHO. *mhGAP: Mental Health Gap Action Programme: scaling up care for mental, neurological and substance use disorders.* Geneva: World Health Organization; 2008.

124. Collins PY, Patel V, Joestl SS, March D, Insel TR, Daar AS. Grand challenges in global mental health. *Nature.* 2011;475:27–30.

125. Benegal V, Chand PK, Obot IS. Packages of care for alcohol use disorders in low- and middle-income countries. *PLoS Med.* 2009;6:e1000170.

126. Mari JdJ, Razzouk D, Thara R, Eaton J, Thornicroft G. Packages of care for schizophrenia in low- and middle-income countries. *PLoS Med.* 2009;6:e1000165.

127. Mbuba CK, Newton CR. Packages of care for epilepsy in low- and middle-income countries. *PLoS Med.* 2009;6:e1000162.

128. Patel V, Simon G, Chowdhary N, Kaaya S, Araya R. Packages of care for depression in low- and middle-income countries. *PLoS Med.* 2009;6:e1000159.

129. Patel V, Thornicroft G. Packages of care for mental, neurological, and substance use disorders in low- and middle-income countries. *PLoS Med.* 2009;6:e1000160.

130. Prince MJ, Acosta D, Castro-Costa E, Jackson J, Shaji KS. Packages of care for dementia in low- and middle-income countries. *PLoS Med.* 2009;6:e1000176.

131. Flisher AJ, Sorsdahl K, Hatherill S, Chehil S. Packages of care for attention-deficit hyperactivity disorder in low- and middle-income countries. *PLoS Med.* 2010;7:e1000235.

132. WHO. *MhGAP Intervention Guide for mental, neurological and substance use disorders in non-specialized health settings: mental health Gap Action Programme (mhGAP).* Geneva: World Health Organization; 2010.

133. Patel V. Why mental health matters to global health. *Transcult Psychiatry.* In press.

134. Kleinman A. Global mental health: a failure of humanity. *Lancet.* 2009;374:603–4.

135. World Health Organization. *Mental health atlas 2011.* Geneva: World Health Organization; 2011.

136. Inter-Agency Standing Committee. *IASC guidelines on mental health and psychosocial support in emergency settings.* Geneva: Inter-Agency Standing Committee; 2007.

137. Eaton J, Radtke B. *Community mental health implementation guidelines.* Bensheim, Germany: CBM; 2010.

138. BasicNeeds. *Mental health and development: A model in practice.* Leamington Spa, UK: BasicNeeds; 2008.

139. Brody EB. *The search for mental health: a history and memoir of WFMH 1948–1997.* Baltimore: Williams & Wilkins; 1998.

140. Patel V, Thara R. *Meeting mental health needs in developing countries.* New Delhi: Sage (India); 2003.

141. de Jong JTVM. Public mental health, traumatic stress, and human rights violations in low-income countries. In: de Jong JTVM (ed.). *Trauma, war, and violence: public mental health in socio-cultural context.* New York: Kluwer Academic/Plenum Publishers; 2002:1–91.

142. de Jong JTVM, Komproe IH, van Ommeren M. Common mental disorders in post-conflict settings. *Lancet.* 2003;361:2128–30.

143. Tol WA, Komproe IH, Susanty D, Jordans MJD, Macy RD, De Jong JTVM. School-based mental health intervention for children affected by political violence in Indonesia: a cluster randomized trial. *JAMA.* 2008;300:655–62.

144. Jordans MJD, Komproe IH, Tol WA, et al. Evaluation of a school based psychosocial inter-vention in conflict-affected Nepal: a randomized controlled trial. *J Child Psychol Psychiatry.* 2010;51:818–26.

145. Jordans MJD, Komproe IH, Tol WA, et al. Practice-driven evaluation of a multi-layered psy-chosocial care package for children in areas of armed conflict. *Community Ment Health J.* 2010;47:267–77.

146. Grand Challenges Canada. *Global Mental Health.* 2010. [cited 2012 November 18]; Available from: http://www.grandchallenges.ca/grand-challenges/gc4-non-communicable-diseases/mentalhealth/.

147. Bash KW, Bash-Liechti J. Studies on the epidemiology of neuropsychiatric disorders among the population of the city of Shiraz, Iran. *Soc Psychiatry.* 1974;9:163–71.

148. WHO. *mhGAP: Mental Health Gap Action Programme: Scaling up care for mental, neurological and substance use disorders.* Geneva: World Health Organization; 2008.

149. Calouste Gulbenkian Foundation. Gulbenkian Global Mental Health Platform 2012.

2 Disorders, Diagnosis, and Classification

Oye Gureje and Dan J. Stein

INTRODUCTION

There is more to health than the absence of a disease, and a prescribed treatment does not necessarily imply the presence of a disorder. For example, the treatment offered to individuals with high cholesterol is not to ameliorate a diseased state but rather to prevent the emergence of a disorder. Nevertheless, the state of having a disease is central to the practice of much of medicine. That is, while health is not just the opposite of ill-health, it is impossible to talk of "global health," either mental or physical, without reference to diseased states or to "disorders."

In general, there is usually less ambiguity about whether a particular condition constitutes a diseased state in physical medicine. However, the definition of what constitutes a "disorder" poses a number of challenges, in mental health in particular. The line between "normality" and abnormal psychological status can be very blurred and difficult to determine. The emotion of anxiety, for example, is common and is normal and understandable in most day-to-day circumstances. Yet, at some level of severity and impairment, the feeling of anxiety acquires the label of a "disorder."

Deciding that level is not a precise science, and this imprecision has been the basis of the controversy about whether psychiatric disorders are moral judgements or reflect real diseases. However, the definitional challenge of deciding what constitutes mental disorders did not start and stop with the controversy between pro-psychiatry and anti-psychiatry forces about the "moral" rather than "medical" nature of mental health conditions[1–3] in which the former had seen mental "disorders" as real medical conditions while the latter contingent regarded them as nothing more than moral deviance. Even today, there are still controversies about the concept of "mental disorder."[4–8]

DEFINING MENTAL DISORDERS

In psychiatry, "mental illness" is often used to describe the presence of a cluster of symptoms that marks a definite change from a previous psychological state for an individual.[9] Generally, when such a change is accompanied by distress and/or a decline in functioning, a disorder is said to occur.[10] In both physical medicine and psychiatry, diseases often have multiple contributing causes, which are not fully understood.[11] While in physical medicine we often have biomarkers for such states, this is not always the case, and psychiatry is characterized by a relative absence of biomarkers for mental disorders. In the absence of precise etiologies and with a reliance on the clustering of symptoms as the basis for defining disorders, defining a case is a challenge. Setting thresholds for "caseness" has therefore involved moving the cutoff points along what is essentially a dimensional spectrum of symptoms. Mental disorders are commonly defined by multiple symptoms, with any given diagnosis requiring a specific combination from a list of possible symptoms.

Given the clinical judgement involved in deciding where to place the cutoff along the symptom dimension, and the likelihood that various cultural factors may affect reporting styles by patients, the key question arises of whether what constitutes a disorder in one cultural setting may be so regarded in another. Thus, for example, it is not enough to show that "depressive disorder" has diagnostic validity and clinical utility in one cultural setting. To make it useful as a concept for "global" health, it has to be shown that the symptom constellation that describes the "disorder" has a measure of cross-cultural validity and utility as well. In this regard, the question of how influential value judgements are in the description of mental disorders is a major one.[12] As noted by Kendell: "The most fundamental issue, and also the most contentious one, is whether disease and illness are normative concepts based on value-free scientific terms; in other words, whether they are biochemical terms or sociopolitical ones."[9] Do mental disorders, as currently conceived and described, reflect social and moral values of the dominant powers within the mental health community, a community that is still essentially Western-dominated, or do they capture universal or global concepts of disordered mental states?

CULTURE AND THE CONCEPT OF MENTAL ILLNESS

This question of whether mental disorders capture universal concepts of disorder, or reflect dominant and social values, has been thoroughly debated in both the philosophical and the clinical literatures.[13,14] On one hand, it seems clear that mental disorders are a different kind of entity than, say, squares, which can be defined in universal terms using necessary and sufficient criteria. However, there is also a good argument that mental disorders are not simply analogous to weeds; which are defined entirely differently from time to time and place to place. Rather, it would seem that judgements about mental disorders do incorporate values (and, thus, are different from time to time and place to place), but are also open to reasonable debate so that universal considerations, such as associated distress and/or impairment, can be brought into consideration. Thus, there is a consistent tension between "medical" and "moral" perspectives on the nature and boundaries of mental disorder.[7]

There is no doubt that the culture and social milieus in which symptoms are experienced affects the presentation of mental disorders. Views about what constitutes an illness are influenced by the norms with which patients and their families are familiar. Such views will affect coping schemas, help-seeking behavior, as well as attitudes about disorder (negative or otherwise). Also, there can be little doubt that the availability of resources devoted to the alleviation of disorder will be relevant to how symptoms are experienced. Indeed, clinical encounters are shaped by the "cultures" of the protagonists. For example, the assessment of mental disorders is often influenced by cultural and social differences between the patient and the physician.[15]

At the same time, immersion in a particular culture may lead to a recognition of universality. For example, it used to be claimed that depression was not a common mental health condition among Africans. Also, when depression was found among Africans, the observation was often made that the features were different from those of depressed patients in the West.[16] Features such as guilt feelings, self-deprecation, psychomotor retardation, and associated suicidal behaviors were often reported to be far less prevalent in Africa than in the Western world. These observations were made by European psychiatrists working in Africa. However, contrary evidence has now been presented by African psychiatrists not only that depression is a common psychiatric disorder in Africa, but that the core symptoms of the illness are common and can be elicited by culturally sensitive assessments.[17-21]

DIAGNOSIS

Diagnosis serves a number of important purposes. Diagnosis facilitates the determination of treatment needs and is predictive of response to treatment or the assessment of prognosis. When clinically useful, diagnosis allows appropriate reimbursement by health insurance schemes (whether public or private). Communication between and within groups can be facilitated when classification is reliable and valid and when it has utility and applicability across diverse clinical settings. In mental health, classification must recognize differences, especially cultural differences. However, because the purpose is to facilitate a "common language,"[22] differences across classification systems must be regarded as the result of works in progress, informing the revision of subsequent versions of classificatory schemes rather than being allowed to impede what is essentially a medium of communication.

Ideally, diagnosis should be based on empirical evidence. Typically, diagnosis is made through a process of acquiring clinical information and eliciting symptoms, organizing the symptoms into plausible syndromes, and confirming the underlying disease process through appropriate biomarkers. However, even though mental disorders are often regarded as brain disorders affecting emotion, higher cognition, and executive function, finding sensitive and specific biomarkers has proved elusive. Most mental health conditions lack validating biological markers. As noted by Hyman, "The existence of only a small number of well-validated biomarkers and the early stage in which our understanding of neurogenetics and pathophysiology finds itself have, reasonably enough, impeded the incorporation of neuroscience into psychiatric diagnosis to date."[23] It is an open question whether or not it will ever be possible to have biomarkers of clinical conditions that are highly heterogenous and influenced by a broad range of etiologies, including psychosocial mechanisms.[11]

It can be argued that a range of empirical evidence other than biomarkers can serve to support the diagnostic validity and clinical utility of disorders. Thus, for example, it turns out that treating cholesterol levels when they exceed certain levels is cost-effective in preventing medical complications; this helps define the boundaries of hypercholesterolemia. Unfortunately, however, such data are often not widely available in the case of mental disorders. For example, clinical trials have typically been confined to academic settings in the West, and there is a dearth of randomized controlled trials in low- and middle-income countries, and a paucity of effectiveness studies in mental health globally.

Important advances in psychiatric epidemiology have been useful in making the argument that many mental disorders are prevalent globally and are universally associated with high levels of distress and/or impairment. Such work has been important in emphasizing the global burden of mental disorders and in helping create the World Health Organization (WHO) rallying cry of "No health without mental health" (see Prince chapter). At the same time, it should be recognized that major problems remain with current epidemiological data. For example, because the tools used to ascertain these disorders lack precision, only approximate rates can be obtained. Also, there are large gaps in existing epidemiological data, especially because of a relative lack of longitudinal studies in low- and middle-income countries.

Most mental disorders are identified and defined within an array of commonly occurring symptoms rather than reflecting distinctly unique cluster of symptoms.[24-26] Therefore, when defining mental disorders categorically within the spectrum of symptoms, a determination has to be made about where to situate the cutoff along the dimension. Consensus needs to be reached on the basis of a range of relevant data concerning diagnostic validity and clinical utility—including, for example, data on associated disability, and response to treatment. Careful judgement is required to weigh data, for example, on whether different numbers of symptoms for the diagnosis of depression optimize diagnostic validity and clinical utility. Such judgements should be informed by an awareness of how the diagnostic construct will be used in different cultures.

CLASSIFYING MENTAL DISORDERS

Classifying mental disorders is not a precise science. Indeed, classifications have often been constructed to reflect national health preferences and needs. Thus, national systems of classification for mental disorders have existed in countries such as China and Cuba for several decades and have served the needs of such countries. However, two major classifications have wider international usage: the *Diagnostic and Statistical Manual of Mental Disorders* (DSM) and the *International Classification of Diseases* (ICD). Even though the DSM is designed by an American organization, it is used widely across the world, especially for research purposes. On the other hand, the ICD is the international standard for health information and is used to monitor mortality, morbidity, and other health parameters by member countries of the World Health Organization.

The number of diagnostic categories for psychiatric disorders was relatively limited until the publication of the third edition of the *Diagnostic and Statistical Manual of Mental Disorders*.[27] The DSM, currently in its fifth edition, and the ICD,[28] currently in its tenth edition, are two classification systems that list and describe criteria for diagnosing mental disorders. DSM-5 has just been published, and ICD-11 will be published soon. It had been hoped that the revisions of the two systems would be strongly influenced by new knowledge about the biological bases of mental disorders. However, that hope has been tempered by the failure of the otherwise remarkable progress in brain research to produce precise biomarkers. While DSM revisions have emphasized diagnostic validity, ICD revisions have emphasized clinical utility.[29-31] As noted by the International Advisory Group for the revision of ICD-10 "Mental and Behavioral Disorders": "If revisions to the classification systems are not going to dramatically alter the structure and descriptions of mental disorders based on biopsychosocial data to improve their validity, an appropriate focus is to improve their clinical utility in order to facilitate identification and treatment of mental disorders by clinicians."[32] Building on earlier articulations of the concept,[30] WHO has offered the following definition of *clinical utility*:

The clinical utility of a classification construct or category for mental and behavioral disorders depends on: a) its value in *communicating* (e.g., among practitioners, patients, families, administrators); b) its *implementation characteristics* in clinical practice, including its goodness of fit (i.e., accuracy of description), its ease of use and the time required to use it (i.e., feasibility); and c) its usefulness in *selecting interventions* and in making *clinical management* decisions.[33]

The goal of seeking clinical utility is of particular importance to the WHO, given its role as a global public health agency. However, even for the American Psychiatric Association

(APA), with its emphasis on scientific validity, improved clinical utility is also one of the main goals of DSM revisions. For example, the APA states in the introduction of the DSM-IV-TR that its "highest priority has been to provide a helpful guide to clinical practice."[10]

While data collected using the DSM-IV and ICD-10 classifications have suggested that many disorders have universal aspects, there is also little doubt that psychiatric nosology is embedded in the cultures of the societies in which it has been formulated and, as such, cultural factors should not be discounted in the classification of mental disorders. In this regard, it is worthy of note that even though evidence such as that provided by the latent structure of common constructs of psychopathology supports the cross-cultural, and thus universal, applicability of these constructs,[34] there is also evidence to suggest significant differences across cultures. Thus, the World Mental Health Surveys initiative, in which similar ascertainment tools were used, found large differences in the prevalence of mental disorders across countries, including those in the same geographical zone or economic group.[35] Such differences possibly attest to the role of context-specific factors, such as culture, in the occurrence and nature of mental disorders. Even so, differences across countries may be useful in revising existing nosologies. For example, in a large survey of mental disorders in Nigeria, a significant number of false positives were apparently found for generalized anxiety disorder (GAD), probably indicating that, against the background of poverty, judgements about whether respondents' worry was "excessive," as required for a diagnosis of GAD by both the DSM-IV and ICD-10, had not been considered.[36] In the United States, however, it has been argued that removal of the "excessive worry" requirement would not decrease diagnostic validity.[37] Nevertheless, any talk about culture in relation to psychiatric nosology is mistaken if it implies an exclusive reference to low- and middle-income countries. These countries are as heterogeneously diverse as high-income countries. There is no more "a culture" that unifies Italians and the British than there is one that unifies Angolans and Gambians. At the same time, and in relation to the classification of mental disorders, it is important to be mindful of the line between an informed consideration of culture and an "exoticization" of cultural differences.

MENTAL DISORDERS AND DISABILITY

The association of mental disorders with disability is a reality that patients and their caregivers, as well as mental health providers, live with on a daily basis. Indeed, it is now widely acknowledged that mental disorders often lead to a greater level of functional disablement, or disability, than do many common chronic physical health conditions.[38] Yet, until recently, the traditional ways of quantifying the impact of health problems, which relied almost exclusively on their likelihood to lead to death, did not permit a full appreciation of the impact of mental health on disability. The entry of disability into the consideration of the impact of diseases through the introduction of the metric of Disability Adjusted Life Years (DALYs) has had a dramatic effect on the estimates of the burden of mental disorders compared to those of physical disorders.[39]

Notwithstanding the importance of the appreciation of the association of disability with mental disorders, the concept of "disability" has not always been presented with consistency and clarity.[40] Thus, it is sometimes used to connote activity limitations that may be associated with a particular mental disorder and sometimes as a way of describing the severity of a mental disorder. Also, in setting thresholds for the presence of a constellation of symptoms to be regarded as constituting a "case" of mental illness, and particularly in response to the concern that estimates of community prevalence of mental disorders obtained through surveys were implausibly high, the DSM introduced the concept of *clinical significance*, within which was subsumed *disability* (or "functional impairment"). The definition of mental disorders produced in this way has conflated what are arguably two different phenomena: disability and clinical syndrome.

Nevertheless, the view that *psychopathology*, or clinical syndrome, is distinct and different from *disability* poses a challenge of its own. As it has been pointed out, a pathological dysfunction can hardly be regarded as a disorder, except when it is associated with some harm, which may be best conceptualized as role impairment.[5] In the area of common mental disorders where the underlying psychopathology is often widely distributed in the community, the point at which to situate the categorical definition of a disorder may be difficult without linking the threshold to some consequence such as disability. The challenge of reliably and validly assessing psychopathology and disability is a pressing one.

These considerations take on greater relevance when mental health is considered within the ambit of global health. The knowledge that reporting styles may be culturally determined will suggest that if symptom expressions are not linked to some clearly defined consequence, having "globally" accepted definitions of what constitutes mental disorders will be problematic.[41] The notion that some such "disorders" reflect "categorical fallacies" will be difficult to refute if a set of symptoms in one setting cannot be demonstrated or shown to have some objectively verifiable consequence in other settings. Even if the measurement of that consequence and its acceptance as a validly defined "harm" may itself be contentious, it is likely to remain an important yardstick for defining "caseness."

CLASSIFICATION OF MENTAL DISORDERS AND GLOBAL MENTAL HEALTH

Global mental health is essentially the mobilization of resources to meet the challenges of population health needs and strive for equity in doing so. Given the large unmet need for mental health services in low- and middle-income countries, it is logical that global mental health will be seen as having a major, if not exclusive, focus on those countries. So, what is the relevance of classification of mental disorders to global mental health?

The pursuit of global mental health does not contradict the development and revision of the classifications of mental disorders. That is, the revisions of both the ICD and the DSM are not processes that should be regarded as distracting luxuries. Indeed, for mental health conditions for which pathognomonic signs and biomarkers are absent, the development of a common language for use across the world is an essential basis for a "global" consideration of what constitutes mental health conditions.

Indeed, in recent years, an important development in the agitation for greater attention to mental health is the demonstration that neuropsychiatric disorders constitute a large proportion of the global burden of disease, as well as information showing, not only the worldwide gap between need and available resources, but also the inequitable distribution of those resources. A basic requirement for these comparative statistics is an agreement about what constitutes a "mental disorder," as well as a demonstration that a particular mental health condition in one setting can be so regarded in another.

While it is important to acknowledge the heuristic value of current definitions of mental disorders and the classifications that organize them into useful groups, it is important that we avoid reification of diagnostic entities, and continually attempt to refine them based on better data.[31] Actors in the field of global mental health cannot and should not support, through the process of classification, the reification of particular conditions or the medicalization of essentially human experiences. It is particularly important to note that different categories may be useful for different purposes. In a research setting in a well-resourced institution, where genetic contributions to variance in psychopathology are being delineated, a more fine-grained diagnostic system may be useful. In a primary care setting in an under-resourced region, where decisions need to be made about whom to refer on for psychiatric treatment, a less fine-grained nosology is more appropriate.

There is now compelling evidence that despite the large global burden of neuropsychiatric disorders, the response to that burden has been grossly inadequate. Thus, across the world, the gap between need for mental health service and available resources is large, so that between 32% and 78% of those with serious mental disorders do not receive any treatment.[42] An important consideration for global mental health is whether the extant classification aids in the effort to bridge the gap between available resources and the burden of mental disorders. It is generally recognized that such an effort has to give a special focus to the delivery of mental health service at the primary care level. This realization is born out of two major observations: most countries, especially low- and middle-income countries where the gap is much larger, do not have the mental health specialist resources to deliver the service that meets the required need; also, across the world, most people with mental health conditions seek care from primary health services rather than from any other level of health service. A classification system that has the potential to expand services must therefore be one that is suitable for use in the non-specialist primary care system. Indeed, in most parts of the world, primary care is delivered by non-physicians.[43] It is in realization of this fact that the WHO recently produced a set of guidelines, the "Mental Health Gap Action Programme Intervention Guide" (mhGAP-IG), which incorporates evidence-based interventions for a list of priority mental health conditions to aid in the recognition and management of such conditions in non-specialist settings. It builds on the knowledge that primary care providers can be trained to deliver both psychological and pharmacological interventions for some of the most common mental disorders with the provision of supervision and support by more highly trained health providers, including specialists.

As noted by the International Advisory Group for the Revision of ICD-10 Mental and Behavioral Disorders, "People are only likely to have access to the most appropriate mental health services when the conditions that define eligibility and treatment selection are supported by a precise, valid, and clinically useful classification system."[32] In order for this purpose to be adequately served, a classification system for mental disorders that will be satisfactory for primary care must capture the complexity of the range of presentations of psychological problems in that setting in which mental health problems are often associated with physical illness and social problems.[44]

Indeed, the diversity of primary care services across the world is another reason why a classificatory system for mental health conditions must be developed through a participatory consensus-based process. While no system will satisfy every need, it is nevertheless important that as many voices as are relevant be heard in the process of arriving at the consensus that engenders the desired common language. Clearly, evidence-based decision-making about diagnostic validity and clinical utility is needed for the ongoing and future refinement of psychiatric nosologies. Nevertheless, it is necessary to incorporate data from different cultures, as well as judgements about diagnostic validity and clinical utility that are informed by real-world experiences in a range of different settings, in order to optimize the classification systems for use in the many settings in which they will ultimately be applied.

COMMON MENTAL DISODERS

Depression, anxiety disorders, and somatoform disorders are often grouped together as "common mental disorders" (CMD). A major reason for this is the frequent co-occurrence of these disorders in clinical samples. Thus, in primary care, different combinations of depressive, anxiety, and somatic symptoms are the norm among patients with mental health conditions seen by clinicians. Therefore, even though described separately in this section, their clinical manifestations are not as distinct in routine clinical practice.

Depression

Depression is one of the most burdensome disorders in the world. Even in low-income countries, it is estimated that depressive disorders will become the third most burdensome health problem after HIV/AIDS and perinatal conditions.

Clinical Features

The core symptoms of depression are low mood (feeling sad), loss of interest and of enjoyment, and reduced energy, usually manifesting as reduced activity or getting easily tired. Other symptoms include change in appetite (reduced appetite is more characteristic), weight loss, disturbed sleep, reduced libido, impaired attention and concentration, feelings of guilt and worthlessness, recurrent thoughts or acts of suicide or self-harm, and pessimistic views about the future. Many patients with depression present with bodily symptoms to clinicians, and it is only after careful questioning that the core symptoms of depression are identified. Symptoms are often worse in the morning. In some cases, patients may present with psychotic symptoms, characterized by hallucinations or delusions, the features of which usually reflect the patient's low mood.

Diagnosis of depression requires a minimum of at least two core symptoms with durations of at least two weeks, as well as several other associated symptoms. In determining severity, clinicians commonly assess the number of symptoms present and the level of disablement that the patient may have.

Anxiety Disorders

These are the most prevalent psychiatric disorders worldwide.[45] Anxiety disorders are more common in females, usually have their onset in adolescence and young adulthood, and tend to be chronic. They often coexist with other psychiatric or physical disorders.

Clinical Features

Anxiety (an unpleasant feeling of apprehension accompanied by autonomic symptoms) is a normal human experience, especially in response to a real or perceived threat. Anxiety disorders are diagnosed when an individual has symptoms of anxiety that are not caused by a physical disease or another psychiatric disorder, and are affecting the person's ability to function. Physical symptoms of anxiety include dry mouth, difficulty with swallowing, feeling bloated, nausea or abdominal distress, frequent loose stools, palpitations, chest pain or discomfort, difficulty breathing, sweating, trembling, muscle tension, and headaches. Psychological symptoms include feeling dizzy, light-headed, or faint; poor sleep; feeling that objects are unreal (derealization) or that the self is distant or "not really there" (depersonalization); fear of losing control or going crazy; and fear of dying. Other symptoms of anxiety include hot flushes, numbness or tingling sensations, and nightmares.

Specific types of anxiety disorders include:

- *Specific phobia*, in which symptoms of anxiety occur predominantly upon exposure to well-defined situations or objects that are perceived as dangerous.
- *Social phobia*, in which the specific fear may be that of being scrutinized by others, of eating or speaking in public, of interacting with the opposite sex, or of any social interaction outside the person's family.
- *Generalized anxiety disorder*, in which there is persistent worry and apprehension about a number of events or activities.

- *Panic disorder,* which is characterized by recurrent, spontaneous, episodic attacks of severe anxiety that are not restricted to any particular situation.
- *Obsessive-compulsive disorder,* in which the essential feature is recurrent intrusive thoughts or compulsive acts or rituals (stereotyped behaviors or mental acts that are repeated over and over).

While DSM-IV included both OCD and post-traumatic disorder in the section on anxiety disorders, ICD-10 differentiated between phobic anxiety disorders, obsessive-compulsive disorders, and stress-related disorders. Both DSM-5 and ICD-11 will have separate chapters on anxiety disorders, obsessive-compulsive and related disorders, and traumatic and stressor-related disorders. These three sets of conditions have a number of overlaps, and together might be termed "anxiety and related disorders."

Somatoform Disorders

Somatoform disorders (formerly "psychosomatic") are characterized by repeated presentation of physical symptoms. Patients frequently request medical examinations and investigations despite prior negative findings and no obvious physical basis for the symptoms. Somatoform disorders are common in primary care settings. Undifferentiated somatoform disorder is the commonest, occurring in up to 10% of primary care patients.[46]

Bipolar Affective Disorder

Clinical Features

Elevation of mood is a central feature of mania, and this often manifests in the form of expansive mood or euphoria or, alternatively, irritability. Patients may experience increased energy and be hyperactive and talkative. There is a marked feeling of well-being, elevated self esteem, and grandiosity. Manic patients have a reduced need for sleep, and the usual social inhibitions are lost, resulting in over-familiarity with strangers, flamboyant dressing, and socially inappropriate behavior. Attention cannot be sustained. Patients make impractical and extravagant plans and spend money or drive recklessly. They may also develop psychotic symptoms, characterized by grossly disturbed behavior, hallucinations, and delusions, often with themes suggestive of their inflated self-worth.

Schizophrenia

Worldwide, the prevalence of schizophrenia is hypothesized to be about 1%. It occurs equally in men and women. The age of onset is usually in late adolescence or young adulthood; however, there is a strong gender effect, with men developing the illness earlier than women. Schizophrenia often follows a chronic or recurrent course, with residual symptoms and incomplete social recovery in many sufferers, causing significant disability and placing a huge burden on their families.

Clinical Features

The clinical presentation of schizophrenia varies, and this diagnosis probably encompasses a heterogeneous group of disorders currently classified together based on the presence of certain clinical signs and symptoms. This heterogeneity is shown by variations in the manifestations, course, and outcome of the disorder.

The appearance and behavior of patients with schizophrenia can range from being almost entirely normal, though having some oddities in dressing and speech, to being grossly agitated or disorganized. Social behavior may deteriorate, resulting in poor grooming, laughing and talking to oneself, or social withdrawal. Patients' speech often reflects underlying disorders of thought; some express strange religious or philosophical ideas. Thought disorder may manifest as reduced stream or content of thought, or loosening of association. Other disorders of thought include various experiences of loss of control over one's thoughts, such as thoughts being "inserted or withdrawn" from the patient's mind by "external influences" (thought insertion or thought withdrawal).

Patients often have persistent delusions that are culturally inappropriate and some-times completely impossible, usually referred to as *bizarre delusions*, or *delusions of control*. More common are persecutory or grandiose delusions, even though the latter may not be congruent with the mood, so-called *mood-incongruent delusions*. Auditory hallucinations are common and may be single words or phrases spoken repeatedly, persistent voices giving a running commentary on the patients' actions, or two or more voices talking about the patient. Hallucinations in other modalities occur less frequently. Some patients may manifest abnormal motor signs, including posturing, mannerisms, or stereotypy, or may be mute. Many patients have poor insight into the nature, severity, and consequences of their illness, and are therefore poorly compliant with treatment.

Substance Use Disorder

The use of psychoactive substances is a major social and public health problem. Substance use disorders worldwide account for 1.8% of DALYs. They comprise disorders of varying severity attributable to the use of one or more psychoactive substances, which may or may not have been medically prescribed. Psychoactive substances include alcohol, tobacco, marijuana, opioids (morphine, heroin, pentazocine, and methadone), cocaine, stimulants (amphetamines, caffeine), hallucinogens (LSD, Ecstasy), sedatives and hypnotic drugs (benzodiazepines, barbiturates), and volatile solvents (glue, petrol/gasoline, polish, cleaning fluids).

Types of Substance Use Disorders

Depending on the specific substance, the following are common problems that may be experienced:

Acute intoxication—This is a transient condition due to the recent ingestion of a psychoactive substance that results in disturbances in the level of consciousness, perception, mood, behavior, and cognition. The characteristic signs and symptoms observed are usually compatible with the known action of the ingested substance. For example, alcohol intoxication is characterized by disinhibition, aggression, impaired attention, impaired judgement, unsteady gait and slurred speech.

Harmful use or abuse—A maladaptive pattern of psychoactive substance use that is causing damage to the patient's health or to social and occupational roles.

Dependence—Usually follows the repeated ingestion of a psychoactive substance. The individual develops a strong desire to use the substance, is unable to control its use, begins to neglect alternative sources of pleasure, and requires increasing doses of the substance to produce the desired effect.

Dementia

Dementia is a clinical syndrome characterized by a generalized impairment of intellectual abilities, memory, and personality, without any disturbance of consciousness. It usually results from diffuse cerebral pathology affecting the cerebral cortex (*cortical dementia*) or subcortical structures (*subcortical dementia*). Some dementias are progressive and irreversible, some are non-progressive, while others are reversible, depending on the underlying cause. The course of the illness typically reflects the cause. Common causes include degenerative disorders (such as Alzheimer's and Parkinson's diseases), vascular disorders, trauma, metabolic disorders (liver failure, uremia), infectious disease (HIV/AIDS, encephalitis), drugs and toxins, and nutritional disorders.

Dementia usually has its onset in old age (above 65 years of age), and its prevalence increases with increasing age. Dementia of the Alzheimer's type is the commonest, accounting for 50% to 60% of cases, followed by vascular dementia.

Clinical Features

Most cases of dementia have an insidious onset. In the early stages, the patient presents with subtle memory changes, fatigue, slowed thinking, and labile mood. Memory impairment is an early and prominent feature of dementia. In the early stages, memory impairment affects recently learnt material such as events of the day, but it gradually involves remoter memory. Orientation is also progressively affected, starting with disorientation with respect to time, place, and (in severe cases) to person. Intellectual deterioration occurs, leading to difficulty with problem-solving and the loss of previously acquired skills. Thinking is slowed and poor in content. Language difficulties manifest initially as vague, imprecise, stereotypical speech, perseveration and difficulty with naming objects; later, patients may become incoherent or aphasic. Judgement, decision-making, and comprehension are impaired. As the illness progresses, behavior becomes disorganized and inappropriate; the patient may be restless, agitated, or wander around aimlessly. Emotional disturbances may manifest as anxiety, depression, suspiciousness, irritability, or hostility. Some patients develop psychotic symptoms characterized by hallucinations and delusions. As disease worsens, patients are unable to care for themselves.

Some Common Childhood Disorders

Childhood psychiatric disorders include disorders that more typically affect children and adolescents, and disorders that are common in adult life but with onset in childhood. Two major examples are developmental disorders and behavioral disorders.

Developmental Disorders

Developmental disorders can be pervasive or specific. *Mental* or *intellectual disability* is an example of pervasive developmental disorder. It is a global defect of intellectual functioning and adaptive skills. It is defined as a score of 70 and below on standardized tests of intelligence, and further sub-classified into *mild* (IQ 50–70), *moderate* (IQ 35–49), *severe* (IQ 20–34), and *profound* (IQ below 20). In settings where the validity of available standardized tests of intelligence has not been established, clinicians may have to base the diagnosis solely on the individual's level of intellectual functioning and adaptive skills, considered in the context of the living environment of the child.

Autistic Disorder Autism is another example of pervasive developmental disorder. It is more common in boys, and usually has its onset within the first three to four years of life. It is characterized by abnormal social development, impaired speech and language development, obsessive desire for sameness, and abnormal stereotyped behaviors and mannerisms.

Other specific developmental disorders are characterized by circumscribed developmental delays that are not attributable to any other disorder or to any lack of opportunity to learn. Specific developmental disorders are further divided into specific disorder of reading, spelling (dyslexia), writing, and motor skills, based on the specific area of scholastic ability that is most affected.

Behavioral Disorders

Children with these disorders often manifest disruptive behavior that make parental control difficult and impair learning. An example is *attention deficit hyperactivity disorder* (ADHD), the features of which are a pervasive, sustained, extreme restlessness, and difficulty in maintaining attention. Children with this disorder are impulsive, have difficulty with task completion, and are easily distracted. The hyperactivity is usually noticed early, by the time the child begins to walk. Another example is *conduct disorder*, which is characterized by persistent antisocial or defiant behavior. Children with this condition manifest features of aggressiveness such as bullying, cruelty to animals and other people; and antisocial behavior such as lying, stealing, truancy, and destructiveness.

CONCLUSION

Mental disorders are real and affect populations across the world, irrespective of their cultures and social organizations. However, classifying these disorders has been a daunting exercise in view of the imprecision of available evidence from neuroscience. With biomarkers still a futuristic hope, international classifications have sought to achieve reliability of communication and wide acceptability in order to serve the goal of clinical utility. Global mental health has benefited from the achievement of this common language, helping to emphasize the considerable burden that these disorders constitute in countries at different stages of development.

REFERENCES

1. Kendell RE. The concept of disease and its implications for psychiatry. *Br J Psychiatry.* 1975;127:305–15.
2. Laing RD. *The divided self.* London: Tavistock; 1960.
3. Szasz TS. The myth of mental illness. *Am Psychol.* 1960;15:113–8.
4. Wakefield JC. The concept of mental disorder: on the boundary between biological facts and social values. *Am Psychol.* 1992;47:73–88.
5. Wakefield JC. The concept of mental disorder: diagnostic implications of the harmful dysfunction analysis. *World Psychiatry.* 2007;6(3):149–56.
6. Jablensky A. Does psychiatry need an overarching concept of "mental disorder"? *World Psychiatry.* 2007;6(3):157–8.
7. Stein DJ. *The philosophy of psychopharmacology: happy pills, smart pills, pep pills.* Cambridge, UK: Cambridge University Press; 2008.
8. Stein DJ, Phillips KA, Bolton D, Fulford KW, Sadler JZ, Kendler KS. What is a mental/psychiatric disorder: from DSM-IV to DSM-V. *Psychol Med.* 2010;20:1–7.
9. Kendell RE. What are mental disorders? In: Freedman AM, Brotman R, Silverman I et al., editors. *Issues in psychiatric classification: science, practice and social policy.* New York: Human Sciences Press; 1986: pp. 23–45.

10. American Psychiatric Association. *Diagnostic and statistical manual of mental disorders*, 4th ed., text revision. Washington: American Psychiatric Association; 2000.

11. Nesse RM, Stein DJ. Towards a genuinely medical model for psychiatric nosology. *BMC Med.* 2012;10:5.

12. Fulford KWM, Broome M, Stanghellini G, Thornton T. Looking with both eyes open: fact and value in psychiatric diagnosis? *World Psychiatry.* 2005;4(2):78–86.

13. Stein DJ, Seedat S, Iversen A, Wessely S. Post-traumatic stress disorder: medicine and politics. *Lancet.* 2007;369:139–44.

14. Fulford KWM, Christodolou G, Stein DJ. Values and ethics: Perspectives on psychiatry for the person. *Int J Person-Centered Med.* 2011;1:161–2.

15. Raguram R, Weiss MG, Channabasavanna SM, Devins GM. Stigma, depression, and somatization in South India. *Am J Psychiatry.* 1996;153(8):1043–9.

16. Gureje O. Psychiatry in Africa: the myths, the exotic and the realities. *S Afr Psychiatry Rev.* 2007;10:11–4.

17. Binitie A. The clinical manifestations of depression in Africans. *Psychopathologie Africaine.* 1981;17:36–40.

18. Majodina MZ, Johnson FYA. Standardized assessment of depressive disorders (SADD) in Ghana. *Br J Psychiatry.* 1983;143:442–6.

19. Odejide AO, Oyewunmi LK, Ohaeri JU. Psychiatry in Africa: an overview. *Am J Psychiatry.* 1989;146:708–16.

20. Rwegellera GGC. Cultural aspects of depressive illnesses: clinical aspects and psychopathology. *Psychopathologie Africaine.* 1981;17:41–63.

21. Gureje O, Kola L, Afolabi E. Epidemiology of major depressive disorder in elderly Nigerians in the Ibadan Study of Ageing: a community-based survey. *Lancet.* 2007;370:957–64.

22. Sartorius N, Kaelber CT, Cooper JE, et al. Progress toward achieving a common language in psychiatry. Results from the field trial of the clinical guidelines accompanying the WHO classification of mental and behavioral disorders in ICD-10. *Arch Gen Psychiatry.* 1993;50(2):115–24.

23. Hyman SE. Can neuroscience be integrated into the DSM-V? *Nat Rev Neurosci.* 2007;8:725–32.

24. Goldberg DP. The heterogeneity of "major depression." *World Psychiatry.* 2011;10(3):226–8.

25. Kendler KS, Gardner COJ. Boundaries of major depression: an evaluation of DSM-IV criteria. *Am J Psychiatry.* 1998;155:172–7.

26. Ruscio J, Ruscio AM. Informing the continuity controversy: a taxometric analysis of depression. *J Abnormal Psychology.* 2000;109:473–87.

27. American Psychiatric Association. *Diagnostic and statistical manual of mental disorders*, 3rd ed. Washington, DC: American Psychiatric Association; 1980.

28. World Health Organization. *International classification of diseases and related health problems, 10th revision.* Geneva: World Health Organization; 1992.

29. Kendell R, Jablensky A. Distinguishing between the validity and utility of psychiatric diagnoses. *Am J Psychiatry.* 2003;160:4–12.

30. First M, Pincus H, Levine JB, Williams JBW, Ustun B, Peele R. Clinical utility as a criterion for revising psychiatric diagnoses. *Am J Psychiatry.* 2004;161(6):946–54.

31. Hyman SE. The diagnosis of mental disorders: the problem of reification. *Annu Rev Clin Psychol.* 2010;6:155–79.

32. International Advisory Group for the Revision of ICD-10 Mental and Behavioral Disorders. A conceptual framework for the revision of the ICD-10 classification of mental and behavioral disorders. *World Psychiatry.* 2011;10:86–92.

33. Reed GM. Toward ICD-11: Improving the clinical utility of WHO's International Classification of Mental Disorders. *Prof Psychol: Res Pract.* 2010;41(6):457–64.

34. Kessler RC, Ormel J, Petukhova M, McLaughlin KA, Green JG, Russo LJ, et al. Development of lifetime comorbidity in the World Health Organization World Mental Health Surveys. *Arch Gen Psychiatry.* 2011;68:90–100.

35. Demyttenaere K, Bruffaerts R, Posada-Villa J, Gasquet I, Kovess V, Lepine JP, et al. Prevalence, severity, and unmet need for treatment of mental disorders in the World Health Organization World Mental Health Surveys. *JAMA.* 2004;291:2581–90.

36. Gureje O, Lasebikan VO, Kola L, Makanjuola VA. The Nigerian Survey of Mental Health and Wellbeing: Lifetime and 12-month prevalence of DSM-IV disorders. *Br J Psychiatry.* 2006;188:465–71.

37. Ruscio AM, Lane M, Roy-Byrne P, Stang PE, Stein DJ, Wittchen HU, et al. Should excessive worry be required for a diagnosis of generalized anxiety disorder? Results from the US National Comorbidity Survey Replication. *Psychol Med.* 2005;35:1761–72.

38. Moussavi S, Chatterji S, Verdes E, Tandon A, Patel V, Ustun B. Depression, chronic diseases, and decrements in health: results from the World Health Surveys. *Lancet.* 2007;370(9590):851–8.

39. Murray CJ, Lopez AD. Global mortality, disability, and the contribution of risk factors: Global Burden of Disease Study. *Lancet.* 1997;349(9063):1436–42.

40. Ustun B, Kennedy C. What is "functional impairment"? Disentangling disability from clinical significance. *World Psychiatry.* 2009;8:82–5.

41. Kirmayer LJ. Culture, context and experience in psychiatric diagnosis. *Psychopathology.* 2005;38:192–6.

42. Wang PS, Aguilar-Gaxiola S, Alonso J, Angermeyer MC, Borges G, Bromet EJ, et al. Use of mental health services for anxiety, mood, and substance disorders in 17 countries in the WHO World Mental Health Surveys. *Lancet.* 2007;370:841–50.

43. Reed GM, Sharan P, Saxena S. Reducing disease burden through the revision of ICD-10 mental and behavioural disorders. *Natl Med J India.* 2009 ICD-10;22(6):285–8.

44. Gask L, Klinkman M, Fortes S, Dowrick C. Capturing complexity: the case for a new classification system for mental disorders in primary care. *Eur Psychiatry.* 2008;7:469–76.

45. Kessler RC, Angermeyer MC, Anthony JC, De Graaf R, Demyttenaere K, Gasquet I, et al. Lifetime prevalence and age-of-onset distributions of mental disorders in the World Health Organization's World Mental Health Initiative. *World Psychiatry.* 2007;6:168–76.

46. Gureje O, Obikoya B, Ikuesan BA. Prevalence of specific psychiatric disorders in an urban primary care setting. *East Afr Med J.* 1992 May;69(5):282–7.

3 Culture and Global Mental Health

Laurence J. Kirmayer and Leslie Swartz

INTRODUCTION

Human beings are fundamentally cultural beings: we acquire our ability to function as adults through developmental processes that are shaped by culture, and we live within culturally constructed systems of meaning that are shared by local and global communities. Clearly, then, culture must be of central concern to global mental health. The discipline of cultural psychiatry aims to bring together insights from anthropology, psychology, sociology, and related fields to understand the social underpinnings and local variability of mental health problems, their prevention and resolution. In this chapter, we outline the contributions of cultural psychiatry to research, training, and clinical practice in global mental health.

Culture matters for global mental health for many reasons:

(a) Along with socioeconomic disparities and multiple forms of discrimination, it contributes to significant health disparities in every society, structuring inequalities and the distribution of health problems and resources in the population.
(b) It influences the symptomatology, course, and outcome of disorders through psychophysiological and sociophysiological processes.
(c) It shapes individual and family coping and adaptation to illness and recovery.
(d) It determines help-seeking and clinical presentations.
(e) It undergirds the clinician–patient relationship and hence the patient's response to medical advice and intervention.
(f) It makes a central contribution to what is at stake in health care by framing the values, alternatives, and outcomes that inform health care decision-making.

Table 3.1 summarizes some of the uses of culture in psychiatry.

Table 3.1 Uses of Culture in Psychiatry

- *For patients*, to allow them to communicate concerns in ways that are intelligible, experience-near, and socially meaningful
- *For clinicians*, to interpret symptoms and signs in ways that lead to appropriate interventions
- *For public health and health systems planners and administrators*, to understand major determinants of help-seeking, coping, and response to illness and interventions
- *For researchers*, to clarify the role of social and cultural factors in psychopathology and treatment

In what follows, we will consider the role of culture in shaping the social determinants of mental health. We then turn to the central role of culture in providing local explanations for suffering and impairment. These explanations and associated systems of knowledge and practice influence the experience of illness, help-seeking behavior, and the social response to mental health problems and interventions. We next consider how culture constitutes modes of coping, adaptation, healing, and recovery. Finally, we discuss how knowledge of culture can be integrated into research, training, and intervention to support the goals of global mental health.

CULTURE IN A GLOBALIZING WORLD

Culture has been conceptualized in different ways at different times and places, reflecting the local history and politics of identity. Early discussions of culture in psychiatry were motivated by colonialist attitudes that generally viewed non-Western peoples as backward, primitive, or uncivilized.[1] "Culture" stood for the civilizing effects of Western tradition. This allowed for the possibility of alternative civilizations, but one set of traditions clearly was valued above all others and used as a tacit measure of health and illness. This Eurocentrism and ethnocentrism was entangled with racist ideologies and systems of domination and exploitation that have left deep wounds and enduring patterns of disadvantage in many places.[2,3] Contemporary views of culture have tried to break free of this troubling history, in part by insisting that all institutions—including those of science, medicine, and psychiatry—are deeply cultural and must be understood in social and historical context.

In its broadest sense, *culture* encompasses all of the humanly constructed and transmitted dimensions of social life. From birth onwards, the process of socialization is a process of enculturation into a system of symbols and values of the social groups and communities to which one belongs. Culture includes both local elements common to a group or community, and global aspects that are transmitted across communities, both locally and through transnational networks. In a narrower sense, culture is also used to refer to the way of life, identity, and traditions of a specific group or community that may be defined in terms of ethnicity, geography, descent, religion, or other social characteristics. Culture in the broader sense gives rise to these local distinctions. For example, race and ethnicity are culturally constructed forms of identity that may be chosen by or assigned to individuals on the basis of their heritage, appearance, or participation in specific communities.[4,5] Although they are culturally constructed, categories like race, ethnicity, religion, and occupational identity are social facts with powerful effects on health and well-being.[3,6,7] The specific aspects of social identity or cultural background that are important considerations for mental health depend on the context, the person, and the nature of the problem.

The rich diversity and complexity of culture and social context poses a challenge for psychiatric theory, research, and practice. In most research studies, culture is reduced to various proxy measures or isolated elements. For example, cross-national epidemiological studies, like those by the WHO[8-11] or the International Consortium for Psychiatric Epidemiology,[12] have generally taken geographic location as a proxy for culture. Of course, there is great cultural variation within any geographic region. Indeed, most cross-national comparative studies occur in more urban, developed settings, where Western education and influence is likely to be greatest. Each country or region has its own ways of configuring identity that may not travel well across borders, hence limiting the generalizability of research findings or clinical approaches. In the United States, for example, most comparative studies have used the ethnoracial blocs established by the U.S. Census (African American, Asian American and Pacific Islander, American Indian and Alaska Native, Latino, and White).[13,14] These categories reflect a very particular history of migration and contemporary politics. As such, they may have utility for framing issues of equity within American society, but in other contexts, different distinctions will be relevant to identify social determinants of health, disparities, and mental health service needs.

Another approach to culture involves unpacking its content to identify cultural factors or variables. For example, a large body of research in cross-cultural psychology examines differences between cultures that emphasize individual autonomy or independence (described as "individualistic" or "egocentric") and those that put more emphasis on interdependence ("collectivistic," "sociocentric").[15] These cultural orientations represent cultural values, but there is wide variation among individuals within any society in the extent to which they adhere to or express these values as personality traits.[16] There is also some evidence that fitting in with cultural norms or values is associated with greater well-being, while those who do not fit in well—whether because of temperament, life experience, or choice—may suffer from this poor fit with their social context and expectations.

Early thinking about culture and cultural differences was heavily influenced by the experiences of explorers from the West who were confronted with cultural practices that felt very alien to them. In this early approach, cultures were seen as bounded entities separate from one another, self-contained, and self-regulating. Contemporary theories, influenced partly by a rapidly diversifying world, recognize that cultures are open, hybrid, fluid systems of meaning contested from both within and without by competing values.[17] Cultures provide systems of meaning that are embodied and embedded in social institutions and practices. Aspects of these practices are inscribed in the brain as they shape individuals over their life span through neurodevelopmental processes.[18,19] Culture is also realized through ongoing cognitive-interactional processes that respond to the social contexts, settings, and predicaments created by social life. Culture is not fully captured in any one person's mental representations, because much of culture resides in networks of relationships, families, communities, and social institutions outside the individual that increasingly involve interactions of the global with the local through global networks, including electronic communication.

Although some have claimed that cultural differences are disappearing with globalization, it appears that increased mobility, telecommunication, and the economic forces of globalization are having more complex effects. While there are aspects of an emerging "global" or "world culture," at the same time, there are reassertions of local identity and reactions to other cultures that serve to consolidate or intensify local cultural identities.[20] There is increasing cultural hybridization with the creation of new cultural forms.[21] Individuals can participate in subcultures that are de-localized through the new forms of networking made possible by the Internet.[22']

CULTURE AND THE SOCIAL DETERMINANTS OF HEALTH

There is increasing recognition that social determinants of health, and mental health specifically, are among the most powerful factors influencing the risk, onset, and course of mental illness. [See Chapter 7][23,24] These determinants include poverty and social inequality, social integration and support, and racism and discrimination. The conditions of social life have powerful effects on well-being, in part because they determine basic physical conditions like nutrition, exposure to infectious agents, toxins or other environmental hazards, and the provision of other essential needs. These needs include a meaningful and coherent social world. We are fundamentally social beings and depend on stable interpersonal bonds, reliable care-giving during our development, social solidarity, and mutual esteem to give our lives meaning and coherence.

Some have argued that cultural considerations are secondary to overriding social and economic forces that lead to poverty, inequality, discrimination, and adversity. But the cultural institutions and practices that constitute local ways of life actually create and maintain the social arrangements that give rise to these social determinants in the first place. Moreover, cultural values and ideologies are used to justify these arrangements, rationalizing inequalities and making them seem natural or inevitable and, at times, even rendering them invisible. For example, the institution of slavery is a cultural practice based on treating some human beings as chattel, who can be owned by others who are considered "free" citizens with agency and autonomy. Without the dehumanizing ideologies of race and racism, there could have been no large-scale system of slavery and no enduring underclass of African Americans in the United States.[25] Similar ideologies rooted in histories of colonization, nation building, and ongoing conflicts serve to maintain systems of social class, caste, privilege, and exclusion in most contemporary societies.

Culture provides the conceptual language, ideological commitments, and institutional practices by which social differences are marked, and determines the consequences these distinctions have for people in terms of exposure to social determinants of health, social positioning, mobility, and access to health care. These have profound effects on every aspect of health. For example, in many countries, indigenous peoples suffer from substantially worse health than the general population.[26] In Canada, Aboriginal youth in some communities have very high rates of suicide.[27] These health disparities reflect a long history of settler colonialism with displacement and marginalization of indigenous peoples, followed by a century of state policies of forced assimilation through residential schools and outlawing of traditional practices.[28] These oppressive policies were rationalized by a view of indigenous peoples as "backward" and in need of education to become similar to Euro-Canadians. With increasing recognition of the damage wrought by these policies, Aboriginal peoples have come to see the restoration, preservation, and strengthening of indigenous cultures as both a human rights and a mental health issue.[29]

Contemporary views of culture emphasize that biomedicine and psychiatry itself are cultural institutions with their own history and implicit values. In general, psychiatry tends to locate problems within the individual as aspects of dysfunctional biology or psychology. Indeed, with the biological turn in the last few decades, psychiatric practice has assumed that mental disorders are fundamentally brain disorders. This justifies the search for biological explanations and the use of psychopharmaceuticals to treat mental and behavioral problems. In fact, there is only limited evidence for specific brain dysfunctions for most psychiatric disorders.[30] The current investment in biologically based diagnoses and treatments in psychiatry reflects cultural values more than scientific evidence per se. Although all behavior undoubtedly has reflections in the brain, many psychiatric problems may have their roots in social-developmental processes, difficult interactions with others, or deleterious environments. This would point toward the need for an *ecosocial* approach that characterizes mental health problems in terms of interactions with the local social environment, including family, community, and other networks. Regardless of their proximal or ultimate cause, systemic interventions based on understanding these interactions may prove most effective for mental health promotion and prevention of mental disorders.

THE NATURE OF MENTAL DISORDERS AND WELLNESS

Culture gives us the concepts we use to think about mental disorders so that psychiatric theory itself is a cultural construction. Indeed, Derek Summerfield, for example, has argued that the whole notion of a psychiatric disorder is culture-bound in ways that make it difficult or impossible to apply uniformly across cultures.[31] As a result, attempts to export psychiatry across cultures end up being forms of neocolonial missionizing, cultural proselytizing, or imposing frames of interpretation and practices of dubious benefit that may also serve to undermine local expertise and competence.

Summerfield's argument holds, to some extent, for common mental disorders (including trauma-related disorders) that have a large "gray zone" of mild or ambiguous cases that can be framed as mental health problems or as everyday problems in living. As summarized in Table 3.2, culture influences illness experience and expression at many levels. Over time, in Europe and North America, languages of distress shaped by psychiatry have displaced local idioms, creating confusion about the boundaries of mental disorder and potentially medicalizing and pathologizing problems like grief or demoralization that may be dealt with more effectively outside the context of mental health services.[32,33] Common mental health problems, including various forms of depression, anxiety, and somatic and dissociative symptoms, are given a wide array of explanations across cultures. Many of these experiences may be viewed, not as health problems, but as personal challenges or moral issues or as consequences of disharmony in family or community.

More severe conditions that consistently cause profound disruptions in social behavior and role performance may share core features across cultures, suggesting the utility of some existing psychiatric categories. However, even though severe mental disorders are recognized as problems in every culture, they also may be explained in very different ways, often appealing to religious, spiritual, or other socio-moral causes, such as malign magic, as is also the case with somatic conditions such as epilepsy and HIV/AIDS.[34-36] Healing interventions within cultural context may play an important role in social reintegration. When healing and recovery fail, the afflicted person may be further stigmatized and marginalized.

What distinguishes mental health problems from other types of illness is that their primary expression is through disturbances of psychological and social functioning, through alterations of processes of sensation, perception, cognition, emotion, and behavioral regulation. While all illnesses can have psychological effects, and many neurological or systemic disorders can impair psychological functioning, if a clear physiological mechanism is identified, illnesses tend to be reclassified as medical rather than psychiatric. This has happened with various forms of dementia, movement disorders like

Table 3.2 Cultural Influences on Mental Health and Illness

- Perception and experience of symptoms, suffering, and well-being
- Modes of expression of distress
- Explanations, interpretations or causal attributions of symptoms and illness
- Patterns of coping and help-seeking
- Strategies for healing and treatment intervention
- Expectations of illness course and outcome
- Social consequences of symptoms, functional impairment, and diagnostic labels

Tourette's syndrome, and some medically unexplained symptoms that are now understood as disturbances of physiological regulation. Despite this, there is always a cultural component to how illness is experienced, viewed, and treated.

The biomedical understanding of psychiatric disorders attributes them to underlying neurophysiological dysfunction. While all behavior has neurobiological substrates, the functioning of the nervous system alone will probably not explain most mental or behavioral disorders. Moreover, efforts to construct a single unifying definition of what constitutes a "mental disorder" fail because the category includes many different kinds of problems.[37] Mental health is not about just one type of problem: some problems may reflect neurodevelopmental problems or other physiological vulnerabilities, and others may arise from maladaptive learning or patterns of interpersonal interaction.[30] Culture and social context may play different roles for different sorts of problems. Advancing global mental health therefore depends crucially on understanding the interaction of psychopathology with diverse types of social structure and process.

CULTURE, PSYCHOPATHOLOGY, AND ILLNESS EXPERIENCE

Culture shapes all illness experience, and this influences the ways in which distress is communicated to others and presented in clinical settings.[34] These experiential and communicative processes may also contribute to pathological processes in their own right and influence the course and outcome of every mental disorder. Recognition of the ubiquitous effects of culture on psychopathology has challenged the notion that current psychiatric nosology describes culture-free universal syndromes. While current nosology points toward some universal patterns, it also includes much that is specific to the contexts where the nosology was developed. Certain problems and patterns of distress that may be common or important in some contexts do not have a prominent place in current diagnostic systems.

In recognition of this ubiquity of culture, the older notion of culture-bound syndromes has given way to more accurate concepts that focus on these processes of cognition and communication. The construct of culture-bound syndromes tended to exoticize other cultural practices, to foster the collection of syndromes based on lists of symptoms or behaviors taken out of context, and to ignore the fact that the categories of international psychiatric nosology are also cultural constructions—built largely on British and American ideas and modestly expanded by international work largely done by clinicians who were trained in Euro-American approaches. In place of culture-bound syndromes, recent research suggests the utility of other constructs, including: *cultural syndromes*—in which specific cultural cognitions, behaviors, or experiences play a role in the pathological mechanisms[38]; *cultural idioms of distress*—in which local codes or styles of expression and communication shape illness behavior[39,40]; and *cultural explanations, models, or attributions*—in which specific concepts are used to explain illness or affliction.[34,41] Some of these explanations may be derived from folk knowledge or the diagnostic categories of indigenous systems of medicine.

Contemporary theories of psychopathology focus on developmental neurobiological processes, including epigenetic mechanisms by which social adversity alters basic regulatory processes that underlie social behavior, affect, and cognition. Cultural variations in development and in the social contexts of everyday life may give rise to distinctive syndromes. Many mental health problems are sustained by vicious circles in which abnormal cognition, emotion, and behavior constitute mutually amplifying positive feedback loops. Specific culturally based explanations or causal attributions may play a role in these loops.[42] For example, Hinton has described several different types of panic attacks among Cambodians (both in Cambodia and immigrants in the United States) in which bodily sensations of dizziness brought on by orthostatic hypotension or sudden twisting of the neck are interpreted culturally as evidence of a "wind" rising in the body that can cause a stroke and so precipitates panic.[38] Many somatic symptoms and syndromes are maintained by specific cultural explanations that direct attention to the body and interpret sensations in ways that aggravate anxiety and increase bodily distress.[42] For example, in India, young men may attribute weakness and fatigue to loss of semen, in what has been termed *dhat syndrome*.[43,44] In equatorial Africa, complaints of heat in the head, a peppery feeling, or sensations of worms crawling in the head are common nonspecific complaints of distress that may be associated with a wide range of mental health problems or concerns.[45]

Around the world, bodily complaints tend to be the most common clinical presentation of mental disorders in primary care.[10] Bodily symptoms of pain, weakness, fatigue, or malaise accompany both severe and common psychiatric disorders. Whether people focus on these somatic symptoms or on emotional feelings and cognitive difficulties reflects the relative salience of these symptoms that is influenced by prevalent models or templates for illness experience. These models come from popular culture, past illness experience, and knowledge of the health care system. Because people recognize that biomedical health care focuses on the body, they may tend to foreground bodily symptoms in their clinical presentations. Moreover, in many settings, emotional distress is viewed as a personal or sociomoral problem that is better dealt with on one's own, within the family, or in religious or other settings. Severe mental disorders that result in disorganized and disruptive or disorganized behavior may be brought to biomedical physicians or psychiatrists. However, less severe problems may not be seen as appropriate to bring to psychiatric attention, which may be associated only with the most severe and highly stigmatized conditions.

Every culture has its own popular idioms of distress—culturally sanctioned modes of expressing suffering that are intelligible to others within a community. In some cases, these idioms may be associated with a coexisting psychiatric disorder, but in many cases they may simply express everyday suffering or concerns. For example, Raymond Prince described a syndrome of *brain fag* in Nigeria in the late 1950s among students who complained of headache, heat in the head, fatigue, and trouble concentrating, which they attributed to mental strain and overwork.[46] The term "brain fag" was popular in the late 1800s in England and traveled to West Africa as part of the colonial exchange.[47] The label persisted in Nigeria and fit the bodily experience and social predicament of young people who were the first in their families to become literate and who faced the challenges of navigating a colonial system that rewarded those pursuing Western education, which, at the same time, may have estranged them from village life.[47,48] Factor-analytic studies of the symptoms of patients with major depression in Nigeria have found a dimension of asthenia and head-related symptoms that may be viewed as similar to brain fag.[49] Scales devised specifically for brain fag include items about burning and crawling sensations in the head.[50,51] While syndromes of depression and brain fag may coexist, brain fag may be better thought of as an idiom of distress that can coexist with a variety of mental disorders.

Cultures provide explanations for affliction derived from local ontologies and ethnophysiological systems. People do not need to know a lot about these systems to make use of them to explain their health problems. For example, around the world, personal misfortune, including illness, may be attributed to the actions of spirits or malign magic. These explanations are caught up in local notions of proper social and moral behavior: observing the moral code, performing the required rites, and maintaining good relations with others, including ancestors. These systems provide explanations for what otherwise might seem inexplicable and satisfy the need to maintain a coherent worldview. They may influence help-seeking and the acceptability of treatments. In some instances, they may contribute directly to the course and outcome of illness by giving positive or negative meanings to affliction and influencing the response of others in ways that maintain social integration or that lead to marginalization, rejection, or ostracism.

These issues of meaning and social response have been invoked to explain the observation that patients with severe mental disorders including schizophrenia may sometimes have a better course in settings where they are less stigmatized.[52,53] While these findings have been challenged,[54] there is little doubt that social factors have an enormous impact on the course and outcome of most psychiatric conditions, including psychotic disorders.[55] The potential benefits of tolerance of unusual behavior and better social integration, however, must be weighed against the consequences of nontreatment and the harsh responses that may occur when people fail to respond to traditional spiritual or religious forms of healing.

CULTURE AND HEALING

Every culture has a variety of healing systems and practices that may be effective for a range of mental disorders.[56] Knowledge of local systems of healing is essential to understanding the logic of local patterns of help-seeking, the pathways people follow, and the goals, benefits, and potential problems associated with specific treatments. In addition to offering symptomatic relief, diagnostic practices and interventions may address issues of personal and social meaning, identify conflicts, and intervene in ways that may improve the social status and position of the patients and their families. This points to the need to consider a broad range of outcomes in assessing the effectiveness of healing. The recovery movement in schizophrenia is an example of an approach to understanding the effectiveness of treatment far more broadly than in terms of symptom relief—issues of social role reintegration and adaptation become central in this model.[57]

Healing practices are embedded in local meaning systems that give them part of their social value and potential efficacy. This is one way of understanding the "placebo effect"—not simply as non-specific positive expectations but as the impact of specific meanings and expectations of the persons coping and responses at physiological, psychological, and social levels.[58,59] Indeed, ritual healing is part of larger religious and sociomoral systems that cannot be simply replaced with psychiatric practices, because, even if symptoms are treated successfully, the existential meanings of the illness and the patient's social predicament are not addressed. This is part of what Kleinman found in his study of patients with neurasthenia in Hunan, China.[60] Although most patients could be diagnosed with major depression and experienced symptomatic improvement with antidepressant medication, many felt their basic problem was not addressed. Their suffering had much to do with losses incurred in the turmoil of Mao's Cultural Revolution. The fractured lives and profound injustices they endured were not resolved despite successful treatment of depression. This is of course an issue for mental health practice worldwide—though it is well known that social, political, and economic factors may contribute to illness and to social exclusion, mental health practitioners do not commonly have the means to intervene in broad social issues.

Most forms of ritual or religious healing occur in communal settings where others close to the patient are actively involved. Janzen has described the help-seeking group that forms around a patient in Africa that organizes the search for treatment.[61] Family and community interactions may be a source of conflict, burden, and suffering as well as support. During healing rituals, issues may be raised that are relevant to others who attend the ritual, and some of the effect of the intervention may be through its ability to change the afflicted person's relationship with family and community. It is essential, therefore, to think about ritual healing in systemic terms as a social network or community intervention. The relevant networks may include relationships with deceased ancestors who remain present in people's lives through acts of worship or commemoration. Healing then works not only to relieve symptoms and resolve illness but also to restore proper relations with the ancestors and within the community. The focus of psychiatry on symptoms or behavioral function does not always assess or address these levels and hence cannot provide some of the benefits associated with traditional, ritual forms of healing.

While traditional healing represents an important resource in global mental health, it is important not to romanticize or uncritically endorse traditional healing. The efficacy of most such forms of healing is unknown. Although people often claim that traditional forms of healing are time-tested, in fact, there is ample evidence from biomedicine as well as other traditions that practices may persist indefinitely even if they not efficacious, or even when they are harmful. There are many frankly harmful practices in common use that can cause serious injury.[62] Ritual and religious healing may also be very expensive, beyond the reach of families and draining the resources of even those who are relatively well off. Finally, all systems of healing have ways of dealing with their intrinsic limitations and failures, and these may involve blaming the patient or reinterpreting the illness in ways that may result in further stigma.

Of course, these critiques of traditional healing apply to biomedicine as well. It is also important to recognize that biomedicine itself takes many different forms. In most parts of the world, the variety of healing practices available reflects the inherent limitations of any one approach and the close links between healing and religious, spiritual, or cultural values. This diversity provides people with many options for treatment, and they tend to consult multiple sources, based on the severity of the problem and their resources.[63] For patients with more severe or persistent mental illness, the diversity of treatments available may also allow patients and their families to find a fit between their needs and expectations and healing practices.

MENTAL HEALTH SERVICES AND INTERVENTIONS

There will never be enough psychiatrists, psychologists, or other specialists in mental health to provide services for the wide range of problems gathered under the rubric of "mental health," so other modes of intervention will remain essential. This may involve collaborative care models, in which mental health providers work closely with primary care clinicians; the use of community mental health workers with less training; or various forms of collaboration with indigenous healers, religious institutions, and other systems of health care and social support.

There has been longstanding interest in the potential integration of biomedical health care with traditional systems of medicine. In the Alma Alta Declaration of 1978, the World Health Organization (WHO) recognized the importance of traditional healers for primary care.[64] This poses many challenges, ranging from the theoretical issues of reconciling illness explanations and interventions based on incompatible ontologies (e.g., molecular pathology versus angry spirits), to the practical issues of identifying skilled practitioners and ensuring access to and quality of care. In most settings, collaboration will be more realistic than integration. There is a risk, though, that in seeking to integrate or collaborate, the more powerful system of biomedicine with its international imprimatur and resources will simply appropriate local forms of healing. This appropriation may undermine the viability of practices that provide meaning and support for patients through modes of intervention that are not primarily symptom-focused. At the same time, recognition by the institutions of biomedicine may provide practitioners of traditional forms of healing with legitimacy without corresponding mechanisms of regulation or quality assurance.

There has been much recent interest in ways of adapting interventions to fit culture and context.[65–69] Table 3.3 lists some of the dimensions along which interventions may be culturally adapted.[70,71] Adaptation may range from simple translation or reformatting of interventions to convey them in local languages and with relevant examples, to

Table 3.3 Dimensions of Cultural Adaptation of Clinical Interventions*

1. Language	Translate intervention into culturally appropriate language.
2. Persons	Consider how ethno-racial and other sociocultural aspects of the identities "patient" and "clinician" can facilitate (or impede) the therapeutic relationship.
3. Metaphors and idioms	Use familiar idioms and evocative metaphors based on concepts shared with the target population.
4. Content	Develop content and examples based on cultural knowledge, values, and traditions of specific groups.
5. Concepts	Identify underlying treatment concepts that are consonant with cultural understandings of "person" and "problem."
6. Goals	Choose goals and outcomes that fit salient social roles, cultural values, and local priorities.
7. Methods	Use specific intervention methods that draw from local cultural traditions, modes of teaching, healing or behavioral change.
8. Context	Adapt intervention to social contexts of assessment, treatment negotiation, and delivery.

* Based on Bernal et al. 1995, 2009.[70,71]

changes in methods (e.g., employing different cognitive strategies, meditation, or relaxation to achieve a specific goal like relaxation, feelings of mastery, etc.), to altering the goals (e.g., aiming for maintenance of a patient within the family rather than encouraging autonomy). The appropriate level of adaptation will depend on the fit of available treatment with local values and resources, as well as on practical considerations. One barrier to effective adaptation may be the assumption that all interventions work by similar mechanisms and can be reduced to the familiar mechanisms invoked by conventional treatments like cognitive-behavior therapy. While there are undoubtedly common mechanisms across diverse treatments, there may be specific mechanisms related to the cultural meaning of the intervention. For example, the acceptability and impact of interventions that promote the expression of suffering, or acceptance and forgiveness as ways to deal with post-traumatic distress may depend on shared religious values that vary widely across traditions.[72]

"Cultural competence" has become a common rubric for attempts to address culture in mental health services and intervention.[73] A culturally competent organization is able to address the needs of its diverse clientele in ways that respect their cultural backgrounds and that support culturally congruent methods of coping and healing. Much of the development of cultural competence has taken place in the United States. An alternative approach, advanced by Maori nurses in New Zealand, has been termed *cultural safety* and emphasizes the need to address the legacy of colonialism and ongoing issues of power and discrimination that make clinical settings unsafe for patients (or clinicians) from particular backgrounds.[74–76] The specific strategies for addressing cultural diversity in public health interventions and mental health services will depend on the types of cultural diversity that are salient in local, regional, or national contexts. Although recognition of culture is a matter of respect and will contribute to acceptability and engagement, it is also essential to ensure effectiveness and to avoid promoting interventions that undermine important local values or modes of community solidarity and social support.[77] Even simple instrumental approaches to providing basic needs like food and shelter may be ineffective or aggravate problems if they are designed in ways that ignore or contradict core cultural values or sources of resilience.[78,79]

Notions of "positive outcomes" or "recovery" may vary across cultures.[78] Whitley and Drake have noted the multiple dimensions or frames within which recovery can be assessed, including: *clinical* (e.g., symptom severity, rehospitalization, treatment adherence); *existential* (hope, emotional well-being); role functioning (employment, housing); adaptation, physical functioning (physical health and activity); and social relationships (social support, integration).[80] Each of these may vary with the social context, and their relative importance depends on culturally defined roles that vary with age, gender, and social status.

CULTURE, ETHICS, AND HUMAN RIGHTS IN HEALTH CARE

There are many areas in bioethics where culture is recognized to be of central importance, including: clinical communication, assessment of competency to make decisions, truth-telling about diagnoses and prognosis, obtaining informed consent, and negotiating treatment.[81] Most of these issues depend centrally on the degree to which clinicians and clients understand each other (see the next section), but in the global context, there are a number of other issues which are crucial to address. Western ideas about ethical practice are commonly premised on the idea that individuals are relatively autonomous beings, able to make independent decisions. As we have discussed earlier, there is an extensive literature in the cross-cultural field on forms of social organization that emphasize collectivity rather than individual agency. In many parts of southern Africa, for example, reference is made to what is termed *ubuntu* (or other forms of this term, such as *umunthu*),[82] an ethic whereby "humanness" is expressed only through interaction with others. Imposition of individualistic norms of practice on societies that embrace collectivist values may constitute an inappropriate form of cultural imperialism. People may seek help and healing as groups rather than as individuals, and decisions about consent and autonomy may be negotiated within a group context.[61] This said, the issue of respecting cultural differences is much more challenging than attempting to respect the practices of different groups. Many practices that are viewed as abhorrent by practitioners of global mental health—from the oppression of women, to the persecution of sexual and other minorities, and even AIDS denialism—have, in various ways, been defended by reference to cultural differences.[83] What is clear is that all practices are embedded in webs of power and control. While it is important to be sensitive to local values and norms, the naïve valorization of the "indigenous" or the local by global mental health practitioners is problematic. Abuse of people with mental disorders, and of people who do not fit in with the social mainstream, remains an international scandal, and abusive practices cannot be excused by reference to "cultural relativism."[84] Ethical behavior, furthermore, is not simply a question of respect of individual and cultural rights, but involves interrogation of practices within frameworks of global and local inequalities in an increasingly unequal world.[85]

Mental health issues are increasingly being viewed within human rights frameworks.[86] The rights of people with mental disorders are enshrined in a number of international documents, the most important of which is the United Nations Convention on the Rights of Persons with Disabilities (UNCRPD; http://www.un.org/disabilities). This convention recognizes the exclusion of people with disabilities (including people with mental disorders) from mainstream cultural life (see Article 30 in particular), and notes the need to create enabling conditions for greater participation. This recognition of social exclusion is an important counterbalance to calls for viewing mental disorder in cultural context. Understanding cultural context is crucial, but it needs to be recognized that cultural practices everywhere may be both inclusive and exclusionary; both facilitative and oppressive.[84]

This recognition of the cultural complexity of ethical issues within a broad context of global inequality makes a further demand on those engaged in global mental health for reflexivity: it is incumbent upon practitioners to examine how their own practices reflect their own prejudices and views of the world. Processes of intercultural negotiation and self-reflection take time and commitment, and can be painful, but they are necessary.

LANGUAGE AND TRANSLATION ISSUES

A common, but often overlooked, feature of much intercultural work in mental health is that of communication across language barriers. It is not unusual for practitioners and researchers in the field of global mental health to be unable to communicate directly with the people who are the recipients of services or the participants in research. Accurate communication in a global mental health context is not just desirable but essential for the best work to take place, and clinical interpreting is a highly skilled task.[87] Though this challenge is widely recognized, much interpreting continues to be conducted on an ad hoc basis, by family members or people with no training in interpreting or mental health, and sometimes even without acceptable proficiency in the languages they are called upon to interpret.[88,89]

These issues make the clinical contexts of diagnostic interviews and treatment interventions challenging. It is well established that interpreters make errors when interpreting in mental health research and practice—including omissions of key material, contraction and inappropriate summarizing of what clinicians and clients say, mistranslations, and even addition of material not mentioned by clinicians or clients[90–92]—but the issue goes far beyond the competence of interpreters.[93] In contemporary research on interpreting, there is now more emphasis on how the complex power relationships among client, interpreter, and clinician affect what happens in interpreted interviews. There are widely differing views on appropriate roles for interpreters. Should interpreters, for example, attempt to be like transparent windows or conduits—simply translating across languages without inserting their own views or opinions (something that is generally impossible to do consistently); should they take on the role of patient advocate; or should they be co-therapists in the clinical encounter?[94] In practice, these questions about how interpreters and clinicians work together are often not addressed by any of the parties, and analysis of interpreted interviews shows that participants in these interviews may move across different roles and role expectations in a single interview. Even in health care settings where there is substantial investment in interpreter services, role confusions and identity issues may affect not just the accuracy of interpretation but even judgments about the mental state of people whose words are (mis)translated.[95] The issues are especially challenging in mental health services, where clinicians are commonly interested not only in what people are saying but also in how they say it.[89] An important contemporary approach to understanding interpreting processes emphasizes the question not of how "good" or "accurate" interpretation is, but whether the clinical goals of an interpreted session are realized.[96]

Recognizing the inevitable limitations of translation, anthropologists have talked about "working misunderstandings."[97] Although it may never be possible to have completely accurate translations across languages and cultures, it is possible to develop ways of working that limit misunderstandings or allow for their correction in order to meet the specific needs of a clinical or research context. Much of this depends on the extent to which both clinician and interpreter understand the complexities of language and interpreting and are able to work together as a team. It is essential to appreciate that these difficulties exist and that they are not easily resolved. Indeed, it is appropriate to be skeptical of any claim that language barriers have been fully overcome in any study in the field and to remain open in clinical encounters to the emergence of new information and meanings that can only be clarified over time. A particular challenge for cross-cultural mental health work is that we are not only interested in the content of what people say (which may include untranslatable idioms of distress), but also in how they say it, including subtle nuances of expression. Tone of voice and the use of particular words or turns of phrase may carry meanings that are difficult to translate. For example, the statements "I feel sad" and "I feel miserable" may commonly be translated into exactly the same words in another language, but some English speakers would understand the word "miserable" as having the connotations of being more troubled and possibly disgruntled than conveyed by the word "sad."[98] Ultimately, the goal for global mental health must be the training of well-qualified clinicians who are native speakers of local languages, so that these important diagnostic and treatment questions can be addressed adequately.

RESEARCH STRATEGIES AND METHODS

The international disparity in the production of knowledge, with 90% of research done on 10% of the world's population, poses a fundamental challenge to global mental health.[99] To take action now, we must assume that the current practices that emerged in the West are applicable to the diverse contexts of low- and middle-income countries (LMIC) or can be readily adapted. Although there is a growing body of research in LMIC, in most cases this work starts from the models and assumptions of Western psychiatry. Guidelines based on expert consensus among practitioners based in LMIC provide a practical short-term solution, although efforts must be made to ensure that the experts themselves—who are usually the product of Western training—are grounded in local realities.[100] There is a need for ongoing research that takes cultural variation seriously, to include local and innovative approaches and establish a stronger evidence base for effective practice.

Evidence-based practice (EBP) aims to provide a firmer footing for mental health practice, and evidence has been crucial in putting global mental health on the agenda.[101] However, there are inherent limitations to EBP, both because of the limitations of the evidence base and because of the complexities of translating general knowledge into locally effective and appropriate interventions. In the search for generalizable knowledge, evidence on mental disorders tends to downplay or ignore cultural variations.[102] Indeed, even within the developed countries where most of the research takes place, studies often are not representative of the cultural diversity of the populations.[103] The selection of topics for research studies tends to be driven by economic interests, so evidence in the public health field is strongest for pharmacological interventions. Clinical trials are designed to maximize positive findings by using placebos, short follow-up periods, and limited outcomes focusing on symptoms, and there has even been some outright misrepresentation, with failure to publish negative results, massaging or misrepresentation of data, and other criminal activities as recognized in recent legal judgments against major pharmaceutical companies.[104,105] Current ethical standards requiring preregistration of trials and declaration of conflicting interests go some distance to rectify these abuses, but researchers and clinicians must remain committed and vigilant to avoid biases with potentially serious consequences for patients. In the global mental health field, it is not uncommon for the interventions to be psychosocial in nature,[106,107] or a combination of psychosocial and pharmacological, and similar ethical standards need to be developed for psychosocial interventions.

Increasing the representativeness of samples in clinical research is crucial to improving the relevance of evidence for diverse populations. In addition to canvassing the diversity within developed countries, this requires studies in LMIC. However, to ensure cultural relevance, these studies need to be not simply replications of extant approaches but to engage with local knowledge and practices to develop innovative interventions.

Establishing Cross-Cultural Equivalence in Research

Cross-cultural research faces special challenges at the level of ensuring the cross-cultural equivalence of diagnostic constructs, interventions, measures, and outcomes. These challenges are both pragmatic and epistemological. The pragmatic issues have to do with how to identify appropriate research questions, sample populations, and develop valid and reliable measures of constructs. The epistemological problems concern the ways in which culture shapes the very categories we use to articulate our ideas about mental health and illness.

In general, research is more likely to address local needs when it is driven by end-users and those with experience "on the ground."[108] For this reason, many advocate community-based participatory research methods as a way to ensure that local priorities are recognized and there is ongoing knowledge exchange during the research process, and greater uptake of results. Community work can also clarify the various stakeholders, identify groups that have been marginalized or excluded, and find ways to reach those most in need.

Translating measures across languages poses additional technical challenges.[92] Though there are many approaches to the translation of measurement instruments,[87] the most commonly accepted method is that of "back-translation," as formulated by Brislin.[109] In this method, an instrument is translated from the source to the target language, and then the translated version is given to independent bilingual people familiar with the target language and culture to "back-translate" into the source language. The original and the back-translated versions are then compared and changes made in an iterative translation and back-translation process. A common error made in back-translation is to use back-translators with extensive knowledge of mental health issues who can often work out the original intention of the instrument and therefore miss translation errors that might affect the target population. The proper translation of instruments can be tedious and costly, but is crucial in order to produce valid instruments. There may be no precise translation for many terms, and even terms that appear similar may have different connotations. The process of translation may reveal differences in the conceptual systems of the two languages, and these should be systematically recorded and reported.[110] Table 3.4 outlines some of the levels of equivalence that must be considered in cross-cultural translation.

Translation may also point to deeper ways in which cultural worlds diverge, organizing experience in terms of categories that simply cannot be mapped onto equivalent categories in other cultures. This divergence may give rise to what the psychiatrist-anthropologist Arthur Kleinman has called a "category fallacy." Kleinman described the category fallacy as the unwarranted assumption that, because we can apply our categories across cultures, they mean the same thing and have the same validity. Here is how Kleinman originally described this problem in the context of work on somatization and depression in China:

[W]e can isolate a depressive syndrome characterized by depressive affect, insomnia, weight loss, lack of energy, diurnal mood changes, constipation, dry mouth, and an apparently limited number of related psychological complaints. Singer is right in suggesting that this syndrome appears to be present in a number of cultural settings. But he is not correct when he uses this fact in support of his conclusion. The depressive syndrome represents a small fraction of the entire field of depressive phenomena. It is a cultural category constructed by psychiatrists in the West to yield a homogenous group of patients. By definition, it excludes most depressive phenomena even in the West because they fall outside its narrow boundaries. Applying such a category to analyze cross-cultural studies or even in direct field research is not a cross-cultural study of depression because by definition it

Table 3.4 Levels of Equivalence in Cross-Cultural Research**

Level	Description	Methodological Strategy	Goal
Content equivalence	Content of each item is relevant to the phenomenon of each culture being studied	Local content experts or participant observation to identify relevant contexts, behaviors, and experiences	Ecological validity of items
Semantic equivalence	Meaning of each item is the same in each culture after translation into the language and idiom of each culture	Blind back-translation, identify discrepancies, seek terms with closest denotations and connotations in everyday usage	Meaning equivalence of text for target population
Technical equivalence	Method of assessment (e.g., written questionnaire or interview) is comparable in each culture with respect to the data that it yields	Experiments on effects of medium	Mode of delivery of measure is acceptable and does not influence response
Criterion equivalence	Interpretation of the measured variable remains the same when compared with the cultural norm	Psychometric standardization; item response analysis	Accurate measure of severity and threshold of caseness
Conceptual equivalence	Instrument measures the same theoretical construct in each culture	Latent variable modeling; correlations with other related constructs	Measure taps a generalizable construct

** Adapted from Flaherty et al.[118]

will find what is "universal" and systematically miss what does not fit its tight parameters. The former is what is defined and therefore "seen" by a Western cultural model, the latter, which is not so defined and therefore not "seen" raises far more interesting questions for cross-cultural research. It is precisely in the latter group that one would expect to find the most striking examples of the influence of culture on depression.[111]

The meaning of a symptom, sign, behavior, or action depends on cultural context. Hence, diagnostic categories and constructs (and their constitutive symptoms and signs) that have meaning in one context cannot be assumed to have the same meaning in another context, even if one believes that there are common illness features. Human perception organizes the world according to preconceived categories. Thus, the study of phenomena with tools sensitive only to certain symptoms and categories will tend to replicate and confirm those categories and not see what is "outside the box."

The way to address this dilemma is to step outside our received categories to investigate other cultural systems of meaning. This involves ethnographic research, using both qualitative and quantitative methods, to explore the meaning systems and practices that constitute a cultural way of life. There is by now a substantial body of ethnographic work illuminating cultural variations in emotional experience and behavior related to major psychiatric categories, including mood disorders, psychoses, anxiety disorders, trauma-related conditions, somatoform disorders, personality disorders, and dementia.[112,113] However, much work remains to be done to understand local idioms of distress, models of illness, and patterns of coping and help-seeking relevant to mental health promotion and intervention. This research can employ the wide range of methods of medical and psychological anthropology, including qualitative research tools developed to specifically address illness experience.[114,115]

This type of ethnographic research, which is largely descriptive, can provide the raw material for constructing quantitative measures of salient dimensions of illness experience, social determinants of health, outcome, and mediators of recovery.[116] These measures need to be validated following standard psychometric methods, adapted to cross-cultural comparison.[117] This requires not only establishing their internal reliability and consistency but also showing that they correlate with other locally validated measures, and with culturally meaningful measures of outcome.[118] In validating culturally generated or adapted measures, it is helpful to compare them with measures that have been validated in other settings. Internationally accepted measures can be supplemented with additional items, scales, or instruments that have been locally generated.[119] This use of both local and global measures will allow cross-cultural comparison and clarify whether the local measures perform better than the existing measures in identifying pathologies and predicting outcomes. This comparison is important because even when categories and constructs can be validated in a new cultural context by showing they have internal consistency and reliability and correlate with expected antecedents and outcomes, they may not be clinically useful. For example, a study in Afghanistan found that while the construct of post-traumatic stress disorder (PTSD) appeared to be valid—in that adults who were exposed to trauma were more likely to have the recognizable symptoms of PTSD—an alternative construct built around general expressions of distress, including depressive and culture-specific symptoms, was more predictive of functional impairment.[120]

CONCLUSION

The profound inequalities in mental health and well-being around the globe present us with an imperative for action. These inequities have arisen in part because of processes of uneven development, colonialism, and exploitation, and current forces of globalization have improved some areas but markedly worsened others. A basic challenge for global mental health concerns how to address these inequities in health without duplicating the hierarchies of power and privilege that gave rise to these injustices in the first place. Will global mental health be a handmaiden of globalization, as some have argued,[31] or can it be a crucial part of building global civil society that strives for human rights and equity for all of humanity while preserving the cultural diversity that is the root of creativity? Can culturally informed contributions to global mental health balance the role of cultural psychiatry as a critique of the mainstream with the urgent need to scale up services in a pragmatic fashion?[121]

Global mental health can be seen, not only as an opportunity to redress profound inequities that reflect a global history of exploitation and domination, but also as an opportunity to benefit from cultural diversity.[122] This perspective would urge us to approach global mental health by engaging in open dialogue and exchange, seeking to learn from different knowledge systems to identify what is most appropriate to promote mental health within a particular way of life, but also to understand the human possibilities opened up by each cultural tradition. This points toward the importance of the overarching value of pluralism.[123–126] Pluralistic forms of political life are compatible with fundamental concerns for human rights. Indeed, the same human rights that motivate the efforts to achieve equity in global mental health also underwrite the protection of social space where people can live out their cultural lifeways and values as members of communities. Pluralism, in the form of a global multiculturalism, would allow the peaceful coexistence and even the promotion of diversity, with the recognition that cultures are constantly undergoing transformation in response to forces from within as well as interactions with each other.

Recognizing the importance of culture in mental health has implications for research, training, and practice. In research, what is needed is not simply replication of studies in samples that represent local diversity, but a more thorough exchange of knowledge that allows researchers and mental health practitioners to learn from other traditions. Training must not simply take the form of experts imparting their knowledge and skills to those with less training, but needs to be an active process of dialogue and co-learning. Clinicians and mental health workers from the same background as the patients they treat are a precious resource in this process. However, for clinicians to make use of their tacit knowledge, they need conceptual models of how culture influences psychopathology and healing. Clinical and public health interventions need not simply scale up best practices identified in wealthy, urban, culturally distinct countries of the North and West, but to work with models that have emerged from local practices. We need more work on the process of cultural adaptation of diagnostic systems, interventions, and health systems to identify practical methods for intervention development and validation in diverse settings.

Global mental health policy faces an inherent paradox: the effort to share resources and scale up practices requires an assumption that more or less standardized interventions will work across contexts. Yet the claim of responding to local needs requires engagement with patients and grass-roots providers and support systems. Global mental health policy therefore must support bottom-up strategies, like those of community-based participatory action research to identify indigenous systems of helping and healing as part of community resilience. Local strategies may not always be optimal and good ideas, and approaches from other places should be widely disseminated. However, it remains important that interventions take local cultural values and perspectives seriously into consideration to ensure the protection and expression of cultural identity and community. Ultimately, this demands pluralistic civil societies, to which mental health services can contribute.

REFERENCES

1. Kirmayer LJ. Cultural psychiatry in historical perspective. In: Bhugra D, Bhui K, editors. *Textbook of cultural psychiatry*. Cambridge, UK: Cambridge University Press; 2007:3–19.
2. Bains J. Race, culture, and psychiatry: a history of transcultural psychiatry. *Hist Psychiatry*. 2005 Jun;16(62 Pt 2):139–54.
3. Fernando S. *Mental health, race, and culture*. 3rd ed. Basingstoke, Hampshire; New York: Palgrave Macmillan; 2010.
4. Gannett L. The biological reification of race. *Br J Philos Sci*. 2004;55:323–45.
5. Smedley A, Smedley BD. Race as biology is fiction, racism as a social problem is real: anthropological and historical perspectives on the social construction of race. *Am Psychol*. 2005 Jan;60(1):16–26.
6. Harris R, Tobias M, Jeffreys M, Waldegrave K, Karlsen S, Nazroo J. Effects of self-reported racial discrimination and deprivation on Maori health and inequalities in New Zealand: cross-sectional study. *Lancet*. 2006 Jun 17;367(9527):2005–9.
7. Smedley BD. The lived experience of race and its health consequences. *Am J Public Health*. 2012 May;102(5):933–5.
8. World Health Organization. *Report of the international pilot study of schizophrenia*. Geneva: WHO; 1973.
9. World Health Organization. *Schizophrenia: An international follow-up study*. Chichester: John Wiley & Sons; 1979.

10. Ustün TB, Sartorius N, editors. *Mental illness in general health care: An international study.* Chichester: John Wiley & Sons; 1995.

11. Wang PS, Aguilar-Gaxiola S, Alonso J, et al. Use of mental health services for anxiety, mood, and substance disorders in 17 countries in the WHO world mental health surveys. *Lancet.* 2007 Sep 8;370(9590):841–50.

12. Andrade L, Caraveo-Anduaga JJ, Berglund P, et al. The epidemiology of major depressive episodes: results from the International Consortium of Psychiatric Epidemiology (ICPE) Surveys. *Int J Methods Psychiatr Res.* 2003;12(1):3–21.

13. Hollinger DA. *Post-ethnic America: Beyond multiculturalism.* New York: Basic Books; 1995.

14. Breslau J, Kendler KS, Su M, Gaxiola-Aguilar S, Kessler RC. Lifetime risk and persistence of psychiatric disorders across ethnic groups in the United States. *Psychol Med.* 2005 Mar;35(3):317–27.

15. Heine SJ, Buchtel EE. Personality: The universal and the culturally specific. *Annu Rev Psychol.* 2009;60:369–94.

16. Oyserman D, Coon H, Kemmelmeier M. Rethinking individualism and collectivism: Evaluation of theoretical assumptions and meta-analyses. *Psychol Bull.* 2002;128:3–72.

17. Kirmayer LJ. Beyond the "new cross-cultural psychiatry": cultural biology, discursive psychology and the ironies of globalization. *Transcult Psychiatry.* 2006 Mar;43(1): 126–44.

18. Worthman CM. *Formative experiences: The interaction of caregiving, culture, and developmental psychobiology.* Cambridge; New York: Cambridge University Press; 2010.

19. Han S, Northoff G, Vogeley K, Wexler BE, Kitayama S, Varnum ME. A cultural neuroscience approach to the biosocial nature of the human brain. *Annu Rev Psychol.* 2013;64:12.1–12.25.

20. Kraidy M. *Hybridity, or the cultural logic of globalization.* Philadelphia, PA: Temple University Press; 2005.

21. Burke P. *Cultural hybridity.* Cambridge, UK: Polity; 2009.

22. Doku PN, Oppong Asante K. Identity: globalization, culture, and psychological functioning. *Int J Hum Sci [Online].* 2011;8(2).

23. Wilkinson R, Marmot M. *Social determinants of health: The solid facts.* Geneva: World Health Organization; 2003.

24. Marmot M. Achieving health equity: from root causes to fair outcomes. *Lancet.* 2007 Sep 29;370(9593):1153–63.

25. Fredrickson GM. *Racism: A short history.* Princeton, NJ: Princeton University Press; 2002.

26. Gracey M, King M. Indigenous health part 1: determinants and disease patterns. *Lancet.* 2009 Jul 4;374(9683):65–75.

27. Kirmayer LJ. Suicide among Canadian aboriginal peoples. *Transcult Psychiatr Res Rev.* 1994;31(1):3–58.

28. King M, Smith A, Gracey M. Indigenous health part 2: the underlying causes of the health gap. *Lancet.* 2009 Jul 4;374(9683):76–85.

29. Kirmayer LJ, Valaskakis GG, editors. *Healing traditions: The mental health of aboriginal peoples in Canada.* Vancouver: University of British Columbia Press; 2008.

30. Kirmayer LJ, Gold I. Re-socializing psychiatry: critical neuroscience and the limits of reductionism. In: Choudhury S, Slaby J, editors. *Critical neuroscience: A handbook of the social and cultural contexts of neuroscience.* Oxford, UK: Blackwell; 2012: 307–30.

31. Summerfield D. Against "global mental health." *Transcult Psychiatry.* 2012;49(3–4).

32. Horwitz AV, Wakefield JC. *The loss of sadness: How psychiatry transformed normal sorrow into depressive disorder.* Oxford; New York: Oxford University Press; 2007.

33. Kirmayer LJ. Psychopharmacology in a globalizing world: the use of antidepressants in Japan. *Transcult Psychiatry.* 2002;39(3):295–312.

34. Kirmayer LJ, Bhugra D. Culture and mental illness: social context and explanatory models. In: Salloum IM, Mezzich JE, editors. *Psychiatric diagnosis: Patterns and prospects.* New York: John Wiley & Sons; 2009:29–37.

35. Okello ES, Neema S. Explanatory models and help-seeking behavior: pathways to psychiatric care among patients admitted for depression in Mulago hospital, Kampala, Uganda. *Qual Health Res.* 2007 Jan;17(1):14–25.

36. Girma E, Tesfaye M. Patterns of treatment seeking behavior for mental illnesses in Southwest Ethiopia: a hospital based study. *BMC Psychiatry.* 2011;11:138.

37. Gold I, Kirmayer LJ. Cultural psychiatry on Wakefield's Procrustean bed. *World Psychiatry.* 2007 Oct;6(3):165–6.

38. Hinton D, Um K, Ba P. *Kyol goeu* ("wind overload") Part I: A Cultural Syndrome of Orthostatic Panic among Khmer Refugees. *Transcult Psychiatry.* 2001;38:403–32.

39. Nichter M. Idioms of distress: alternatives in the expression of psychosocial distress: a case study from South India. *Cult Med Psychiatry.* 1981 Dec;5(4):379–408.

40. Nichter M. Idioms of distress revisited. *Cult Med Psychiatry.* 2010 Jun;34(2):401–16.

41. Weiss MG, Somma D. Explanatory models in psychiatry. In: Bhugra D, Bhui K, editors. *Textbook of cultural psychiatry.* Cambridge, UK: Cambridge University Press; 2007:127–40.

42. Kirmayer LJ, Sartorius N. Cultural models and somatic syndromes. *Psychosom Med.* 2007 Dec;69(9):832–40.

43. Ranjith G, Mohan R. *Dhat* syndrome as a functional somatic syndrome: developing a sociosomatic model. *Psychiatry.* 2006 Summer;69(2):142–50.

44. Sumathipala A, Siribaddana SH, Bhugra D. Culture-bound syndromes: the story of *dhat* syndrome. *Br J Psychiatry.* 2004 Mar;184:200–9.

45. Ebigbo PO, Ihezue UH. Some psychodynamic observations on the symptom of heat in the head. *Afr J Psychiatry.* 1981 Jan–Apr;7(1–2):25–30.

46. Prince R. The "brain fag" syndrome in Nigerian students. *J Ment Sci.* 1960 Apr;106:559–70.

47. Ola BA, Morakinyo O, Adewuya AO. Brain fag syndrome—a myth or a reality? *Afr J Psychiatry (Johannesbg).* 2009 May;12(2):135–43.

48. Guinness EA. Social origins of the brain fag syndrome. *Br J Psychiatry Suppl.* 1992 Apr(16):53–64.

49. Okulate GT, Olayinka MO, Jones OB. Somatic symptoms in depression: evaluation of their diagnostic weight in an African setting. *Br J Psychiatry.* 2004 May;184:422–7.

50. Ebigbo PO. A cross sectional study of somatic complaints of Nigerian females using the Enugu Somatization Scale. *Cult Med Psychiatry.* 1986 Jun;10(2):167–86.

51. Ola BA, Igbokwe DO. Factorial validation and reliability analysis of the Brain Fag Syndrome Scale. *Afr Health Sci.* 2011 Sep;11(3):334–40.

52. Leff J, Sartorius N, Jablensky A, Korten A, Ernberg G. The international pilot study of schizophrenia: Five-year follow-up findings. *Psychol Med.* 1992;22:131–45.

53. Sartorius N, Gulbinat W, Harrison G, Laska E, Siegel C. Long-term follow-up of schizophrenia in 16 countries. A description of the international study of schizophrenia conducted by the World Health Organization. *Soc Psychiatry Psychiatr Epidemiol.* 1996;31:249–58.

54. Cohen A, Patel V, Thara R, Gureje O. Questioning an axiom: better prognosis for schizophrenia in the developing world? *Schizophr Bull.* 2008 Mar;34(2):229–44.

55. Morgan C, McKenzie K, Fearon P. *Society and psychosis.* Cambridge; New York: Cambridge University Press; 2008.

56. Kirmayer LJ. The cultural diversity of healing: meaning, metaphor, and mechanism. *Br Med Bull.* 2004;69:33–48.

57. Davidson L, Rakfeldt J, Strauss J. *The roots of the recovery movement in psychiatry: Lessons learned.* New York: Wiley; 2010.

58. Thompson JJ, Ritenbaugh C, Nichter M. Reconsidering the placebo response from a broad anthropological perspective. *Cult Med Psychiatry.* 2009 Mar;33(1):112–52.

59. Kirmayer LJ. Unpacking the placebo response: Insights from ethnographic studies of healing. *J Mind-Body Reg.* 2011;1(3):112–24.

60. Kleinman A. *Social origins of distress and disease: Depression, neurasthenia, and pain in modern China.* New Haven, CT: Yale University Press; 1986.

61. Janzen JM. *The quest for therapy in lower Zaire.* Berkeley: University of California; 1978.

62. Qureshi NA, Al-Amri AH, Abdelgadir MH. Traditional cautery among psychiatric patients in Saudi Arabia. *Transcult Psychiatry.* 1998;35(1):75–83.

63. Halliburton M. Finding a fit: psychiatric pluralism in south India and its implications for WHO studies of mental disorder. *Transcult Psychiatry.* 2004 Mar;41(1):80–98.

64. World Health Organization. *From Alma-Ata to the year 2000: Reflections at the midpoint.* Geneva: World Health Organization; 1988.

65. Ferrer-Wreder L, Sundell K, Mansoory S. Tinkering with perfection: theory development in the intercultural adaptation field. *Child Youth Care Forum.* 2012;41:149–71.

66. Lau AS. Making the case for selective and directed cultural adaptations of evidence-based treatments: Examples form parent training. *Clin Psychol Sci Pract.* 2006;13:295–310.

67. Wendt DC, Gone JP. Rethinking cultural competence: insights from indigenous community treatment settings. *Transcult Psychiatry.* 2012 Apr;49(2):206–22.

68. Hinton DE, Rivera EI, Hofmann SG, Barlow DH, Otto MW. Adapting CBT for traumatized refugees and ethnic minority patients: examples from culturally adapted CBT (CA-CBT). *Transcult Psychiatry.* 2012 Apr;49(2):340–65.

69. Verdeli H, Clougherty KF, Bolton P, et al. Adapting group interpersonal psychotherapy for a developing country: experience in rural Uganda. *World Psychiatry.* 2003;2(2):114–20.

70. Bernal G, Bonilla J, Bellido C. Ecological validity and cultural sensitivity for outcome research: issues for the cultural adaptation and development of psychosocial treatments with Hispanics. *J Abnorm Child Psychol.* 1995 Feb;23(1):67–82.

71. Bernal G, Jimenez-Chafey MI, Domenech Rodriguez MM. Cultural adaptation of treatments: A resource for considering culture in evidence-based practice. *Prof Psychol Res Pract.* 2009;40(4):361–8.

72. Kirmayer LJ, Kienzler H, Afana AH, Pedersen D. Trauma and disasters in social and cultural context. In: Bhugra D, Morgan C, editors. *Principles of social psychiatry.* 2nd ed. New York: Wiley-Blackwell; 2010:155–77.

73. Kirmayer LJ. Rethinking cultural competence. *Transcult Psychiatry.* 2012 Apr;49(2):149–64.

74. Papps E, Ramsden I. Cultural safety in nursing: the New Zealand experience. *Int J Qual Health Care.* 1996 Oct;8(5):491–7.

75. Brascoupé S, Waters C. Cultural safety: exploring the applicability of the concept of cultural safety to aboriginal health and community wellness. *J Aboriginal Health.* 2009;7(1):6–40.

76. Koptie S. Irihapeti Ramsden: The public narrative on cultural safety. *First Peoples Child & Fam Rev.* 2009;4(2):30–43.

77. Jordans MJ, Tol WA, Komproe IH, De Jong JVTM. Systematic review of evidence and treatment approaches: Psychosocial and mental health care for children in war. *Child & Adolesc Ment Health.* 2009;14:2–14.

78. Kirmayer LJ, Sedhev M, Dandeneau S, Whitley R. *Community resilience: Models, metaphors and measures.* Montreal: Culture and Mental Health Research Unit; 2008.

79. Kirmayer LJ, Dandeneau S, Marshall E, Phillips MK, Williamson KJ. Rethinking resilience from indigenous perspectives. *Can J Psychiatry.* 2011 Feb;56(2):84–91.

80. Whitley R, Drake RE. Recovery: a dimensional approach. *Psychiatr Serv.* 2010 Dec;61(12):1248–50.

81. Turner L. From the local to the global: bioethics and the concept of culture. *J Med Philos.* 2005 Jun;30(3):305–20.

82. Mji G, Gcaza S, Swartz L, MacLachlan M, Hutton B. An African way of networking around disability. *Disabil & Soc.* 2011;26:365–8.

83. Nattrass N. *The AIDS conspiracy: Science fights back.* New York: Columbia University Press; 2012.

84. Kirmayer LJ. Culture and context in human rights. In: Dudley M, Silove D, Gale F, editors. *Mental health and human rights: Vision, praxis, and courage.* Oxford, UK: Oxford University Press; 2012:95–112.

85. Benatar S, Brock G. *Global health and global health ethics.* Cambridge, UK: Cambridge University Press; 2011.

86. Dudley M, Silove D, Gale F. *Mental health and human rights: Vision, praxis, and courage.* 1st ed. Oxford, UK: Oxford University Press; 2012.

87. Swartz L. *Culture and mental health: A southern African view.* Cape Town, South Africa: Oxford University Press; 1998.

88. Kilian S, Swartz L, Joska J. Linguistic competence of interpreters in a South African hospital. *Psychiatr Serv.* 2010;61:310–2.

89. Swartz L, Rohleder P. Cultural psychology. In: Willig C, Stainton-Rogers W, editors. *Handbook of qualitative research methods in psychology.* London: Sage; 2008:541–53.

90. Tribe R, Lane P. Working with interpreters across language and culture in mental health. *J Ment Health.* 2009;18:233–41.

91. Westermeyer J. Working with an interpreter in psychiatric assessment and treatment. *J Nerv Ment Dis.* 1990 Dec;178(12):745–9.

92. Westermeyer J, Janca A. Language, culture, and psychopathology: conceptual and methodological issues. *Transcult Psychiatry.* 1997;34(3):291–311.

93. Hsieh E, Ju H, Kong H. Dimensions of trust: the tensions and challenges in provider–interpreter trust. *Qual Health Res.* 2010 Feb;20(2):170–81.

94. Swartz L, Drennan G, Crawford A. Changing language policy in mental health services: a matter of interpretation? In: Foster D, Freeman M, Pillay Y, editors. *Mental health policy issues for South Africa.* Cape Town: MASA Multimedia; 1997:166–80.

95. Krog A, Mpolweni-Zantsi N, Ratele K. *There was this goat: Investigating the truth commission testimony of Notrose Nobomvu Konile.* Pietermartizburg, South Africa: University of KwaZulu-Natal Press; 2009.

96. Penn C, Watermeyer J. When asides become central: small talk and big talk in interpreted health interactions. *Patient Educ Couns.* 2012 Sep;88(3):391–8.

97. Sahlins M. Two or three things that I know about culture. *J R Anthropological Inst.* 1999;5:399–421.

98. Andreasen NC. Scale for the assessment of thought, language, and communication (TLC). *Schizophr Bull.* 1986;12(3):473–82.

99. Summerfield D. How scientifically valid is the knowledge base of global mental health? *BMJ.* 2008 May 3;336(7651):992–4.

100. Minas H, Jorm AF. Where there is no evidence: use of expert consensus methods to fill the evidence gap in low-income countries and cultural minorities. *Int J Ment Health Syst.* 2010;4(1):33.

101. Dua T, Barbui C, Clark N, et al. Evidence-based guidelines for mental, neurological, and substance use disorders in low- and middle-income countries: summary of WHO recommendations. *PLoS Med.* 2011 Nov;8(11):e1001122.

102. Kirmayer LJ. Cultural competence and evidence-based practice in mental health: epistemic communities and the politics of pluralism. *Soc Sci Med.* 2012 Apr 23;75:249–56.

103. Whitley R, Rousseau C, Carpenter-Song E, Kirmayer LJ. Evidence-based medicine: opportunities and challenges in a diverse society. *Can J Psychiatry.* 2011 Sep;56(9):514–22.

104. Moller HJ, Maier W. Evidence-based medicine in psychopharmacotherapy: possibilities, problems, and limitations. *Eur Arch Psychiatry Clin Neurosci.* 2010 Feb;260(1):25–39.

105. Angell M. The epidemic of mental illness: why? *New York Review of Books.* June 23, 2011.

106. Chatterjee S, Pillai A, Jain S, Cohen A, Patel V. Outcomes of people with psychotic disorders in a community-based rehabilitation programme in rural India. *Br J Psychiatry.* 2009 Nov;195(5):433–9.

107. Rahman A, Malik A, Sikander S, Roberts C, Creed F. Cognitive behaviour therapy-based intervention by community health workers for mothers with depression and their infants in rural Pakistan: a cluster-randomised controlled trial. *Lancet.* 2008 Sep 13;372(9642):902–9.

108. Campbell C, Burgess R. The role of communities in advancing the goals of the Movement for Global Mental Health. *Transcult Psychiatry.* 2012 Jul;49(3–4):379–95.

109. Brislin RW. The wording and translation of research instruments. In: Lonner WJ, Berry JW, editors. *Field methods in cross-cultural research.* Beverly Hills, CA: Sage; 1986:137–64.

110. Van Ommeren M, Sharma B, Thapa SB, et al. Preparing instruments for transcultural research: use of the translation monitoring form with Nepali-speaking Bhutanese refugees. *Transcult Psychiatry.* 1999;36(3):285–301.

111. Kleinman AM. Depression, somatization, and the "new cross-cultural psychiatry." *Soc Sci Med.* 1977;11:3–10.

112. Kleinman A. Anthropology and psychiatry: The role of culture in cross-cultural research on illness. *Br J Psychiatry.* 1987;151:447–54.

113. Gone JP, Kirmayer LJ. On the wisdom of considering culture and context in psychopathology. In: Millon T, Krueger RF, Simonsen E, editors. *Contemporary directions in psychopathology: Scientific foundations of the DSM-V and ICD-11.* New York: Guilford; 2010:72–96.

114. Weiss M. Explanatory model interview catalogue (EMIC): framework for comparative study of illness. *Transcult Psychiatry.* 1997;34(2):235–63.

115. Groleau D, Young A, Kirmayer LJ. The McGill illness narrative interview (MINI): an interview schedule to elicit meanings and modes of reasoning related to illness experience. *Transcult Psychiatry.* 2006 Dec;43(4):671–91.

116. De Jong JTVM, Van Ommeren M. Toward a culture-informed epidemiology: combining qualitative and quantitative research in transcultural contexts. *Transcult Psychiatry.* 2002;39(4):422–33.

117. van de Vijver F, Leung K. *Methods and data analysis for cross-cultural research.* Thousand Oaks, CA: Sage Publications; 1997.

118. Flaherty JA, Gaviria FM, Pathak D, et al. Developing instruments for cross-cultural psychiatric research. *J Nerv & Ment Dis.* 1988;176(5):257–63.

119. Canino G, Lewis-Fernandez R, Bravo M. Methodological challenges in cross-cultural mental health research. *Transcult Psychiatry.* 1997;34(2):163–84.

120. Miller KE, Omidian P, Kulkarni M, Yaqubi A, Daudzai H, Rasmussen A. The validity and clinical utility of post-traumatic stress disorder in Afghanistan. *Transcult Psychiatry.* 2009 Jun;46(2):219–37.

121. Swartz L. An unruly coming of age: the benefits of discomfort for global mental health. *Transcult Psychiatry.* 2012 Jul;49(3–4):531–8.

122. Page SE. *Diversity and complexity.* Princeton, NJ: Princeton University Press; 2011.

123. Lassman, P. Pluralism. Cambridge: Polity Press, 2011.

124. Talisse RB. Pluralism and Liberal Politics. New York: Taylor & Francis, 2011.

125. Marshall PA. Human rights, cultural pluralism, and international health research. *Theor Med Bioeth*, 2005, 26(6):529–557.

126. Kirmayer LJ. Multicultural medicine and the politics of recognition. *J Med Philos*, 2011, 36(4):410–423.

4 Cross-Cultural Research Methods and Practice

Martin J. Prince

Much "cross-cultural" mental health research involves the adaptation and application of concepts and methods developed in one cultural setting (usually the United Kingdom or the United States) to another, typically a non–English speaking low- or middle-income country (LAMIC) in Latin America, Africa, or Asia. The existence of such research is, in the main, a reflection of the dominance of Western biomedical and social science in terms of academic institutions, human resource, research funding, and access to outlets for dissemination. British researchers, after all, do not generally conduct cross-cultural research in the United States. True cross-cultural comparative research is less common, much of it in the past having been carried out under the aegis of the World Health Organization (WHO); the International Pilot Study of Schizophrenia[1,2]; the Collaborative Study on Strategies for Extending Mental Health Care[3]; and the Collaborative Project on Psychological Problems in General Health Care (PPGHC).[4] More recent examples include the World Mental Health Survey of over 200,000 participants in two dozen countries,[5,6] and the 10/66 Dementia Research Group's studies of dementia and aging in ten LAMIC.[7]

The purpose of this chapter is to review the necessary procedures to establish measurement equivalence across cultures, including some recent methodological developments in the quantitative assessment of cross-cultural construct validity. We shall then examine some of the potential applications for cross-cultural research.

ESTABLISHING MEASUREMENT EQUIVALENCE ACROSS CULTURES

In all cross-cultural research, the need to establish the relevance of the constructs studied to the diverse settings, to use bicultural and bilingual translators to arrive at an appropriate local language version of the assessment, and to make all necessary cultural adaptations, is well established; the methods and procedures have been extensively described, with a fairly clear emerging consensus.[8] Early descriptions of the process defined parameters by which a translated or adapted questionnaire should be evaluated[9]:

1. *Content equivalence:* Is the construct meaningful, acknowledged, recognized in the culture?
2. *Semantic equivalence:* Does the meaning of each item remain the same after translation?
3. *Technical equivalence:* Does the method of data collection affect results differentially between two cultures?
4. *Criterion equivalence:* What is an instrument's relationship with previously established and independent criteria for the same phenomena?
5. *Conceptual equivalence:* Does the instrument measure the same construct in different cultures?

This framework has helped to raise awareness of cultural influences on idioms of distress, explanatory models, help-seeking behavior, and clinical responses—all of which have clear implications for nosology and measurement. The five subcategories can be linked to three research activities that are necessary to demonstrate measurement equivalence—the investigation, through formative research of the cultural relevance of the concept (content equivalence); the process of adaptation and translation of an existing measure (semantic and technical equivalence); and the local and cross-cultural validation of the measure at the end of the instrument adaptation and development process (criterion and conceptual equivalence). These are now considered, in turn.

Formative Research to Investigate the Construct Under Study

Kleinman first drew attention to the danger of committing a "category fallacy," which he defined as "the reification of a nosological category developed for a particular cultural group that is applied to members of another culture for whom it lacks coherence."[10] To use his evocative example, the syndrome of "soul loss" identified in some non-Western settings could be operationalized and applied to an urban middle-class North American population, and prevalence data would be generated, although clearly without validity. Kleinman's contention was that such fallacies were common but, given the dominance of the Western cultural perspective, tended to proceed in the opposite cultural direction. Errors might arise through the confusion of culturally distinctive behavior with psychopathology on the basis of superficial phenomenological similarities. Hence, dysthymic disorder, he argued, might be inappropriately diagnosed in a low-income-country setting among those with chronic physical disorders—for example, anemia, nutritional or parasitic diseases—that were common in those settings but rare in North America where the DSM classification had been devised.

The coherence of Western diagnostic paradigms was investigated in the seminal WHO Collaborative Study on Strategies for Extending Mental Health Care in Sudan, northern India, and the Philippines.[11] Skeleton vignettes representing epilepsy, mental retardation, acute psychosis, mania, depressive psychosis, "process" schizophrenia, and depressive neurosis were constructed and embellished by local teams using local idiom, events, and customs. These were presented to multiple key informants. Each condition was widely recognized, with epilepsy, mental retardation, psychosis, and depressive neurosis being most commonly cited. All tended to be rated as serious, while the psychoses were thought particularly likely to lead to social and occupational disability. This study did not explore illness perceptions—similar vignette-based[12] and qualitative studies[13] in

India indicated that, while something resembling the dementia syndrome was widely recognized and indeed named, it was viewed as a normal part of aging rather than as a medical condition that might lead to help-seeking. More "bottom-up" ethnographic explorations of illness models include Manson's extension of the Western "Diagnostic Interview Schedule" to include an operationalized list of symptoms and categories, from Hopi indigenous nosology with a prima facie resemblance to depression,[14] the work of Patel and colleagues on Shona idioms for psychological distress in Zimbabwe,[15] and the work of Betancourt and colleagues on the development of scales to assess depression-like (*two tam, par,* and *kumu*), anxiety-like (*ma lwor*), and conduct problems (*kwo maraco*) among war-affected adolescents in northern Uganda.[16]

The decision as to whether to develop a locally valid assessment *de novo*, or to put resources into adapting existing Western measures, can be difficult. Clearly this will depend first upon the similarity of the construct's definitions in different cultures. Locally developed assessments that tap into local idioms should in principle have superior measurement properties with respect to local feasibility, validity, and sensitivity to change. However, the process of instrument development is highly technical, and costly in time and resources. If those resources are limited, then the local assessment may not live up to expectations, and adaptation of an existing measure from another culture may be more cost-effective. The notion that Western assessments are intrinsically more generalizable, favoring cross-cultural comparative research, is probably false. For example, the Shona Symptom Questionnaire has been shown to match U.K.-developed screening assessments for the identification of common mental disorders in primary care settings in Wales.[17] The key issue is that when an assessment developed in one cultural setting is to be used in another, particularly careful attention must be given to translation and need for adaptation.

Process of Translation and Adaptation of Instruments

The World Health Organization has developed a protocol for translations of its English-language assessments to be approved for use in other settings.[18] This probably represents the "state of the art" at present. WHO defines the overall goal succinctly as

to achieve different language versions of the English instrument that are conceptually equivalent in each of the target countries/cultures. That is, the instrument should be equally natural and acceptable and should practically perform in the same way. The focus is on cross-cultural and conceptual, rather than on linguistic/literal equivalence.[18]

Forward Translation

The translator should be bilingual. Their mother tongue should be that of the target culture, but they should also have knowledge of the culture from which the assessment originated. They should have technical expertise in the area covered by the instrument. Translators should consider the meaning of the original term and attempt to translate it, aiming for conceptual equivalence rather than a word-for-word translation. They should strive to be simple, clear, and concise. Fewer words are better. Long sentences with many clauses should be avoided. They should consider the typical respondent for the instrument being translated and what the respondent will understand when they hear the question, avoiding jargon and technical terms that cannot be understood clearly. They should consider gender and age applicability and avoid any terms that might be considered offensive.

Expert Panel

A bilingual expert panel should be convened to identify and resolve inadequate expressions, as well as any discrepancies between the forward translation and the original. The expert panel may question words or expressions and suggest alternatives. In general, the panel should include the original translator, experts in health, as well as experts with experience in instrument development and translation. The result of this process will be a complete translated version of the questionnaire.

Back-Translation

The instrument is translated back to English by an independent translator, whose mother tongue is English but who has no knowledge of the original questionnaire. Emphasis is again on conceptual rather than linguistic equivalence. Discrepancies require further work—forward translations, discussion by the bilingual expert panel, and back-translation, iterated as necessary until a satisfactory version is reached.

Pre-Testing and Cognitive Interviewing

Pre-test respondents should include individuals representative of those who will be administered the questionnaire, with purposive recruitment to ensure that both sexes, all relevant age groups, and different socioeconomic groups are included. An experienced interviewer administers the instrument, and the respondent is then systematically debriefed. In the debriefing (sometimes referred to as "cognitive interviewing"), respondents are asked what they thought each question was asking, whether they could paraphrase the question in their own words, and their rationale for the answer that they gave. Any difficulties with comprehension are noted, together with requests for clarification. Any words or expressions that were found to be unacceptable or offensive are noted.

Final Version

Each stage should be appropriately documented, including the initial forward version, the recommendations by the expert panel, the back-translation, a summary of problems found during the pre-testing, and the modifications proposed; and the final version.

Other approaches have been advocated. Sumathipala and Murray[19] used a panel of nine to independently translate items from the Bradford Somatic Inventory into Sinhala, and then to rate these for conceptual and semantic equivalence. Translations failing to reach consensus were discussed by the group for modifications and subjected to further discussion to achieve consensus. This combined the processes of forward translation and expert panel review. The authors argued that no single forward translation could hope to address satisfactorily the complexities of rendering problematic items into the new language, and that the consensus element did away with the need for back-translation to ensure content and semantic equivalence. The utility of back-translation has been questioned, since misjudgement on the part of forward or back translators can result in a lack of sensitivity and specificity for the identification of problematic items. Moreover, while back-translation may help identify problems, it cannot generate solutions.

Occasionally, extensive and important modifications of items are required for linguistic or cultural reasons, while still retaining the essence of the symptom or construct being assessed. Thus, in a validation of three different assessments for common mental disorder among post-natal women in rural Ghana,[20] since, in the local Twi language it is unusual to ask questions in the negative, seven items in the WHO's Self-Reporting Questionnaire,[21] which were perceived as being particularly culturally dissonant, were converted from negatively worded to positively worded items. For example, the question "Do you sleep badly?" was changed to "Do you sleep well?" and then reverse-scored so that a negative answer scored one point and a positive answer zero. The impact of these modifications upon scale performance could not be estimated directly, but the discrim-inability of the modified items (as measured by their likelihood ratios) and the item–total correlations were, if anything, somewhat higher than those for the unmodified items.[20]

Technical equivalence is an important issue where, for example, the mode of admin-istration differs from that originally intended. This is likely to arise when adapting a self-completion assessment intended for educated Western participants to participants in LAMIC, many of whom may be illiterate. The questionnaire could be administered by an interviewer instead, but this might change its measurement properties. Complex response formats may need to be simplified or broken down into components for verbal administration. Thus, for example, in the validation of the nine-item Patient Health Questionnaire in the rural Ghana study described in the previous paragraph, partici-pants found it difficult to map their experience of depression symptoms onto the pre-cise proportions of time in the last two weeks used as response options in the original questionnaire (*not at all, several days, more than half the days, nearly every day*).[20] Hence the administration was broken down into two stages. Respondents were asked if they had experienced the symptom, *yes* or *no*. If yes, they were further asked if the problem had been bothering them "some of the time, most of the time or all the time." Technical equivalence was not formally established—while it might have been assessed by com-paring the original self-administered and modified interviewer-administered approach among literate participants, this would not have been possible for the majority of the sample, who had little education and low literacy.

In reality, few translations and adaptations aspire to, let alone achieve, the level of sophistication and rigor recommended by the WHO. The nature of the modifications and the rationale for making them are often poorly documented. Mumford's careful translation of the Hospital Anxiety and Depression Questionnaire into Urdu is an excel-lent example of good practice.[22]

Cross-Cultural Measurement Validation

Criterion Validity

Testing criterion validity requires a "gold standard," technically the very thing that one is setting out to measure. The most commonly used gold standard in psychiatric research is a clinician semi-structured interview, generally the Schedules for Clinical Assessment in Neuropsychiatry (SCAN) or the Structured Clinical Interview for DSM Disorders (SCID), applying ICD-10 or DSM-IV diagnoses. Kessler, describing the validation pro-cedures planned for the World Mental Health Survey, highlights several problems, most of which are not particular to cross-cultural research.[23] First, the reliability of clinician semi-structured interviews is by no means perfect, particularly in community-based research, and this random error will set an upper limit on the validity coefficients that are likely to be observed. Secondly, repetition of comprehensive mental-state assessments is associated with systematic underreporting of symptoms on the second interview com-pared with the first, again tending towards an underestimate of true validity. Thirdly, the DSM and ICD diagnostic criteria are not fully operationalized, and differing judgements made in the diagnostic algorithms for the test assessment and gold standard research interviews may be another source of discrepancy. Fourth, Cohen's kappa varies with the prevalence of the disorder even when specificity and sensitivity are constant, limit-ing the utility of this validity coefficient in comparing the validity of a measure across different populations—Kessler proposes instead the area under the Receiver Operating

Characteristic (ROC) curve, which in the special case of a dichotomous test variable is the average of sensitivity and specificity.[23] Youden's index ((sensitivity + specificity) − 1) performs the same function and is much better-established.[24]

For all of these reasons, Kessler suggested that it would be more appropriate instead to "calibrate" the lay-structured World Mental Health Composite International Diagnostic Interview (WMH-CIDI) against the clinician semi-structured SCID.[23] Prediction equations were developed in a clinical calibration sub-sample, with WMH-CIDI symptom-level data used to predict SCID diagnoses, and these coefficients were then used to assign predicted probabilities of SCID diagnoses to each respondent in the remainder of the sample. It was then possible to investigate whether estimates of prevalence and associations based on WMH-CIDI diagnoses were consistent with those based on predicted SCID diagnoses. With data from WMH surveys in France, Italy, Spain, and the United States, this was the case for 12-month prevalence estimates of anxiety and mood disorder, while lifetime prevalence estimates from the CIDI were conservative with respect to the SCID.[25] Diagnostic concordance was also good for any anxiety disorder (Area Under ROC curve (AUROC) = 0.88) and any mood disorder (AUROC = 0.83).

The 10/66 Dementia Research Group (10/66 DRG) used a similar calibration approach to arrive at a "10/66 Dementia" diagnosis. However, the calibration algorithm was first developed and tested in an international pilot study conducted in 26 centers in Latin America, Africa, India, and China.[26] The assessments that contributed to the algorithm were selected empirically on the basis of "culture-fair" characteristics (capable of discriminating equivalently between DSM-IV dementia cases and non-cases across a variety of settings) and "education-fair" characteristics (capable of discrimination across the full range of educational abilities, and with a minimal false positive rate among those with little or no education). The predictive algorithm was developed on one random half of the pilot data set, and tested on the other. The resulting probabilistic 10/66 diagnosis showed similar validity in all world regions, with 94% sensitivity overall, and false positive rates of 6% and 3% in low- and high-education controls, respectively.[26] The algorithm was then applied in the subsequent population-based studies, at which stage it was subject to further concurrent and predictive validation.[7,27,28]

A more fundamental concern with respect to cross-cultural research is whether it is ever really possible to identify a single "gold standard" that could be meaningfully applied across a wide variety of countries and cultures. This is not properly addressed in either the WMH or 10/66 DRG studies. The SCID, for example, has not itself been validated against locally appropriate criteria, and the universal applicability of DSM-IV nosologies has also been challenged.[29] The demonstration of equivalent validity against a universal external criterion does not exclude the commission of a category fallacy as described by Kleinman. There are examples in the literature of the use of external criteria that may more accurately reflect local diagnostic practice. For example, clinician checklists can be used that are consistent with standard nosologies, but at least allow local clinicians to use culturally appropriate interview techniques to elicit and rate symptoms that they consider to be relevant. This approach was used successfully in Sri Lanka to validate the Revised Clinical Interview Schedule (CIS-R) at the symptom-cluster level.[30] In Ethiopia, the Comprehensive Psychopathological Rating Scale (CPRS) was used as the gold standard to validate the Self-Reporting Questionnaire and the Edinburgh Postnatal Depression Scale, after its inter-rater and test-retest reliability had first had been assessed and improved through training.[31,32] In an innovative approach, Patel used recognition by local practitioners (both allopathic and traditional healers), when confirmed by a Western structured psychiatric interview (the CIS-R), as the gold standard against which to validate the Shona Symptom Questionnaire as an assessment of common mental disorders.[15] There are no examples yet of such approaches' being used in validation studies across a variety of countries and cultures. One possible approach would be to use both a common "etic" criterion (a universalist approach, assuming internationally common criteria and measurement, such as the SCAN) together with "emic" criteria (locally culturally relevant and valid) that could be selected for each cultural setting. The reliability of the "emic" criterion is clearly a key consideration.

Construct Validity

Construct validity is generally not well understood, but it is highly relevant to establishing the validity of constructs and assessments across populations and cultures. The term was proposed by the APA Committee on Psychological Tests in 1954, including Meehl and Cronbach, who wrote a classic paper defining the term.[33] Pre-existent concepts of validity had focused on content validity and criterion-related validity, where a gold standard for the construct was already established. *Construct validity*, as defined by Meehl and Cronbach, referred to a situation in which "the tester has no definite criterion measure of the quality with which he is concerned, and must use indirect measures. Here the (elucidation of the) trait or quality underlying the test is of central importance."[33] Meehl and Cronbach considered that expert ratings of these matters would be of limited, if any, value. Construct validity would be involved in answering such questions as: "To what extent is this test culture-free?" "Does this test measure reading ability, quantitative reasoning, or response sets?" "How does a person with a high score differ from a person with a low score?" The answers to these questions would be derived from quantitative research, essentially through a series of hypothesis-driven investigations aimed at identifying the "nomological net" or theoretical framework consisting of more or less proximate identifiers for the construct, at least some of which would need to be observable.

Meehl and Cronbach described the investigation of a test's construct validity as comparable to that for developing and confirming theories in observational research. This was particularly the case for test-"criterion" correlations used to define the nomological net (in quotation marks since the construct validity of the criteria themselves is also under investigation, and, as with a hypothesis in observational research, the construct that is intended to be measured can be refined on the basis of findings). Other quantitative procedures for establishing construct validity included inter-item correlations and internal consistency, factor analysis, and test-retest reliability. Methodological developments in recent years have led to the introduction of more sophisticated, hypothesis-driven approaches to testing construct validity across cultures. Confirmatory factor analysis (CFA) and Rasch models can be used to assess whether a scale measures the same trait dimension, in the same way, when applied in qualitatively distinct groups; this is referred to as "measurement invariance." In a worked example, Reise et al. illustrated these approaches with respect to mood symptoms assessed in Minnesota and China.[34] The demonstration of measurement invariance across countries, cultures, and ethnic groups provides strong evidence to support the construct validity of an assessment for the purposes of comparative research. Despite their evident applicability to cross-cultural validity of assessments of mental health status, there are relatively few examples in the literature.

Principal component analysis (PCA) is an exploratory technique based on a covariance matrix of tetrachoric correlations to estimate factor loadings of items upon underlying latent traits.[35] PCA has been widely used to demonstrate similar patterns of factor loadings when a measure is used in different cultural contexts—for example, the Bradford Somatic Inventory used on patients with medically unexplained symptoms in general healthcare settings in Pakistan and the United Kingdom.[36] In confirmatory factor analysis, a model is tested that specifies in advance the relations between observed variables and latent factors. Testing for measurement invariance involves an assessment of whether the best factor solution relates to the latent trait or traits in the same way in each of several populations. CFA has been used to validate the Parental Bonding Interview across European centers participating in the World Mental Health Survey,[37] providing strong evidence for the invariance of a three-factor solution suggested by exploratory factor analysis, across six countries, both sexes, and all age groups. The general approach is to compare two models in which all item loadings are (a) constrained and (b) not constrained to be identical between countries. Partial measurement invariance may be tested for, if full measurement is not supported. Partial measurement invariance occurs if a majority of the non-fixed values are still invariant across groups and if these invariant loadings define a meaningful latent trait. The absolute fit of a CFA model can be evaluated by means of a $\chi 2$ statistic. Several other absolute and relative indices of fit are recommended. Akaike's Information Criterion (AIC)[38] adjusts the model chi-square to penalize for model complexity. The lower the AIC value, the better the fit of the model. The Tucker-Lewis index (TLI)[39] indicates the proportion of covariation among indicators explained by the model relative to a null model of independence, and is independent of sample size. Values near zero indicate poor fit, whereas values near 1.0 indicate good fit; those greater than 0.90 are considered satisfactory. In contrast, the root mean square error of approximation (RMSEA) assesses badness of fit per degree of freedom in the model, and is zero if the model fits perfectly; RMSEA values of less than 0.05 indicate close fit, and 0.05 to 0.08, reasonable fit of a model.

Rasch analysis belongs to a family of statistical models developed from item response theory (IRT).[34] Whereas CFA models account for the covariance between test items, IRT models account for patterns of item responses. The Rasch model suggests that the responses to a set of items can be justified by a person's position on the underlying trait that is being measured and by the item severity (also referred to as "item calibration"). Item calibrations are measured on the same scale as the severity of the underlying trait. Participants with severity scores below the calibration for the given item are more likely to deny than endorse the item, while those with severity scores above the calibration for the item are more likely to endorse it. It follows that the items with higher calibrations are less frequently endorsed. Also, a participant who endorses an item of middling severity is likely to have endorsed all items with lower calibrations. Infit (Information weighted fit) assesses the extent to which observed response patterns were consistent, or inconsistent with the item calibrations. Mean square (MNSQ) infit statistics of less than 1.3 indicate that the subscale items contribute to a single hierarchical underlying construct (unidimensionality). While there can be no single satisfactory test of model adequacy, techniques can be used to assess different aspects of goodness of fit of Rasch models.

Rasch analysis was used in the WHO international study of psychological problems in general health care settings (PPGHC).[40] Strong evidence was provided to support a common hierarchy for CIDI symptoms (in increasing order of item severity: sleep, mood, concentration fatigue, loss of interest, suicidality, guilt, agitation/ retardation, appetite change) across three groups of countries categorized by the prevalence of major depression (low, intermediate, or high). Despite measurement invariance, threshold effects arising from culturally determined differences in norms or expectations or expressions of mood and mental health may still be a problem, and may explain much of the observed difference in prevalence. In the PPGHC study, this possibility was addressed through a formal test for differential item functioning; the goodness-of-fit for a model allowing different symptom thresholds for the three prevalence groups was not significantly better than that for a simpler model assuming identical symptom thresholds (Chi sq 19.4, df 18, $P = 0.38$). The authors concluded from these findings that there was no evidence that prevalence differences were explained by cross-cultural differences in the form or validity of the depressive syndrome, and that therefore the apparent differences in depression prevalence could not be attributed to "category fallacy." Where threshold differences are identified (as, for example, in the case of self-reported global health), the use of anchoring vignettes has been advocated to identify and adjust for the consequent response bias.[41]

An Example of Cross-Cultural Construct Validation—The EURO-D

Background

The EURO-D scale[42] was developed to harmonize data on late-life depression from population-based studies in 11 European countries as part of the EURODEP collaboration. EURO-D items were all taken from the Geriatric Mental State clinical interview,[43] but were selected on the basis that they were also common to four other depression scales used in some of the EURODEP studies. Thus, the EURO-D has intrinsically strong face validity. The initial validation showed adequate internal consistency, and a cutoff point of 3/4 was optimal for the identification of clinically significant depression in most countries.[42] Principal components analysis generated two factors ("affective suffering" and "motivation") that were common to nearly every participating country.[42] The same factor structure was also identified for Indian, Latin-American, and Caribbean sites in the 10/66 Dementia Research Group pilot studies.[46]

Cross-Cultural Measurement Invariance

A more detailed investigation of the cross-cultural validity of the EURO-D and its measurement properties[44] was carried out using data from the Survey of Health, Ageing and Retirement in Europe (SHARE) 2004 baseline study, comprising cross-sectional surveys of representative samples of community residents aged 50 years and over from 10 European countries (Denmark, Sweden, Austria, France, Germany, Switzerland, the Netherlands, Spain, Italy, and Greece).

Principal component analysis again suggested a two-factor solution (affective suffering and motivation) in nine of the 10 countries. In all countries, the full EURO-D scale was moderately internally consistent with Cronbach's alpha ranging from 0.62 to 0.78. However, in confirmatory factor analysis, the fit of the two-factor solution was always superior to that of the one-factor solution.[44] The two-factor solution was tested for measurement invariance across countries by comparing three measurement models; (a) with no constraints, (b) with both factors constrained to load equally across all countries (full measurement invariance), and (c) where only items from the affective suffering factor were constrained to load equally across all countries (partial measurement invariance). The fit of Model 1 was clearly superior to that of Model 2; therefore, the full invariance model did not hold across countries, and was rejected. However, the three absolute goodness-of-fit indices provided strong evidence that the partial invariance model was adequate and did not clearly differ from Model 1. Therefore, there was evidence to suggest that the affective suffering factor represented a stable latent trait, measured in a similar way by its indicator items across European countries and cultures. The same could not be claimed for the motivation factor.

The Rasch model indicated that the EURO-D was a hierarchical scale.[44] The rank ordering of EURO-D item calibration values was similar for all countries. Depression (followed by sleep disturbance) had the lowest item calibrations overall, while guilt and suicidality had the highest. The intraclass correlation coefficient (ICC) for agreement in item calibrations across all 10 countries was 0.89 (0.78–0.95). There was therefore strong evidence for measurement invariance with respect to item calibration. However, there was more heterogeneity in item calibration between countries for the motivation than for the affective suffering items. For the subset of items loading on affective suffering, the ICC was 0.94 (0.85–0.99), whereas for the four motivation items it was only 0.65 (0.30–0.96).

What Are the Factors Measuring? The Nomological Net

It had been previously noted in both the EURODEP[45] and the 10/66 pilot studies[46] that the affective suffering factor was associated with female sex, while the motivation factor scores, but not affective suffering scores, increased with increasing age. Did this correlation between motivation and age, considered in the context of the orthogonal relationship with affective suffering, suggest that an expressed lack of interest and enjoyment, together with pessimism, might be affectively neutral statements representing an adaptive cognitive appraisal of activity limitation in older age? An alternative hypothesis was that the motivation factor might be capturing some of the clinical features of vascular depression[47]—impaired executive functioning associated with vascular damage to subcortical brain structures. In the SHARE data set, the previously observed pattern of association with age and sex was confirmed to be consistent across all 10 SHARE countries.[48] The earlier hypothesis regarding impaired executive functioning was tested formally, and higher motivation factor scores were indeed associated with poorer performance on animal-naming (executive function), while there was no association with 10-word recall (memory). The affective suffering factor was not associated with either cognitive test. Again, the pattern of association between the cognitive tests and the EURO-D factors was highly consistent across all countries.[48]

Summary of Findings

1. In all settings, the EURO-D held up well as a unidimensional scale, as evidenced by the moderately high Cronbach's alpha and the reasonable fit of the one-factor solution.
2. However, there was also evidence that it may be measuring two underlying factors, *affective suffering* (well characterized and invariant across cultures) and *motivation* (less well characterized and variable across cultures).
3. The affective suffering factor showed excellent cross-cultural measurement properties, with strong evidence for measurement invariance with respect both to item loadings onto a common underlying latent trait, and to item calibrations. It also has strong face validity as a depression measure.
4. The motivation factor exhibited heterogeneity in factor loading patterns and item calibrations between countries, suggesting some limitations for use in cross-cultural research.

POTENTIAL APPLICATIONS FOR CROSS-CULTURAL RESEARCH

Comparative Studies of Disease Frequency

Clusters of low or high prevalence for a disorder are of interest to epidemiologists, since they may give important clues about etiology. The simplest studies are those of single populations. The high prevalence of motor neuritides in Guam,[49] and the rarity of multiple sclerosis in Southern Africa,[50] have led to the formulation of etiological hypotheses.[51,52] Early studies of schizophrenia have reported clusters of strikingly low prevalence (e.g., among the Hutterite Anabaptist sect in the United States)[53] and high prevalence (e.g., in parts of Croatia).[54]

Some research collaborations were established with the explicit aim of making much broader comparisons of the frequency of mental disorders between countries and cultures. The conclusion from WHO's Collaborative Study on Determinants of Outcome of Severe Mental Disorders[55] was that, when both clinical interview techniques and case criteria were standardized, there was little variability in incidence rates between different centers, in North and South America, Europe, Africa, Asia, and the far East. That having been said, using narrow criteria, there was a twofold variation in the annual incidence of schizophrenia. Subsequent meta-analyses of incidence studies confirm a wide variation in rates.[56] Prognosis also seemed to be better in some of the developing country Determinants of Outcome of Severe Mental Disorders study (DOSMED) centers,[55,57] although the interpretation of this finding has been contested.[58] In the 15-site WHO International Study of Psychological Problems in General Health Care (PPGHC), there was a 15-fold variation in the prevalence of major depression (assessed using the lay-administered Composite International Diagnostic Instrument [CIDI-PC]), with the lowest prevalence in Asia, the highest prevalence in Latin America, and intermediate prevalence in Europe and North America.[40] Preliminary findings from the World Mental Health Survey from 15 surveys in 14 countries in the Americas (Colombia, Mexico, the United States), Europe (Belgium, France, Germany, Italy, the Netherlands, Spain, Ukraine), the Middle East and Africa (Lebanon, Nigeria), and Asia (Japan and China) indicates considerable between-center heterogeneity in the prevalence of all common mental disorders.[5] The prevalence of any DSM-IV mental disorder varies from 4.3% to 26.4% (interquartile range 9.1% to 16.9%), with strikingly low prevalence in Shanghai (4.3%) and Nigeria (4.9%), and strikingly high prevalence in the United States (26.4%). Even within Europe, there was a more than twofold variation in prevalence among countries.

Interpreting Differences Observed Across Cultures

Any observed differences in disease frequency between regions, countries, cultures, and ethnicities need to be interpreted with care, for the following reasons.

1. The history of psychiatric epidemiology has demonstrated that much of the heterogeneity in reported disease frequency is attributable to methodological differences between studies. Relevant factors include sampling, inclusion and exclusion criteria, assessments used to identify mental disorder (scale-based versus diagnostic interview, lay- versus clinician-administered), and particularly, diagnostic criteria. As operationalized criteria are established, diagnostic interview technologies are developed, and study methodologies increasingly standardized, so is this source of heterogeneity between estimates minimized.[55,59]

2. Standardized methodologies are desirable in comparative cross-cultural research to the extent that the approach can be assumed, or, ideally, demonstrated, to be measuring the same thing in the same way across cultures. Consistent identification across cultures by the standardized methodology may represent a category fallacy and should not therefore be interpreted as supporting universal applicability. Attempts to validate and calibrate standard assessments across countries and cultures are few and far between.[23,26,60] Use of identical, and valid diagnostic methods may yet identify different levels of disease severity in different language or cultural groups.[40]

3. As prevalence is the product of incidence and duration, low prevalence may indicate a high recovery rate or a low survival rate for those with the disorder, rather than a true difference in incidence. Longitudinal studies measuring disease incidence and duration are needed if valid comparisons are to be made between settings.[61,62]

4. Differing response rates between studies make it very difficult to make valid comparisons of disease frequency—in the World Mental Health Survey, the proportions of non-responders varied from 46% (France) to 88% (Colombia), with a weighted average of just 70%.[5]

5. In unstable populations, low prevalence may be accounted for either by selective out-migration of susceptible persons, or by in-migration of those unlikely to

develop the disorder, and vice versa for high prevalence. This has been an important issue in schizophrenia research (see below).

Assessing the Contribution of Compositional and Contextual Factors

If genuine, differences in disease frequency may be explained by compositional or contextual factors. Compositional factors relate to variation in the makeup of the populations under study. Factors that are already known to influence prevalence and incidence, such as age and gender, are often controlled for through standardization to permit a more informative comparison of disease frequency between populations. However, compositional differences can also be used to generate hypotheses about etiology—for example: a disease is common in population x, exposure y is also common in population x; therefore exposure y is hypothesized as a cause of the disease. Compositional explanations for differences in disease frequency between populations may arise from the main effect of genetic factors or environmental exposures, or by interactions between genes and environment, genes and other genes, or between different environmental factors.[63]

Contextual factors are characteristics of the population, rather than the individuals that make up the population. Where populations are defined as countries, these might include, for example, the political system under which people live, the structure of the health system, the extent of income inequalities, and the dominant culture.

Study Designs to Attribute Differences Observed Across Populations

While international studies can be used to generate hypotheses regarding etiology, it is not generally possible to adduce direct evidence to support genetic or environmental explanations. We shall consider the potential contribution of four broad types of study designs: ecological correlational studies, migration studies, genetic admixture studies, and multilevel study designs. In brief, ecological correlational studies can help generate hypotheses regarding etiology, but hypothesis testing needs to be carried out with samples of individuals. Migration studies and admixture studies can help determine the relative contribution of genes and environment to between population differences in disease frequency. Multilevel study designs can be used to apportion and study compositional and contextual effects.

Ecological Correlational Studies

Ecological correlational studies provide a crude quantitative framework for analyzing factors that might contribute to variations in disease frequency. An aggregate measure of the hypothesized exposure at population level (the proportion exposed, or the mean level of the exposure in the population) is correlated with an aggregate measure of the outcome (population prevalence or incidence) across centers. For example, in sub-Saharan Africa, there was noted to be a general inverse association at the country level between the prevalence of male circumcision and the seroprevalence of HIV, leading to the suggestion that male circumcision may reduce the risk of sexual transmission.[64] However, an ecological correlation need not imply a correlation at the level of individuals within populations, a problem referred to as the "ecological fallacy." Put simply, we cannot confirm that those individuals living with HIV are less likely to be circumcised. Many other factors of direct relevance to HIV risk may covary at the country level with circumcision practices, and it is not possible to control for confounding at the individual level. Reverse causality also cannot be excluded. For these reasons, it is difficult to make causal inferences from ecological correlational studies. A more definitive test of an ecological hypothesis can be carried out using traditional analytical study designs (cohort or case-control studies) on individuals within a single population where there is variance in the exposure—this work has now been carried out on the association between male circumcision and HIV risk,[65] confirming an inverse association at the individual level, with yet stronger evidence coming from randomized controlled trials of circumcision of HIV-negative men.[66] Where an ecological correlation is demonstrated with a contextual-level variable—for example, associations between own-group ethnic density[67] or inequality[68] and the treated incidence of schizophrenia—individual-level analysis cannot be used. However, multilevel study designs (see below) can be used to control for compositional variation; for example, to check that the increased incidence in areas of high inequality was not accounted for by the high proportion of low-income individuals that might be found in those areas.

Understanding the Roles of Genes and Environment—Migration and Genetic Admixture Studies

Genetic explanations for population differences in disease frequency have fallen into disfavor, given that as little as 10% of genetic variation is among, as opposed to within, continents. Cooper asserts that "race, at the continental level, has not been shown to provide a useful categorization of genetic information about the response to drugs, diagnosis, or causes of disease."[69] However, evidence suggests that the genetic variability among populations seems to include relatively recent population-specific adaptations to environmental changes and cultural innovations[70]; the genes most strongly affected by recent population-specific selection appear to be those associated with skin color, bone structure, and the metabolism of different foods. Several of these genes have already been identified as implicated in disease processes.[70] Both genetic and environmental explanations for regional differences in disease frequency are, therefore, tenable in most cases.

In migration studies, the health outcomes of migrants from a high-prevalence setting to a low-prevalence setting (or vice versa) are compared with those of the population at origin. Such studies can offer insights into the likely genetic or environmental contributions to observed differences in disease frequency. Sustained high or low prevalence despite dietary acculturation, as is seen, for example, with type II diabetes among South Asian migrants to the United Kingdom,[71] suggests that genetic factors may be relevant. Convergence of disease frequency with that of the host population, as has been noted for cardiovascular disease among Japanese Americans,[72] suggests that environmental (lifestyle) risk factors were involved.

Studies of ethnic minority groups in the United Kingdom consistently report a particularly high incidence of schizophrenia and bipolar disorder among those of African and African Caribbean ancestry. The AESOP studies of first-onset psychosis indicate that high incidence rates are relatively specific to these diagnoses and these ethnic groups, although more modest elevations of risk for psychosis are also seen in white and Asian migrants.[73] Risk in second-generation migrants seems to be higher than for first-generation migrants. There are similar findings from other European countries.[74] These are effectively migration studies without a comparison group in the country of origin. Findings from Trinidad suggest a higher incidence of psychosis among islanders with African compared with Indian ancestry.[75] Comparative studies between migrants to the Netherlands and France, and their source populations in the Caribbean, give inconsistent findings on relative frequencies of psychosis.[74] Selective migration is considered to be an unlikely explanation for the higher rates seen in Caribbean migrants to Europe, particularly given the higher risk among second-generation migrants.[74] Much research to date has focused upon the interaction between the process of migration and the experience of racism and disadvantage as a plausible explanation for these findings.[74]

Studying the relationship of disease risk to individual admixture within admixed populations (for example, the proportion of an individual's genome that is inherited from African versus Caucasian ancestors) is the most direct way to distinguish genetic from environmental explanations for ethnic differences.[76] This approach has been used to explore the influence of genes linked to African ancestry on dementia prevalence and the effect of the Apolipoprotein E (APOE) genotype on dementia risk in the racially admixed Cuban population.[77] Where there is an association with admixture, admixture mapping can be used to identify chromosomal regions that might include the genes linked to ancestry that may be responsible for ethnic differences.

Multilevel Study Designs

For contextual factors, multilevel study designs offer a sophisticated approach, allowing the simultaneous study of compositional and contextual effects. Multiple communities are selected to ensure variance in the contextual factors under study (such as social capital or income inequality); individuals are then surveyed within each community cluster so that information can be collected on compositional individual-level risk factors and mental health outcomes. The independent and interactive effects of compositional and contextual variables can then be assessed in a statistically and methodologically robust fashion.[78] In the United Kingdom, very little of the variance in psychological morbidity scores seemed to occur at the area level, particularly after adjusting for compositional factors, in contrast with the variance at the household level, which was substantial and statistically significant.[79] This finding implied that individual and household factors might be more important than the contextual effects of place on risk for common mental disorder (CMD). Furthermore, the effects of income inequality (at the regional level) upon prevalence of CMDs depended upon individual-level socioeconomic status; living in a high income-inequality area was a risk factor for those with high incomes, but protective for those with low incomes.[80] However, in an analysis of data from another nationally representative data set that oversampled black and ethnic minority populations, there were substantial protective small-area effects of own-group ethnic density upon the prevalence of CMD, which were not mediated by the compositional effects of reduced experiences of racism or increased social support.[81]

Cross-Cultural Issues in Intervention Research

The evidence base for psychological and psychopharmacological interventions needs to be extended to countries and cultures beyond Europe and North America, where the vast majority of trials have been carried out. Patel identifies four reasons for potential non-generalizability for trial evidence from developed countries.[82]

1. The explanatory models of common mental disorders in many developing countries are unlikely to acknowledge a role for biomedical interventions, which would influence the acceptability of psychiatric interventions.
2. Cultural factors are unlikely to influence treatment response for physical treatments such as antidepressants, but there may be genetically mediated effects on the pharmacokinetics and pharmacodynamics of drug therapies, affecting dosage and therapeutic windows. Culture may also impact the acceptability and tolerance of side-effects.
3. Widely varying and rapidly changing health system–related factors can profoundly influence the applicability of treatment research.
4. While efficacy of treatments may vary relatively little, the cost of drugs is strongly influenced by regional economic factors, such as the differing interpretations of

drug patent rules, the production of generic drugs, and the variable dose strengths of pharmaceutical preparations. The cost of psychological interventions will depend more on the cost (and availability) of therapists to implement them. The relative cost-effectiveness and cost–benefit ratios associated with treatments are therefore likely to vary between settings.

Most importantly, the prioritization of mental health care will be much more heavily influenced by locally conducted research. The drug policies in many countries require at least Phase IV trials before new medications are licensed for use, even if they are being widely used elsewhere. Trials in developing countries might also usefully focus also on the interface between mental health and established health priorities, such as, for example, the management of common mental disorders in those presenting for treatment of HIV/AIDS. Despite the paucity of experimental evidence from low- and middle-income countries, recently conducted good-quality randomized controlled trials already indicate effectiveness for selective serotonin-reuptake inhibitor (SSRI) antidepressants,[83] psychological interventions,[84,85] and stepped care psychological and pharmacological interventions[86,87] for the treatment of depression and other common mental disorders in sub-Saharan Africa, South Asia, and Latin America. A key feature of all of these trials was that the intervention was administered by nonspecialists working in the community or in primary care, hence providing proof of principal of the feasibility of task-sharing to promote efforts to close the sizeable treatment gap for those disorders in resource-poor settings with few mental health specialist professionals.

Important and controversial issues for intervention research in novel cultural settings are the inclusion criteria for the trial and the definition of outcome. It may not be appropriate, for reasons already described, simply to use Western diagnostic nosologies to identify cases for treatment. Thus Bolton and colleagues, in their trial of group interpersonal therapy in Uganda, included the individuals who were self-identified and confirmed by key informants as suffering from depression-like syndromes, *yo'kwekyawa* (loosely translated as "self-loathing") and *okwekubazida* ("self-pity"). However, to enter the trial, these persons also had to meet all, or all but one, of the criteria for DSM-IV major depression, identified using a culturally adapted version of the Hopkins Symptom Checklist (HSCL), and have at least some functional impairment, identified using a locally developed scale with separate versions for male and female participants.[88] The locally developed functional impairment scale was also then used as a secondary outcome to judge the efficacy of the intervention, in addition to the HSCL.

Cultural and local health system and health service issues also need to be considered carefully in the development of any intervention strategy. The systematic process of developing an intervention and critically evaluating plans for its implementation is carefully described and documented for the Manashanti Sudar Shodh (MANAS) trial, integrating an evidence-based package of treatments for depression and anxiety into routine public and primary care settings in Goa, India.[89]

CONCLUSION

Valid assessment across cultures requires qualitative research to investigate the cultural relevance of a construct, a careful translation and adaptation of a common measure, followed by pre-testing and cognitive interviews on the populations to be tested. Full criterion validation across diverse cultures may be a chimera, given the difficulty in establishing a universally applicable "gold standard." Quantitative analyses can, however, have a part to play in establishing construct validity across cultures. Scale internal consistency, inter-item and item-total correlations, and test-retest reliability provide basic support for the viability of a measure in a new cultural setting. Exploratory factor analysis can be used to compare factors and factor loadings. The hypothesis of "measurement invariance" across countries and cultures can be tested explicitly using confirmatory factor analysis (common underlying factors and factor loadings) and Rasch models (common hierarchy of items). Despite measurement invariance, threshold effects arising from cultural differences in norms, expectations, or expressions of mental distress may still be a problem. Comparative mental health research has identified significant variations in the prevalence and incidence of mental disorders worldwide, including common mental disorders, psychoses, and dementia. The interpretation of such differences, and in particular their attribution to underlying etiological factors, is much more problematic, particularly given the difficulty of excluding the role of methodological factors, chief amongst these being measurement validity. There are few examples in the cross-cultural mental health literature of demonstrably valid, culture-fair comparison. Much more could, in principle, be done to demonstrate measurement invariance, and to identify and explore sources of heterogeneity.

REFERENCES

1. Sartorius N, Jablensky A, Shapiro R. Two-year follow-up of patients included in the WHO International Pilot Study of Schizophrenia. *Psychol Med*. 1977;7:529–41.
2. Sartorius N, Shapiro R, Kimura M, Barrett K. WHO International Pilot Study of Schizophrenia. *Psychol Med*. 1972 Nov;2(4):422–5.
3. Harding TW, Climent CE, Diop M, et al. The WHO collaborative study on strategies for extending mental health care, II: the development of new research methods. *Am J Psychiatry*. 1983 Nov;140(11):1474–80.
4. Sartorius N, Ustun TB, Costa ESJ, et al. An international study of psychological problems in primary care. Preliminary report from the World Health Organization Collaborative Project on "Psychological Problems in General Health Care." *Arch Gen Psychiatry*. 1993;50(10):819–24.
5. Demyttenaere K, Bruffaerts R, Posada-Villa J, et al. Prevalence, severity, and unmet need for treatment of mental disorders in the World Health Organization World Mental Health Surveys. *JAMA*. 2004 Jun 2;291(21):2581–90.
6. Kessler RC, Haro JM, Heeringa SG, Pennell BE, Ustun TB. The World Health Organization World Mental Health Survey Initiative. *Epidemiol Psychiatr Soc*. 2006 Jul;15(3):161–6.
7. Prince M, Ferri CP, Acosta D, et al. The protocols for the 10/66 Dementia Research Group population-based research programme. *BMC Public Health*. 2007 Jul;7(1):165.
8. Patel V. Cultural issues in measurement and research. In: Prince M, Stewart R, Ford T, Hotopf M, editors. *Practical Psychiatric Epidemiology*. Oxford, UK: Oxford University Press; 2003: 43–64.
9. Flaherty JA, Gaviria FM, Pathak D, et al. Developing instruments for cross-cultural psychiatric research. *J Nerv Ment Dis*. 1988 May;176(5):257–63.
10. Kleinman A. Anthropology and psychiatry. The role of culture in cross-cultural research on illness. *Br J Psychiatry*. 1987 Oct;151:447–54.
11. Wig NN, Suleiman MA, Routledge R, et al. Community reactions to mental disorders. A key informant study in three developing countries. *Acta Psychiatr Scand*. 1980 Feb;61(2):111–26.
12. Patel V, Prince M. Ageing and mental health in a developing country: who cares? Qualitative studies from Goa, India. *Psychol Med*. 2001;31(1):29–38.
13. Shaji KS, Smitha K, Praveen Lal K, Prince M. Caregivers of patients with Alzheimer's disease: a qualitative study from the Indian 10/66 Dementia Research Network. *Int J Geriatr Psychiatry*. 2002;18:1–6.
14. Manson SM, Shore JH, Bloom JD. The depressive experience in American Indian communities. A challenge for psychiatric theory and diagnosis. In: Kleinman A, Good B, editors. *Culture and Depression*. Berkeley: University of California Press; 1985:331–68.
15. Patel V, Simunyu E, Gwanzura F, Lewis G, Mann A. The Shona Symptom Questionnaire: the development of an indigenous measure of common mental disorders in Harare. *Acta Psychiatr Scand*. 1997 Jun;95(6):469–75.
16. Betancourt TS, Bass J, Borisova I, et al. Assessing local instrument reliability and validity: a field-based example from northern Uganda. *Soc Psychiatry Psychiatr Epidemiol*. 2009 Aug;44(8):685–92.

17. Winston M, Smith J. A trans-cultural comparison of four psychiatric case-finding instruments in a Welsh community. *Soc Psychiatry Psychiatr Epidemiol.* 2000 Dec;35(12):569–75.

18. World Health Organization. *Process of translation and adaptation of instruments.* 2008.

19. Sumathipala A, Murray J. New approach to translating instruments for cross-cultural research: a combined qualitative and quantitative approach for translation and consensus generation. *Int J Methods Psychiatr Res.* 2001;9(2):85–97.

20. Weobong B, Akpalu B, Doku V, et al. The comparative validity of screening scales for postnatal common mental disorder in Kintampo, Ghana. *J Affect Disord.* 2009 Feb;113(1-2):109–17.

21. Beusenberg M, Orley J. *User's guide to the Self Reporting Questionnaire.* 1994. Geneva, World Health Organization. Ref. type: Generic.

22. Mumford DB, Tareen IA, Bajwa MA, Bhatti MR, Karim R. The translation and evaluation of an Urdu version of the Hospital Anxiety and Depression Scale. *Acta Psychiatr Scand.* 1991 Feb;83(2):81–5.

23. Kessler RC, Abelson J, Demler O, et al. Clinical calibration of DSM-IV diagnoses in the World Mental Health (WMH) version of the World Health Organization (WHO) Composite International Diagnostic Interview (WMH-CIDI). *Int J Methods Psychiatr Res.* 2004;13(2):122–39.

24. Youden WJ. Index for rating diagnostic tests. *Cancer.* 1950;3:32–5.

25. Haro JM, Rbabzadeh-Bouchez S, Brugha TS, et al. Concordance of the Composite International Diagnostic Interview Version 3.0 (CIDI 3.0) with standardized clinical assessments in the WHO World Mental Health surveys. *Int J Methods Psychiatr Res.* 2006 Dec;15(4):167–80.

26. Prince M, Acosta D, Chiu H, Scazufca M, Varghese M. Dementia diagnosis in developing countries: a cross-cultural validation study. *Lancet.* 2003;361:909–17.

27. Prince MJ, de Rodriguez JL, Noriega L, et al. The 10/66 Dementia Research Group's fully operationalised DSM-IV dementia computerized diagnostic algorithm, compared with the 10/66 dementia algorithm and a clinician diagnosis: a population validation study. *BMC Public Health.* 2008;8:219.

28. Jotheeswaran AT, Williams JD, Prince MJ. The predictive validity of the 10/66 dementia diagnosis in Chennai, India: a 3-year follow-up study of cases identified at baseline. *Alzheimer Dis Assoc Disord.* 2010 Jul;24(3):296–302.

29. Mezzich JE, Kirmayer LJ, Kleinman A, et al. The place of culture in DSM-IV. *J Nerv Ment Dis.* 1999 Aug;187(8):457–64.

30. Wickramasinghe SC, Rajapakse L, Abeysinghe R, Prince M. The Clinical Interview Schedule–Revised (CIS-R): modification and validation in Sri Lanka. *Int J Methods Psychiatr Res.* 2002;11(4):169–77.

31. Hanlon C, Medhin G, Alem A, et al. Detecting perinatal common mental disorders in Ethiopia: Validation of the self-reporting questionnaire and Edinburgh Postnatal Depression Scale. *J Affect Disord.* 2008;108(3):251–62.

32. Hanlon C, Medhin G, Alem A, et al. Measuring common mental disorders in women in Ethiopia: Reliability and construct validity of the comprehensive psychopathological rating scale. *Soc Psychiatry Psychiatr Epidemiol.* 2008;43(8):653–9.

33. Cronbach LE, Meehl PE. Construct validity in psychological tests. *Psychol Bull.* 1955;52:281–302.

34. Reise SP, Widaman KF, Pugh RH. Confirmatory factor analysis and item response theory: two approaches for exploring measurement invariance. *Psychol Bull.* 1993;114(3):552–66.

35. Olsson U. Maximum likelihood estimation of the polychoric correlation coefficient. *Psychometrika.* 1979;44:443–60.

36. Mumford DB, Bavington JT, Bhatnagar KS, Hussain Y, Mirza S, Naraghi MM. The Bradford Somatic Inventory. A multi-ethnic inventory of somatic symptoms reported by anxious and depressed patients in Britain and the Indo-Pakistan subcontinent. *Br J Psychiatry.* 1991 Mar;158:379–86, 379–86.

37. Heider D, Matschinger H, Bernert S, et al. Empirical evidence for an invariant three-factor structure of the Parental Bonding Instrument in six European countries. *Psychiatry Res.* 2005 Jun 30;135(3):237–47.

38. Akaike H. Factor analysis and AIC. *Psychometrika.* 1987;52:317–32.

39. Tucker L, Lewis C. A reliability coefficient for maximum likelihood factor analysis. *Psychometrika.* 1973;38:1–10.

40. Simon GE, Goldberg DP, Von KM, Ustun TB. Understanding cross-national differences in depression prevalence. *Psychol Med.* 2002 May;32(4):585–94.

41. Salomon JA, Tandon A, Murray CJL. World Health Survey pilot study collaborating group. Comparability of self rated health: cross sectional multi-country survey using anchoring vignettes. *BMJ.* 2004;328(333).

42. Prince M, Reischies F, Beekman ATF, et al. Development of the EURO-D scale—a European Union initiative to compare symptoms of depression in 14 European centres. *Br J Psychiatry.* 1999;174:330–8.

43. Copeland JR, Dewey ME, Griffiths-Jones HM. Computerised psychiatric diagnostic system and case nomenclature for elderly subjects: GMS and AGECAT. *Psychol Med.* 1986;16:89–99.

44. Castro-Costa E, Dewey M, Stewart R, et al. Ascertaining late-life depressive symptoms in Europe: an evaluation of the survey version of the EURO-D scale in 10 nations. The SHARE project. *Int J Methods Psychiatr Res.* 2008;17(1):12–29.

45. Prince M, Beekman A, Fuhrer R, et al. Depression symptoms in late-life assessed using the EURO-D scale. Effect of age, gender and marital status in 14 European centres. *Br J Psychiatry.* 1999;174:339–45.

46. Prince M, Acosta D, Chiu H, et al. Effects of education and culture on the validity of the Geriatric Mental State and its AGECAT algorithm. *Br J Psychiatry.* 2004 Nov;185:429–36.

47. Alexopoulos GS, Meyers BS, Young RC. Vascular depression hypothesis. *Arch Gen Psychiatry.* 1997;54:915–22.

48. Castro-Costa E, Dewey M, Stewart R, et al. Prevalence of depressive symptoms and syndromes in later life in ten European countries: the SHARE study. *Br J Psychiatry.* 2007 Nov;191:393–401.:393–401.

49. Zhang ZX, Anderson DW, Mantel N, Roman GC. Motor neuron disease on Guam: temporal occurrence, 1941–1985. *Acta Neurol Scand.* 1995;92(4):299–307.

50. Dean G, Bhigjee AI, Bill PL, et al. Multiple sclerosis in black South Africans and Zimbabweans. *J Neurol Neurosurg Psychiatry.* 1994;57(9):1064–9.

51. Spencer PS. Guam ALS/Parkinsonism dementia: a long-latency neurotoxic disorder caused by "slow toxin(s)" in food? *Can J Neurol Sci.* 1987;14(3 Suppl):347–57.

52. Alter M, Zhen Xin Z, Davanipour Z, Sobel E, Min Lai S, LaRue L. Does delay in acquiring childhood infection increase risk of multiple sclerosis? *Ital J Neurol Sci.* 1987;8(1):23–8.

53. Nimgaonkar VL, Fujiwara TM, Dutta M, et al. Low prevalence of psychoses among the Hutterites, an isolated religious community. *Am J Psychiatry.* 2000 Jul;157(7):1065–70.

54. Folnegovic Z, Folnegovic-Smalc V. Schizophrenia in Croatia: interregional differences in prevalence and a comment on constant incidence. *J Epidemiol Commun Health.* 1992 Jun;46(3):248–55.

55. Sartorius N, Jablensky A, Korten A, et al. Early manifestations and first-contact incidence of schizophrenia in different cultures. *Psychol Med.* 1986;16:909–28.

56. McGrath J, Saha S, Chant D, Welham J. Schizophrenia: a concise overview of incidence, prevalence, and mortality. *Epidemiol Rev.* 2008;30:67–76.

57. Leff J, Sartorius N, Jablensky A, Korten A, Ernberg G. The International Pilot Study of Schizophrenia: five-year follow-up findings. *Psychol Med.* 1992 Feb;22(1):131–45.

58. Cohen A, Patel V, Thara R, Gureje O. Questioning an axiom: better prognosis for schizophrenia in the developing world? *Schizophr Bull.* 2008 Mar;34(2):229–44.

59. Beekman ATF, Copeland JRM, Prince MJ. Review of community prevalence of depression in later life. *Br J Psychiatry.* 1999;174:307–11.

60. Goldberg DP, Gater R, Sartorius N, et al. The validity of two versions of the GHQ in the WHO study of mental illness in general health care. *Psychol Med.* 1997;27(1):191–7.

61. Hendrie HC, Ogunniyi A, Hall KS, et al. Incidence of dementia and Alzheimer disease in two communities: Yoruba residing in Ibadan, Nigeria, and African Americans residing in Indianapolis, Indiana. *JAMA.* 2001 Feb 14;285(6):739–47.

62. Perkins AJ, Hui SL, Ogunniyi A, et al. Risk of mortality for dementia in a developing country: the Yoruba in Nigeria. *Int J Geriatr Psychiatry.* 2002 Jun;17(6):566–73.

63. Cooper RS, Kaufman JS. Race and hypertension: science and nescience. *Hypertension.* 1998 Nov;32(5):813–6.

64. Moses S, Bradley JE, Nagelkerke NJ, Ronald AR, Ndinya-Achola JO, Plummer FA. Geographical patterns of male circumcision practices in Africa: association with HIV seroprevalence. *Int J Epidemiol.* 1990 Sep;19(3):693–7.

65. Bailey RC, Plummer FA, Moses S. Male circumcision and HIV prevention: current knowledge and future research directions. *Lancet Infect Dis.* 2001 Nov;1(4):223–31.

66. Siegfried N, Muller M, Deeks JJ, Volmink J. Male circumcision for prevention of heterosexual acquisition of HIV in men. *Cochrane Database Syst Rev.* 2009;(2):CD003362.

67. Boydell J, van OJ, McKenzie K, et al. Incidence of schizophrenia in ethnic minorities in London: ecological study into interactions with environment. *BMJ.* 2001 Dec 8;323(7325):1336–8.

68. Boydell J, van OJ, McKenzie K, Murray RM. The association of inequality with the incidence of schizophrenia—an ecological study. *Soc Psychiatry Psychiatr Epidemiol.* 2004 Aug;39(8):597–9.

69. Cooper RS, Kaufman JS, Ward R. Race and genomics. *N Engl J Med.* 2003 Mar 20;348(12):1166–70.

70. Voight BF, Kudaravalli S, Wen X, Pritchard JK. A map of recent positive selection in the human genome. *PLoS Biol.* 2006 Mar;4(3):e72.

71. Dhawan J, Bray CL, Warburton R, Ghambhir DS, Morris J. Insulin resistance, high prevalence of diabetes, and cardiovascular risk in immigrant Asians. Genetic or environmental effect? *Br Heart J.* 1994 Nov;72(5):413–21.

72. Worth RM, Kato H, Rhoads GG, Kagan K, Syme SL. Epidemiologic studies of coronary heart disease and stroke in Japanese men living in Japan, Hawaii and California: mortality. *Am J Epidemiol.* 1975 Dec;102(6):481–90.

73. Kirkbride JB, Fearon P, Morgan C, et al. Heterogeneity in incidence rates of schizophrenia and other psychotic syndromes: findings from the three-center AeSOP study. *Arch Gen Psychiatry.* 2006 Mar;63(3):250–8.

74. Selten JP, Cantor-Graae E, Kahn RS. Migration and schizophrenia. *Curr Opin Psychiatry.* 2007 Mar;20(2):111–5.

75. Morgan C, Dazzan P, Morgan K, et al. First episode psychosis and ethnicity: initial findings from the AESOP study. *World Psychiatry.* 2006 Feb;5(1):40–6.

76. McKeigue PM, Carpenter JR, Parra EJ, Shriver MD. Estimation of admixture and detection of linkage in admixed populations by a Bayesian approach: application to African-American populations. *Annu Hum Genet.* 2000 Mar;64(Pt 2):171–86.

77. Teruel BM, Rodriguez JJ, McKeigue P, et al. Interactions between genetic admixture, ethnic identity, APOE genotype and dementia prevalence in an admixed Cuban sample; a cross-sectional population survey and nested case-control study. *BMC Med Genet.* 2011;12:43.

78. Veenstra G. Location, location, location: contextual and compositional health effects of social capital in British Columbia, Canada. *Soc Sci Med.* 2005 May;60(9):2059–71.

79. Weich S, Holt G, Twigg L, Jones K, Lewis G. Geographic variation in the prevalence of common mental disorders in Britain: a multilevel investigation. *Am J Epidemiol.* 2003 Apr 15;157(8):730–7.

80. Weich S, Lewis G, Jenkins SP. Income inequality and the prevalence of common mental disorders in Britain. *Br J Psychiatry.* 2001 Mar;178:222–7.

81. Das-Munshi J, Becares L, Dewey ME, Stansfeld SA, Prince MJ. Understanding the effect of ethnic density on mental health: multi-level investigation of survey data from England. *BMJ.* 2010;341:c5367.

82. Patel V. The need for treatment evidence for common mental disorders in developing countries. *Psychol Med.* 2000 Jul;30(4):743–6.

83. Patel V, Chisholm D, Rabe-Hesketh S, as-Saxena F, Andrew G, Mann A. Efficacy and cost-effectiveness of drug and psychological treatments for common mental disorders in general health care in Goa, India: a randomised, controlled trial. *Lancet.* 2003 Jan 4;361(9351):33–9.

84. Bolton P, Bass J, Neugebauer R, et al. Group interpersonal psychotherapy for depression in rural Uganda: a randomized controlled trial. *JAMA.* 2003 Jun 18;289(23):3117–24.

85. Rahman A, Malik A, Sikander S, Roberts C, Creed F. Cognitive behaviour therapy-based intervention by community health workers for mothers with depression and their infants in rural Pakistan: a cluster-randomised controlled trial. *Lancet.* 2008 Sep 13;372(9642):902–9.

86. Araya R, Rojas G, Fritsch R, et al. Treating depression in primary care in low-income women in Santiago, Chile: a randomised controlled trial. *Lancet.* 2003 Mar 22;361(9362):995–1000.

87. Patel V, Weiss HA, Chowdhary N, et al. Effectiveness of an intervention led by lay health counsellors for depressive and anxiety disorders in primary care in Goa, India (MANAS): a cluster randomised controlled trial. *Lancet.* 2010 Dec 18;376(9758):2086–95.

88. Bolton P, Tang AM. An alternative approach to cross-cultural function assessment. *Soc Psychiatry Psychiatr Epidemiol.* 2002 Nov;37(11):537–43.

89. Chatterjee S, Chowdhary N, Pednekar S, et al. Integrating evidence-based treatments for common mental disorders in routine primary care: feasibility and acceptability of the MANAS intervention in Goa, India. *World Psychiatry.* 2008 Feb;7(1):39–46.

5 The Epidemiology and Impact of Mental Disorders[*]

Ronald C. Kessler, Jordi Alonso, Somnath Chatterji, and Yanling He

This chapter reviews the literature on the worldwide epidemiology and adverse effects of mental disorders. Interest in adverse effects of health problems—not only direct treatment costs, but the human costs as well—has increased dramatically over the past two decades as part of the larger movement to rationalize the allocation of treatment resources and maximize the benefits of treatment in relation to costs. Indeed, much of the current interest in mental disorders among health policymakers is based on the fact that these disorders have consistently been found in cost-of-illness studies to be among the most burdensome health problems in the population.[1] A number of factors account for these results: that mental disorders are commonly occurring, often begin at an early age, often are quite persistent throughout the life course, and often have substantial adverse effects on a wide range of functional outcomes. This chapter reviews the detailed epidemiological evidence regarding these points. For a summary of the global burden of mental and neurological disorder, relative to that of other conditions, see Chapter 6—Mental Health and the Global Health and Development Agendas.

METHODS OF ASSESSING MENTAL DISORDERS IN EPIDEMIOLOGICAL SURVEYS

Information about the epidemiology of mental disorders has proliferated over the past two decades. The reason for this can be traced to the development of fully structured research diagnostic interviews appropriate for use by trained lay interviewers. The first of these interviews was the Diagnostic Interview Schedule (DIS), an instrument developed for use in a large community epidemiological survey in the United States and subsequently used in a number of similar surveys in other parts of the world.[2] WHO subsequently developed the Composite International Diagnostic Interview (CIDI), which was based on the DIS, to generate reliable diagnoses according to the definitions of both the

DSM and ICD systems throughout the world.[3] General population surveys were carried out in a number of countries with the first version of the CIDI. WHO created a cross-national research consortium to carry out systematic comparisons of these CIDI surveys.[4] Results based on these comparisons led to the expansion and refinement of the CIDI and to a new generation of cross-national CIDI surveys in the WHO World Mental Health (WMH) Survey Initiative. The latter is an ongoing initiative to carry out and analyze community epidemiological surveys and provide information about the results to health policymakers in countries throughout the world. Twenty-eight countries have completed WMH surveys as of the time this chapter is being written. We draw heavily on the results of these surveys in this chapter. A complete list of WMH survey reports can be found at www.hcp.med.harvard.edu/wmh.

As the CIDI has become so predominant in psychiatric epidemiological surveys throughout the world, a few words need to be said about the accuracy of diagnoses based on the CIDI. Clinical reappraisal studies of the original version of the CIDI were quite mixed in showing concordance of diagnoses of common mental disorders based on the CIDI and on independent clinical evaluations.[3] Concordance is considerably better, though, for the more recent version of the CIDI used in the WMH surveys in Western countries.[5] However, much less is known about the clinical relevance of diagnoses based on fully structured diagnostic interviews in developing countries. Prevalence estimates in epidemiological surveys in some developing countries seem implausibly low, raising concerns that the diagnoses based on research diagnostic interviews like the CIDI are not valid in such countries, or that the Western diagnostic constructs embedded in these interviews have low relevance to those countries. Methodological studies to investigate these possibilities are only beginning to be carried out, but show preliminarily that modifications to the CIDI can be made that yield reliable and valid diagnoses in countries where the vocabulary of distress is different from Western countries, but that extensive developmental work is needed to make these modifications.[6] Based on the fact that this kind of work has not been carried out in most CIDI cultural adaptations, caution is needed in interpreting the results of epidemiological studies carried out in such countries.

LIFETIME PREVALENCE OF COMMON MENTAL DISORDERS

With these cautions as a backdrop, we consider the prevalence estimates of common mental disorders reported in published community epidemiological surveys. The vast majority of these surveys used DSM-IV criteria, so those criteria will be used throughout our review of the literature. A number of recent literature reviews presented detailed summary tables of prevalence estimates for individual DSM-IV disorders across a number of epidemiological surveys.[7,8] Several consistent patterns emerge from these summaries. One is that lifetime prevalence of having any clinically significant mental disorder is generally high, but also quite variable across countries. In the WMH surveys, for example, the proportion of respondents who met lifetime criteria for one or more of the core disorders (which included anxiety, mood, disruptive behavior, and alcohol and illicit-drug disorders) ranged from a high of 47.4% in the United States to a low of 12.0% in Nigeria, with an inter-quartile range (IQR; 25th–75th percentiles across countries) of 18.1% to 36.1%.[7] More than one-third of respondents met criteria for at least one disorder in five countries (Colombia, France, New Zealand, Ukraine, United States), more than one-fourth in six other countries (Belgium, Germany, Lebanon, Mexico, Netherlands, South Africa), and more than one-sixth in four other countries (Israel, Italy, Japan, Spain). Lower estimates were obtained in surveys carried out in the cities of Beijing and Shanghai in the People's Republic of China (13.2%)[9] and Nigeria (12.0%),[10] while prevalence estimates in other low/middle-income countries were all above the lower bound of the between-country inter-quartile range in country-level prevalence (25.8%–39.1%).

Another consistent pattern in the epidemiological literature is that anxiety disorders (generalized anxiety disorder, obsessive-compulsive disorder, panic disorder with or without agoraphobia, post-traumatic stress disorder, social phobia, specific phobia) are usually found to be the most prevalent class of mental disorders, and mood disorders (major depressive disorder or dysthymia, bipolar I–II disorder) the next most prevalent. In the WMH surveys, for example, anxiety disorders were the most prevalent in roughly two-thirds of countries assessed, with prevalence estimates in the range 4.8% to 31.0% (IQR 9.9%–16.7%), while mood disorders had highest prevalence in all but one other country (prevalence 3.3%– 21.4%, IQR: 9.8%–15.8%).[7] Disruptive behavior disorders (attention-deficit/hyperactivity disorder, conduct disorder, intermittent explosive disorder, oppositional-defiant disorder) were the least prevalent of the four broad classes of disorders considered in the majority of countries surveyed (prevalence 0.3%–25.0%, IQR: 3.1%–5.7%), while substance use disorders (alcohol or illicit drug abuse or dependence) were least prevalent in the remaining countries (prevalence 1.3%–15.0%, IQR: 4.8–9.6). Substance dependence was assessed incompletely in some countries, though, in that substance dependence was not assessed in the absence of a history of abuse, presumably reducing estimated prevalence. It should be noted, in addition, that these relative prevalence estimates apply to adults, not to children or adolescents, as disruptive behavior disorders are much more prominent among in childhood[11] but diminish in late adolescence and early adulthood.[12]

It is important to note that these prevalence estimates are, if anything, conservative, as the diagnostic criteria in the DSM and ICD systems are considered by some critics to be overly conservative[13] and considerable evidence exists for clinically significant sub-threshold manifestations of many mental disorders.[14] In addition, two less common types of disorders were not included in the above estimates, as these disorders are typically not considered in the community epidemiological surveys reviewed above. These two are dementia (Alzheimer's disease and other subtypes) and non-affective psychosis (NAP; including schizophrenia, schizophreniform disorder, schizoaffective disorder, and delusional disorder). Although lifetime prevalence of these disorders is low in relation to the more common mental disorders reviewed above, the severity and burden of dementia[15] and NAP[16] make them important to acknowledge in this review.

It is more difficult to estimate prevalence of dementia due to the fact that epidemiological data are sparse in most parts of the world. An international group of experts attempted to address this problem in the early 2000s by using a Delphi consensus panel method to review the available epidemiological literature and estimate worldwide prevalence.[17] The panel concluded that prevalence was in the range 0.3% to 1.2% among people in their 60s, 1.3% to 7.6% among those in their 70s, and 25% or more among people in their 80s and older. However, these estimates were limited by the absence of good-quality data from low- and middle-income countries[17] and by the fact that the aging of the world population is occurring at such a rapid pace that estimates are needed not only for point prevalence, but also for trends.[18]

More recent research from the 10/66 Dementia Research Group surveys has addressed the problem of weak data from low- and middle-income countries[19] and suggests that age-specific dementia prevalence in low- and middle-income countries may be similar to in high-income countries. Based on these new data, a systematic review of the global evidence found that age-standardized prevalence estimates were in the range of 5% to 8% among people aged 60 years and over across all world regions other than sub-Saharan Africa (where estimates were in the 2%–4% range).[20] Onset of dementia before the age of 60 was found in these studies to be rare, accounting for less than 10% of all prevalent cases; thereafter, prevalence was found to roughly double with every five-year age increment, from around 1% to 2% at ages 60 to 64 years to as many as 33% to 50% of those aged 90 and older. Systematic review also suggests that dementia incidence roughly doubles with every six years of increased age, from approximately three per 1000 person years at age 60 to 64, to 175 per

1000 person years at age 95 and older. Based on these patterns, numbers of people with dementia worldwide are forecast to increase sharply (7.7 million new cases are anticipated each year[21]) in the coming years driven by global patterns of population aging. Based on the estimate that there were more than 35 million people with dementia in the world in 2010, and with projections of numbers nearly doubling every 20 years, it is anticipated that there will be approximately 65 million worldwide in 2030 and more than 115 million in 2050. The total estimated worldwide costs of dementia were estimated to be over US$600 billion in 2010, accounting for around 1% of the world's gross domestic product, varying from an estimated roughly 0.25% in low-income countries to 1.25% in high-income countries.[22]

In the case of NAP, most epidemiological research focuses on schizophrenia. An exhaustive review of this literature concluded that the lifetime morbid risk (i.e., the proportion of the population that will ever develop the disorder at some time in their life) of schizophrenia in the general population is 0.7% (10th/90th centile 0.3%/2.7%).[23] The median annual incidence of schizophrenia was 15/100,000 (10th/ 90th centile 8/43). As the centile distributions indicate, there was considerable variation in both prevalence and incidence estimates. Incidence was generally higher among men than women (median m/f incidence ratio 1.4), but no significant gender difference was observed in prevalence. Both prevalence and incidence were markedly higher among migrant groups. While prevalence (both genders) and incidence (males) were higher at higher latitudes, there was also a tendency for a lower prevalence and incidence in less developed countries.

Although evidence is considerably sparser on other types of NAP, it has been suggested that lifetime prevalence of overall NAP might be three to four times as high as that of schizophrenia.[24] In addition, a surprisingly high proportion of people in the general population report a history of isolated hallucinations and delusions that do not qualify for a diagnosis of NAP. The latter are often referred to as "psychotic-like experiences" (PLEs). A meta-analysis of 35 community epidemiological surveys found a median lifetime prevalence of PLEs of 5.3%.[25] Although, as one would expect, PLEs are powerful predictors of later conversion to full NAP, they are also associated with a much wider range of mental disorders, including anxiety, mood, and substance use disorders.[26]

AGE-OF-ONSET DISTRIBUTIONS

It is important to examine age-of-onset (AOO) distributions (the distributions across people with a lifetime history of specific disorders of when these disorders first occur) for two reasons. First, commonly occurring lifetime disorders might have much less effect if they only occur late in life. Second, an understanding of AOO is important for targeting research on prevention of mental disorders, early intervention with prodromal or incipient mental disorders, and primary prevention of secondary disorders. Despite the wide cross-national variation in estimated lifetime prevalence of mental disorders, estimates of AOO distributions are highly consistent.[27] The WMH AOO results, which are based on retrospective reports, are quite typical in this regard[7] in showing disruptive behavior disorders to have the earliest AOO distributions and mood disorders the latest among the common mental disorders and dementia to have by far the latest AOO distribution overall.

In terms of disruptive behavior disorders, median AOO across WMH surveys was estimated to be seven to nine years of age for attention-deficit/hyperactivity disorder (ADHD), seven to 15 for oppositional-defiant disorder (ODD), nine to 14 for conduct disorder (CD), and 13 to 21 for intermittent explosive disorder (IED). There is an extremely narrow age range of onset risk for these disorders, with 80% of all lifetime ADHD estimated to begin in the age range four to 11, and the vast majority of ODD and CD in the age range of five to 15. Although the IED AOO distribution was found to be less concentrated, fully half of all lifetime cases had onsets in childhood and adolescence.

The situation is more complex with anxiety disorders, as the estimated AOO distributions fall into two distinct sets. The phobias and separation anxiety disorder (SAD) all were estimated in the WMH surveys to have very early AOO (medians 7–14, IQR 8–11). (Figure 5.1) Generalized anxiety disorder (GAD), panic disorder (PD), and post-traumatic stress disorder (PTSD), in comparison, were estimated to have much later AOO (medians 24–50, IQR 31–41), (Figure 5.2) as well as much wider cross-national variation in AOO than the disruptive behavior disorders, phobias or seasonal affective disorder (SAD). No significant ecological associations were found in the WMH data between the position of the curves in the swarm of either figure and either prevalence of the disorders in the country or the county's level of economic development.

The mood disorder AOO distributions in the WMH surveys were found to be quite similar to those of the later-onset anxiety disorders, with consistently low prevalence until the early teens followed by a roughly linear increase through late middle age and a declining increase thereafter. However, median AOO of mood disorders was found to have a very wide range across countries (25–45) and an even wider IQR (17–65), but again without any consistent ecological association between the shape of the curve and either prevalence of the disorders in the country or the county's level of economic development. Although epidemiological survey data on the AOO distribution of NAP are not widely available, treatment studies and long-term prospective population cohort studies suggest that NAP seldom begins before age 14, has a median AOO in the early 20s, has an IQR ranging from the late teens to the late 20s, and has somewhat earlier aggregate onset for males than females (28–30).

THE COURSE OF COMMON MENTAL DISORDERS

Course of illness, like AOO, has been much less well studied in epidemiological surveys than has prevalence. However, the fact that mental disorders are seen as being quite persistent adds to the judgment that they have highly adverse effects. The small number of long-term prospective studies that have charted course of common mental disorders

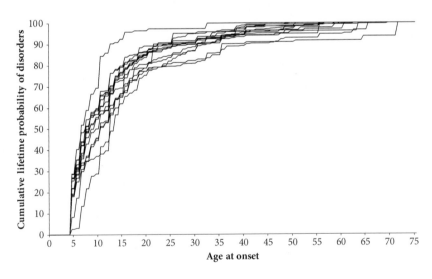

FIGURE 5.1

Standardized age-of-onset distributions of DSM-IV/CIDI phobias and separation anxiety disorder in the WMH surveys.[1] (Originally published in: Kessler RC, Wang PS, Wittchen H-U. The societal costs of anxiety and mood disorders: An epidemiological perspective. In Preedy VR & Watson RR, editors. Handbook of Disease Burdens and Quality of Life Measures. New York: Springer Publishing; 2010. p. 1516. © 2010 Springer Publishing; Used with permission.)

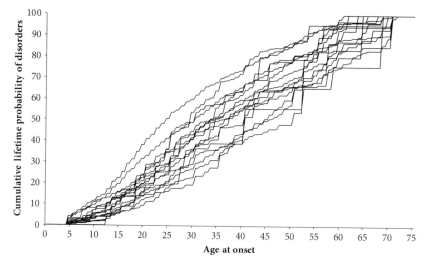

FIGURE 5.2

Standardized age-of-onset distributions of DSM-IV/CIDI generalized anxiety disorder, panic disorder, and post-traumatic stress disorder in the WMH surveys.[1] (Originally published in: Kessler RC, Wang PS, Wittchen H-U. The societal costs of anxiety and mood disorders: An epidemiological perspective. In Preedy VR & Watson RR, editors. Handbook of Disease Burdens and Quality of Life Measures. New York: Springer Publishing; 2010. p. 1517. © 2010 Springer Publishing; Used with permission.)

shows, consistent with this impression, that these disorders often have a chronic-recurrent course. However, most of these studies are based on clinical samples that almost certainly include a higher proportion of persistent cases than in the general population.[31]

Indirect information about course of illness can also be obtained in representative samples by comparing estimates of recent prevalence (variously reported for the year, six months, or one month before interview) with estimates of lifetime prevalence. High ratios of recent-to-lifetime prevalence in such studies would suggest indirectly that these disorders have a persistent course.

Such data were obtained in the WMH surveys by beginning with estimates of 12-month prevalence and then comparing them to estimates of lifetime prevalence. The proportion of respondents estimated to have any DSM-IV/CIDI disorder in the 12 months before interview averaged (mean) 16.7% across surveys, with a median of 13.6% and IQR of 10.0% to 20.7% (Table 5.1). Relative prevalence estimates were quite consistent across surveys. The ratios obtained by comparing these 12-month prevalence estimates to lifetime prevalence estimates were for the most part in the range of 0.5 to 0.6 for anxiety disorders, somewhat lower for mood disorders (0.4–0.6), and lower still for disruptive behavior disorders and substance use disorders (0.2–0.4). Ratios as high as these strongly imply that a meaningful proportion of mental disorders are persistent throughout the life course. More detailed analyses of these ratios could be carried out by breaking them down separately for sub-samples defined by age at interview or by time since first onset, although we are unaware of any published research that has reported such data. Preliminary WMH analyses of this sort suggest that although 12-month to lifetime prevalence ratios decline with increasing age, this decline is fairly modest, suggesting that mental disorders are often quite persistent over the entire life course. The few long-term longitudinal studies that exist in representative samples of people with lifetime mental disorders yield results consistent with these and suggest that persistence is due to a recurrent-intermittent course that often features waxing and waning of episodes of different comorbid disorders.[32]

Table 5.1 Twelve-Month Prevalence of DSM-IV/CIDI Disorders[1] in the WMH Surveys[2]

	Any disorder		Anxiety disorders		Mood disorders		Disruptive behavior disorders[3]		Substance disorders	
	%	(se)	%	(se)	%	(se)	%	(se)	%	(se)
I. Low/lower-middle income countries										
Colombia	21.0	(1.0)	14.4	(1.0)	6.9	(0.4)	4.4	(0.4)	2.8	(0.4)
India—Pondicherry	20.0	(1.1)	10.5	(0.8)	5.5	(0.5)	4.3	(0.7)	5.3	(0.6)
Iraq	13.6	(0.8)	10.4	(0.7)	4.1	(0.4)	1.7	(0.3)	0.3	(0.1)
Nigeria	6.0	(0.6)	4.2	(0.5)	1.2	(0.2)	0.1	(0.0)	0.9	(0.2)
PRC—Beijing, Shanghai	7.1	(0.9)	3.0	(0.5)	2.2	(0.4)	2.7	(0.6)	1.6	(0.4)
PRC—Shenzhen	16.0	(0.9)	11.4	(0.9)	4.8	(0.4)	2.9	(0.3)	0.0	(0.0)
Ukraine	21.4	(1.3)	6.8	(0.7)	10.0	(0.8)	5.1	(0.8)	6.4	(0.8)
Total	14.8	(0.4)	9.2	0.3	4.8	(0.2)	2.7	(0.2)	1.9	(0.1)
II. Upper-middle income countries										
Brazil—São Paulo	29.6	(1.0)	19.9	(0.8)	11.8	(0.7)	5.3	(0.7)	3.8	(0.4)
Bulgaria	11.2	(0.8)	7.6	(0.7)	3.2	(0.3)	0.8	(0.3)	1.2	(0.3)
Lebanon	17.9	(1.6)	12.1	(1.2)	7.0	(0.8)	2.6	(0.7)	1.3	(0.8)
Mexico	13.4	(0.9)	8.4	(0.6)	5.0	(0.4)	1.6	(0.3)	2.5	(0.4)
Romania	8.2	(0.7)	4.9	(0.5)	2.5	(0.3)	1.9	(0.7)	1.0	(0.2)
South Africa	16.9	(0.9)	8.4	(0.6)	4.9	(0.4)	1.9	(0.3)	5.7	(0.6)
Total	16.7	(0.4)	10.2	(0.3)	5.8	(0.2)	2.5	(0.2)	3.2	(0.2)

III. High income countries

Belgium	13.2	(1.5)	8.4	(1.4)	6.1	(0.8)	1.7	(1.0)	1.3	(0.4)
France	18.9	(1.4)	13.7	(1.1)	6.8	(0.7)	2.4	(0.6)	0.8	(0.3)
Germany	11.0	(1.3)	8.3	(1.1)	3.4	(0.3)	0.6	(0.3)	1.2	(0.4)
Israel	10.0	(0.5)	3.6	(0.3)	6.4	(0.4)	0.0	(0.0)	1.3	(0.2)
Italy	8.8	(0.7)	6.5	(0.6)	3.6	(0.3)	0.4	(0.2)	0.1	(0.1)
Japan	8.0	(0.7)	4.8	(0.6)	2.8	(0.4)	0.2	(0.1)	1.0	(0.3)
Netherlands	13.6	(1.0)	8.9	(1.0)	5.5	(0.7)	1.9	(0.7)	1.7	(0.5)
New Zealand	20.7	(0.6)	15.0	(0.5)	8.0	(0.4)	0.0	(0.0)	3.4	(0.3)
Northern Ireland	23.1	(1.4)	14.6	(1.0)	10.6	(0.9)	4.5	(1.0)	3.5	(0.5)
Portugal	22.9	(1.0)	16.5	(1.0)	8.3	(0.6)	3.5	(0.4)	1.6	(0.3)
Spain	9.7	(0.8)	6.6	(0.9)	4.4	(0.4)	0.5	(0.2)	0.3	(0.2)
United States	27.0	(0.9)	19.0	(0.7)	9.8	(0.4)	10.5	(0.7)	3.8	(0.4)
Total	17.7	(0.3)	11.9	(0.2)	7.2	(0.2)	2.7	(0.2)	2.2	(0.1)
IV. Total	16.7	(0.2)	10.8	(0.2)	6.2	(0.1)	2.6	(0.1)	2.4	(0.1)

[1] The disorders included DSM-IV/CIDI anxiety disorders (generalized anxiety disorder, panic disorder, agoraphobia, specific phobia, social phobia, post-traumatic stress disorder, and separation anxiety disorder), mood disorders (major depressive disorder, dysthymic disorder, bipolar disorder), disruptive behavior disorders (attention–deficit/hyperactivity disorder, oppositional–defiant disorder, conduct disorder, intermittent explosive disorder), and substance disorders (alcohol and drug abuse with or without dependence).

[2] Between-country differences in prevalence are significant both for any disorder ($\chi^2_{24} = 1401.2$, p <.001) and for each class of disorder ($\chi^2_{24} = 715.4 - 1099.9$, p <.001).

[3] Prevalence of disruptive behavior disorders was estimated in the sub-sample of respondents who were 44 years of age or younger at the time of the interview.

A version of this table was originally published in: Kessler RC, Aguilar-Gaxiola S, Alonso J, et al. The burden of mental disorders worldwide: Results from the World Mental Health surveys. In: Cohen N & Galea S, editors. *Population mental health: Evidence, policy, and public health practice.* Abingdon, UK: Routledge; 2011:18–19. © 2011 Routledge; used with permission.

COMORBIDITY AMONG MENTAL DISORDERS

Comorbidity among mental disorders is quite common, with up to half of people who meet criteria for any given lifetime disorder meeting criteria for at least one other disorder.[33] It is important to note that some of this comorbidity may be arti-factual, arising from artificial nosological distinctions (for a further discussion, see Chapter 2—Disorders, Diagnosis, and Classification). Numerous factor analysis stud-ies have been carried out in recent years to study the structure of common mental disorders.[34] Two main factors of internalizing (anxiety and mood disorders) and externalizing (disruptive behavior and substance disorders) disorders are consis-tently found in these studies. Two recent studies also documented that inclusion of a broader range of disorders leads to a third factor consisting of thought disorders (non-affective psychosis, bipolar disorder, Cluster A personality disorders).[35,36] Clear AOO hierarchies exist in each of these three clusters of comorbid disorders, with specific phobias and SAD the internalizing disorders with the earliest AOO, ADHD and ODD the externalizing disorders with the earliest AOO, and PLEs the thought disorders with the earliest AOO.

This evidence of high comorbidity among mental disorders is interesting for a number of reasons, but perhaps the most important of these is that comorbidity is strongly associated with disorder progression, persistence, and severity.[37,38] This raises the possibility that early effective interventions to treat temporally primary disorders in each comorbid cluster might be effective in reducing risk of later disorders. Although only a small amount of research has been carried out on this possibility with regard to either internalizing[39] or externalizing[40] disorders, preliminary results are promising, and there is increasing recognition of the potential value of expanding such interventions.[41] Promising studies have also been carried out to determine whether diverse interventions aimed at PLEs might prevent onset of psychotic disorders, although these studies have so far been small, and the results have been mixed.[42]

SEVERITY OF COMMON MENTAL DISORDERS

It is important to recognize that many mental disorders, like many physical disorders, are relatively mild and self-limiting. This is an important observation in light of the fact that the high prevalence of mental disorders far exceeds the capacity of the health-care system to provide treatment.[43] Indeed, some healthcare provider organizations have imposed restrictions on treatment for mental disorders based on disorder sever-ity. Federal block grant funds in the United States, for example, can be used only to treat *serious* mental illness (SMI), which is defined as a DSM disorder that exceeds one of several thresholds defined by the cross-classification of severity of distress, severity of role impairment, and duration (see http://www.odmhsas.org/eda/advancedquery/smi.htm).

Based on these kinds of restrictions, it is interesting to examine not only the preva-lence of overall mental disorders but also the severity of mental disorders. Although little systematic epidemiological research has been carried out on the severity of mental disor-ders, the WMH surveys included information designed explicitly to determine if disor-ders present in the 12 months before interview met criteria for SMI. SMI was defined for these purposes as having either NAP or bipolar I disorder or having any other 12-month DSM-IV/CIDI disorder along with evidence of serious role impairment. "Serious role impairment," in turn, was defined as either having a score in the severe range on one or more of the Sheehan Disability Scales (SDS)[44] or attempting suicide at some time in the 12 months before the interview.

Roughly one-fourth (24.5%) of all WMH respondents with 12-month mental disorders were classified as having SMI based on the above definition (Table 5.2). The median proportion of 12-month cases with SMI across surveys was 22.3%, the range was 6.2% to 36.9%, and the IQR was 18.6% to 25.8%. Higher proportions of cases were classified as moderate (mean 37.8%, median 38.7%, range 12.5%–50.6%, IQR 32.7%–42.9%), which was defined as not meeting criteria for SMI but reporting at least moderate role impairment on the SDS. The remainder of 12-month cases were classified residually as mild (mean and median both 37.7%, range 28.3%–74.8%, IQR 34.9%–42.1%). Between-country variation in the severity distribution was relatively modest in substantive terms, with a Pearson contingency coefficient of only .06 for the association between country income level and disorder severity. Much more substantial positive associations (Pearson correlations) of overall disorder prevalence were found, though, with both the proportion of cases classified as serious (.30) and the proportion of cases classified as either serious or moderate (.40).

The finding of a *positive* association between estimated prevalence and severity across countries is important because it speaks to an issue that has been raised in the methodological literature regarding the possibility of biased prevalence estimates. Two previous studies by other research groups using different instruments to assess depression found the opposite: that is, that the average amount of impairment associated with depression across countries was inversely proportional to the estimated prevalence of depression in those countries. One of those two studies compared results in an epidemiological survey in Korea with the world literature,[45] while the other compared results in primary care samples screened for major depression across a number of different countries.[46] The authors of both reports argued that the substantial cross-national variation in estimated prevalence of depression might be at least partly due to cross-national differences in diagnostic thresholds. However, the more broadly representative WMH findings argue against that interpretation with regard to prevalence estimates based on the improved version of CIDI used in the WMH surveys.

ADVERSE EFFECTS OF COMMON MENTAL DISORDERS ON ROLE INCUMBENCY

A recently published volume in the Cambridge University Press book series on the WMH Surveys is devoted to an investigation of the adverse effects of common mental disorders.[47] The papers in that volume present extensive data showing that mental disorders are significant predictors of a wide array of adverse outcomes that might be conceptualized as individual and societal burdens of these disorders. The remainder of the current chapter reviews these results.

The first class of outcomes considered involve role incumbency. Given their typically early AOO, mental disorders might be expected to have adverse effects on critical developmental transitions, such as educational attainment and timing of marriage. A number of epidemiological studies have examined these effects, with a focus on four domains: education, marital timing and stability, childbearing, and occupation.

Education

Several studies have shown that early-onset mental disorders are associated with premature termination of education.[48] Disruptive behavior disorders and bipolar disorder tend to have the strongest associations in these studies, although major depressive disorder and anxiety disorders also have been linked to elevated odds of failure to complete secondary school as well as failure to go on to higher education after graduating from secondary school.

Table 5.2 Twelve-Month Prevalence of DSM-IV/CIDI Disorders by Severity in the WMH Surveys[1]

	Unconditional prevalence[2]						Conditional prevalence[2]					
	Serious		Moderate		Mild		Serious		Moderate		Mild	
	%	(se)	%	(se)	%	(se)	%	(se)	%	(se)	%	(se)
I. Low/lower-middle income countries												
Colombia	4.9	(0.5)	8.6	(0.7)	7.5	(0.5)	23.3	(2.1)	41.2	(2.6)	35.5	(2.1)
India—Pondicherry	4.3	(0.3)	7.8	(0.7)	7.9	(0.8)	21.7	(1.6)	39.0	(3.1)	39.3	(2.8)
Iraq	3.0	(0.4)	4.9	(0.4)	5.7	(0.6)	21.9	(2.3)	36.0	(2.6)	42.1	(2.9)
Nigeria	0.8	(0.3)	0.8	(0.2)	4.5	(0.5)	12.8	(3.8)	12.5	(2.6)	74.8	(4.2)
PRC—Beijing, Shanghai	1.0	(0.3)	2.3	(0.5)	3.8	(0.6)	13.8	(3.7)	32.2	(4.9)	54.0	(4.6)
PRC—Shenzhen	1.0	(0.3)	5.2	(0.5)	9.8	(0.8)	6.2	(1.6)	32.7	(2.9)	61.2	(3.6)
Ukraine	4.9	(0.4)	8.4	(0.8)	8.1	(1.0)	22.9	(1.8)	39.4	(2.9)	37.7	(3.5)
Total	2.8	(0.2)	5.3	(0.2)	6.7	(0.3)	18.8	(0.9)	35.9	(1.2)	45.3	(1.3)
II. Upper-middle income countries												
Brazil—São Paulo	10.0	(0.6)	9.8	(0.5)	9.8	(0.6)	33.9	(1.4)	33.0	(1.8)	33.2	(1.4)
Bulgaria	2.3	(0.3)	3.6	(0.5)	5.4	(0.5)	20.3	(2.8)	32.1	(3.6)	47.7	(2.7)
Lebanon	4.0	(0.7)	7.7	(1.0)	6.2	(1.2)	22.3	(3.1)	42.9	(4.9)	34.9	(5.6)
Mexico	3.5	(0.4)	4.7	(0.4)	5.2	(0.5)	26.3	(2.4)	34.8	(2.2)	38.9	(2.5)
Romania	2.3	(0.4)	2.4	(0.3)	3.5	(0.5)	27.9	(3.4)	29.3	(3.7)	42.8	(3.5)
South Africa	4.3	(0.4)	5.3	(0.5)	7.2	(0.6)	25.7	(1.8)	31.4	(2.1)	43.0	(2.1)
Total	4.7	(0.2)	5.5	(0.2)	6.5	(0.3)	28.0	(0.9)	33.1	(1.1)	39.0	(1.0)

III. High income countries

Belgium	4.3 (0.8)	5.1 (0.8)	3.8 (0.6)	32.6 (4.2)	38.7 (3.4)	28.8 (4.8)
France	3.5 (0.5)	8.1 (0.8)	7.2 (0.9)	18.6 (2.5)	43.1 (3.0)	38.3 (3.6)
Germany	2.4 (0.4)	4.8 (0.8)	3.9 (0.7)	21.6 (2.5)	43.2 (4.5)	35.2 (4.1)
Israel	3.7 (0.3)	3.5 (0.3)	2.8 (0.2)	36.9 (2.4)	34.8 (2.3)	28.3 (2.1)
Italy	1.4 (0.2)	4.2 (0.5)	3.2 (0.5)	15.9 (2.7)	47.8 (3.9)	36.3 (3.9)
Japan	1.3 (0.4)	3.8 (0.5)	2.9 (0.4)	16.1 (4.5)	47.2 (4.8)	36.7 (3.7)
Netherlands	4.2 (0.6)	4.2 (0.5)	5.2 (0.8)	31.1 (3.5)	31.1 (3.6)	37.8 (4.7)
New Zealand	5.3 (0.3)	8.6 (0.4)	6.7 (0.3)	25.8 (1.0)	41.7 (1.4)	32.5 (1.2)
Northern Ireland	6.7 (0.7)	7.7 (0.7)	8.7 (1.1)	28.8 (3.0)	33.4 (2.6)	37.8 (3.3)
Portugal	4.0 (0.4)	11.6 (0.6)	7.3 (0.5)	17.5 (1.5)	50.6 (2.0)	31.9 (1.9)
Spain	1.9 (0.2)	4.2 (0.5)	3.6 (0.6)	19.9 (2.4)	43.5 (4.1)	36.6 (4.8)
United States	6.9 (0.4)	10.7 (0.5)	9.4 (0.6)	25.5 (1.4)	39.7 (1.2)	34.8 (1.4)
Total	4.5 (0.1)	7.2 (0.2)	6.0 (0.2)	25.4 (0.6)	40.7 (0.7)	33.9 (0.7)
IV. Total	4.1 (0.1)	6.3 (0.1)	6.3 (0.1)	24.5 (0.5)	37.8 (0.5)	37.7 (0.6)

[1] See Table 5.1, footnote 1, for a list of the disorders. See the text for a description of how severity was defined.

[2] "Unconditional prevalence" is prevalence in the total sample. "Conditional prevalence" is prevalence among cases. For example, the 4.9% of respondents in the Colombia survey with a 12-month serious disorder represent 23.3% of the 21.0% of respondents in the Colombia survey who had any 12-month DSM-IV/CIDI disorder. (The 21.0% total prevalence is reported in Table 5.1.)

[3] Between-country differences in prevalence are significant both for unconditional prevalence for each class of disorders ($\chi^2_{24} = 377.9 - 741.6$, p <.001) and for conditional prevalence for each class of disorders ($\chi^2_{24} = 146.8 - 187.2$, p <.001).

A version of this table was originally published in: Kessler RC, Aguilar-Gaxiola S, Alonso J, et al. The burden of mental disorders worldwide: Results from the World Mental Health surveys. In: Cohen N, Galea S, editors. *Population mental health: Evidence, policy, and public health practice.* Abingdon, UK: Routledge; 2011:22–23. © 2011 Routledge; used with permission.

Marital Timing and Stability

Several studies examined associations of premarital mental disorders with subsequent marriage.[49] Early-onset mental disorders were shown in these studies to predict low probability of ever marrying, to be either positively associated or unrelated with early (before age 18) marriage (which is known to be associated with a number of adverse outcomes), and to be negatively associated with later marriage (which is known to be associated with a number of benefits, such as financial security and social support). These associations are largely the same for men and women and across countries. A separate set of studies has shown that premarital history of mental disorders predicts divorce,[50] again with associations quite similar for husbands and wives across all countries. A wide range of mental disorders are implicated in these associations, although early-onset disruptive behavior disorders with problems of impulse-control are the dominant predictors of early marriage.

Teen Childbearing

We are aware of only one study that examined the association between child-adolescent mental disorders and subsequent teen childbearing.[51] A number of early-onset mental disorders, most of them externalizing disorders, were significant predictors of increased teen childbearing in that study. Disaggregation found that the overall associations were due to disorders predicting increased sexual activity rather than decreased use of contraception.

Employment Status

Although mental disorders are known to be associated with unemployment, most research on this association has emphasized the impact of job loss on these disorders rather than effects of mental disorders on job loss.[52] A recent WMH analysis, though, documented the latter association by showing that history of a wide range of mental disorders as of the subject's age of completing schooling predicted current (at the time of interview) unemployment and work disability.[53] However, these associations were only significant in high-income countries, raising the possibility that mental disorders become more detrimental to work performance as the substantive complexity of work increases.

ADVERSE EFFECTS OF COMMON MENTAL DISORDERS ON ROLE PERFORMANCE

A considerably larger amount of research has been carried out on the associations of mental disorders with various aspects of role performance, with a special focus on marital quality, work performance, and financial success.

Marital Quality

It has long been known that marital dissatisfaction and discord are strongly related to depressive symptoms and that this association is bidirectional.[54] Fewer studies have considered the effects of clinical depression or other DSM-IV disorders on marital functioning,[55] but the latter studies consistently document significant adverse effects. A number of other studies document significant associations of mental disorders with physical violence in marital relationships, although these studies generally focus on presumed mental health *consequences* of relationship violence.[56] A growing body of research now suggests, though, that marital violence is partly a consequence of preexisting mental disorders. Indeed, longitudinal studies consistently find that premarital history of a wide range of mental disorders predicts elevated risk of subsequent marital violence perpetration[57] and victimization.[58] Disruptive behavioral disorders and substance-use disorders appear to be the most important mental disorders in this regard.[59]

Parental Functioning

A number of studies have documented significant associations of both maternal[60] and paternal[61] mental disorders with negative parenting behaviors. These associations are found throughout the age range of children, but are most pronounced for the parents of young children. Although only an incomplete understanding exists of pathways, both laboratory and naturalistic studies of parent–infant micro-interactions have documented subtle ways in which parent mental disorders, especially depression, lead to maladaptive interactions that impede infant affect-regulation and later child development.[62]

Days Out of Role

Considerable research has examined days out of role associated with various physical and mental disorders. These studies typically find that mental disorders are significant predictors of days out of role.[63] In the WMH surveys, for example, 62,971 respondents across 24 countries were studied to assess the associations of a wide range of common physical disorders as well as mental disorders with a measure of days out of role in the 30 days before interview.[37] Mental disorders were associated with one-sixth of all days out of role at the population level and included three of the five disorders with the highest individual-level mean numbers of days out of role (bipolar disorder, panic disorder, and post-traumatic stress disorder, the other two being neurological disorders and chronic pain disorders).

Financial Success

The personal earnings and household income of people with mental disorders are substantially lower than those of other people.[64,65] However, it is unclear whether mental disorders are primarily causes, consequences, or both in these associations due to the possibility of reciprocal causation (for further details see also Chapter 7—Social Determinants of Mental Health). Although causal effects of low income on anxiety, depression, and substance disorders have been documented in quasi-experimental studies of job loss,[52] studies of the effects of mental disorders on reductions in income have not controlled for these reciprocal effects, making the size of the adverse effects of mental disorders on income-earnings uncertain. One way to sort out this temporal order is to take advantage of the fact that many mental disorders start in childhood or adolescence, and to use prospective epidemiological data to study long-term associations between early-onset disorders and subsequent income-earnings. Several such studies exist, all of them suggesting that mental disorders in childhood-adolescence predict significantly reduced income-earnings in adulthood.[66] To put the magnitude of these associations in perspective, WMH analyses estimated that lifetime mental disorders with AOO prior to age of completing education were associated with a population-level 1.1% reduction in gross household income (GHI) worldwide (i.e., a 1.1% reduction in the overall income in the *entire population*, not only among people with mental disorders), including 0.5% in low/lower-middle income countries, 1.0% in upper-middle income countries, and 1.4% in high-income countries.[53] A decrement of 1% GHI in the United States is equal to roughly $79 billion, which is roughly equivalent to the entire annual budget of the U.S. Department of Health and Human Services.

Comparative Impairments

A number of community surveys, most of them carried out in the United States, examined the comparative effects of diverse health problems on various aspects of role functioning.[67] Results typically show that musculoskeletal disorders and major depression are associated with the highest levels of disability at the individual level among all commonly occurring disorders assessed. The most compelling cross-national study of this sort was based on the WMH surveys.[68] Disorder-specific disability scores were compared across people who experienced each of ten chronic physical disorders and ten mental disorders in the year before interview, leading to 100 mental versus physical disorder comparisons. The proportion of disability ratings in the severe range was higher for the mental than physical disorder in 76 of these 100 comparisons in high-income countries and in 84 of 100 in low/middle-income countries (Table 5.3). Nearly all of these higher mental-than-physical disability ratings were statistically significant at the .05 level and held in within-person comparisons (i.e., comparing the reported disabilities associated with a particular mental-physical disorder pair in the sub-sample of respondents who had both disorders). A similar pattern was found when treated physical disorders were compared with all (i.e., treated or not) mental disorders to address the concern that the more superficial assessment of physical than mental disorders might have led to the inclusion of sub-threshold cases of physical disorders with low disability. Major depressive disorder (MDD) and bipolar disorder (BPD) were the mental disorders most often rated severely impairing in both developed and developing countries. None of the 10 physical disorders in the analysis had impairments as high as those of MDD or BPD despite the physical disorders, including such severe conditions as cancer, diabetes, and heart disease.

ADVERSE EFFECTS OF COMMON MENTAL DISORDERS ON PHYSICAL MORBIDITY AND MORTALITY

It is well established that common mental disorders are significantly associated with a wide variety of chronic physical disorders such as arthritis, asthma, cancer, cardiovascular disease, diabetes, hypertension, chronic respiratory disorders, and a variety of chronic pain conditions[69] (for a broader account of interactions with other health conditions, see also Chapter 6—Mental Health and the Global Health and Development Agendas). These associations have considerable individual and public health significance and can be thought of as representing costs of mental disorders in at least two ways. First, to the extent that mental disorders are causal risk factors, they lead to an increased prevalence of these physical disorders, with all their associated financial costs, impairments, and increased mortality risk. Evidence about mental disorders as causes of physical disorders is spotty, though, although we know from longitudinal studies that some mental disorders, especially major depression, are significant predictors of the subsequent first onset of coronary artery disease, stroke, diabetes, heart attacks, and certain types of cancer.[70] A number of biologically plausible mechanisms have been proposed to explain these associations, including a variety of poor health behaviors known to be linked to mental disorders (e.g., smoking, drinking, obesity, low compliance with treatment regimens) and a variety of biological dysregulations (e.g., HPA hyperactivity and impaired immune function). Based on these observations, there is good reason to believe that common mental disorders might be causal risk factors for at least some chronic physical disorders. Second, even if mental disorders are more consequences than causes of chronic physical disorders, as they appear to be for some disorders, comorbid mental disorders are often associated with a worse course of the physical disorder.[71] A number of reasons could be involved here involving lifestyle factors and non-adherence to treatment regimens.

Table 5.3 Disorder-Specific Impairment Ratings in the WHO World Mental Health Surveys

| | Proportion rated severely impaired | | | | |
| | High income countries | | Low/middle income countries | | |
	%	(se)	%	(se)	χ^2
	I. Physical disorders				
Arthritis	23.3	(1.5)	22.8	(3.0)	0.1
Asthma	8.2*	(1.4)	26.9	(5.4)	9.0*
Back/neck	34.6*	(1.5)	22.7	(1.8)	27.0*
Cancer	16.6	(3.2)	23.9	(10.3)	0.0
Chronic pain	40.9*	(3.6)	24.8	(3.8)	12.9*
Diabetes	13.6	(3.4)	23.7	(6.1)	1.4
Headaches	42.1*	(1.9)	28.1	(2.1)	15.7*
Heart disease	26.5	(3.9)	27.8	(5.2)	0.3
High blood pressure	5.3*	(0.9)	23.8	(2.6)	50.0*
Ulcer	15.3	(3.9)	18.3	(3.6)	0.1
	II. Mental disorders				
ADHD	37.6	(3.6)	24.3	(7.4)	0.8
Bipolar	68.3*	(2.6)	52.1	(4.9)	7.9*
Depression	65.8*	(1.6)	52.0	(1.8)	30.4*
GAD	56.3*	(1.9)	42.0	(4.2)	7.9*
IED	36.3	(2.8)	27.8	(3.6)	2.0
ODD	34.2	(6.0)	41.3	(10.3)	1.2
Panic disorder	48.4*	(2.6)	38.8	(4.7)	4.3*
PTSD	54.8*	(2.8)	41.2	(7.3)	4.2*
Social phobia	35.1	(1.4)	41.4	(3.6)	2.6
Specific phobia	18.6	(1.1)	16.2	(1.6)	1.9

*Significant difference between high and low/middle income countries at the .05 level, two-sided test.
A version of this table was originally published in Ormel J, Petukhova M, Chatterji S, et al. Disability and treatment of specific mental and physical disorders across the world. *Br J Psychiatry.* 2008;192(5):372. © 2008 The Royal College of Psychiatrists, used with permission.

Based on these considerations, it should not be surprising that common mental disorders are associated with significantly elevated risk of early death.[72] This is true partly because people with mental disorders have high suicide risk, but also because mental disorders are is associated with elevated risk of the many types of physical disorders. Common mental disorders are also associated with elevated mortality risk among people with certain kinds of physical disorders as part of a larger pattern of associations of mental disorders with the severity of physical disorders. There has been particular interest in major depression as a risk factor for cardiovascular mortality due to heart attack and stroke among people with cardiovascular disease (CVD).[73] Indeed, a number of interventions have been developed to detect and treat depression among people with CVD in an effort to prolong life, although these studies have so far shown only modest effects.[74]

DISCUSSION

The combination of high prevalence, early age-of-onset, high persistence, and significant adverse effects in the many countries where epidemiological surveys have been administered confirm the worldwide importance of mental disorders. Although evidence is not definitive that mental disorders play a causal role in their associations with the many adverse outcomes reviewed here, there is clear evidence that mental disorders have causal effects on a number of important mediators, making it difficult to assume anything other than that mental disorders are likely to have strong causal effects on many types of burden. These results have been used to argue for the likely cost-effectiveness from a societal perspective of expanded outreach, detection, and treatment of common mental disorders.[75] Yet the proportion of people with mental disorders who receive treatment remains low throughout the world.[76] Randomized controlled trials are needed to increase our understanding of the effects of expanded detection and treatment of common mental disorders. Detection is feasible in school-based screening programs, workplace health-risk-appraisal surveys, and screening programs in healthcare settings. Controlled effectiveness trials with long-term follow-ups are needed in all those settings to increase our understanding of the effects of the resulting treatment on changes in life-course role trajectories of youth, on the performance of workers, and on the physical health of patients with comorbid physical and mental disorders.

* Preparation of this chapter was supported, in part, by the following grants from the U.S. Public Health Service: U01MH060220, R01DA012058, R01MH070884 and R01DA016558. Portions of this paper appeared previously in the following publications: Kessler RC, Aguilar-Gaxiola S, Alonso J, et al. The burden of mental disorders worldwide: results from the World Mental Health surveys. In: Cohen N, Galea S, editors. *Population mental health: Evidence, policy, and public health practice*. Abingdon: Routledge; 2011:9–37, © 2011 Routledge; Kessler RC, Wang PS, Wittchen H-U. The societal costs of anxiety and mood disorders: an epidemiological perspective. In Preedy VR, Watson RR, editors. *Handbook of disease burdens and quality of life measures*. New York: Springer Publishing; 2010:1509–1525, © 2010 Springer Publishing; Kessler RC, Angermeyer M, Anthony JC, et al. Lifetime prevalence and age-of-onset distributions of mental disorders in the World Health Organization's World Mental Health Survey Initiative. *World Psychiatry* 2007;6(3):168–76, © 2007 World Psychiatric Association; Kessler RC. The costs of depression. *Psychiatr Clin North Am.* 2012;35(1):1–14, © 2012 Elsevier Inc.; Ormel J, Petukhova M, Chatterji S, et al. Disability and treatment of specific mental and physical disorders across the world. *Br J Psychiatry.* 2008;192(5):368–75, © 2008 The Royal College of Psychiatrists. All are used here with permission of the publishers. The views and opinions expressed in this report are those of the authors and should not be construed to represent the views of any of the sponsoring organizations, agencies, or governments.

Declaration of Interest: In the past three years, Kessler has been a consultant for GlaxoSmithKline Inc., Sanofi-Aventis, and Shire Pharmaceuticals.

REFERENCES

1. Ezzati M, Lopez AD, Rodgers A, Vander Hoorn S, Murray CJ. Selected major risk factors and global and regional burden of disease. *Lancet.* 2002;360(9343):1347–60.
2. Horwath E, Weissman MM. The epidemiology and cross-national presentation of obsessive-compulsive disorder. *Psychiatr Clin N Am.* 2000;23(3):493–507.
3. Wittchen HU. Reliability and validity studies of the WHO-Composite International Diagnostic Interview (CIDI): a critical review. *J Psychiatr Res.* 1994;28(1):57–84.
4. WHO International Consortium in Psychiatric Epidemiology. Cross-national comparisons of the prevalences and correlates of mental disorders. *Bull WHO.* 2000;78(4):413–26.
5. Haro JM, Arbabzadeh-Bouchez S, Brugha TS, et al. Concordance of the Composite International Diagnostic Interview version 3.0 (CIDI 3.0) with standardized clinical assessments in the WHO World Mental Health surveys. *Int J Methods Psychiatr Res.* 2006;15(4):167–80.

6. Ghimire DJ, Chardoul S, Kessler RC, Axinn WG, Adhikari BP. Modifying and validating the Composite International Diagnostic Interview (CIDI) for use in Nepal. *Int J Methods Psychiatr Res*. 2013;22(1):71–81.

7. Kessler RC, Angermeyer M, Anthony JC, et al. Lifetime prevalence and age-of-onset distributions of mental disorders in the World Health Organization's World Mental Health Survey Initiative. *World Psychiatry*. 2007;6(3):168–76.

8. Somers JM, Goldner EM, Waraich P, Hsu L. Prevalence and incidence studies of anxiety disorders: a systematic review of the literature. *Can J Psychiatry*. 2006;51(2):100–13.

9. Shen YC, Zhang MY, Huang YQ, et al. Twelve-month prevalence, severity, and unmet need for treatment of mental disorders in metropolitan China. *Psychol Med*. 2006;36(2):257–67.

10. Gureje O, Lasebikan VO, Kola L, Makanjuola VA. Lifetime and 12-month prevalence of mental disorders in the Nigerian Survey of Mental Health and Well-Being. *Br J Psychiatry*. 2006;188:465–71.

11. Belfer ML. Child and adolescent mental disorders: the magnitude of the problem across the globe. *J Child Psychol Psychiatry*. 2008;49(3):226–36.

12. Costello EJ, Foley DL, Angold A. 10-year research update review: the epidemiology of child and adolescent psychiatric disorders: II. Developmental epidemiology. *J Am Acad Child Adolesc Psychiatry*. 2006;45(1):8–25.

13. Ruscio AM, Chiu WT, Roy-Byrne P, et al. Broadening the definition of generalized anxiety disorder: effects on prevalence and associations with other disorders in the National Comorbidity Survey Replication. *J Anxiety Disord*. 2007;21(5):662–76.

14. Matsunaga H, Seedat S. Obsessive-compulsive spectrum disorders: cross-national and ethnic issues. *CNS Spectrums*. 2007;12(5):392–400.

15. Kalaria RN, Maestre GE, Arizaga R, et al. Alzheimer's disease and vascular dementia in developing countries: prevalence, management, and risk factors. *Lancet Neurol*. 2008;7(9):812–26.

16. Awad AG, Voruganti LN. The burden of schizophrenia on caregivers: a review. *Pharmacoeconomics*. 2008;26(2):149–62.

17. Ferri CP, Prince M, Brayne C, et al. Global prevalence of dementia: a Delphi consensus study. *Lancet*. 2005;366(9503):2112–7.

18. Larson EB. Prospects for delaying the rising tide of worldwide, late-life dementias. *Int Psychogeriatr*. 2010;22(8):1196–202.

19. Llibre Rodriguez JJ, Ferri CP, et al. Prevalence of dementia in Latin America, India, and China: a population-based cross-sectional survey. *Lancet*. 2008;372(9637):464–74.

20. Prince M, Bryce R, Albanese E, Wimo A, Ribeiro W, Ferri C. The global prevalence of dementia: A systematic review and metaanalysis. *Alzheimer's & Dementia*. 2013;9(1):63–75.e2.

21. World Health Organization. *Dementia: A public health priority*. Geneva: World Health Organization; 2012.

22. Prince MJ, Wimo A, editors. *World Alzheimer report, 2010*. London: Alzheimer's Disease International; 2010.

23. McGrath J, Saha S, Chant D, Welham J. Schizophrenia: a concise overview of incidence, prevalence, and mortality. *Epidemiol Rev*. 2008;**30**:67–76.

24. Kendler KS, Gallagher TJ, Abelson JM, Kessler RC. Lifetime prevalence, demographic risk factors, and diagnostic validity of nonaffective psychosis as assessed in a U.S. community sample. The National Comorbidity Survey. *Arch Gen Psychiatry*. 1996;53(11):1022–31.

25. van Os J, Linscott RJ, Myin-Germeys I, Delespaul P, Krabbendam L. A systematic review and meta-analysis of the psychosis continuum: evidence for a psychosis proneness-persistence-impairment model of psychotic disorder. *Psychol Med*. 2009;39(2):179–95.

26. Kelleher I, Keeley H, Corcoran P, et al. Clinicopathological significance of psychotic experiences in non-psychotic young people: evidence from four population-based studies. *Br J Psychiatry*. 2012;201:26–32.

27. de Girolamo G, Dagani J, Purcell R, Cocchi A, McGorry PD. Age of onset of mental disorders and use of mental health services: needs, opportunities and obstacles. *Epidemiol Psychiatr Sci*. 2012;21(1):47–57.

28. Eranti SV, Maccabe JH, Bundy H, Murray RM. Gender difference in age at onset of schizophrenia: a meta-analysis. *Psychol Med*. 2013;43(1):155–67.

29. Lauronen E, Miettunen J, Veijola J, Karhu M, Jones PB, Isohanni M. Outcome and its predictors in schizophrenia within the Northern Finland 1966 Birth Cohort. *Eur Psychiatry*. 2007;22(2):129–36.

30. Thomsen PH. Schizophrenia with childhood and adolescent onset—a nationwide register-based study. *Acta Psychiatr Scand.* 1996;94(3):187–93.

31. Leon AC, Solomon DA, Mueller TI, et al. A 20-year longitudinal observational study of somatic antidepressant treatment effectiveness. *Am J Psychiatry.* 2003;160(4):727–33.

32. Bruce SE, Yonkers KA, Otto MW, et al. Influence of psychiatric comorbidity on recovery and recurrence in generalized anxiety disorder, social phobia, and panic disorder: a 12-year prospective study. *Am J Psychiatry.* 2005;162(6):1179–87.

33. Kessler RC, Petukhova M, Zaslavsky AM. The role of latent internalizing and externalizing predispositions in accounting for the development of comorbidity among common mental disorders. *Curr Opin Psychiatry.* 2011;24(4):307–12.

34. Krueger RF, Markon KE. Reinterpreting comorbidity: a model-based approach to understanding and classifying psychopathology. *Annu Rev Clin Psychol.* 2006;2:111–33.

35. Kotov R, Chang SW, Fochtmann LJ, et al. Schizophrenia in the internalizing-externalizing framework: a third dimension? *Schizophr Bull.* 2011;37(6):1168–78.

36. Kotov R, Ruggero CJ, Krueger RF, Watson D, Yuan Q, Zimmerman M. New dimensions in the quantitative classification of mental illness. *Arch Gen Psychiatry.* 2011;68(10):1003–11.

37. Alonso J, Petukhova M, Vilagut G, et al. Days out of role due to common physical and mental conditions: results from the WHO World Mental Health surveys. *Mol Psychiatry.* 2011;16(12):1234–46.

38. Borges G, Nock MK, Haro Abad JM, et al. Twelve-month prevalence of and risk factors for suicide attempts in the World Health Organization World Mental Health Surveys. *J Clin Psychiatry.* 2010;71(12):1617–28.

39. Trudeau L, Spoth R, Randall GK, Mason WA, Shin C. Internalizing symptoms: effects of a preventive intervention on developmental pathways from early adolescence to young adulthood. *J Youth Adolesc.* 2012;41(6):788–801.

40. Mason WA, Spoth RL. Sequence of alcohol involvement from early onset to young adult alcohol abuse: differential predictors and moderation by family-focused preventive intervention. *Addiction.* 2012;107(12):2137–48.

41. Rothenberger A. One problem is the risk of the next: a vote for early detection and preventive intervention of coexisting psychopathology. *Eur Child Adolesc Psychiatry.* 2012;21(8):417–9.

42. Marshall M, Rathbone J. Early intervention for psychosis. *Cochrane Database Syst Rev.* 2011;(6): CD004718.

43. Regier DA, Kaelber CT, Rae DS, et al. Limitations of diagnostic criteria and assessment instruments for mental disorders. Implications for research and policy. *Arch Gen Psychiatry.* 1998;55(2):109–15.

44. Leon AC, Olfson M, Portera L, Farber L, Sheehan DV. Assessing psychiatric impairment in primary care with the Sheehan Disability Scale. *Int J Psychiatry Med.* 1997;27(2):93–105.

45. Chang SM, Hahm BJ, Lee JY, et al. Cross-national difference in the prevalence of depression caused by the diagnostic threshold. *J Affect Disord.* 2008;106(1–2):159–67.

46. Simon GE, Goldberg DP, Von Korff MR, Üstün TB. Understanding cross-national differences in depression prevalence. *Psychol Med.* 2002;32(4):585–94.

47. Alonso J, Chatterji S, He Y, editors. *The burdens of mental disorders in the WHO World Mental Health Surveys.* New York: Cambridge University Press; 2013.

48. Lee S, Tsang A, Breslau J, et al. Mental disorders and termination of education in high-income and low- and middle-income countries: epidemiological study. *Br J Psychiatry.* 2009;194(5):411–7.

49. Breslau J, Miller E, Jin R, et al. A multinational study of mental disorders, marriage, and divorce. *Acta Psychiatr Scand.* 2011;124(6):474–86.

50. Butterworth P, Rodgers B. Mental health problems and marital disruption: is it the combination of husbands and wives' mental health problems that predicts later divorce? *Soc Psychiatry Psychiatr Epidemiol.* 2008;43(9):758–63.

51. Kessler RC, Berglund PA, Foster CL, Saunders WB, Stang PE, Walters EE. Social consequences of psychiatric disorders, II: Teenage parenthood. *Am J Psychiatry.* 1997;154(10):1405–11.

52. Dooley D, Fielding J, Levi L. Health and unemployment. *Ann Rev Public Health.* 1996;17:449–65.

53. Kawakami N, Abdulghani EA, Alonso J, et al. Early-life mental disorders and adult household income in the World Mental Health Surveys. *Biol Psychiatry.* 2012;72(3):228–37.

54. Whisman MA, Uebelacker LA. Prospective associations between marital discord and depressive symptoms in middle-aged and older adults. *Psychol Aging.* 2009;24(1):184–9.

55. Kronmuller KT, Backenstrass M, Victor D, et al. Quality of marital relationship and depression: results of a 10-year prospective follow-up study. *J Affect Disord.* 2011;128(1–2):64–71.

56. Afifi TO, MacMillan H, Cox BJ, Asmundson GJ, Stein MB, Sareen J. Mental health correlates of intimate partner violence in marital relationships in a nationally representative sample of males and females. *J Interpers Violence.* 2009;24(8):1398–417.

57. Kessler RC, Molnar BE, Feurer ID, Appelbaum M. Patterns and mental health predictors of domestic violence in the United States: results from the National Comorbidity Survey. *Int J Law Psychiatry.* 2001;24(4–5):487–508.

58. Riggs DS, Caulfield MB, Street AE. Risk for domestic violence: factors associated with perpetration and victimization. *J Clin Psychol.* 2000;56(10):1289–316.

59. Miller E, Breslau J, Petukhova M, et al. Premarital mental disorders and physical violence in marriage: cross-national study of married couples. *Br J Psychiatry.* 2011;199(4):330–7.

60. Lovejoy MC, Graczyk PA, O'Hare E, Neuman G. Maternal depression and parenting behavior: a meta-analytic review. *Clin Psychol Rev.* 2000;20(5):561–92.

61. Wilson S, Durbin CE. Effects of paternal depression on fathers' parenting behaviors: a meta-analytic review. *Clin Psychol Rev.* 2010;30(2):167–80.

62. Tronick E, Reck C. Infants of depressed mothers. *Harv Rev Psychiatry.* 2009;17(2):147–56.

63. Wang PS, Beck A, Berglund P, et al. Chronic medical conditions and work performance in the health and work performance questionnaire calibration surveys. *J Occup Environ Med.* 2003;45(12):1303–11.

64. Lund C, Breen A, Flisher AJ, et al. Poverty and common mental disorders in low and middle income countries: A systematic review. *Soc Sci Med.* 2010;71(3):517–28.

65. McMillan KA, Enns MW, Asmundson GJ, Sareen J. The association between income and distress, mental disorders, and suicidal ideation and attempts: findings from the collaborative psychiatric epidemiology surveys. *J Clin Psychiatry.* 2010;71(9):1168–75.

66. Goodman A, Joyce R, Smith JP. The long shadow cast by childhood physical and mental problems on adult life. *Proc Natl Acad Sci.* 2011;108(15):6032–7.

67. Stewart WF, Ricci JA, Chee E, Morganstein D. Lost productive work time costs from health conditions in the United States: results from the American Productivity Audit. *J Occup Environ Med.* 2003;45(12):1234–46.

68. Ormel J, Petukhova M, Chatterji S, et al. Disability and treatment of specific mental and physical disorders across the world. *Br J Psychiatry.* 2008;192(5):368–75.

69. Dew MA. Psychiatric disorder in the context of physical illness. In: Dohrenwend BP, editor. *Adversity, stress, and psychopathology.* New York: Oxford University Press; 1998: 177–218.

70. Von Korff MR. Global perspectives on mental-physical comorbidity. In: Von Korff MR, Scott KM, Gureje O, editors. *Global perspectives on mental-physical comorbidity in the WHO World Mental Health Surveys.* New York: Cambridge University Press; 2009: 1–11.

71. Gillen R, Tennen H, McKee TE, Gernert-Dott P, Affleck G. Depressive symptoms and history of depression predict rehabilitation efficiency in stroke patients. *Arch Phys Med Rehabil.* 2001;82(12):1645–9.

72. Cuijpers P, Schoevers RA. Increased mortality in depressive disorders: a review. *Curr Psychiatry Rep.* 2004;6(6):430–7.

73. Barth J, Schumacher M, Herrmann-Lingen C. Depression as a risk factor for mortality in patients with coronary heart disease: a meta-analysis. *Psychosom Med.* 2004;66(6):802–13.

74. Thombs BD, de Jonge P, Coyne JC, et al. Depression screening and patient outcomes in cardiovascular care: a systematic review. *JAMA.* 2008;300(18):2161–71.

75. Wang PS, Patrick A, Avorn J, et al. The costs and benefits of enhanced depression care to employers. *Arch Gen Psychiatry.* 2006;63(12):1345–53.

76. Wang PS, Aguilar-Gaxiola S, Alonso J, et al. Use of mental health services for anxiety, mood, and substance disorders in 17 countries in the WHO World Mental Health surveys. *Lancet.* 2007;370(9590):841–50.

6 Mental Health and the Global Health and Development Agendas

Martin J. Prince, Atif Rahman,
Rosie Mayston, and Benedict Weobong

"No health without mental health" is now a very widely adopted slogan. The reasons why there can be "no health without mental health" provide much of the core evidence-based case for increased investment in mental health, and for greater integration of mental health awareness, knowledge, and skills into health policymaking and practice. These can be summarized under three main headings.[1]

1. The considerable burden arising from mental disorders in all world regions, both in absolute terms, and relative to other health conditions
2. The important contribution of mental disorders to mortality, greatly under-estimated in the Global Burden of Disease estimates
3. The many connections between mental and physical disorders, the resulting comorbidity complicating help-seeking, diagnosis, and treatment, and adversely affecting the outcomes of treatment for physical conditions.

In this chapter, we review evidence to support these arguments and the implications for policy and practice in the development context. Mental health is too often either ignored or underemphasized in pro-development agendas; in establishing donor priorities; in setting the policy framework for health improvement; in operational research; and as a factor to be addressed in the pursuit of several UN Millennium Development Goals—particularly, the promotion of gender equality and the empowerment of women, the reduction of child mortality, the improvement of maternal health, and the combating of HIV/ AIDS, malaria, and other diseases.[1,2] More broadly, sound mental health is an important economic and social resource for communities and nations.[3] Poverty and social disadvantage are prominent among both the determinants and consequences of mental disorder and, by extension, interventions that promote better mental health and reduce the duration of illness episodes may help prevent and alleviate poverty (see Chapter 7).

The most recent estimates for the global burden of disease (GBD) released by the World Health Organization are for the year 2005, with projections through to 2030. A further wholesale revision was recently published by the Institute for Health Metrics and Evaluation (IHME),[4] and its ratification by the World Health Organization is pending. Estimates provided here are from the WHO sources, with some indications of how these may be modified in the light of the IHME revision. The Global Burden of Disease estimates provide evidence of the relative impact of health problems worldwide.[5,6] Patterns of morbidity seem to be globalizing, with non-communicable diseases (NCD) rapidly becoming the dominant causes of ill health in all developing regions except sub-Saharan Africa (Table 6.1). Within this wider health transition, the GBD reports showed for the first time the true scale of the contribution of mental disorders: this revelation can be attributed to the use of the Disability-Adjusted Life Year (DALY), the sum of Years Lived with Disability (YLD), and Years of Life Lost (YLL) as a single integrated measure of disease burden.

Neuropsychiatric conditions (comprising, in descending order of DALY contribution: mental disorders, substance and alcohol use disorders, other neuropsychiatric disorders, dementia, mental retardation, migraine, epilepsy, Parkinson's disease, and multiple sclerosis) account for 14% of all DALYs and 28% of all DALYs attributed to non-communicable disease (Table 6.1).[6] They are the chief contributor to burden among the non-communicable diseases (Figure 6.1), more than either cardiovascular disease (22% of NCD DALYs) or cancer (11%). According to the new IHME estimates, mental, and behavioral, and neurological disorders collectively accounted for 7% of all DALYs and 17% of all NCD DALYs in 1990, rising to 10% of all DALYs and 19% of all NCD DALYs by 2010.[4] Among the NCDs, mental and neurological disorders (MND) make a larger contribution than cancer (14% of NCD DALYs) but a slightly lesser contribution than cardiovascular diseases (22% of NCD DALYs).[4]

Proportionately, mental disorders account for just 9% of the burden in low-income countries (LIC), compared with 18% in middle-income (MIC) and 27% in high-income countries (HIC). The reason for this discrepancy becomes apparent when the same data are presented in a different way; as per capita DALYs (DALYs per 1000 population—Figure 6.2). The per capita burden of disease is greater in lower compared with higher income countries (323 DALYs per 1000 in low-income countries and 126 DALYs per 1000 in high-income countries) because the burden of communicable, perinatal, and maternal conditions remains high in many low- and low–middle-income countries. However, the absolute burden of mental disorder varies little between world regions, from 29 to 39 DALYs per 1000 population (Figure 6.2).

Mental disorders are a leading cause of long-term disability and dependency. According to the GBD, mental disorders account for 31.7% of all years lived with disability, the five major contributors being unipolar depression (11.8%), alcohol-use disorder (3.3%), schizophrenia (2.8%), bipolar depression (2.4%), and dementia (1.6%).[7] In the new IHME estimates, mental and neurological disorders account for a similar 28.2% of all YLDs in 2010.[8] However, the relative contributions of individual disorders are rather different, explained mainly by the significant changes to the disability weights applied to them; the five leading contributors were unipolar depressive disorders (9.6%), anxiety disorders (3.5%), drug use disorders (2.1%), schizophrenia (1.9%), and alcohol use disorders (1.8%). These chronic diseases impose an immense societal burden, particularly in low- and middle-income countries. Depressive and anxiety disorders account for between one quarter and one third of all primary health care visits worldwide.[9] *Somatization*, defined as medically unexplained somatic symptoms coupled with psychological distress and help-seeking, is present in around 15% of patients seen in primary care.[10] It is highly disabling,[10] and those affected consult professionals frequently and make an important independent contribution to health care costs.[11] In 2010, the annual

Table 6.1 Number ('000s) and Proportion of Total Disability Adjusted Life Years (DALYs) Contributed By Different Groups of Health Conditions By Country Income-Level in 2005 and (Projected) 2030[5]

	2005				2030			
	World	*HIC*	*MIC*	*LIC*	*World*	*HIC*	*MIC*	*LIC*
Total DALYs	*1,483,060*	*119,361*	*492,549*	*871,141*	*1,650,629*	*118,309*	*528,066*	*1,004,236*
I. Communicable, maternal, perinatal, and nutritional conditions	572,292	6,647	99,696	465,948	494,384	4,060	79,623	410,698
	38.6%	5.6%	20.2%	53.5%	30.0%	3.4%	15.1%	40.9%
II. Non-communicable diseases	725,506	102,311	318,415	304,773	938,468	105,716	380,324	452,416
	48.9%	85.7%	64.7%	35%	56.9%	89.4%	72%	45.1%
III. Injuries	185,262	10,403	74,439	100,420	217,777	8,533	68,120	141,122
	12.5%	8.7%	15.1%	11.5%	13.2%	7.2%	12.9%	14.1%
Neuropsychiatric conditions	199,606	32,717	87,398	79,490	237,962	34,798	92,590	110,571
	13.5%[1]	27.4%[1]	17.7%[1]	9.1%[1]	14.4%[1]	29.4%[1]	17.5%[1]	11.0%[1]
	27.5%[2]	32.0%[2]	27.5%[2]	26.1%[2]	25.4%[2]	32.9%[2]	24.3%[2]	24.4%[2]

1. As a percentage of all DALYs
2. As a percentage of all non-communicable disease DALYs

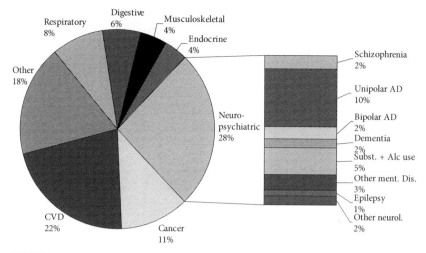

FIGURE 6.1

The proportion of Disability Adjusted Life Years (DALYs) arising from non-communicable disease in 2005, attributed to particular disease groups and specific neuropsychiatric disorders.[5]

global economic cost of dementia was estimated at over US$ 600 billion,[12] with nearly two-thirds of the estimated 36 million people affected living in low- or middle-income countries, rising to three-quarters by 2050.[13] The prevalence of epilepsy is at least two to three times higher in low-income countries than in industrialized countries, and with a substantially higher mortality.[14]

MENTAL DISORDERS AND MORTALITY

According to the WHO GBD estimates, neuropsychiatric disorders account for 1.2 million deaths per annum and just 1.4% of all years of life lost, the majority arising from

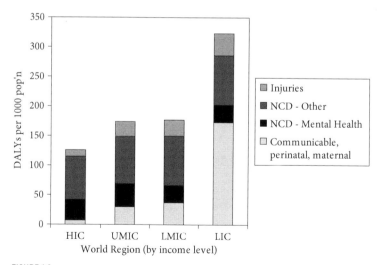

FIGURE 6.2

Disability Adjusted Life Years per 1000 population, attributed to different GBD disease categories (I—Communicable, perinatal, and maternal conditions; II—Non-communicable diseases, subdivided into "neuropsychiatric" and "other"; III—Injuries) by country income status.

dementia, Parkinson's disease, and epilepsy. Only 40,000 deaths are directly attributed to mental disorder (unipolar and bipolar depression, schizophrenia, and PTSD) and 182,000 to drug and alcohol use. The new IHME estimates are similar, with an estimated 232,000 deaths from mental and behavioral disorder and a further 1.2 million deaths from neurological disorders in 2010.[15] This is almost certainly a gross underestimate, given that deaths from suicide are listed separately under "injuries" in both the WHO and IHME estimates. Each year at least 800,000 people commit suicide, 86% in low- and middle-income countries (LMIC), and over half involving young people.[5] A recent comprehensive nationally representative verbal autopsy study in India estimated there were 187,000 suicide deaths annually, with a marked peak among those aged 15 to 29 years, particularly among women.[16] The authors estimated that, in India, suicide caused about twice as many deaths as HIV/AIDS, and, among young women, about the same number of deaths as maternal causes. Mental disorder is overwhelmingly the most important preventable factor.[17,18] As well as strengthening mental health services, effective preventive strategies need to target the means of suicide, which, in South Asia, would involve restricting access to poisons, principally pesticides, the method used in around half of all cases.[16]

The burden of mental disorders is also probably underestimated in the Global Burden of Disease estimates, given the strong associations between serious mental disorder and non-suicide mortality. Mortality from causes other than suicide is substantially elevated in psychosis,[19] depression,[20,21] and dementia.[22,23] These mortality effects have recently been summarized as reduced life expectancies for those with serious mental disorders: these are substantial, generally in the range of 10 to 15 years, depending on diagnosis, and somewhat greater for psychosis and substance use disorder than for depressive episode.[24-26] The impact of mental disorder on life expectancy is comparable to, and at worst substantially greater than, that of more widely appreciated contributors such as smoking, diabetes, and obesity.[25] Aside from increased exposure to cardiovascular risk factors and the side effects of psychotropic medication, limited access to healthcare, and the poor quality of general healthcare received by those with mental disorders, are likely to explain some of the excess mortality.[1,27]

INTERACTIONS BETWEEN MENTAL AND PHYSICAL HEALTH CONDITIONS

Much of the burden of mental ill health may be mediated through complex interactions with other health conditions, including infectious disease, and reproductive, maternal, and child health.[1] Mental disorders are risk factors for the development of communicable and non-communicable diseases, and many physical health conditions increase the risk for mental disorder. For example, in population-based studies, depression is a prospective risk factor for cardiovascular diseases (CVD), including angina, myocardial infarction,[28] and stroke.[29,30] In the case of HIV, mental health problems have been found to be associated with infection among some high-risk populations.[31] Among high-risk groups, there is evidence to suggest that depression, substance use and risk-taking behaviors may interact synergistically to heighten the risk of infection.[32,33]

Living with a disease often increases the risk for mental disorder, through a variety of mechanisms. For example, for those living with HIV, apart from the psychological trauma of the diagnosis, the stigma of the condition, and its impact on life roles and relationships, HIV infection[34] and highly active antiretroviral therapy (HAART) treatment[35] have direct effects on the central nervous system. Infection with HIV is consistently associated with a high prevalence of affective disorder.[31] HIV-associated dementia has a prevalence of 15% to 30% in untreated populations, and a prevalence of 10% and an annual incidence of 1% among those receiving HAART.[36,37] Beyond HIV-associated dementia, HIV-associated neurocognitive disorder (HAND) has a prevalence of

20% to 30%. Higher prevalences have been seen among people accessing HIV care in high-HIV-seroprevalence sub-Saharan African countries; for example, 42% with HAND and 25% with HIV-associated dementia in those starting HAART in primary care centers in Cape Town, South Africa.[38]

Comorbidity and Its Impact on the Management of Physical Disease

Comorbidity complicates help-seeking, diagnosis, and treatment, and affects the outcomes of treatment for physical conditions, including disease-related mortality. Thus, comorbid depression predicts re-infarction and death after myocardial infarction.[28] Post-stroke depression is associated with poor functional outcomes[39] and increased mortality over 10 years.[40] In diabetes, depression is associated with poor glycemic control,[41] complications,[42] and death.[43] In the United States and in Tanzania, chronic depressive symptoms were associated with increased AIDS-related mortality[44-46] and more rapid disease progression[44,46] independent of receipt of treatment. Cognitive impairment in HIV is associated with greatly increased mortality.[47] Schizophrenia complicates HIV treatment and is associated with worse prognosis.[35]

A common underlying mechanism may be the poor adherence to treatment regimes that has been demonstrated for behavior change in cardiovascular disease,[48] for oral hypoglycemic therapy among people with schizophrenia,[49] and for diet, exercise recommendations, and oral hypoglycemic medication among diabetics with depression.[50] Adherence to HAART is adversely affected by depression,[51] cognitive impairment,[52] and alcohol and substance use.[53] Depression may also adversely impact initial help-seeking for treatment after a HIV diagnosis has been received.[54]

Mental Disorders, Maternal and Child Health

Mental disorders in women are important, given links to reproductive, maternal, and child health. Women are at heightened risk for common mental disorders, with a typical female to male gender ratio of 1.5 to 2.0.[55] Abuse, anxiety, depression, substance, and alcohol use are all robustly associated with dysmenorrhea, dyspareunia, and pelvic pain.[56] In Asian cultures, explanatory models of reproductive and mental health experiences may enhance these associations: in a study in south India, the complaint of vaginal discharge was associated with common mental disorder rather than reproductive tract infection.[57] Maternal mental health may also have important implications for perinatal outcomes, infant growth and survival. Maternal schizophrenia is consistently associated with pre-term delivery,[58,59] low birth weight,[58-60] still birth, and infant mortality.[61] Meta-analyses of studies of the prevalence of postpartum depression suggest a slightly higher prevalence in sub-Saharan Africa countries (18.3%, 95% CI 17.5%–19.1%)[62] than in high-income-country settings (12.9%, 95% CI 10.6%–15.8%),[63] but even higher prevalences have been recorded in studies in south Asia (19%–28%),[64,65] and Latin America (35%–50%).[66] In developed countries, there are adverse consequences for the early mother–infant relationship and for the child's psychological development.[67] In Asia, two prospective studies suggest an independent association between antenatal CMD and low birth weight,[68,69] and associations between perinatal CMD and infant under-nutrition at six months have been consistently demonstrated.[68,70-72] With occasional exceptions,[73] these findings have generally not been replicated in cohort or cross-sectional studies in sub-Saharan Africa.[74-77] However, as in Pakistan,[78] persistent common mental disorder was associated with infant diarrheal episodes in Ethiopia,[79] suggesting one possible mediating mechanism for the associations with infant growth. Maternal depression also reduces adherence to child-health promotion and disease-prevention interventions;

for example, immunization.[68] There is good evidence from developed countries[80] and LMIC[73,81] that maternal depression is associated with sub-optimal breastfeeding.

Links Between Mental Health, Accidents, and Injuries

Injury and violence are important causes of death and disability worldwide. According to the 2005 GBD estimates, there were 5.4 million injury deaths globally, accounting for 9% of deaths and 12% of the burden of disease.[5] The burden of injury is expected to increase substantially by the year 2030. Mental health problems are both a cause and a consequence of injury. Injury and mental disorder also have many determinants in common; for example, poverty,[82,83] conflict, violence, and alcohol use. Mental health considerations must be integral to any public health approach to injury control.

TREATMENT OF MENTAL DISORDERS IN THE CONTEXT OF PHYSICAL DISORDERS

There is ample evidence that treatment of comorbid mental disorder is highly effective in improving mental health and quality of life across a range of disorders, including cancer,[84] diabetes,[85] heart disease,[86,87] and HIV.[88]

The evidence on whether mental health interventions can improve physical disease outcomes is more mixed. Psychological interventions have been shown to improve diabetic control in Type 1[89] and Type 2 diabetes.[90] Pharmacological treatments are effective for depression, but do not improve glycemic control[85] or diabetic self-care.[91] Antidepressants and cognitive behavioral therapy (CBT) are safe and moderately effective treatments for depression post-MI,[87,92] but do not reduce re-infarction rates or overall mortality.[87] The evidence base for the effectiveness of antidepressants post-stroke is weak, both for prevention[93] and treatment.[94] A randomized controlled trial (RCT) of a cognitive behavior therapy–based intervention for depressed mothers integrated into the routine work of community-based primary health workers in rural Pakistan was effective in increasing immunization rates and reducing diarrheal episodes in their infants, as well as much improving the mental health outcome for the mothers, but it did not reduce infant stunting.[95] Non-randomized evaluations of psychotherapeutic interventions integrated with tuberculosis treatment suggest possible improvements in treatment completion and cure, in Peru,[96] India,[97] and Ethiopia.[98] The picture now emerging is complex and requires careful interpretation. Despite clear and apparently independent associations between comorbid mental disorders and adverse treatment outcomes across a range of disorders, successful intervention targeting the mental disorder seems often to be relatively ineffective in improving the outcome of the physical disorder.

In the case of HIV, for example, a large, randomized controlled trial of directly observed treatment with fluoxetine for homeless persons living with HIV in California showed a clear treatment benefit with a 2.5 times greater odds of treatment response (adjusted odds ratio [AOR] 2.40; 95% CI 1.86–3.10) and a three-fold increase in odds of remission of depression (AOR 2.97, 95% CI 1.29–3.87).[88] However, there was no statistically significant effect of the antidepressant treatment on secondary HIV outcomes, including antiretroviral therapy (ART) uptake, ART adherence, and viral suppression. Conversely, results from the U.S. Health Living Project RCTs indicate that a 15-session cognitive behavioral therapy intervention targeting stress, coping, and adjustment; safer behaviors; and health behaviors (including an emphasis on ART adherence) was successful in increasing adherence to ART[99] and in reducing risk behaviors (unprotected sex acts with people who were HIV-negative or of unknown status).[100] However, the CBT intervention across these three trials was not associated with any discernible or statistically significant impact on psychosocial adjustment, including among the subgroup of individuals who had mild to moderate depressive symptoms at baseline.[101]

Therefore, despite evidence from observational cohort studies, depression in HIV may not be causally related to poor adherence and other adverse HIV-related outcomes. Such findings may, instead, have been accounted for by uncontrolled confounding. The same may apply to associations between maternal depression and infant stunting[95] and depression post-myocardial infarction and subsequent re-infarction and death.[87] Negative illness perceptions, which, in turn, influence health behaviors may be important mediators or confounders of the relationship between mental comorbidity and physical health outcomes, and may not have been directly addressed in the interventions. For HIV, these may include internalized stigma,[102] and attitudes regarding the treatability of the illness and the necessity for medication[103,104] While the treatment of serious comorbid mental disorder is always indicated, interventions may need to have a broader focus, addressing underlying psychosocial factors and health psychology, if they are to have an impact on downstream health outcomes. For example, a randomized controlled trial that addressed adherence (including barriers to adherence) as well as depression among people living with HIV/AIDS yielded promising results, with better outcomes for both adherence and depression in the intervention arm as compared to the enhanced "usual care" group.[105] A "vertical" focus on psychiatric treatment of the mental disorder alone may not be enough to improve physical disease outcomes: interventions that address mental health in the context of other psychological factors related to illness and treatment may be more effective.

CONCLUSION

In summary, mental disorders make an important independent contribution to the overall burden of disease in all world regions, which may, hitherto, have been underestimated. Furthermore, mental disorders are risk factors for the development of communicable and non-communicable diseases, and a contributory factor to accidental and non-accidental injuries. Many health conditions increase the risk for mental disorder, or lengthen episodes of mental illness. The resulting comorbidity complicates help-seeking, diagnosis, and treatment, and affects the outcomes of treatment for physical conditions, including disease-related mortality. Hence, there can be "no health without mental health."

Mental health awareness needs to be incorporated into health and social policy, health system planning, and health care delivery. When mental disorders are seen as a distinct health domain, with separate services and budgets, then investing in mental health is perceived as having an unaffordable opportunity cost. More research is needed to assess the macroeconomic consequences of scaling up of mental health care.[106] The evidence presented in this chapter makes a compelling case for the greater integration of mental health care into general health care at all levels of the health system. The goal of integration tends to be interpreted in different ways. In one sense, this can refer simply to the provision of mental health care in general health care settings, by non-specialist health professionals. This is an important objective, maximizing the impact of the small number of mental health professionals, by task-sharing and mobilizing the forces of public and community health to work for better mental health. Without this step, little progress will be made in closing the sizeable treatment gap for all priority mental and neurological conditions.[107] Other benefits could include a preference among patients and families for local care, which is more cheaply and easily accessed, and may be less stigmatizing than attending a specialist mental health unit. "Integration" can also refer to the horizontal integration of mental health care into existing health programs, and care for other priority disorders. This remains a significant challenge, with few if any successful examples to date. However, there could be substantial benefits.

1. The care for individuals with serious mental illnesses such as schizophrenia, dementia, and epilepsy is long-term, often lifelong. Therefore, care is best delivered within a facility and health system structure that attends to the principles of good chronic disease care—these include, *inter alia*, case registers, health information systems, a paradigm shift towards extended regular health care contact, centering care on patients and families, and supporting patients in the community. This would be a radical shift in perspective for most services in low- and middle-income countries, where primary care facilities have been oriented to providing single episodes of care for acute conditions. WHO, in proposing the Innovative Care for Chronic Conditions (ICCC) framework, called for a dialogue to build consensus and political commitment for health system–level change.[108] Clearly these changes are as necessary for effective care of diabetes and hypertension, or for frail older people with multiple morbidities, as they are for chronic serious mental illnesses. Integrating care of those with serious mental disorders into the generic strengthening of facilities and systems to provide chronic disease care programs would minimize organizational inefficiencies, and may also ensure better attention to the physical health care needs of those with mental disorder. For example, people with schizophrenia need to have their weight and blood sugar monitored, and attention paid to cardiovascular risk factors.[107] For those with dementia, attention should be paid to under-nutrition, mobility, visual and auditory impairment, and bowel and bladder function.[109]

2. Given the lack of a prior culture of help-seeking and treatment for serious mental disorders in general health care settings, it is envisaged that community sensitization and case-finding may be necessary to increase illness detection and access to care.[109,110] However, this is not the case for common mental disorders, which frequently present in primary care; often, as we have seen, comorbid with other health conditions that constitute the primary indication for attendance. Here, the strengthening of health care systems to deliver mental health care should focus where possible upon the detection and management of depression, anxiety, and alcohol and substance use disorders integrated within existing prioritized programs and activities[111]; for example, HIV prevention, the roll-out of antiretroviral treatment, TB treatment, gender-based violence campaigns, perinatal care, and new chronic disease management programs.

Better attention to mental health may be relevant to the achievement of all three of the health-related Millennium Development Goals.[2] Improvements in maternal mental health are likely to benefit child growth and development, and may even contribute to enhanced child survival. There is extensive evidence now in the HIV field to suggest that mental ill health, alcohol, and substance use and cognitive impairment make an important contribution to risk of transmission, timely detection, and engagement with HIV services, adherence, and treated outcome. With concern growing regarding the epidemic of chronic non-communicable diseases, it is important that mental health is accorded due priority, both as a significant contributor to chronic disease burden in its own right, and as an important comorbidity in the treatment and control of other chronic conditions. As we have seen (Chapter 7) important social determinants of adverse mental health include poverty, gender, and unsatisfactory living conditions. Poverty is both a likely cause and a consequence of mental ill health.[112] A recent review identified stronger evidence for mental health interventions' being pro-poor than for the mental health benefits of poverty-alleviation interventions.[106] However, the consequences for mental health of, on one hand, progressive-income and wealth redistribution policies, and on the other, the impact of economic shocks and market failures, are poorly understood.[106] Women are at greater risk of common mental disorders, an association that is probably mediated through a raft of potentially modifiable factors, including lack of autonomy, limited education, socioeconomic disadvantage, marital dissatisfaction, and intimate-partner violence. The promotion of gender equality and empowerment of women are therefore important strategies for mental health promotion. Population mental health is clearly germane to development, leading some to call for this to be recognized as a global development priority for the remainder of the MDG period and beyond.[113] The new UN focus on "social, economic, and environmental well-being," as enunciated at the Rio+20 United Nations Conference on Sustainable Development in 2012 is likely to inform priorities post-2015. This would seem to leave the door open for further advocacy for mental health promotion, coupled with more attention to prevention, treatment, and care.

REFERENCES

1. Prince M, Patel V, Saxena S, et al. No health without mental health. *Lancet.* 2007 Sep 8;370(9590):859–77.
2. Miranda JJ, Patel V. Achieving the Millennium Development Goals: does mental health play a role? *PLoS Med.* 2005 Oct;2(10):e291.
3. Beddington J, Cooper CL, Field J, et al. The mental wealth of nations. *Nature.* 2008 Oct 23;455(7216):1057–60.
4. Murray CJ, Vos T, Lozano R, et al. Disability-adjusted life years (DALYs) for 291 diseases and injuries in 21 regions, 1990–2010: a systematic analysis for the Global Burden of Disease Study 2010. *Lancet.* 2013 Dec 15;380(9859):2197–223.
5. World Health Organization. WHO Statistical Information System. Working paper describing data sources, methods, and results for projections of mortality and burden of disease for 2005, 2015, and 2030. 2006. Geneva: WHO.
6. World Health Organization. *The global burden of disease. 2004 update.* Geneva: World Health Organization; 2008.
7. Mathers CD, Loncar D. Projections of global mortality and burden of disease from 2002 to 2030. *PLoS Med.* 2006 Nov;3(11):e442.
8. Vos T, Flaxman AD, Naghavi M, et al. Years lived with disability (YLDs) for 1160 sequelae of 289 diseases and injuries 1990–2010: a systematic analysis for the Global Burden of Disease Study 2010. *Lancet.* 2013 Dec 15;380(9859):2163–96.
9. Ustun TB, Sartorius N. *Mental illness in general health care: An international study.* Chichester, UK: John Wiley & Sons; 1995.
10. Gureje O, Simon GE, Ustun TB, Goldberg DP. Somatization in cross-cultural perspective: a World Health Organization study in primary care. *Am J Psychiatry.* 1997 Jul;154(7):989–95.
11. Barsky AJ, Orav EJ, Bates DW. Somatization increases medical utilization and costs independent of psychiatric and medical comorbidity. *Arch Gen Psychiatry.* 2005 Aug;62(8):903–10.
12. Wimo A, Prince M. World Alzheimer Report 2010; *The global economic impact of dementia.* London: Alzheimer's Disease International; 2010.
13. Alzheimer's Disease International. *World Alzheimer report 2009.* London: Alzheimer's Disease International; 2009.
14. Newton CR, Garcia HH. Epilepsy in poor regions of the world. *Lancet.* 2012 Sep 29;380(9848):1193–201.
15. Lozano R, Naghavi M, Foreman K, et al. Global and regional mortality from 235 causes of death for 20 age groups in 1990 and 2010: a systematic analysis for the Global Burden of Disease Study 2010. *Lancet.* 2013 Dec 15;380(9859):2095–128.
16. Patel V, Ramasundarahettige C, Vijayakumar L, et al. Suicide mortality in India: a nationally representative survey. *Lancet.* 2012 Jun 23;379(9834):2343–51.
17. Cavanagh JT, Carson AJ, Sharpe M, Lawrie SM. Psychological autopsy studies of suicide: a systematic review. *Psychol Med.* 2003 Apr;33(3):395–405.
18. Phillips MR, Yang G, Zhang Y, Wang L, Ji H, Zhou M. Risk factors for suicide in China: a national case-control psychological autopsy study. *Lancet.* 2002 Nov 30;360 (9347):1728–36.
19. Saha S, Chant D, McGrath J. A systematic review of mortality in schizophrenia: is the differential mortality gap worsening over time? *Arch Gen Psychiatry.* 2007 Oct;64(10):1123–31.

20. Saz P, Dewey ME. Depression, depressive symptoms and mortality in persons aged 65 and over living in the community: a systematic review of the literature. *Int J Geriatr Psychiatry.* 2001 Jun;16(6):622–30.

21. Mogga S, Prince M, Alem A, et al. Outcome of major depression in Ethiopia: population-based study. *Br J Psychiatry.* 2006 Sep;189:241–6.:241–6.

22. Dewey ME, Saz P. Dementia, cognitive impairment and mortality in persons aged 65 and over living in the community: a systematic review of the literature. *Int J Geriatr Psychiatry.* 2001 Aug;16(8):751–61.

23. Prince M, Acosta D, Ferri CP, et al. Dementia incidence and mortality in middle-income countries, and associations with indicators of cognitive reserve: a 10/66 Dementia Research Group population-based cohort study. *Lancet.* 2012 Jul 7;380(9836):50–8..

24. Kodesh A, Goldshtein I, Gelkopf M, Goren I, Chodick G, Shalev V. Epidemiology and comorbidity of severe mental illnesses in the community: findings from a computerized mental health registry in a large Israeli health organization. *Soc Psychiatry Psychiatr Epidemiol.* 2012 Nov;47(11):1775–82.

25. Chang CK, Hayes RD, Perera G, et al. Life expectancy at birth for people with serious mental illness and other major disorders from a secondary mental health care case register in London. *PLoS ONE.* 2011;6(5):e19590.

26. Hannerz H, Borga P, Borritz M. Life expectancies for individuals with psychiatric diagnoses. *Public Health.* 2001 Sep;115(5):328–37.

27. Lawrence DM, Holman CD, Jablensky AV, Hobbs MS. Death rate from ischaemic heart disease in Western Australian psychiatric patients 1980–1998. *Br J Psychiatry.* 2003 Jan;182:31–6.:31–6.

28. Albus C. Psychological and social factors in coronary heart disease. *Ann Med.* 2010 Oct;42(7):487–94.

29. Larson SL, Owens PL, Ford D, Eaton W. Depressive disorder, dysthymia, and risk of stroke: thirteen-year follow-up from the Baltimore epidemiologic catchment area study. *Stroke.* 2001 Sep;32(9):1979–83.

30. Everson SA, Roberts RE, Goldberg DE, Kaplan GA. Depressive symptoms and increased risk of stroke mortality over a 29-year period. *Arch Intern Med.* 1998 May 25;158(10):1133–8.

31. Ciesla JA, Roberts JE. Meta-analysis of the relationship between HIV infection and risk for depressive disorders. *Am J Psychiatry.* 2001 May;158(5):725–30.

32. Safren SA, Thomas BE, Mimiaga MJ, et al. Depressive symptoms and human immunodeficiency virus risk behavior among men who have sex with men in Chennai, India. *Psychol Health Med.* 2009 Dec;14(6):705–15.

33. Koblin BA, Husnik MJ, Colfax G, et al. Risk factors for HIV infection among men who have sex with men. *AIDS.* 2006 Mar 21;20(5):731–9.

34. Dube B, Benton T, Cruess DG, Evans DL. Neuropsychiatric manifestations of HIV infection and AIDS. *J Psychiatry Neurosci.* 2005 Jul;30(4):237–46.

35. Cournos F, McKinnon K, Sullivan G. Schizophrenia and comorbid human immunodeficiency virus or hepatitis C virus. *J Clin Psychiatry.* 2005;66 Suppl 6:27–33.:27–33.

36. McArthur JC, Steiner J, Sacktor N, Nath A. Human immunodeficiency virus-associated neurocognitive disorders: mind the gap. *Ann Neurol.* 2010 Jun;67(6):699–714.

37. Sacktor N. The epidemiology of human immunodeficiency virus-associated neurological disease in the era of highly active antiretroviral therapy. *J Neurovirol.* 2002 Dec;8 Suppl 2:115–21.

38. Joska JA, Westgarth-Taylor J, Myer L, et al. Characterization of HIV-associated neurocognitive disorders among individuals starting antiretroviral therapy in South Africa. *AIDS Behav.* 2011 Aug;15(6):1197–203.

39. Chemerinski E, Robinson RG, Kosier JT. Improved recovery in activities of daily living associated with remission of poststroke depression. *Stroke.* 2001 Jan;32(1):113–7.

40. Morris PL, Robinson RG, Andrzejewski P, Samuels J, Price TR. Association of depression with 10-year poststroke mortality. *Am J Psychiatry.* 1993 Jan;150(1):124–9.

41. Lustman PJ, Anderson RJ, Freedland KE, de GM, Carney RM, Clouse RE. Depression and poor glycemic control: a meta-analytic review of the literature. *Diabetes Care.* 2000 Jul;23(7):934–42.

42. de GM, Anderson R, Freedland KE, Clouse RE, Lustman PJ. Association of depression and diabetes complications: a meta-analysis. *Psychosom Med.* 2001 Jul;63(4):619–30.

43. Katon WJ, Rutter C, Simon G, et al. The association of comorbid depression with mortality in patients with type 2 diabetes. *Diabetes Care.* 2005 Nov;28(11):2668–72.

44. Ickovics JR, Hamburger ME, Vlahov D, et al. Mortality, CD4 cell count decline, and depressive symptoms among HIV-seropositive women: longitudinal analysis from the HIV Epidemiology Research Study. *JAMA*. 2001 Mar 21;285(11):1466–74.

45. Cook JA, Grey D, Burke J, et al. Depressive symptoms and AIDS-related mortality among a multisite cohort of HIV-positive women. *Am J Public Health*. 2004 Jul;94(7):1133–40.

46. Antelman G, Kaaya S, Wei R, et al. Depressive symptoms increase risk of HIV disease progression and mortality among women in Tanzania. *J Acquir Immune Defic Syndr*. 2007 Apr 1;44(4):470–7.

47. Wilkie FL, Goodkin K, Eisdorfer C, et al. Mild cognitive impairment and risk of mortality in HIV-1 infection. *J Neuropsychiatry Clin Neurosci*. 1998;10(2):125–32.

48. Ziegelstein RC, Fauerbach JA, Stevens SS, Romanelli J, Richter DP, Bush DE. Patients with depression are less likely to follow recommendations to reduce cardiac risk during recovery from a myocardial infarction. *Arch Intern Med*. 2000 Jun 26;160(12):1818–23.

49. Dolder CR, Lacro JP, Jeste DV. Adherence to antipsychotic and nonpsychiatric medications in middle-aged and older patients with psychotic disorders. *Psychosom Med*. 2003 Jan;65(1):156–62.

50. Lin EH, Katon W, Von KM, et al. Relationship of depression and diabetes self-care, medication adherence, and preventive care. *Diabetes Care*. 2004 Sep;27(9):2154–60.

51. Springer SA, Dushaj A, Azar MM. The impact of DSM-IV mental disorders on adherence to combination antiretroviral therapy among adult persons living with HIV/AIDS: a systematic review. *AIDS Behav*. 2012 Nov;16(8):2119–43.

52. Hinkin CH, Hardy DJ, Mason KI, et al. Medication adherence in HIV-infected adults: effect of patient age, cognitive status, and substance abuse. *AIDS*. 2004 Jan 1;18 Suppl 1:S19–25.

53. Chander G, Himelhoch S, Moore RD. Substance abuse and psychiatric disorders in HIV-positive patients: epidemiology and impact on antiretroviral therapy. *Drugs*. 2006;66(6):769–89.

54. Ramirez-Avila L, Regan S, Giddy J, et al. Depressive symptoms and their impact on health-seeking behaviors in newly-diagnosed HIV-infected patients in Durban, South Africa. *AIDS Behav*. 2012 Nov;16(8):2226–35.

55. Kuehner C. Gender differences in unipolar depression: an update of epidemiological findings and possible explanations. *Acta Psychiatr Scand*. 2003 Sep;108(3):163–74.

56. Latthe P, Mignini L, Gray R, Hills R, Khan K. Factors predisposing women to chronic pelvic pain: systematic review. *BMJ*. 2006 Apr 1;332(7544):749–55.

57. Patel V, Pednekar S, Weiss H, Rodrigues M, Barros P, Nayak B, et al. Why do women complain of vaginal discharge? A population survey of infectious and pyschosocial risk factors in a South Asian community. *Int J Epidemiol*. 2005 Aug;34(4):853–62.

58. Nilsson E, Lichtenstein P, Cnattingius S, Murray RM, Hultman CM. Women with schizophrenia: pregnancy outcome and infant death among their offspring. *Schizophr Res*. 2002 Dec 1;58(2–3):221–9.

59. Bennedsen BE, Mortensen PB, Olesen AV, Henriksen TB. Preterm birth and intra-uterine growth retardation among children of women with schizophrenia. *Br J Psychiatry*. 1999 Sep;175:239–45.

60. Jablensky AV, Morgan V, Zubrick SR, Bower C, Yellachich LA. Pregnancy, delivery, and neonatal complications in a population cohort of women with schizophrenia and major affective disorders. *Am J Psychiatry*. 2005 Jan;162(1):79–91.

61. Webb R, Abel K, Pickles A, Appleby L. Mortality in offspring of parents with psychotic disorders: a critical review and meta-analysis. *Am J Psychiatry*. 2005 Jun;162(6):1045–56.

62. Sawyer A, Ayers S, Smith H. Pre- and postnatal psychological wellbeing in Africa: a systematic review. *J Affect Disord*. 2010 Jun;123(1–3):17–29.

63. Gavin NI, Gaynes BN, Lohr KN, Meltzer-Brody S, Gartlehner G, Swinson T. Perinatal depression: a systematic review of prevalence and incidence. *Obstet Gynecol*. 2005 Nov;106(5 Pt 1):1071–83.

64. Rahman A, Iqbal Z, Harrington R. Life events, social support and depression in childbirth: perspectives from a rural community in the developing world. *Psychol Med*. 2003 Oct;33(7):1161–7.

65. Gausia K, Fisher C, Ali M, Oosthuizen J. Magnitude and contributory factors of postnatal depression: a community-based cohort study from a rural subdistrict of Bangladesh. *Psychol Med*. 2009 Jun;39(6):999–1007.

66. Wolf AW, De A, I, Lozoff B. Maternal depression in three Latin American samples. *Soc Psychiatry Psychiatr Epidemiol*. 2002 Apr;37(4):169–76.

67. Murray L, Cooper PJ. Intergenerational transmission of affective and cognitive processes associated with depression: infancy and the pre-school years. In: Goodyer IM, editor. *Unipolar depression: A lifespan perspective*. Oxford, UK: Oxford University Press; 2003:17–46.

68. Rahman A, Iqbal Z, Bunn J, Lovel H, Harrington R. Impact of maternal depression on infant nutritional status and illness: a cohort study. *Arch Gen Psychiatry.* 2004 Sep;61(9):946–52.

69. Patel V, Prince M. Maternal psychological morbidity and low birth weight in India. *Br J Psychiatry.* 2006 Mar;188:284–5.

70. Rahman A, Lovel H, Bunn J, Iqbal Z, Harrington R. Mothers' mental health and infant growth: a case-control study from Rawalpindi, Pakistan. *Child Care Health Dev.* 2004 Jan;30(1):21–7.

71. Patel V, DeSouza N, Rodrigues M. Postnatal depression and infant growth and development in low income countries: a cohort study from Goa, India. *Archives of Disease in Childhood.* 2003 Jan;88(1):34–7.

72. Patel V, Rahman A, Jacob KS, Hughes M. Effect of maternal mental health on infant growth in low income countries: new evidence from South Asia. *BMJ.* 2004 Apr 3;328(7443):820–3.

73. Adewuya AO, Ola BO, Aloba OO, Mapayi BM, Okeniyi JA. Impact of postnatal depression on infants' growth in Nigeria. *J Affect Disord.* 2008 May;108(1–2):191–3.

74. Hanlon C, Medhin G, Alem A, et al. Impact of antenatal common mental disorders upon perinatal outcomes in Ethiopia: the P-MaMiE population-based cohort study. *Trop Med Int Health.* 2009 Feb;14(2):156–66.

75. Medhin G, Hanlon C, Dewey M, et al. The effect of maternal common mental disorders on infant undernutrition in Butajira, Ethiopia: the P-MaMiE study. *BMC Psychiatry.* 2010;10:32.

76. Servili C, Medhin G, Hanlon C, et al. Maternal common mental disorders and infant development in Ethiopia: the P-MaMiE Birth Cohort. *BMC Public Health.* 2010;10:693.

77. Tomlinson M, Cooper PJ, Stein A, Swartz L, Molteno C. Post-partum depression and infant growth in a South African peri-urban settlement. *Child Care Health Dev.* 2006 Jan;32(1):81–6.

78. Rahman A, Bunn J, Lovel H, Creed F. Maternal depression increases infant risk of diarrhoeal illness: —a cohort study. *Arch Dis Child.* 2007 Jan;92(1):24–8.

79. Ross J, Hanlon C, Medhin G, et al. Perinatal mental distress and infant morbidity in Ethiopia: a cohort study. *Arch Dis Child Fetal Neonatal Ed.* 2011 Jan;96(1):F59–64.

80. Paulson JF, Dauber S, Leiferman JA. Individual and combined effects of postpartum depression in mothers and fathers on parenting behavior. *Pediatrics.* 2006 Aug;118(2):659–68.

81. Galler JR, Harrison RH, Biggs MA, Ramsey F, Forde V. Maternal moods predict breastfeeding in Barbados. *J Dev Behav Pediatr.* 1999 Apr;20(2):80–7.

82. Patel V, Kleinman A. Poverty and common mental disorders in developing countries. *Bull WHO.* 2003;81(8):609–15.

83. Edwards P, Roberts I, Green J, Lutchmun S. Deaths from injury in children and employment status in family: analysis of trends in class specific death rates. *BMJ.* 2006 Jul 15;333(7559):119.

84. Osborn RL, Demoncada AC, Feuerstein M. Psychosocial interventions for depression, anxiety, and quality of life in cancer survivors: meta-analyses. *Int J Psychiatry Med.* 2006;36(1):13–34.

85. Katon WJ, Von KM, Lin EH, et al. The Pathways Study: a randomized trial of collaborative care in patients with diabetes and depression. *Arch Gen Psychiatry.* 2004 Oct;61(10):1042–9.

86. Rees K, Bennett P, West R, Davey SG, Ebrahim S. Psychological interventions for coronary heart disease. *Cochrane Database Syst Rev.* 2004;(2):CD002902.

87. Berkman LF, Blumenthal J, Burg M, et al. Effects of treating depression and low perceived social support on clinical events after myocardial infarction: the Enhancing Recovery in Coronary Heart Disease Patients (ENRICHD) randomized trial. *JAMA.* 2003 Jun 18;289(23):3106–16.

88. Tsai AC, Karasic DH, Hammer GP, et al. Directly observed antidepressant medication treatment and HIV outcomes among homeless and marginally housed HIV-positive adults: a randomized controlled trial. *Am J Public Health.* 2013 Feb;103(2):308–15.

89. Winkley K, Ismail K, Landau S, Eisler I. Psychological interventions to improve glycaemic control in patients with type 1 diabetes: systematic review and meta-analysis of randomised controlled trials. *BMJ.* 2006 Jul 8;333(7558):65.

90. Ismail K, Winkley K, Rabe-Hesketh S. Systematic review and meta-analysis of randomised controlled trials of psychological interventions to improve glycaemic control in patients with type 2 diabetes. *Lancet.* 2004 May 15;363(9421):1589–97.

91. Lin EH, Katon W, Rutter C, et al. Effects of enhanced depression treatment on diabetes self-care. *Ann Fam Med.* 2006 Jan;4(1):46–53.

92. Glassman AH, O'Connor CM, Califf RM, et al. Sertraline treatment of major depression in patients with acute MI or unstable angina. *JAMA.* 2002 Aug 14;288(6):701–9.

93. Hackett ML, Anderson CS, House A, Halteh C. Interventions for preventing depression after stroke. *Cochrane Database Syst Rev*. 2008 Jul 16;(3):CD003689.

94. Hackett ML, Anderson CS, House A, Xia J. Interventions for treating depression after stroke. *Cochrane Database Syst Rev*. 2008;(4):CD003437.

95. Rahman A, Malik A, Sikander S, Roberts C, Creed F. Cognitive behaviour therapy-based intervention by community health workers for mothers with depression and their infants in rural Pakistan: a cluster-randomised controlled trial. *Lancet*. 2008 Sep 13;372(9642):902–9.

96. Acha J, Sweetland A, Guerra D, Chalco K, Castillo H, Palacios E. Psychosocial support groups for patients with multidrug-resistant tuberculosis: five years of experience. *Glob Public Health*. 2007;2(4):404–17.

97. Janmeja AK, Das SK, Bhargava R, Chavan BS. Psychotherapy improves compliance with tuberculosis treatment. *Respiration*. 2005 Jul;72(4):375–80.

98. Demissie M, Getahun H, Lindtjorn B. Community tuberculosis care through "TB clubs" in rural North Ethiopia. *Soc Sci Med*. 2003 May;56(10):2009–18.

99. Johnson MO, Charlebois E, Morin SF, Remien RH, Chesney MA. Effects of a behavioral intervention on antiretroviral medication adherence among people living with HIV: the healthy living project randomized controlled study. *J Acquir Immune Defic Syndr*. 2007 Dec 15;46(5):574–80.

100. Healthy Living Project Team. Effects of a behavioral intervention to reduce risk of transmission among people living with HIV: the healthy living project randomized controlled study. *J Acquir Immune Defic Syndr*. 2007 Feb 1;44(2):213–21.

101. Carrico AW, Chesney MA, Johnson MO, et al. Randomized controlled trial of a cognitive-behavioral intervention for HIV-positive persons: an investigation of treatment effects on psychosocial adjustment. *AIDS Behav*. 2009 Jun;13(3):555–63.

102. Peltzer K, Ramlagan S. Perceived stigma among patients receiving antiretroviral therapy: a prospective study in KwaZulu-Natal, South Africa. *AIDS Care*. 2011 Jan;23(1):60–8.

103. Gonzalez JS, Penedo FJ, Llabre MM, et al. Physical symptoms, beliefs about medications, negative mood, and long-term HIV medication adherence. *Ann Behav Med*. 2007 Aug;34(1):46–55.

104. Cooper V, Gellaitry G, Hankins M, Fisher M, Horne R. The influence of symptom experiences and attributions on adherence to highly active anti-retroviral therapy (HAART): a six-month prospective, follow-up study. *AIDS Care*. 2009 Apr;21(4):520–8.

105. Safren SA, O'Cleirigh CM, Bullis JR, Otto MW, Stein MD, Pollack MH. Cognitive behavioral therapy for adherence and depression (CBT-AD) in HIV-infected injection drug users: a randomized controlled trial. *J Consult Clin Psychol*. 2012 Jun;80(3):404–15.

106. Lund C, De SM, Plagerson S, et al. Poverty and mental disorders: breaking the cycle in low-income and middle-income countries. *Lancet*. 2011 Oct 22;378(9801):1502–14.

107. Dua T, Barbui C, Clark N, et al. Evidence-based guidelines for mental, neurological, and substance use disorders in low- and middle-income countries: summary of WHO recommendations. *PLoS Med*. 2011 Nov;8(11):e1001122.

108. Epping-Jordan JE, Pruitt SD, Bengoa R, Wagner EH. Improving the quality of health care for chronic conditions. *Qual Saf Health Care*. 2004 Aug;13(4):299–305.

109. Prince MJ, Acosta D, Castro-Costa E, Jackson J, Shaji KS. Packages of care for dementia in low- and middle-income countries. *PLoS Med*. 2009 Nov;6(11):e1000176.

110. de Jesus MJ, Razzouk D, Thara R, Eaton J, Thornicroft G. Packages of care for schizophrenia in low- and middle-income countries. *PLoS Med*. 2009 Oct;6(10):e1000165.

111. Patel V, Thornicroft G. Packages of care for mental, neurological, and substance use disorders in low- and middle-income countries: PLoS Medicine Series. *PLoS Med*. 2009 Oct;6(10):e1000160.

112. Lund C, Breen A, Flisher AJ, et al. Poverty and common mental disorders in low and middle income countries: A systematic review. *Soc Sci Med*. 2010 Aug;71(3):517–28.

113. Skeen S, Lund C, Kleintjes S, Flisher A. Meeting the Millennium Development Goals in sub-Saharan Africa: what about mental health? *Int Rev Psychiatry*. 2010;22(6):624–31.

7 Social Determinants of Mental Health

Crick Lund, Stephen Stansfeld, and
Mary De Silva

INTRODUCTION

The role of social factors in determining public health outcomes is now widely accepted internationally.[1] Mental health is no exception. However, the precise manner in which mental health is socially determined is complex, and there are many features of the social determinants of mental health that distinguish it from other illnesses. Consequently, there is a growing international field of research dedicated to studying the social determinants of mental health and the interventions that may be required to address these determinants and improve the mental health of populations.

Understanding the social determinants of mental health is important for a number of reasons. First, it is essential to understand the etiology of mental disorders, not only from a genetic or individual perspective, but also from a social perspective. Social factors play a major role in determining the mental health status of individuals, interacting with more proximal genetic factors and individual experiences across the life course. Second, understanding this social etiology opens up opportunities for interventions at a population level. In particular, these can target the promotion of mental health and primary and secondary prevention of mental illness, with the aim of reducing social and health inequities. Third, with a better understanding of social determinants, population-level interventions that target these determinants can be planned more effectively and efficiently. This is particularly important, as tackling social determinants of mental health is likely to require the coordination of a range of social, health, education, and justice sectors.[2] Fourth, with the large body of international research and policy regarding the UN Millennium Development Goals (MDGs), and more recently, sustainable development goals (SDGs),[3] it is essential to link mental health with international development targets. As some have argued, mental health is crucial, both as a means and an end of global development, and there is substantial and growing evidence regarding these links[4-6] (see Chapter 6).

The purpose of this chapter is to review the current evidence on the associations between a variety of social determinants and mental health, to discuss some theoretical perspectives on the potential causal pathways that may link social factors and mental health, to summarize the evidence for interventions that may address both the social causes and consequences of mental illness, and to suggest avenues for policy development, implementation, and future research.

DEFINING AND MEASURING SOCIAL DETERMINANTS AND POVERTY

Addressing the social determinants of mental health immediately raises questions: What are social determinants, and how can they be measured? How do we define poverty? To what extent is poverty a composite measure of a range of more specific measures such as income, education, social class, material deprivation, and food insecurity? The WHO Commission on the Social Determinants of Health (CSDH) defines social determinants in very broad terms as follows: "The social determinants of health are the circumstances in which people are born, grow up, live, work, and age, and the systems put in place to deal with illness. These circumstances are in turn shaped by a wider set of forces: economics, social policies, and politics."[7] As health systems and services are discussed extensively in other chapters, in this chapter we will focus on the social and economic structures of society and the manner in which these influence the life circumstances and mental health of people across their life course.

There are many challenges with measuring social determinants. To illustrate, "absolute" poverty has traditionally been measured by the level of income of an individual or household. For example, the World Bank has in the past identified people living on less than $1 per day, or more recently, less than $2 per day, as living in "absolute poverty."[8] This approach is limited because it does not take into account inequalities in income within a society; it is often difficult to accurately assess income in informal low resource economies; and international comparisons are difficult because there are substantial differences between societies in what a dollar can purchase. Subsequently, approaches have focused on "relative poverty," which defines income in relation to the mean or median income within a given society.[8] This approach, while partially addressing issues of inequality, still does not resolve other limitations of income as a proxy for poverty. More recently, attempts have been made to develop multidimensional approaches to poverty; for example, through the use of "multiple deprivation" indices.[9] These build on Townsend's distinction between *deprivation* as the unmet needs people have for a number of basic commodities, and *poverty* as the lack of resources that are required to meet those needs.[10,11] Multiple deprivation indices include a number of indicators of social and economic deprivation and exclusion, such as income, education, housing, assets, and food insecurity, some of which may be combined in composite indices. Examples include the Index of Multiple Deprivation[9,12] and the Human Development Index.[13] These latter approaches carry advantages of being more explicit about their definitions, and when composite indicators are developed, it is possible to be more specific about weighting and measurement of various constructs.

The issue of definition is important, both for poverty studies and for understanding the social determinants of mental health. Social factors and their relationship with the prevalence and incidence of mental disorders have not been clearly conceptualized or measured in low- and middle-income countries (LMIC). Cooper and colleagues conducted a systematic review of psychiatric epidemiology studies that reported the relationship between poverty and common mental disorders (depression, anxiety, and somatoform disorders) in low- and middle-income countries from 1990 to 2008, and found diverse measures of poverty being employed.[14] Most of the

139 articles, representing 123 studies from 33 countries, did not provide a definition of the concept of poverty being used, and very few used validated or standardized measures. This inconsistent and weak conceptualization of poverty contributes to highly heterogeneous findings, and difficulties in understanding the causal pathways that may underpin the social determinants of mental health.

In a review of socioeconomic status in health research subtitled "One Size Does Not Fit All," Braveman and colleagues stressed the importance of considering plausible explanatory pathways and mechanisms, specifying the particular socioeconomic factors being measured, rather than measuring overall socioeconomic status (SES), and considering how unmeasured social and economic factors may potentially influence outcomes.[15] We will adopt this approach in this chapter, attempting to identify specific social and economic factors and their relationship with mental health throughout.

RELATIONSHIPS BETWEEN SOCIAL DETERMINANTS AND MENTAL HEALTH: WHAT DO WE KNOW FROM OBSERVATIONAL STUDIES?

A wide range of social determinants have been found to influence mental health. These may be conceptualized within an overall framework, as illustrated in Figure 7.1. The framework depicts the social determinants of mental health across five domains: demographic, social, economic, environmental structures, environmental events. Each of these is broken down into distal and proximal factors. These domains interact in multiple and complex ways. In the discussion that follows, we will attempt to document the evidence of associations of these factors with mental health outcomes.

Social and Economic Factors

Although social and economic factors are conceptually separate, they are often assessed using composite measures of SES, or socioeconomic position (SEP), in the psychiatric epidemiology literature.[14] Studies have shown that a range of mental disorders are associated with less-advantaged SEP. These include schizophrenia, depressive illness, substance misuse, and personality disorders.[16] In studies, SEP has been measured by a variety of indicators, such as social class (based on occupation), income, housing tenure, debt, financial problems, and educational attainment. In this section, we will report findings according to these specific indicators where they are identified in the research or in relation to composite indicators (e.g., SES), as they are defined in the studies we cite.

Socioeconomic Position in Childhood

Low SEP in childhood is associated with a higher risk of internalizing and externalizing disorders in childhood as well as depressive symptoms in later adulthood, adjusting for childhood socio-demographic factors, family history of mental illness, and adult SEP.[17] Social gradients in depression have also been found in adolescents in U.S. studies[18] but in some U.K. studies, there is an equalization of SEP effects of health in adolescence.[19]

Socioeconomic Position in Adulthood

Depressive illnesses show a strong association with less advantaged socioeconomic position.[20] A meta-analysis of 51 prevalence studies, five incidence studies, and four persistence studies, mostly from high-income countries (HIC), found that low SEP individuals had a higher risk of being depressed than high SEP individuals (unadjusted

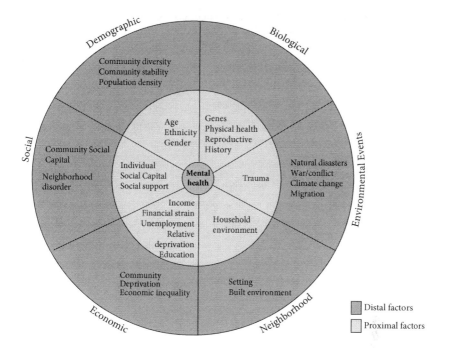

FIGURE 7.1

Social determinants of mental health: A conceptual framework.

OR = 1.81, p < 0.001).[20] In minor depressive and anxiety disorders, the social gradient tends to be shallower and less consistent. This may represent different social gradients for different types of common mental disorder (CMD). It may also reflect the less certain validity of milder categories of CMD in the global cross-cultural context. In addition, SEP, often measured by occupational social class, is only a distal determinant of depression, and financial disadvantage, unemployment, low income, low education, or low material standard of living have a more proximal effect on risk of disorder.[21–23] Living in rented accommodation,[24,25] financial strain,[26] and receiving welfare[27] have been associated with CMD. Financial and physical assets have been inversely associated with mood, anxiety, alcohol, and drug use disorders in the U.S. National Co-morbidity Study.[28] Living in a single adult household, which may be an indicator of poverty, is also consistently related to subsequent CMD.[29–31]

Some studies in HIC find associations between educational attainment and CMD,[32–34] while some do not.[35–37] In LMIC, a systematic review of associations between education and CMD found that 20 of 30 studies published between 1990 and 2008 showed a significant association between lower educational attainment and increased prevalence of CMD, while nine studies reported a null association, and one study reported unclear findings.[38] The evidence for occupational grade and CMD is mixed, with two studies finding an association[39,40] and another not.[41] The direction of evidence for the association between adult income and CMD appears to indicate that lower income is associated with greater risk for CMD, but there are exceptions, particularly when controlling for other variables. In one study, low income in African American women was predictive[36,42]; in another study, higher earning in African American males was found to be protective,[32,36] while Marmot and colleagues found an association in males but not in females in an ethnically heterogeneous sample.[36] Similarly, the findings from LMIC for associations between adult income and mental health determined that most bivariate analyses showed an association between lower income and CMD, but this was less evident in multivariate analysis.[38,43] These findings seem to indicate that income alone is unlikely to account entirely for population-level mental health disparities.

There is evidence of a short-term negative effect of unemployment on CMD, over one or two years,[21,44–47] either directly or through financial strain.[48] There is also evidence for longer-term effects; for example, in unemployed young adults there was increased risk of CMD at seven years[49] at 14 years,[50] and at 22 years.[51] In those that explored the effects of unemployment in adults of a broader age range, one found an association,[33] and one did not.[52]

There is some evidence that low SEP, and factors related to it such as poverty, may have stronger effects on maintaining depression than on the onset of depression. In Lorant's meta-analysis, the odds ratio for onset (OR = 1.24) were lower than the odds ratio for persistent depression (OR = 2.06).[20] Poverty, financial difficulties, and low income may thus prevent recovery once a person is depressed.[21] The most consistent evidence is that sustained or cumulative impoverishment (either measured by more than one indicator such as income or occupational class and poor material conditions at one time-point, or one indicator measured over several time-points) is associated with CMD.[17,25,30,53–56] In a Dutch aging study, older adults with high lifetime SEP had a lower risk for depression than older adults with a low lifetime level of SEP,[57] consistent with long-term income's being more important for health than current income and persistent poverty's being more noxious than occasional episodes of poverty.[54] There is also the possibility that this may be evidence of social drift in depression (see further discussion of social drift and social causation, below).

Social Capital

Popularized by Robert Putnam in the1990s,[58] *social capital*, or the "value" of social relationships, provides an explanation of how the social environment affects health, and is increasingly seen as a central construct in social policy and health, particularly in high-income countries.[59]

Measurement of Social Capital

There is a consensus that social capital consists of cognitive (perceptions of the quality of social relationships, such as trust and social harmony), structural (the quantity of social relationships, such as membership in groups), bonding (links between people of similar status), bridging (links between people of dissimilar status), and linking (links between different power levels) components.[60,61] There is also debate as to whether social capital is the property of both individuals (individual social capital—the impact of an individual's participating in a network and their perceptions about the quality of social relationships), and groups (most commonly a community, termed *ecological social capital*). Some authors argue that social capital can be both the property of individuals and groups, thereby recognizing the complex relationship between compositional and contextual factors.[62,63]

Critiques of Social Capital

The development of social capital theory has been extensively critiqued (see, for example[61,64–66]). A primary criticism is that social capital as a concept is too broad, essentially encompassing all social relationships at any level, be they within families or between state-level organizations.[64,67–69] While individual measures, such as the number of groups that an individual belongs to, have been criticized as "old wine in new bottles,"[70] ecological measures such as the percentage of non-voters show little commonality with such measures, and yet are included under the same term. The second major criticism levied against social capital is that the measurement does not match up to the theory.[71–73] A number of theorists stress that social capital is a multidimensional concept whose complexity cannot be accurately captured by a single question.[72–75] Yet a number of studies retrofit concepts of social capital onto existing survey data, resulting in measures such as newspaper readership or census response rates, which bear little relation to the theoretical concepts,[76–78] while other studies use only one indicator of social capital,[77,79] or collapse several indicators into one scale of low, medium, or high social capital.[78,80] Nevertheless, in recent years, progress has been made towards more theoretically informed and multidimensional measures,[75] although the debate about the level at which social capital should be measured persists.

Association Between Social Capital and Mental Illness

Despite the valid critiques about the definition and measurement of social capital, a growing body of research has explored the impact of social capital on mental illness. A systematic review found 21 studies of this possible relationship, only two of which were set in LMIC.[62] Though the studies showed fairly consistent associations between higher individual level cognitive social capital and reduced risk of mental illness, no clear pattern of association was found with individual level structural or ecological measures of social capital, largely due to the small number of studies in these areas. Since then, a number of largely cross-sectional studies in both HIC and LMIC have been conducted that generally confirm the positive association between individual and ecological-level cognitive social capital and mental health, including suicide rates and common mental disorders[43,81] and common mental disorders,[82–84,85] and more inconsistent associations with individual and ecological-level structural social capital.[62,86–89,85]

However, there is evidence that community-level social capital may not have the same effect for all people in a community. There is evidence from both high- and low-income countries that community-level cognitive social capital is associated with better mental health in individuals with a low socioeconomic status, but has no effect in those of a high socioeconomic status.[62,90] It is plausible that, in deprived populations, social capital acts to buffer an individual against the stressors that would otherwise cause mental ill health, and therefore that social capital could be used as an intervention to prevent vulnerable people from developing mental illness.

With no clear consensus on the definition and measurement of social capital, the relationship of each type of social capital to mental illness should be considered independently. In light of this, three conclusions can be drawn from the literature: both individual and ecological measures of social capital predict mental illness; cognitive social capital is consistently associated with better mental health, and structural social capital has more context-dependent effects as they relate to participation in the structures of a society; and social capital may be more important in deprived groups by acting to buffer the stress and negative life events associated with deprivation.

Economic Inequalities and Mental Health

Absolute levels of poverty are undoubtedly deleterious to mental health, but many studies suggest that there is a stepwise gradient of increasing ill health with increasingly disadvantaged economic position. One explanation for this is relative deprivation, which suggests that the magnitude of the difference between those in the most affluent and least affluent sections of a society has a powerful effect on mental health.[91] Wilkinson and colleagues have shown that levels of adult mental health and childhood well-being, as well as indicators of other social problems such as levels of hostility and homicides, vary by the degree of social inequality in a society.[92] Thus there are lower rates of these health and other social problems in more equal societies. This is a persuasive hypothesis demonstrated in many different data sets,[92] although some authors dispute the psychosocial explanation underlying the effects of inequality as too simplistic.[93] The convincing evidence for the association between national level economic inequality and mental ill-health is found largely in HIC. In LMIC there are not sufficiently robust nationally representative epidemiological studies to draw similar conclusions.

Environmental Structure: Area-Level Determinants of Mental Health

Area-level indicators of less advantaged SES have been associated with mental ill-health even after adjustment for individual SES.[94] This suggests that living in a poor neighborhood may have an influence on mental health independent of individual SES. Fear of crime, witnessing violence, poor neighborhood quality, and lack of access to social resources may all contribute to mental ill-health. In a classic study published in 1939, Faris and Dunham showed that the prevalence of psychosis was higher in the poor slum neighborhoods of Chicago than the wealthier neighborhoods.[95] This finding has received at least partial support from a meta-analysis of the incidence of schizophrenia, which shows higher rates in urban settings.[96] In relation to CMD, Ostler and colleagues have shown the negative influence of area level socioeconomic deprivation (as measured by Jarman under-privileged area scores) on the prevalence and outcomes of depression in adults attending primary care services in Hampshire, U.K.[29] In this study, under-privileged area scores accounted for 48.3% of the variance between primary care practices in the prevalence of depressive symptoms, measured using the Hospital Anxiety and Depression Scale. This trend has also been shown for suicidal ideation in older adult populations: in Monroe County, New York, residents of census tracts with median household income of less than $30,000 per annum were more likely to report suicidal ideation than residents of higher income census tracts (unadjusted odds ratio [OR] 4.60; 95% confidence interval [CI] 1.64–12.86), and this association was not eliminated after adjustment for demographic and baseline clinical factors.[30]

Environmental Events

A range of negative life events which occur as a result of natural disasters, war, and conflict have been identified as strong determinants of mental illness (see Chapter 17, Mental Health and Humanitarian Settings). In this context, climate change is likely to have a major influence on population mental health, although further research is clearly needed.[97] Evidence of the link between negative life events, economic adversity, and mental illness has been clearly conceptualized in Aneshensel's "stress-process" model of disparities, based on work from the Los Angeles depression study[98] (see Social Causation Mechanisms, below).

Demographic Factors: Vulnerable Groups

Ethnicity

Experiences of racism, exclusion, and alienation by ethnic minorities are likely to increase risk for a range of mental disorders. In a large case-control study of cumulative social disadvantage, ethnicity, and first episode psychosis in the United Kingdom, there was a clear linear association between cumulative disadvantage and odds of psychosis, with black Caribbeans experiencing greater social disadvantage and isolation than white

British subjects.[24] In studies of this nature, it may be difficult to disentangle the effects of migration and acculturation (discussed further below) from experiences of racism. In a meta-analysis of schizophrenia and migration, migrants from areas where the majority population is black, compared to white or neither black nor white showed a relative risk for schizophrenia of 4.8 (95% CI = 3.7–6.2).[99] However, findings from this review appear to indicate that ethnicity and not migration may have a more powerful effect, as the relative risk was higher in second-generation migrants: the mean weighted relative risk for developing schizophrenia among first-generation migrants was 2.7 (95% CI = 2.3–3.2) from 40 effect sizes, but in the same review, a separate analysis of second-generation migrants using seven effect sizes yielded a relative risk of 4.5 (95% CI = 1.5–13.1).

Findings about the influence of ethnicity on CMDs are complex and do not always follow the predicted pattern that disadvantaged minority ethnic groups are more vulnerable. In a large national household probability sample from the United States, lifetime prevalence of major depressive disorder was highest for whites (17.9%), followed by Caribbean blacks (12.9%), and African Americans (10.4%), and estimates were similar across groups for 12-month major depressive disorder.[100] However, the chronicity of major depressive disorder was higher for both black groups, and blacks were less likely to access treatment for depression than whites. This finding was confirmed by Breslau and colleagues, who reported that disadvantaged ethnic groups in the United States (specifically non-Hispanic blacks and Hispanics) had lower risk for anxiety and depression, but more persistent anxiety and depression.[101] In South Africa, there was reported to be no significant difference between ethnic groups in the 12-month prevalence of psychiatric disorders in a nationally representative survey, except that Africans had a lower risk of intermittent explosive disorder, and Indians had a lower risk of substance use disorder.[102,103] For lifetime prevalence, there was similarly no difference, except that whites had an increased risk of intermittent explosive disorder, and coloreds had an increased risk of substance use disorder.[103]

Gender

There is substantial evidence to indicate that women are at greater risk of developing common mental disorders, and men are at increased risk of substance abuse, with the effects of gender being frequently interconnected with social determinants of mental health.[104] Research has examined the effect of gender on how people respond to stressors,[105] and the different patterns of psychological distress among women compared to men.[106] For example, multiple roles, such as child-rearing, caring for sick relatives, and earning an income, are thought to put an increased burden and stress on women. Violence against women, in particular domestic violence, contributes significantly to women's stress and mental ill-health.[43,107–109] Low income and low levels of education make it more likely that women who suffer domestic violence will remain in abusive relationships.[110] Physical health problems also place a great burden on women with respect to their role as carers. This is of importance in the context of HIV/AIDS, where women may have to cope, not only with their families' ill health, but their own failing health as well.[105] Thus, poor women are a particularly at risk for common mental disorders, and conversely, women with poor mental health are particularly vulnerable to increasing levels of poverty (see Chapter 16—Gender).

Globalization

Globalization (defined by Wikipedia as "the process of international integration arising from the interchange of world views, products, ideas, and other aspects of culture"), economic restructuring, and the revolution in information and communication technology are crucial contextual considerations for the social determinants of mental health.[111] The economic and social changes associated with globalization have been linked with mental disorder in HICs and to a lesser extent in LMICs.[43,112–118] Globalization is likely to influence mental health through increased social and economic inequalities, partly driven by changing global trade regulations and the reduction of tariff and non-tariff restrictions on international trade.[119] There is evidence that trade fluctuations may negatively affect vulnerable groups such as small farmers in India, among whom the resulting high levels of debt have driven up rates of suicide.[43,120] In these settings, pesticides have been found to be a means of suicide or acts of deliberate self-harm.

In addition, globalization affects idioms of distress and pathways to care,[112] as people in LMICs adopt Western explanatory models as well as treatments.[117] For example, people who suffer from what might be diagnosed as a mental disorder using a Western nosological system may understand their condition using a complex combination of traditional and Western explanatory models, and this may affect both their attribution of causality and their treatment-seeking behavior. Increased rural to urban migration has occurred as a result of globalization, with the rural poor migrating to cities in search of work. This may lead to a reduction in support for mothers as traditional family structures are disrupted, and fathers and other family members migrate to cities. This also affects the elderly and mentally ill, who are less likely to be cared for. Social networks and community cohesiveness are also disrupted as whole families migrate in search of work.[117] Some authors argue that globalization is likely to be influenced by a range of contextual factors (described elsewhere in this chapter) and therefore may have heterogeneous effects on mental health[119] (see Chapter 8, Global Concerns).

THEORIES OF THE SOCIAL DETERMINANTS OF MENTAL HEALTH

Epidemiological studies on the social and economic correlates of mental illness have been largely cross-sectional, making it difficult to draw conclusions regarding causal pathways, particularly in LMIC. However, a growing number of longitudinal studies and RCTs, supplemented by qualitative research, are contributing to a burgeoning theoretical literature on the social determinants of mental health.

The excess of people with schizophrenia in less advantaged SES groups has traditionally been explained by the "social drift hypothesis" (sometimes known as the "social selection hypothesis") according to which people developing mental illness become unemployed, withdraw from social relationships, move to less expensive neighborhoods, and thus descend the social scale.[16] In this case, the social decline is secondary to the illness, and understood to be driven by reduced income and employment associated with the disability and stigma of the illness, together with increased health care expenditure. By contrast, the association between depressive illness or personality disorder and lower socioeconomic status is explained in terms of the "social causation hypothesis" where exposure to poverty, debt, unemployment, poor educational opportunities, substandard housing, frequent adverse life events, childhood neglect, and dangerous and impoverished environments contribute to the etiology of depression.

Some authors argue that these relationships are complex and that social causation factors may also influence people living with schizophrenia and conversely social drift factors may determine more adverse economic outcomes for people living with depression and anxiety disorders.[121] For example, the AESOP study has demonstrated that rates of psychosis may also be determined by social factors.[122] The dual action of these causal pathways has sometimes been referred to as a "vicious cycle" of poverty and mental illness.[123]

To refine these two broad pathways further, there are many possible mechanisms for the effects of social inequalities on mental health. We will present these according to each of the overall pathways described above.

Social Selection Mechanisms

The theory of *social selection* suggests that a person's health may determine their social position. As mentioned above, the major mechanisms implicated here appear to be reduced income and employment associated with the disability and stigma of mental illness, and increased health expenditure on both mental health care and general health care.[121] There is some intra-generational evidence for social drift occurring in schizophrenia and to a smaller extent in depression.[16] There is evidence that childhood psychological distress may lead to health selection into lower adult social class through interfering with social and educational development and hence upward social mobility.[124] However, in general, this has not been found to have a sizeable effect in mental or physical health. Health behaviors as an explanation are probably more relevant to physical illness. For example, in the case of cardiovascular morbidity, social gradients in disease may be explained by differences in smoking, blood pressure, cholesterol, glucose intolerance, and diet.[125]

Social Causation Mechanisms

Aneshensel has elaborated on the social causation pathways for depression through her *"stress process"* model (mentioned above).[98] According to this model, differential access to resources leads to lower SES household members' mental health being more sensitive to resource fluctuations than higher SES households, as they have less of a financial "buffer" to protect themselves from adverse events. In addition, lower SES households have more stressful life events, further increasing risk for common mental disorders such as depression and anxiety. This is borne out in some LMIC studies, for example in South Africa, where low SES groups had both increased negative life events and increased psychological distress, and the occurrence of recent life events appeared to partially mediate the association between SES and psychological distress ($p = 0.035$).[126]

Access to medical care has been put forward as a possible explanation of social class differentials in health. However, studies of mortality suggest that improvements in mortality have largely been among non-treatment amenable causes amongst higher social classes in the United Kingdom, thus not supporting a view that medical care is a major contributor to social class differentials.[127] Even with equal access to high quality care, there are social inequalities in response to treatment for depression.[128]

A *materialist explanation* focuses on environmental factors people are exposed to according to their socioeconomic status. Standard of housing, occupational hazards such as damaging chemical exposures, and psychosocial factors may be important. It is likely that these factors cluster in people of low SES where low-status jobs, poor incomes, inadequate housing in dangerous and rundown neighborhoods, exposure to high levels of pollution, and more psychosocial stress both at home and work may have a deleterious effect on mental as well as physical health. Although *psychosocial* and materialist explanations have been pitted against each other as explanations, this makes little sense as they are usually intertwined.[129] For instance, hazardous working conditions are associated with poor work-management, and household poverty is often, but not inevitably, associated with poor parenting.

Finally there are potential *biological mechanisms* for the social causation pathway. It is hypothesized that social inequalities "get under the skin" through the stress hypothesis where exposure to social disadvantage stimulates the hypothalamic-pituitary-adrenal (HPA) axis to secrete excessive levels of cortisol (a steroid hormone frequently released in response to stress) that lead to increased risk of illness. This was confirmed in the Mexican *Oportunidades* study, in which children in households in receipt of a social grant displayed significantly lower levels of salivary cortisol than children in households without grants.[130] This effect was more pronounced in households in which mothers scored higher on the Center for Epidemiological Studies—Depression (CES-D) scale. Exposure to stressors in adult life, such as financial strain, job insecurity, low control, and monotony at work, stressful life events, poor social networks, low self-esteem, and fatalism may have effects on health through neuroendocrine pathways.[131] Excessive production of glucocorticoids resulting from stimulation of the HPA axis is also related to increased risk of depression. Studies have shown links between C-reactive protein and depressive symptoms,[132] and baseline measures of high C-reactive protein and interleukin-6 have been shown to predict cognitive symptoms of depression at 12-year follow-up in the U.K. Whitehall II study.[133] Furthermore, there is evidence from human studies that social status is associated with increased HPA activity. Perceptions of control are an indicator of level in the social hierarchy. Low control at work has been related to risk of coronary heart disease and also to clotting factors such as fibrinogen. Prolonged exposure to stressful experiences may have a physiological adaptive cost in which there is a resetting of physiological parameters through a process defined as *allostasis*.[134]

These biological mechanisms are felt across the life course: childhood socioeconomic disadvantage may be linked to adult psychiatric disorder by either "critical period," pathway, or risk accumulation models.[135,136] In *critical period* models, there is exposure to socioeconomic disadvantage in childhood whose effects, sometimes on biological systems such as the HPA axis, remain latent until adulthood, and whose effects are independent of adult exposure to adversity. Sensitization of cortisol receptors related to exposure to adversity during early childhood may be related to exaggerated HPA responses in adulthood.

INTERVENTIONS THAT AIM TO BREAK THE CYCLE

Evidence presented above, regarding the two principle causal pathways of the social determinants of mental health (social causation and social drift/selection) raises the question: What interventions are required to break the cycle? More specifically, should interventions target the social causes of mental illness, for example by providing poverty alleviation through financial instruments such as grants and conditional cash transfers; improving nutrition, particularly in children; increasing food and water security in vulnerable communities; reducing socioeconomic inequality; and promoting safer and more secure living environments? Or should they target the social drift or social selection pathway by treating mental illness, reducing stigma and promoting recovery? Or, indeed, should both causal pathways be targeted? In this section we review some of the evidence regarding interventions that address the social causation and social selection/drift pathways. These are illustrated in Figure 7.2.

Social Causation Interventions

Financial Interventions

A recent systematic review of studies in LMIC found that the evidence for financial interventions targeting the social causation pathway was equivocal: while there was some support for the benefits of conditional cash transfers on childhood developmental and behavioral outcomes, as well as the benefits of asset promotion programs for self-esteem, there was no evidence of benefit from unconditional cash transfers or loans.[137] However, the absence of evidence does not necessarily indicate evidence of absence, as was shown in two subsequent studies not included in the review. Participation in the Mexican *Oportunidades* conditional cash-transfer program was shown to significantly reduce symptoms of maternal depression, while controlling for maternal age, education, and household demographic, ethnic, and socioeconomic

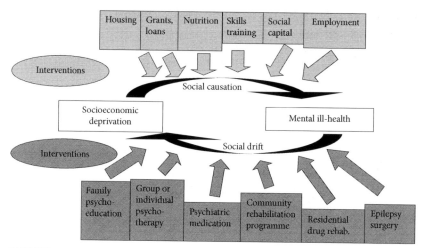

FIGURE 7.2

Interventions targeting the social causation and social drift pathways. Adapted with permission from Elsevier (Lund et al., 2011).

variables.[138] Similarly, in the *Bono de Desarrollo Humano* (BDH) unconditional cash transfer program in Ecuador, young children in households in receipt of a social grant in rural areas showed significant improvements in language development, although this was not shown in urban areas.[139] In relation to high-income countries, in the landmark Smoky Mountains study, Costello and colleagues evaluated the outcomes of the introduction of guaranteed income for families on an American Indian reservation as a result of the establishment of a casino in the area. In a four-year follow-up, Costello and colleagues reported that the Indian children whose family income was no longer below the poverty line showed a significant reduction in behavioral symptoms of oppositional defiant disorder and conduct disorder, although there was no effect on anxiety and depression symptoms.[140] The findings support a reasonably strong inference in support of the social causation hypothesis.[139]

Nutrition

A range of nutrition interventions (e.g., iodine supplementation) have been shown to yield improvements in cognitive and emotional development in children, alongside the well-documented physical health benefits.[141,142] Childhood undernutrition is generally associated with cognitive, motor, and behavioral deficits, and although the relationship is likely to be confounded by socioeconomic factors, nutrition supplementation trials have consistently shown concurrent benefits from pregnancy up to 24 months of age, suggesting a causal relationship.[43,141]

Skills Training, Employment, and Housing

There is a substantial literature on the mental health effects of skills training, employment generation, and housing improvements, although this evidence is predominantly from HICs. Such interventions may not have the improvement of mental health as their primary objective, but the fact that improvements in mental health have been shown to occur seems to indicate that the evaluation of mental health outcomes is an important line of enquiry. Much of this research is located within the growing field of mental health promotion and mental illness prevention research,[143,144] including in low-resource settings,[143–145] which indicates that such interventions can carry mental health and economic benefits (see Chapter 11—Mental Health Promotion and Prevention of Disorders). In particular, interventions that target infants and children through primary and secondary prevention and mental health promotion, have shown promise, including in LMIC, as highlighted in a recent *Lancet* series article on child mental health by Kieling and colleagues.[146]

Social Capital Interventions

The use of social capital as a health-promotion tool is tantalizing,[147] and strengthening social capital has been suggested as a way to improve various mental health outcomes, including reducing suicide[148] and improving the mental health of young people.[149] There is some evidence that social capital can be built through targeted interventions, though whether this has subsequent effect on mental health remains unknown. A randomized controlled trial of group-based microfinance with participatory gender and HIV training in South Africa showed significantly greater levels of cognitive and structural social capital generated in the intervention group, but this study did not assess the effect on mental health.[150] Similarly, a non-randomized study in Nicaragua showed that interventions promoting management and leadership in post-conflict communities significantly increased levels of cognitive social capital, and also higher levels of civic participation and political empowerment. Though these improvements in social capital were associated with positive individual health behaviors, such as a willingness to use modern medicine to treat childhood illnesses, their effect on mental health was not tested.[151] Only one non-randomized experimental study has demonstrated that a large-scale psychosocial intervention primarily aimed at creating social bonding caused a lasting improvement in mental health in survivors of the mass violence in Rwanda, though this intervention was primarily designed to improve mental health rather than build social capital.[152] Thus while it may be possible to have targeted interventions to build social capital, it remains untested whether social capital can be used as an intervention to prevent mental illness.

Social Drift/Selection Interventions

There is relatively strong evidence from LMIC that economic outcomes for people living with mental illness can be improved by successfully treating mental health problems. A recent systematic review of all intervention studies (including randomized and non-randomized intervention designs) assessing the effect of any intervention designed to treat any type of mental disorder in a low- or middle-income country showed that treatment interventions can lead to improvements in the economic status of both the individual suffering from mental health problems and their families and carers, thereby preventing a social drift into poverty.[137] The review identified nine studies from six countries assessing the effect of various mental health treatments for depression, psychosis, substance abuse, and epilepsy. The studies included three types of economic status: measures of employment status, family finances, and health care costs. Of the 19 associations tested, ten showed the interventions to have significant positive effects on economic status and nine had non-significant positive effects (or no tests of significance were provided). No study showed a mental health intervention to have a significant negative effect on economic status.

The three studies on interventions for depression were all randomized controlled trials. Group interpersonal psychotherapy for depression was associated with significant improvements in women's ability, but not men's, to perform daily tasks in Uganda.[153] Family-based community rehabilitation including drug treatment and psycho-education significantly decreased family economic burden, increased family employment, and increased the working ability of the patient in China.[43,154] Antidepressant treatment showed a non-significant reduction, and individual psychological therapy a non-significant increase, in family out-of-pocket payments for treatment in India.[155] Two of the three studies on interventions for psychosis were randomized controlled trials, one of which showed a significant positive effect of the intervention on economic status. Community-based rehabilitation in China including drug treatment and family psycho-education had a significant positive effect on duration of employment and the burden on family finances, but no effect on non-ill family members' working patterns or the patients' ability to work.[43,156] A non-randomized intervention study in India showed a reduction in work-related disability among participants who were prescribed antipsychotic drugs.[157] The two cohort studies that evaluated the effect of residential treatment programs for substance misuse in Iran[158,159] and Nigeria[158] showed improvements in employment status as a result of the intervention, but no tests of significance were provided, and both studies had biases that might have affected their results. The cohort study evaluating the effect of successful epilepsy surgery on multiple dimensions of employment status identified very large significant increases in productive work, average income, and job status.[160]

The findings of this review showed a clear trend in which mental health interventions are associated with improved economic outcomes in LMIC. All studies showed an economic benefit, although the difference was not statistically significant in every study. While some of the interventions may be too costly or technical to be suitable for delivery at scale by non-specialist health workers in LMIC (e.g., epilepsy surgery),[160] three studies did evaluate fairly simple and brief interventions that either were or could be delivered by non-specialist health workers.[153,155,157] Two of these studies showed significant improvements in functioning and economic status for small investments,[43,153,157] and the third showed a significant cost-effectiveness benefit of antidepressant treatment in improving clinical symptoms.[155]

Improvements in economic status go hand in hand with improvements in clinical symptoms, creating a virtuous cycle of increasing returns. All of the studies that showed a significant effect on economic status also showed a significant improvement in clinical status. These clinical improvements could also account for improvements in family economic status. Both randomized trials that explored the effect on family burden showed that patients in the intervention group had significantly fewer readmissions to hospital, shorter duration of hospital stay, and longer time in gainful employment compared with the control group, accounting for the reduced effect on the family finances in the intervention group.[43,154,156]

CONCLUSION: RECOMMENDATIONS FOR POLICY AND FUTURE RESEARCH

The findings of the systematic reviews outlined above suggest that certain interventions can have an impact in addressing the social determinants of mental health and breaking the cycle of poverty and mental ill-health. The current evidence base appears to be most robust for interventions that address the social drift pathway by providing treatment and rehabilitation interventions for people with mental illness. This evidence supports the call to scale up mental health services,[161] not only as a public health and human rights priority, but also a development priority. The evidence for poverty alleviation interventions addressing the social causation pathway is weaker, and there is an urgent need for further research, particularly to include methodologically sound mental health outcomes in evaluations of poverty alleviation interventions.

There are a number of potentially fruitful avenues for research on the social determinants of mental health in both HICs and LMICs. These include more robust studies to

(a) evaluate the mental health consequences of poverty alleviation interventions, including social grants, social capital, nutrition, improved food security, housing, and employment, as well as interventions to improve working conditions; and (b) evaluate the social and economic consequences of mental health interventions, particularly low cost community-based interventions that can be brought up to scale in low-resource settings. In addition, longitudinal observational studies are necessary to identify the relationships between more distal economic and structural forces and more proximal factors such as social capital and adverse life events, and their impact on mental health across the life course.

To conclude, several recent international developments have highlighted the global importance of the social determinants of mental health. The WHO Mental Health and Development report, published in 2010, makes a compelling case for targeting people with mental disorders in LMIC as a vulnerable group who require development assistance.[162] In the same year, the United Nations adopted a resolution on global health and foreign policy in which it recognized that mental ill-health has "huge social and economic consequences."[163] A review—Equity, Social Determinants and Public Health Programs—part of the WHO Commission on the Social Determinants of Health, also included a chapter on the social determinants of mental health (focusing on depression and attention deficit/hyperactivity disorder [ADHD]).[164] In addition, the World Health Assembly (WHA65.8) recently endorsed the Rio Political Declaration on Social Determinants of Health and called on member states to implement the pledges made in the Rio declaration. It also has proposed a global action plan for mental health, as set out in the recent World Health Assembly Resolution on mental health (WHA65.4). If these developments are to lead to substantial action to address the social determinants of mental health, it is vital that a combination of political will and robust research evidence be employed. Based on the evidence in this chapter, there are encouraging indications of growing understanding regarding these determinants, and growing evidence for interventions that can address upstream factors and ultimately improve the mental health and well-being of populations.

REFERENCES

1. Blas E, Kurup AS. *Equity, social determinants and public health programmes.* Geneva: WHO; 2010.
2. Skeen S, Kleintjes S, Lund C, et al. "Mental health is everybody's business": Roles for an intersectoral approach in South Africa. *Int Rev Psychiatry.* 2010;22(6):611–23.
3. Sachs JD. From millennium development goals to sustainable development goals. *Lancet.* 2012;379(9832):2206–11.
4. Lund C. Poverty and mental health: a review of practice and policies. *Neuropsychiatry.* 2012;2(3):213–9.
5. Miranda JJ, Patel V. Achieving the Millennium Development Goals: does mental health play a role? *PLoS Med.* 2005;2(10):0962–5.
6. Skeen S, Lund C, Kleintjes S, Flisher AJ. Meeting the Millennium Development Goals in sub-Saharan Africa: what about mental health? *Int Rev Psychiatry.* 2010;22(6):624–31.
7. WHO. *Closing the gap in a generation: Health equity through action on the social determinants of health.* Geneva: WHO; 2008.
8. Toye M, Infanti J. *Social inclusion and community economic development: Literature review.* Victoria, BC, Canada: The Canadian CED Network; 2004.
9. Barnes H, Wright G, Noble M, Dawes A. *The South African index of multiple deprivation for children: Census 2001.* Cape Town, SA: HSRC Press; 2007.
10. Townsend P. *Poverty in the United Kingdom.* Harmondsworth, Middlesex, UK: Penguin Books; 1979.
11. Townsend P. Deprivation. *J Soc Policy.* 1987;16:125–46.
12. Department of the Environment T, the R. *Measuring multiple deprivation at the small area level the indices of deprivation 2000.* London: DETR; 2000.
13. United Nations Development P. *Human Development Report 2006. Beyond scarcity: power, poverty and global water crisis.* New York: Macmillan; 2006.

14. Cooper S, Lund C, Kakuma R. The measurement of poverty in psychiatric epidemiology in LMICs: critical review and recommendations. *Soc Psychiatry Psychiatr Epidemiol.* 2011.

15. Braveman PA, Cubbin C, Egerter S, et al. Socioeconomic status in health research: one size does not fit all. *JAMA.* 2005;294(22):2879–88.

16. Dohrenwend BP, Levav I, Shrout PE, et al. Socioeconomic status and psychiatric disorders: the causation-selection issue. *Science.* 1992;255(5047):946–52.

17. Gilman SE. Childhood socioeconomic status, life course pathways and adult mental health. *Int J Epidemiol.* 2002;31(2):403–4.

18. Goodman E. The role of socioeconomic status gradients in explaining differences in US adolescents' health. *Am J Public Health.* 1999;89(10):1522–8.

19. Sweeting PW. Evidence on equalisation in health in youth from the West of Scotland. *Soc Sci Med.* 2004.

20. Lorant V, Deliege D, Eaton W, Robert A, Philippot P, Ansseau M. Socio-economic inequalities in depression: a meta-analysis. *Am J Epidemiol.* 2003;157:98–112.

21. Weich S, Lewis G. Poverty, unemployment, and common mental disorders: Population based cohort study. *BMJ.* 1998;317:115–9.

22. Fryers T, Melzer D, Jenkins R. Social inequalities and the common mental disorders: a systematic review of the evidence. *Soc Psychiatry Psychiatr Epidemiol.* 2003;38(5):229–37.

23. Melzer D, Fryers T, Jenkins R. *Social inequalities and the distribution of the common mental disorders.* Maudsley Monographs 44. Hove, UK: Psychology Press Ltd.; 2004.

24. Morgan C, Kirkbride J, Hutchinson G, et al. Cumulative social disadvantage, ethnicity and first-episode psychosis: a case-control study. *Psychol Med.* 2008;38(12):1701–15.

25. Power C, SA S, Matthews R, O M, S H. Childhood and adulthood risk factors for socio-economic differentials in psychological distress: evidence from the 1958 British birth cohort. *Soc Sci Med.* 2002.

26. Weich S, Sloggett A, Lewis G. Social roles and gender difference in the prevalence of common mental disorders. *Br J Psychiatry.* 1998;173:489–93.

27. Ahmed S, Rana A, Chowdhury M, Bhuiya A. Measuring perceived health outcomes in non-western culture: does SF-36 have a place? *J Health Pop & Nutr.* 2002 Dec;20(4):334–42.

28. Muntaner C, WW E, C D, RC K, PD S. Social class, assets, organizational control and the prevalence of common groups of psychiatric disorders. *Soc Sci Med.* 1998.

29. Ostler K, Thompson C, Kinmonth AL, Peveler RC, Stevens L, Stevens A. Influence of socio-economic deprivation on the prevalence and outcome of depression in primary care: the Hampshire Depression Project. *Br J Psychiatry.* 2001;178(1):12–7.

30. Cohen A, Chapman BP, Gilman SE, et al. Social inequalities in the occurrence of suicidal ideation among older primary care patients. *Am J Geriatr Psychiatry.* 2010;18(12):1146–54.

31. Ibrahim F, Cohen CI, Ramirez PM. Successful aging in older adults with schizophrenia: prevalence and associated factors. *Am J Geriatr Psychiatry.* 2010;18(10):879–86.

32. Neighbors HW, Caldwell C, Williams DR, et al. Race, ethnicity, and the use of services for mental disorders: results from the National Survey of American Life. *Arch Gen Psychiatry.* 2007;64(4):485–94.

33. K K, L P, M P. Selection into long-term unemployment and its psychological consequences. *Int J Behav Dev.* 2000.

34. Armstrong S. Rape in South Africa: an invisible part of apartheid's legacy. *Focus on Gender.* 1994;2(2):35–9.

35. Jokela M, Singh-Manoux A, Ferrie JE, et al. The association of cognitive performance with mental health and physical functioning strengthens with age: the Whitehall II cohort study. *Psychol Med.* 2010;40(5):837–45.

36. Marmot M, Shipley M, Brunner E, Hemingway H. Relative contribution of early life and adult socioeconomic factors to adult morbidity in the Whitehall II study. *J Epidemiol & Commun Health.* 2001;55(5):301–7.

37. Jaffee SR. Pathways to adversity in young adulthood among early childbearers. *J Fam Psychol.* 2002;16(1):38–49.

38. Lund C, Breen A, Flisher AJ, et al. Poverty and common mental disorders in low and middle income countries: a systematic review. *Soc Sci Med.* 2010;71(3):517–28.

39. SA S, Head J, Fuhrer R, Wardle J, V C. Social inequalities in depressive symptoms and physical functioning in the Whitehall II study: Exploring a common cause explanation. *J Epidemiol & Commun Health.* 2003.

40. Poulton R, Caspi A, Milne BJ, et al. Association between children's experience of socioeconomic disadvantage and adult health: a life-course study. *Lancet.* 2002;360(9346):1640–5.

41. Lindblad F, Hjern A, Vinnerljung B. Intercountry adopted children as young adults—a Swedish cohort study. *Am J Orthopsychiatry.* 2003;73(2):190–202.

42. Fernandez ME, Mutran EJ, Reitzes DC, Sudha S. Ethnicity, gender, and depressive symptoms in older workers. *Gerontologist.* 1998;38(1):71–9.

43. Araya R, Lewis G, Rojas G, Fritsch R. Education and income: which is more important for mental health? *Journal of Epidemiology and Community Health.* 2003;57:501–505.

44. Morrell S, Taylor R, Quine S, Kerr C, Western J. A cohort study of unemployment as a cause of psychological disturbance in Australian youth. *Soc Sci Med.* 1994;38(11):1553–64.

45. Hammarstrom A, Janlert U. Nervous and depressive symptoms in a longitudinal study of youth unemployment—selection or exposure? *J Adolescence.* 1997;20(3):293–305.

46. Breslin FC, Mustard C. Factors influencing the impact of unemployment on mental health among young and older adults in a longitudinal, population-based survey. *Scand J Work Environ & Health.* 2003;29(1):5–14.

47. Dooley D, Catalano R, Wilson G. Depression and unemployment: panel findings from the Epidemiologic Catchment Area study. *Am J Commun Psychol.* 1994;22(6):745–65.

48. Vuori J, Silvonen J, Vinokur AD, Price RH. The Tyohon job search program in Finland: benefits for the unemployed with risk of depression or discouragement. *J Occup Health Psychol.* 2002;7:5–19.

49. Pevalin DJ, Goldberg DP. Social precursors to onset and recovery from episodes of common mental illness. *Psychol Med.* 2003;33(2):299–306.

50. Hammarstrom A, Janlert U. Early unemployment can contribute to adult health problems: results from a longitudinal study of school leavers. *J Epidemiol & Commun Health.* 2002;56(8):624–30.

51. Upmark M, Lundberg I, Sadigh J, Allebeck P, Bigert C. Psychosocial characteristics in young men as predictors of early disability pension with a psychiatric diagnosis. *Soc Psychiatry Psychiatr Epidemiol.* 1999;34(10):533–40.

52. Montgomery SM, Cook DG, Bartley MJ, Wadsworth ME. Unemployment pre-dates symptoms of depression and anxiety resulting in medical consultation in young men. *Int J Epidemiol.* 1999;28(1):95–100.

53. Lynch JW, Kaplan GA, Shema SJ. Cumulative impact of sustained economic hardship on physical, cognitive, psychological, and social functioning. *N Engl J Med.* 1997;337(26):1889–95.

54. Benzeval M, Judge K. Income and health: the time dimension. *Soc Sci Med.* 2001;52(9):1371–90.

55. Everson SA, Maty SC, Lynch JW, Kaplan GA. Epidemiologic evidence for the relation between socioeconomic status and depression, obesity, and diabetes. *J Psychosom Res.* 2002;53(4):891–5.

56. Schoon I, Sacker A, Bartley M. Socio-economic adversity and psychosocial adjustment: a developmental-contextual perspective. *Soc Sci Med.* 2003;57(6):1001–15.

57. Grouse BV. [Unequal chances for reaching "a good old age." Socio-economic health differences among older adults from a life course perspective]. *Tijdschr Gerontol Geriatr.* 2003.

58. Putnam R. *Making democracy work: Civic traditions in modern Italy.* Princeton, NJ: Princeton University Press; 1993.

59. McKenzie K, Harpham T. *Social capital and mental health.* London: Jessica Kingsley; 2006.

60. Bain K, Hicks N. *Building social capital and reaching out to excluded groups: the challenge of partnerships.* Paper presented at CELAM meeting on The Struggle Against Poverty Towards the Turn of the Millennium; Washington, DC; 1998.

61. Szreter S, Woolcock M. Health by association? Social capital, social theory, and the political economy of public health. *Int J Epidemiol.* 2004;33:1–18.

62. De Silva MJ, McKenzie K, Huttly SR, Harpham T. Social capital and mental illness: a systematic review. *J Epidemiol & Commun Health.* 2005;59(8):619–27.

63. De Silva M. The methods minefield: a systematic review of the methods used in studies of social capital and mental health. In: McKenzie K, Harpham T, editors. *Social capital and mental health.* London: Jessica Kingsley Publishers; 2006.

64. Macinko J, Starfield B. The utility of social capital in research on health determinants. *Milbank Q.* 2001;79(3):387–427, IV.

65. Van Deth J, W. Measuring social capital: orthodoxies and continuing controversies. *Int J Social Res Method.* 2003;6(1):79–92.

66. Whitley R, McKenzie K. Social capital and psychiatry: review of the literature. *Harv Rev Psychiatry*. 2005;13(2):71–84.

67. Muntaner C, Lynch J, Smith GD. Social capital, disorganized communities, and the third way: understanding the retreat from structural inequalities in epidemiology and public health. *Int J Health Services*. 2001;31(2):213–37.

68. Fine B. They f**k you up those social capitalists. *Antipode*. 2002;34(4):796–9.

69. McKenzie K. Concepts of social capital—authors reply. *Br J Psychiatry*. 2003;182:458.

70. Lochner K, Kawachi I, Kennedy BP. Social capital: a guide to its measurement. *Health & Place*. 1999;5(4):259–70.

71. Woolcock M. Social capital and economic development: toward a theoretical synthesis and policy framework. *Theory & Society*. 1998;27:151–208.

72. Stone W. *Measuring social capital: Towards a theoretically informed measurement framework for researching social capital in family and community life*. Working paper. Melbourne: Australian Institute of Family Studies; Feb 2001. Report No.: 24.

73. McKenzie K, Whitley R, Weich S. Social capital and mental health. *Br J Psychiatry*. 2002;181(4):280–3.

74. Lynch J. *Is social capital relevant to population health?* Michigan; 2002.

75. Harpham T, Grant E, Thomas E. Measuring social capital within health surveys: key issues. *Health Policy & Planning*. 2002;17(1):106–11.

76. Harper S, Yang S, Angell S, et al. Is social capital associated with all causes of death? Unpublished manuscript, 2003.

77. Weitzman E, R, Kawachi I. Giving means receiving: the protective effect of social capital on binge drinking on college campuses. *Am J Public Health*. 2000;90:1936–9.

78. Rosenheck R, Morrissey J, Lam J, et al. Service delivery and community: social capital, service systems integration, and outcomes among homeless persons with severe mental illness. *Health Serv Res*. 2001;36(4):691–710.

79. McCulloch A. Social environments and health: cross-sectional national survey. *BMJ*. 2001;323:208–9.

80. Desai RA, Dausey DJ, Rosenheck RA. Mental health service delivery and suicide risk: the role of individual and facility factors. *Am J Psychiatry*. 2005;162(2):311–8.

81. Kelly BD, Davoren M, Mhaolain AN, Breen EG, Casey P. Social capital and suicide in 11 European countries: an ecological analysis. *Soc Psychiatry Psychiatr Epidemiol*. 2009;44(11):971–7.

82. Giordano GN, Lindstrom M. Social capital and change in psychological health over time. *Soc Sci Med*. 2011;72(8):1219–27.

83. Fitzsimon N, Shiely F, Corradino D, Friel S, Kelleher CC. Predictors of self-reported poor mental health at area level in Ireland: a multilevel analysis of deprivation and social capital indicators. *Ir Med J*. 2007;100(8): suppl 49–52.

84. Hamano T, Fujisawa Y, Ishida Y, Subramanian SV, Kawachi I, Shiwaku K. Social capital and mental health in Japan: a multilevel analysis. *PLoS One*. 2010;5(10):e13214.

85. De Silva MJ, Huttly SR, Harpham T, Kenward MG. Social capital and mental health: A comparative analysis of four low income countries. *Soc Sci Med*. 2007;64(1):5–20.

86. Araya R, Dunstan F, Playle R, Thomas H, Palmer S, Lewis G. Perceptions of social capital and the built environment and mental health. *Soc Sci Med*. 2006;62(12):3072–83.

87. Forsman AK, Nyqvist F, Wahlbeck K. Cognitive components of social capital and mental health status among older adults: a population-based cross-sectional study. *Scand J Public Health*. 2011;39(7):757–65.

88. Phongsavan P, Chey T, Bauman A, Brooks R, Silove D. Social capital, socio-economic status and psychological distress among Australian adults. *Soc Sci Med*. 2006;63(10):2546–61.

89. Poblete FC, Sapag JC, Bossert TJ. [Social capital and mental health in low income urban communities in Santiago, Chile]. *Rev Med Chil*. 2008;136(2):230–9.

90. Stafford M, De Silva M, Stansfeld S, Marmot M. Neighbourhood social capital and common mental disorder: testing the link in a general population sample. *Health & Place*. 2008;14(3):394–405.

91. Wilkinson RG. Socioeconomic determinants of health. Health inequalities: relative or absolute material standards? *BMJ*. 1997;314(7080):591–5.

92. Pickett KE, Wilkinson RG. Greater equality and better health. *BMJ*. 2009;339: b4320.

93. Lynch J. Income inequality and health: expanding the debate. *Soc Sci Med*. 2000;51(7):1001–5; discussion 9–10.

94. Fone D, Dunstan F, Lloyd K, Williams G, Watkins J, Palmer S. Does social cohesion modify the association between area income deprivation and mental health? A multilevel analysis. *Int J Epidemiol*. 2007;36(2):338–45.

95. Faris RE, Dunham HW. *Mental disorders in urban areas: an ecological study of schizophrenia and other psychoses*. Chicago: University of Chicago Press; 1939.

96. McGrath J, Saha S, Welham J, El Saadi O, MacCauley C, Chant D. A systematic review of the incidence of schizophrenia: the distribution of rates and the influence of sex, urbanicity, migrant status and methodology. *BMC Med*. 2004;2:13.

97. Berry HL, Bowen K, Kjellstrom T. Climate change and mental health: a causal pathways framework. *Int J Public Health*. 2010;55(2):123–32.

98. Aneshensel C. Toward explaining mental health disparities. *J Health & Soc Behav*. 2009;50:377–94.

99. Cantor-Graae E, Selten JP. Schizophrenia and migration: a meta-analysis and review. *Am J Psychiatry*. 2005;162(1):12–24.

100. Williams DR, Gonzalez HM, Neighbors H, et al. Prevalence and distribution of major depressive disorder in African Americans, Caribbean blacks, and non-Hispanic whites: results from the National Survey of American Life. *Arch Gen Psychiatry*. 2007;64(3):305–15.

101. Breslau J, Kendler KS, Su M, Gaxiola-Aguilar S, Kessler RC. Lifetime risk and persistence of psychiatric disorders across ethnic groups in the United States. *Psychol Med*. 2005;35(3):317–27.

102. Williams DR, Herman A, Stein DJ, et al. Prevalence, service use and demographic correlates of 12-month psychiatric disorders in South Africa: the South African Stress and Health Study. *Psychol Med*. 2008;38(2):211–20.

103. Stein DJ, Seedat S, Herman A, et al. Lifetime prevalence of psychiatric disorders in South Africa. *Br J Psychiatry*. 2008;192:112–7.

104. Harpham T, Snoxell S, Grant E, Rodriguez C. Common mental disorders in a young urban population in Colombia. *Br J Psychiatry*. 2005;187:161–7.

105. Patel V, Araya R, de Lima M, Ludermir A, Todd C. Women, poverty and common mental disorders in four restructuring societies. *Soc Sci Med*. 1999;49(11):1461.

106. Desjarlais R, Eisenberg L, Good B, Kleinman A. *World mental health: Problems and priorities in low-income countries*. New York: Oxford University Press; 1995.

107. Bowman C. Domestic violence: does the African context demand a different approach? *Int J Law & Psychiatry*. 2003;26(5):473–91.

108. Ceballo R, Ramirez C, Castillo M, Caballero GA, Lozoff B. Domestic violence and women's mental health in Chile. *Psychol Women Q*. 2004;28(4):298–308.

109. Jewkes R, Levin J, Penn-Kekana L. Risk factors for domestic violence: findings from a South African cross-sectional study. *Soc Sci Med*. 2002;55(9):1603–18.

110. Miller G. Poor countries, added perils for women. *Science*. 2005;308(5728 (Electronic)):1576–.

111. National Academies Press. *Cities transformed: Demographic change and its implications in the developing world*. 2003 2005/10/07/ [cited; Available from:

112. Bhugra D, Mastrogianni A. Globalisation and mental disorders: overview with relation to depression. *Br J Psychiatry*. 2004;184(10):20.

113. Chan KP, Hung SF, Yip PS. Suicide in response to changing societies. *Child & Adolesc Psychiatr Clin North Am*. 2001;10:777–95.

114. Dech H, Ndetei D, Machleidt W. Social change, globalization and transcultural psychiatry: some considerations from a study on women and depression. *Seishin Shinkeigaku Zasshi*. 2003;105(1):17–27.

115. Lewis G, Araya R. Globalization and mental health. In: Sartorius N, Gaebel W, editors. *Psychiatry in society*. 2002:57–78.

116. Mastrogianni A, Bhugra D. Editorial: Globalization, cultural psychiatry and mental distress. *Int J Soc Psychiatry*. 2003;49(3):163.

117. Swartz L. Globalisation and mental health. *Insights Health*. 2005;6.

118. Yang MJ. Globalization and mental health status in Taiwan. *Int Med J*. 2004;11:203–11.

119. Corrigall J, Plagerson S, Lund C, Myers J. Global trade and mental health. *Global Social Policy*. 2008;8(3):335–58.

120. Chowdhury AN, Banerjee S, Brahma A, Weiss MG. Pesticide practices and suicide among farmers of the Sundarban region in India. *Food & Nutrition Bull*. 2007;28(2 Suppl): S381–91.

121. Saraceno B, Itzhak L, Kohn R. The public mental health significance of research on socio-economic factors in schizophrenia and major depression. *World Psychiatry*. 2005;4(3):181–5.

122. Morgan C, Hutchinson G. The social determinants of psychosis in migrant and ethnic minority populations: a public health tragedy. *Psychol Med.* 2009:1-5.

123. Patel V. Poverty, inequality, and mental health in developing countries. In: Leon DA, Walt G, editors. *Poverty, inequality and health: An international perspective.* Oxford, UK: Oxford University Press; 2001:247-62.

124. Stansfeld SA, Clark C, Rodgers B, Caldwell T, Power C. Repeated exposure to socioeconomic disadvantage and health selection as life course pathways to mid-life depressive and anxiety disorders. *Soc Psychiatry Psychiatr Epidemiol.* 2011;46(7):549-58.

125. Link BG, Phelan J. Social conditions as fundamental causes of disease. *J Health & Soc Behav.* 1995;35:80-94.

126. Myer L, Stein DJ, Grimsrud A, Seedat S, Williams DR. Social determinants of psychological distress in a nationally representative sample of South African adults. *Soc Sci Med.* 2008;66(8):1828-40.

127. Marmot M. Social differentials in health within and between populations. *Daedalus.* 1994;123(4):197-216.

128. Cohen A, Houck PR, Szanto K, Dew MA, Gilman SE, Reynolds CF, III. Social inequalities in response to antidepressant treatment in older adults. *Arch Gen Psychiatry.* 2006;63(1):50-6.

129. Gilman SE, Kawachi I, Fitzmaurice GM, Buka SL. Socioeconomic status in childhood and the lifetime risk of major depression. *Int J Epidemiol.* 2002;31(2):359-67.

130. Fernald L, Gunnar M. Poverty-alleviation program participation and salivary cortisol in very low-income children. *Soc Sci Med.* 2009;68(12):2180-9.

131. Brunner E. Stress and the biology of inequality. *BMJ.* 1997;314(7092):1472-6.

132. Pikhart H, Hubacek JA, Kubinova R, et al. Depressive symptoms and levels of C-reactive protein: a population-based study. *Soc Psychiatry Psychiatr Epidemiol.* 2009;44(3):217-22.

133. Gimeno D, Kivimaki M, Brunner EJ, et al. Associations of C-reactive protein and interleukin-6 with cognitive symptoms of depression: 12-year follow-up of the Whitehall II study. *Psychol Med.* 2009;39(3):413-23.

134. McEwen BS, Magarinos AM. Stress effects on morphology and function of the hippocampus. *Ann NY Acad Sci.* 1997;821:271-84.

135. C H, C P. Child development as a determinant of health across the life course. *Current Paediatrics.* 2004.

136. D K, Ben-Shlomo Y. A life course approach to chronic disease epidemiology. 2004.

137. Lund C, De Silva M, Plagerson S, et al. Poverty and mental disorders: breaking the cycle in low-income and middle-income countries. *Lancet.* 2011;378(9801):1502-14.

138. Ozer EJ, Fernald LC, Weber A, Flynn EP, VanderWeele TJ. Does alleviating poverty affect mothers' depressive symptoms? A quasi-experimental investigation of Mexico's *Oportunidades* program. *Int J Epidemiol.* 2011;40(6):1565-76.

139. Fernald LC, Hidrobo M. Effect of Ecuador's cash transfer program (*Bono de Desarrollo Humano*) on child development in infants and toddlers: a randomized effectiveness trial. *Soc Sci Med.* 2011;72(9):1437-46.

140. Costello E, Compton S, Keeler G, Angold A. Relationship between poverty and psychopathology: A natural experiment. *JAMA.* 2003;290(15):2023-9.

141. Grantham-McGregor S, Baker-Henningham H. Review of the evidence linking protein and energy to mental development. *Public Health Nutr.* 2005;8(7A):1191-201.

142. Grantham-McGregor SM, Cheung YN, Cueto S, Glewwe P, Richter L, Strupp B. Developmental potential in the first 5 years for children in developing countries. *Lancet.* 2007;369:60-70.

143. WHO. *Prevention of mental disorders: Effective interventions and policy options.* Geneva: WHO; 2004.

144. WHO. *Promoting mental health: Concepts, emerging evidence, practice.* Geneva: WHO; 2005.

145. Petersen I, Bhana A, Flisher A, Swartz A, Richter L. *Promoting mental health in scarce-resource contexts.* Cape Town, SA: HSRC; 2010.

146. Kieling C, Baker-Henningham H, Belfer M, et al. Child and adolescent mental health worldwide: evidence for action. *Lancet.* 2011;378(9801):1515-25.

147. Eriksson M. Social capital and health—implications for health promotion. *Global Health Action.* 2011;4.

148. Patel V. Building social capital and improving mental health care to prevent suicide. *Int J Epidemiol.* 2010;39(6):1411-2.

149. Boyd CP, Hayes L, Wilson RL, Bearsley-Smith C. Harnessing the social capital of rural communities for youth mental health: an asset-based community development framework. *Aust J Rural Health*. 2008;16(4):189–93.

150. Pronyk PM, Harpham T, Busza J, et al. Can social capital be intentionally generated? a randomized trial from rural South Africa. *Soc Sci Med*. 2008;67(10):1559–70.

151. Brune NE, Bossert T. Building social capital in post-conflict communities: evidence from Nicaragua. *Soc Sci Med*. 2009;68(5):885–93.

152. Scholte WF, Verduin F, Kamperman AM, Rutayisire T, Zwinderman AH, Stronks K. The effect on mental health of a large scale psychosocial intervention for survivors of mass violence: a quasi-experimental study in Rwanda. *PLoS One*. 2011;6(8):e21819.

153. Bolton P, Bass J, Neugebauer R, et al. Group interpersonal psychotherapy for depression in rural Uganda: a randomized controlled trial. *JAMA*. 2003;289(23):3117–24.

154. Hu X, Wang YL, Fu HP. [Synthetical family treatment for depression: a randomized-controlled single-blind study among 76 cases]. *J Clin Rehabil Tissue Engineering Res*. 2007;11:7787–90.

155. Patel V, Chisholm D, Rabe-Hesketh S, Dias-Saxena F, Andrew G, Mann A. Efficacy and cost-effectiveness of drug and psychological treatments for common mental disorders in general health care in Goa, India: a randomised, controlled trial. *Lancet*. 2003;361(9351):33–9.

156. Xiong W, Phillips MR, Hu X, et al. Family-based intervention for schizophrenic patients in China. A randomised controlled trial. *Br J Psychiatry*. 1994;165(2):239–47.

157. Thirthalli J, Venkatesh BK, Kishorekumar KV, et al. Prospective comparison of course of disability in antipsychotic-treated and untreated schizophrenia patients. 2009;119(3):209–17.

158. Lawal RA, Adelekan ML, Ohaeri JU, Orija OB. Rehabilitation of heroin and cocaine abusers managed in a Nigerian psychiatric hospital. 1998;75(2):107–12.

159. Abdollahnejad MR. Follow-up evaluation of Tehran therapeutic community. *Therapeutic Communities*. 2008;29(1):57–75.

160. Locharernkul C, Kanchanatawan B, Bunyaratavej K, et al. Quality of life after successful epilepsy surgery: evaluation by occupational achievement and income acquisition. 2005.

161. Group. LGMH. Scale up services for mental disorders: a call for action. *Lancet*. 2007;370:1241–52.

162. WHO. *Mental Health and Development: Targeting people with mental health conditions as a vulnerable group*. Geneva: World Health Organization and Mental Health and Poverty Project;2010.

163. United Nations. *United Nations General Assembly Resolution on Global Health A/65/L.27*. New York: United Nations; 2010.

164. Patel V, Lund C, Hatherill S, et al. Mental disorders: equity and social determinants. In: Blas E, Sivasankara Kurup A, editors. *Equity, social determinants and public health programmes*. Geneva: WHO; 2010:115–34.

8 Human Security, Complexity, and Mental Health System Development

Harry Minas

Good health, like so many things, is inequitably distributed. Entering the twenty-first century, about half the world's people had been left behind, unable to achieve their full health potential. World health today spotlights the paradox of unprecedented achievement among the privileged and a vast burden of preventable diseases among those less privileged, the majority of humankind. Differing risks and vulnerabilities to avoidable health insults are found among people of different ages, sexes, communities, classes, races and nations. No surprise then that the poor, marginalized, and excluded have a higher risk of dying than other groups. Especially vulnerable are children and women across all groups. These disparities are found not only among countries—but within countries, rich and poor.

—Commission on Human Security[1]

We stress the right of people to live in freedom and dignity, free from poverty and despair. We recognize that all individuals, in particular vulnerable people, are entitled to freedom from fear and freedom from want, with an equal opportunity to enjoy all their rights, and fully develop their human potential. To this end, we commit ourselves to discussing and defining the notion of human security in the General Assembly.

—UN General Assembly Resolution 60/1[2]

Mental illness is a major public health problem. The high prevalence of mental disorders[3]; the staggering annual loss of life from suicide,[4] the most common cause of death among young adults; the premature all-cause mortality of people with schizophrenia and other mental disorders; the high disability burden attributable to mental disorders;[5] the massive loss of economic productivity; and the abject poverty[6-10] and misery of so many people with mental disorders, most of whom have no access to treatment and care in low- and middle-income countries; would suggest that mental disorders should be a high priority for governments and for health services. And yet mental health has, until recent years, been largely ignored by governments, bilateral aid agencies and other major development funders, international development NGOs, researchers, and educators. This situation has begun to change. Evidence for action has been effectively marshalled,[11–25] effective intervention packages are available,[26–32] and the global mental health community is becoming better organized[13,33–35] and is engaging more effectively in the global development agenda.

Australia is committed to reducing poverty and achieving sustainable development in developing countries, and improving responses to people with mental illness is an important building block towards achieving this....Unless the needs of people with disability, including those with mental illness, are met, it will not be possible to achieve the targets of the Millennium Development Goals by 2015.[36]

There is a renewed commitment to focus attention on the mental health of populations and on the scaling up of mental health services that have the capacity to respond to mental health service needs.[15,37–45] There is general agreement that scaling up activities must be evidence-based and that the effectiveness of such activities must be evaluated. If these requirements are to be realized, it will be essential to strengthen capacity in countries to conduct rigorous monitoring and evaluation of system development projects and to demonstrate sustained benefit to populations. Failure to sustain long-term gains from even well designed and implemented community mental health system development projects is a source of serious concern and is all too common.

GLOBAL CONCERNS

At every point in history, including now, the world has been beset by troubles. Armed conflict is currently raging in Mali, Afghanistan, Syria, and many other places. Asylum seekers and refugees from the world's conflicts are being increasingly viewed with suspicion, and ever-tighter border control measures are being put in place by receiving countries. Civil unrest has again broken out in Egypt, and, unexpectedly, on the streets of Belfast, Ireland. Preoccupation with the threat of global terrorism and the ill-conceived "war on terror" have resulted in the readiness of democracies to engage in flagrant human rights abuses in pursuit of the objectives of this "war." Economic catastrophe in Greece and other countries of southern Europe, with unemployment among the young at over 50% in Spain, and ineffectual wrangling over economic policy in the Congress of the United States, demonstrate that there is no clear end in sight for what is already the longest and most severe economic crisis in decades. Widespread poverty, particularly in Africa and Asia, with all of its attendant miseries has been reduced in the past two decades, but hundreds of millions still live in debilitating poverty.

Sexual violence against women, resulting in global public attention (and widespread demonstrations in India following the brutal rape and murder of a student on a bus in New Delhi) occurs everywhere and in most instances goes unremarked. Abuse of children in families and by trusted institutions such as the Catholic Church, has resulted finally in the announcement of a Royal Commission in Australia.[46]

Less spectacular but no less important than these dramatic events for mental health is the daily and widespread structural discrimination experienced by multiple population sub-groups, indigenous and ethnic minorities, religious minorities, gay and lesbian men and women, people with disabilities, people with mental disorders, and many others. Discrimination that blights lives by oppression, exclusion and marginalization.

Climate change and the future horrors that are being predicted in the absence of coordinated global action to deal with this current and looming threat is perhaps the greatest challenge facing humanity, resulting in observable increases in the number and severity of extreme weather events and natural disasters resulting in devastation, particularly for increasingly densely populated coastal communities.

HUMAN SECURITY

Human security in its broadest sense embraces far more than the absence of violent conflict. It encompasses human rights, good governance, access to education and health care and ensuring that each individual has opportunities and choices to fulfill his or her own potential. Every step in this direction is also a step towards reducing poverty, achieving economic growth and preventing conflict. Freedom from want, freedom from fear and the freedom of future generations to inherit a healthy natural environment— these are the interrelated building blocks of human, and therefore national, security. (Kofi Annan[1])

The concept of human security[47,48] is a shift in focus from the security of states to the security of people. It recognizes that, while the state remains the main guarantor of the security of its citizens, states frequently fail to fulfill their security obligations, and sometimes become the key source of threat, to their own people. The Commission on Human Security's definition of *human security* is "to protect the vital core of all human lives in ways that enhance human freedoms and human fulfillment."[1] Human security means protecting fundamental freedoms and protecting people from severe and pervasive threats. It also means building on people's strengths and aspirations, and creating political, social, environmental, economic, military, and cultural systems that protect human survival, livelihood, and dignity. The concept of human security broadens the focus from security of state borders to focus on the lives of people within and across state borders. Human security connects several kinds of freedoms: freedom from want, freedom from fear, and freedom to take action on one's own behalf. The overriding goal of human security is to expand the real freedoms that people must have to live a long, fulfilling, and productive life.

The enlargement of freedoms requires action from above and from below. It requires protection from threats that are outside the control of individuals and communities, and empowerment strategies that will strengthen resilience and reduce vulnerabilities.

Protection. People are deeply threatened by menaces that are beyond their control, threats such as violent conflict, climate change, financial crisis, poverty and destitution, environmental degradation, infectious diseases epidemics, natural and man-made disaster, lack of access to essential services such as health, education, and clean water. All of these threats reduce freedoms and erode capabilities. Effective protection requires a clear understanding of the threats, preparation, and prevention, effective response and recovery, and minimizing of harms.

Empowerment involves fostering the ability of people and communities to act on their own behalf, and on behalf of others. This requires access to education and information that enables scrutiny of social arrangements and individual and collective action. It requires access to health care and basic social services and protections. It encourages plurality, and engagement in discussion and decision-making. It builds capability and the resilience necessary to creatively and adaptively respond to risk and threats.

Human Rights

Attention to the human rights of people with mental illness has a long history. Resolution 33/53 of the United Nations General Assembly requested of the UN Commission on

Human Rights that "the study of the question of the protection of those detained on the grounds of mental ill health be undertaken as a matter of priority by the Sub-Commission on Prevention of Discrimination and Protection of Minorities."[49] The outcome of this work was General Assembly Resolution 46/119, adopted in December 1991, which established principles for the protection of persons with mental illness and the improvement of mental health care.[50] The first of the 25 principles enunciated in Resolution 46/119 is headed *Fundamental Freedoms and Basic Rights*, asserting that all persons have the right to the best available mental health care, which shall be part of the health and social care system. All persons with mental illness shall be treated with humanity and respect for the inherent dignity of the human person, and have the right to protection from exploitation, abuse, and degrading treatment. All persons with mental illness have the right to freedom from discrimination, and freedom to exercise all civil, political, economic, social, and cultural rights, as recognized by the Universal Declaration of Human Rights;[51] the International Covenant on Economic, Social and Cultural Rights;[52] the International Covenant on Civil and political Rights;[53] and other relevant instruments.

Table 8.1 is not a complete but an indicative listing of global and regional instruments relevant to the protection of the rights of persons with mental illness. Despite this impressive international legal architecture designed to protect human rights, most low- and middle-income countries (LAMICs) have not signed or ratified these instruments. Of the LAMICs that have ratified UN instruments, most do not have the institutional arrangements, financial resources, and technical capabilities that are required to give effect to these clearly articulated citizen's rights and state obligations. The consequence is a widespread abuse of the basic human rights of people with mental disorders.[37,54–56]

Implementation of the core principles of human security—protection and empowerment—is one of the most urgent and important imperatives of global mental health.

THREATS

Threats are events or circumstances that[1] are likely to degrade the quality of life of individuals, communities or whole populations, or[2] significantly narrow the range of policy choices available to governments or to private, nongovernmental entities (persons, groups, corporations). In addition to military actions or civil disorder, events such as population growth, urbanization, and migration should be considered as security threats.

Risks and threats may be sudden—such as conflict or economic or political collapse. But they need not be, for what defines a menace to human security is its depth, not only its swift onset. And many threats and disastrous conditions are pervasive—affecting many people, again, and again. Some causes of human insecurity are deliberately orchestrated, and some are inadvertent, the unexpected downside risks. Some, such as genocide or discrimination against minorities, threaten people's security directly. Others are indirect threats: when military overinvestment causes under-investment in public health, when the international community does not provide sufficient resources to protect refugees in a deprived area. But these menaces must be identified and prioritized in an empowering way.[1]

Violent conflict

Wars between states, internal conflicts and transnational terrorism pose major risks to people's survival, livelihoods, and dignity—and thus to human security. An estimated 190 million people were killed directly or indirectly as a result of the 25 largest violent conflicts in the twentieth century, often in the name of religion, politics, ethnicity or racial superiority. In many societies, violent conflict suffocates daily life, adding to pervasive feelings of insecurity and hopelessness. During conflict, groups may engage in gross

Table 8.1 Human Rights and Instruments

Year	Organization	Instrument
1948	UN	Universal Declaration of Human Rights, Article 25[51]
1950	Council of Europe	Convention for the Protection of Human Rights and Fundamental Freedoms
1966	UN	Convention on Economic, Social and Cultural Rights, Article 12[52]
1966	UN	International Covenant on Civil and Political Rights, Article 7[53]
1966	UN	International Covenant on the Elimination of All Forms of Racial Discrimination
1966	Council of Europe	Revised European Social Charter (Article 15—The right of persons with disabilities to independence, social integration, and participation in the life of the community)
1975	UN	Declaration on the Rights of Disabled Persons
1977	Council of Europe	Recommendation on the Situation of the Mentally Ill
1979	UN	Convention on the Elimination of all Forms of Discrimination against Women, Article 12
1982	UN	World Programme of Action concerning Disabled Persons
1987	Council of Europe	European Convention for the Prevention of Torture and Inhuman or Degrading Treatment or Punishment, Article 18
1988	UN	Body of Principles for the Protection of all Persons Under Any Form of Detention or Imprisonment
1988	Organization of American States	Additional Protocol to the American Convention on Human Rights in the Area of Economic, Social, and Cultural Rights
1989	UN	Convention on the Rights of the Child, Article 25
1991	UN	Principles for the Protection of Persons with Mental Illness and the Improvement of Mental Health Care
1992	Council of Europe	Recommendation 1185 on Rehabilitation Policies for the Disabled
1992	Council of Europe	A Coherent Policy for People with Disabilities
1993	UN	Standard Rules on Equalisation of Opportunities for Persons with Disabilities
1996	European Parliament	Resolution on the Human Rights of Disabled People
1999	Organization of American States	Organization of American States Inter-American Convention on the Elimination of All Forms of Discrimination Against Persons with Disabilities
2000	European Union	Charter of Fundamental Rights of the European Union, Articles 21 and 26
2007	UN	Convention on the Rights of Persons with Disabilities

violations of human rights and war crimes, including torture, genocide, and the use of rape as a weapon of war.[1]

There is a clear link between poverty, low levels of human development, and violent conflict. In 2002, 16 of the 20 countries with the lowest Human Development Index were in the midst of violent conflict (mostly internal) or had just emerged from such a conflict. Among the factors that make violent conflict more likely are the following: competition over land and resources; sudden and profound political, social, and economic transitions, particularly rapid economic decline; growing and obvious economic gap between the rich and the poor; increasing crime, corruption in government and business; weak and unstable, and therefore vulnerable, political regimes and institutions; and ethnic, religious, and communal antipathies and competition for influence. Internal violent conflict can frequently spill over borders into neighboring countries. Conflicts are frequently financed by illegal activities, including arms smuggling, and drug trafficking and money laundering. They breed criminal syndicates that stand to make huge profits. In some cases, government, and opposition groups are themselves not much more than criminal syndicates, fighting over the spoils of power. Areas of conflict are also perfect environments for the organization of terrorist organizations and the training and deployment of terrorists. State-sponsored terrorism and the oppression of citizens and the torture of opponents is widely practiced.

The poor, the elderly, women and children, the disabled, and people with mental illness are among the most vulnerable in the context of violent conflict. Gender-based violence, including rape, forced prostitution, and trafficking, are not infrequently used as tools of war, although they are clearly identified as crimes against humanity.[57–58]

Natural Disasters

The public health impacts of natural disasters are now well understood. In recent years, these disasters—earthquakes and tsunamis, volcanic eruptions, extreme weather events such as hurricanes Katrina and Sandy, and heat waves and bushfires—have affected millions of people in many countries, causing substantial loss of life and wreaking social and economic devastation on communities. People with mental illness, who are more likely to be poor and socially isolated, more likely to have physical health problems, and less likely to have the individual resilience and capabilities necessary to deal effectively with specific or pervasive threats to their well-being, are more likely to suffer the multiple negative impacts[59,60] of such threats.

A study[61] of mental health response following the massive December 2004 earthquake and tsunami was carried out in affected areas of Aceh and Nias, Indonesia. As well as exploring the effect on mental health of direct exposure to the tsunami, the study examined the effect on mental health of immediate post-disaster changes in life circumstances (impact) in a sample of 783 people aged 15 years and over. High rates of psychopathology, including symptoms of anxiety and affective disorders and post-traumatic stress syndrome, were recorded in the overall sample, particularly among internally displaced persons (IDPs) who experienced more substantial post-disaster changes in life circumstances (impact). The IDP group experienced significantly more psychological symptoms than did the non-IDP group. Demographic factors alone accounted for less two percent of variance in psychological symptom scores. Higher psychological symptom scores were observed among women, those with lower education, those with diminished resilience, those experiencing high scores on disaster impact, those experiencing direct exposures to the disaster, and due to (unmeasured) conditions related to being an IDP. The greatest effect among these was due to disaster impacts—that is, changes in life circumstances as a result of the disaster. The pattern was similar when considering post-traumatic stress symptoms separately. It was suggested that ameliorating the extent and duration of post-disaster negative changes in life circumstances may play an important role in prevention of post-disaster psychological morbidity.

Both natural disasters and violent conflict represent also an opportunity to strengthen human development. The transition from disaster or conflict generally begins with humanitarian response[58] to rehabilitation and reconstruction and then to development. As a result of the conflict or disaster, governance and other arrangements are frequently severely disrupted, in flux and amenable to change.[62] The frequent presence in these circumstances of international funds and expertise and the creation of new relationships makes innovation possible and there are frequently funds available for innovation and scaling up of health, mental health, education, and other social systems.

Poverty

When people's livelihoods are deeply compromised—when people are uncertain where the next meal will come from, when their life savings suddenly plummet in value, when their crops fail and they have no savings—human security contracts. People eat less and some starve. They pull their children out of school. They cannot afford clothing, heating or health care. Repeated crises further increase the vulnerability of people in absolute or extreme poverty.[63]

There is a clear relationship between poverty, mental illness and disability,[6,7,25,65] with the presence of any one factor increasing the likelihood of the others.[6-10] Reducing mental illness and disability, and the poverty that is so commonly a consequence, requires strengthening of human rights protections and development of mental health systems that ensure equitable access to skilled treatment, rehabilitation, social support, housing, and employment.

Poverty is the clearest focus of development programs.[65] In recent years, it has been recognized that it is not possible to focus on poverty alleviation programs without paying particular attention to the most vulnerable in poor communities, especially people living with disabilities.[66] People with mental disorders are increasingly being recognized as a particularly vulnerable group that warrants the attention of development agencies and programs.[36] It is also now being recognized that people with mental disorders living in poor communities, particularly rural and remote communities in low- and middle-income countries, are most likely to experience the most severe forms of human rights abuses.[54-56] This is also true for people with mental disorders whose families are too poor to house and look after them, who are homeless, and who find themselves in state-run social protection centers and or religious healing shrines.[37,67]

National economic data (as with many other types of national level data) can conceal as much as they reveal. It is important to be aware of the very uneven distribution of resources within countries, across geographic regions, and across ethnic and other population sub-groups. Figure 8.1, showing the geographic distribution of multidimensional poverty in Kenya, illustrates the very stark differences in poverty that can be found in different areas and among different sub-populations within a country.

Efforts to reduce poverty and to deal with the mental health associations of poverty must be carefully targeted to those most in need. It will generally be true, particularly in low- and middle-income countries without effective social and income protection arrangements for people with disabilities, that people with severe and persistent mental disorders will be among the poorest of the country's citizens.

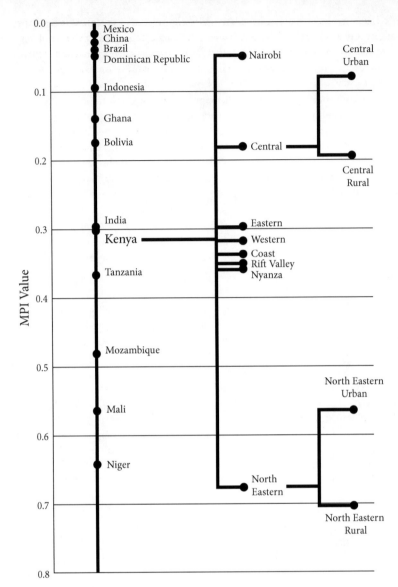

FIGURE 8.1

Within-country variation in multidimensional poverty in Kenya.[88] *Source:* Alkire. *Human Development*, p. 5.

Financial and Economic Crises

A fifth of the world's people—1.2 billion—experience severe income poverty and live on less than $1 a day, nearly two-thirds of them in Asia and a quarter in Africa. Another 1.6 billion live on less than $2 a day. Together, 2.8 billion of the world's people live in a chronic state of poverty and daily insecurity, a number that has not changed much since 1990. About 800 million people in the developing world and 24 million in developed and transition economies do not have enough to eat.[63]

The world has been dealing with the global financial crisis for a number of years, the most serious and prolonged global economic downturn since the 1930s. An important feature of the crisis is that all countries have been affected, but that some are affected more than others. In earlier crises, in the 1980s and 1990s, which started in the developing world, more than 100 million people were tipped back into poverty, often as a result of structural adjustment programs mandated by the International Monetary Fund (IMF). There is in this crisis, which began in the industrialized world, a very active debate about the wisdom and the short- and long-term consequences for human security, including mental health, of the severe austerity measures that are in some places being applied. There is no question that these measures are resulting in significant resentment and some civil unrest. There is also the question of whether the crisis and the austerity measures are a breeding ground for extremist political groups and a rise in racism and xenophobia. There is an emerging examination of the values that underpin societies worldwide.

Economic crises, and increases in unemployment rates, are a well-known risk to the mental well-being of populations, particularly to those who are already poor and marginalized. It is expected that the crisis will result, and some evidence that it has already resulted, in increased suicides and increased alcohol-related deaths.[68,69] In several countries that are in particular economic difficulty, such as Greece, there have been substantial reductions in health budgets and health services, particularly mental health services.

There is an increasing need for income and social protection measure in the context of decreasing capacity to provide such protection. Targeted investment in mental health services that are crucial for people's well-being can reduce the damaging impact of the crisis. There is a clear need for active labor market, housing, and family support programs, particularly for people with preexisting mental disorders.

Climate Change

As I wrote this (mid-January 2013), the east coast of Australia was in flames.[70] There were more than 200 bushfires across several states, destroying all in their paths and displacing mostly people from small rural communities and from the outskirts of urban centers. Thousands of firefighters and logistics and strategic command personnel were battling these infernos, with great courage and often with spectacular success. It is noteworthy that the great majority who risked their lives to fight these fires were volunteers in rural fire brigades. Most were defending their own communities, but it is a regular occurrence that one state will send firefighters and equipment to help another that is under extreme threat. With considerable good luck, we got through the summer without great bushfire-related loss of life and with economic and social costs minimized as much as possible.

Australia, like many countries, regularly experiences natural disasters—floods, fire, and storms. Although Australia has the resources to prepare for and to respond effectively to these calamities, as in all countries experiencing disasters it is the most economically and socially vulnerable who suffer the most adverse consequences and the greatest challenges in recovery. Disasters are more likely to be experienced by poorer rural communities. Losses that are easily borne by those with personal financial means or adequate insurance coverage destroy the lives of those without such means.

Massive floods affecting Brisbane and large parts of rural Queensland, New South Wales, and Victoria, increased storms and cyclones, and greatly increased risk of summer bushfires generated an active debate about whether the apparently increased risk of these events may be attributed to climate change. A report published by the Australian Climate Commission in January 2013 conveys the following key messages.

The length, extent, and severity of the current heatwave are unprecedented in the measurement record; although Australia has always had heatwaves, hot days and bushfires, climate change is increasing the risk of more frequent and longer heatwaves and more extreme hot days, as well as exacerbating bushfire conditions; climate change has contributed to making the current extreme heat conditions and bushfires worse; and good community understanding of climate change risks is critical to ensure we take appropriate action to reduce greenhouse gas emissions and to put measures in place to prepare for, and respond to, extreme weather.[71]

The current and expected mental health impacts of climate change are outlined in Panel 8.1.

Panel 8.1 Climate Change and Mental Health[98]

Grant Blashki

When exploring the complex determinants of mental health in a global context it is essential for those working in the field of global mental health to consider the implications of climate change. It is clear from leading climate scientists that the global temperature is steadily rising and that it will have substantial implications for human health. However, the implications for global mental health are not straightforward and present with a mix of direct impacts on mental well-being and indirect causal pathways.

Given the controversy that has surrounded climate change in the popular press, it is worth briefly reiterating the robust scientific case form the Intergovernmental Panel on Climate Change (IPCC)[99] that climate change is indeed occurring. There is a vast body of evidence that the earth is warming from multiple lines of evidence including ground level temperature monitoring, satellite measurements, ocean measurements and importantly a globally coherent fingerprint amongst biological systems such as tree rings and changes in animal migrations indicative of a warming signal.[100] The IPCC also indicates that it is "very likely" (greater than 90%) that this warming has been caused by human activities, predominantly the emission of greenhouse gases into the atmosphere.[99]

The evidence for *the health impacts* of climate change is also very strong. Key reports from the World Health Organization,[101] the 2012 Rio Convention Health report,[102] and influential systematic reviews[103] together paint a picture that climate change is indeed one of the greatest threats to global public health in this century.

The *direct* effects of climate change on health are fairly well understood. Perhaps the most obvious is the substantial morbidity and mortality associated with heat waves, which are already occurring with greater frequency and are predicted to dramatically increase in the coming century.[71,103] Around the globe new record high heat waves are occurring with increasing frequency. Another direct impact of climate change is the health effects of more severe and frequent floods and storms, which are also predicted to continue to escalate in the coming decades.[103] Changes in the distribution of vector-borne diseases, in particular malaria and dengue fever are also forecast, although there is some debate about exactly what bearing this will have on human populations.[103]

Concurrently, in the background of these extreme weather events, is perhaps the more important and dramatic *indirect* impacts of climate change that will play out via an array of complex causal pathways.[98] Gradual reductions in grain production and agriculture will cause immense socio economic pressures and communities especially in the developing countries who rely on subsistence farming.[99] The loss of livelihood and food security have a plethora of follow-on effects such as forced migration, stress on families, and setting the scene for conflicts.[99] Environmental refugees, especially those who are fleeing from low lying areas, which are predicted to be inundated with rising sea level, are anticipated to number in the tens to hundreds of millions of people, with enormous public health implications.[99]

In the context of these dramatic movements of human populations from environmental pressures, especially changes in climate, it is important for the global mental health practitioner to contemplate the challenges for the next century. As we know from decades of experience in non-climate change related extreme weather events, severe floods, fires, storms and other extreme weather events will cause major mental health problems for those communities that are caught affected by such events.[98] Post traumatic stress disorder, anxiety disorders, depression and of course grief are inevitable for some people caught up in such life threatening events.[98]

In the longer term, its important to consider the psychosocial implications for communities where entire populations may need to be relocated, as is being planned for some populations on low-lying islands in the Asia-Pacific such as Kiribas.[21] Notably, it is the vulnerable members of communities such as children and adolescents and those with existing mental disorders that are particularly at risk.[21]

Measuring the mental health consequences of climate change poses some particular challenges. Notably, the high baseline prevalence of mental disorders in most populations means that detecting increases due to a particular etiology is not always possible. But perhaps more importantly, it is the complex chains of causation, the interrelated and overlapping stresses and strains on human populations, that mean that climate change's contributions are often not easy to measure.

Nevertheless in contemplating responses to the mental health impacts of climate change, a practical approach needs to be taken. It is clear that the broader context of global health and global mental health cannot be ignored. The reality is that throughout the world great deficiencies in global health continue to exist- consider for example, the Millennium Development Goals and the worldwide effort to achieve basic standards in water and sanitation, improvements in child health, maternal mortality and the like. At the same time, even though mental disorders make up five of the top 10 contributors to the global burden of disease, currently mental health services around the world, particularly at a community level are still very basic in many developing countries. Therefore current efforts to strengthen mental health services globally is very much part of a growing human rights movement in its own right (with or without climate change).

Having said this, there are hotspots where viewing global mental health through a climate change lens does highlight some particularly vulnerable populations. For example people who are living in environmentally sensitive areas that are vulnerable to climate change, for example those in low-lying islands, or those who are living on the deltas of some of the great rivers that track through Asia, or subsistence farmers who are living in sub-Saharan Africa and are vulnerable to droughts.[104] And even within those populations we know that it is the young and the elderly and those who have disabilities who are particularly at risk.

Climate change is now under way and substantial health impacts are already occurring and are predicted to worsen. In regions particularly affected by climate change mental disorders are likely to increase in prevalence and severity, and are most likely to emerge in particular configurations of illness—increased post-traumatic stress disorder for those affected by acute events, and the well known constellation of mental health problems seen in refugees and forced population movements throughout the ages. In the coming decades, global mental health practitioners can help strengthen mental health services through having an awareness of the likely impacts of climate change in these vulnerable regions and vulnerable populations.

Used with permission from Springer Science + Business Media.

170 million people live outside their country of origin, and every year more than 700 million people cross national boundaries.[11] The money that migrants send back to families in the country of origin is often a major part of external revenue for poor countries. In fact the total amount of overseas remittances by temporary and permanent migrants is larger than the total global development assistance budget. The public-health importance of this massive movement of people is apparent for communicable diseases, and, although less visible, is no less important for mental health.

Many factors that lead to permanent and temporary migration, such as violent conflict and poverty, are also important determinants of mental health and illness. Complex emergencies and human-rights abuses produce large flows of asylum seekers and refugees, mostly into neighboring low-income countries that have little capacity to receive and to care for them. Poverty fuels the deadly trade of human trafficking, and is the major engine for undocumented immigration. The decline of rural economies everywhere and rapidly escalating global ecological problems will substantially increase the pressure on people to move. Temporary labor migrants, often women from rural areas with poor education who have been separated from their family, have access to few legal protections, and are vulnerable to exploitation and abuse. High-income countries with declining and aging populations need immigrants, but are often ambivalent about them when they come. The power of institutional or individual racism over the mental health of immigrants must not be ignored. Fragmentation and erosion of identity, the loss associated with displacement from familiar contexts and support networks, the difficulties of settlement, and the pressures on accustomed family structures and relationships can increase vulnerability to mental illness.

Violent conflicts are one of the most common causes of large-scale internal displacement of people, and the commonest reason for people to flee and to seek asylum outside of a country's borders. 2011 was a record year for forced displacement across borders, with more people becoming asylum seekers and refugees than in any year since 2000, with 4.3 million newly displaced and 800,000 fleeing their countries and becoming refugees. 42.5 million ended 2011 as refugees (15.2 million), internally displaced (26.4 million) or in the process of seeking asylum. The biggest producers of refugees were Afghanistan (2.7 million), Iraq (1.4 million), Somalia (1.1 million), Sudan (500,000), and the Democratic Republic of Congo 491,000). Table 8.2, showing the number of refugees produced by these countries and some human development indicators, starkly illustrates the link between conflict, forced displacement of people, and low human development.

Table 8.2 Number of Refugees Produced and Some Human Development Indicators

Country	Number of refugees from the country	Country's Human Development Index	Country's Human Development Index rank*	Life expectancy at birth (years)
Afghanistan	2,700,000	0.398	172	48.7
Iraq	1,400,000	0.573	132	69.0
Somalia	1,100,000	Unavailable	Unranked	51.2
Sudan	500,000	0.408	169	61.5
Democratic Republic of Congo	491,000	0.286	187	48.4

* In a total of 187 countries

The countries hosting the largest numbers of refugees are Pakistan (1.7 million), Iran (886,500), and Syria (775,400). Of course Syria is now a refugee-producing country as a result of the brutal civil war that is still in progress. Eighty percent of the world's refugees continue to be in developing countries.

A global problem that is testing the capacity and will of countries to uphold the provisions of the Refugee Convention is the phenomenon of people-smuggling. This lucrative trade in desperation and misery is resulting in ever tighter immigration controls and greater suspicion of asylum seekers. Over the past decade in Australia, "unauthorized boat arrivals"—asylum seekers from some of the world's most protracted and brutal conflicts—have been subjected to a harsh regime of detention while their claim for asylum has been assessed and other measures intended to deter future asylum seekers from paying people-smugglers to get them by boat to Australia. This issue has produced a deep divide within Australian society and a toxic political debate that is causing substantial and long-term harm to asylum seekers.[72]

VULNERABILITIES

Development agencies have recognized that their development aid should focus on ensuring that vulnerable groups receive particular attention and assistance, and that the vulnerable will not benefit from development assistance unless they are identified and specific strategies are developed to reach them. Aid effectiveness[73,74] cannot be achieved without a focus on the most vulnerable.

Funk and colleagues[36] have persuasively presented the argument that people with mental disorders constitute a specific vulnerable group that should attract the attention and support of development agencies and programs in ways similar to the traditional focus of development efforts targeting people living in poverty, people living with HIV/AIDS, asylum seekers and refugees, trafficked children and adults, commercial sex workers, and people with disabilities. People with mental disorders have been largely neglected despite the fact of their vulnerability. However "vulnerability should not be confused with incapacity, nor should vulnerable groups be regarded as passive victims. Ways must be found to empower vulnerable groups to participate fully in society."[36]

Factors contributing to vulnerability[36] and the specific rights conferred by the Convention on the Rights of Persons with Disabilities[75] are summarized in Table 8.3.

DEVELOPMENT

When bombs were still raining on London, John Maynard Keynes was preparing the blueprint for the Bretton Woods institutions. When Europe was still at war, Jean Monnet was dreaming about a European Economic Community. When the dust of war still had not begun to settle, the Marshall Plan for the reconstruction of Europe was taking shape. When hostility among nations was still simmering, the hopeful design of a United Nations was being approved by the leaders of the world....[76]

—Mahbub ul Haq, *Reflections on Human Development*

People are the real wealth of a nation. The basic objective of development is to create an enabling environment for people to live long, healthy, and creative lives. This may appear to be a simple truth. But it is often forgotten in the immediate concern with the accumulation of commodities and financial wealth.

—UNDP Human Development Report 1990[77]

Table 8.3 Threats and Vulnerabilities and Rights of People with Mental Disorders

Threats and Vulnerabilities[36,97]	The Convention on the Rights of People with Disabilities (CRPD)[75]
Stigma and discrimination	*States Parties shall prohibit all discrimination on the basis of disability and guarantee to persons with disabilities equal and effective legal protection against discrimination on all grounds.* —Article 5, United Nations Convention on the Rights of Persons with Disabilities
Violence and abuse	*No one shall be subjected to torture or to cruel, inhuman or degrading treatment or punishment…. States Parties shall take all appropriate… measures to protect persons with disabilities, both within and outside the home, from all forms of exploitation, violence and abuse….* —Articles 15 and 16, United Nations Convention on the Rights of Persons with Disabilities
Restrictions in exercising civil and political rights	*States Parties shall recognize that persons with disabilities enjoy legal capacity on an equal basis with others in all aspects of life…. States Parties shall… (e)nsure that persons with disabilities can effectively and fully participate in political and public life on an equal basis with others….* —Articles 12 and 29, United Nations Convention on the Rights of Persons with Disabilities
Exclusion from participating fully in society	*… persons with disabilities should have the opportunity to be actively involved in decision-making processes about policies and programmes, including those directly concerning them….* Preamble, United Nations Convention on the Rights of Persons with Disabilities
Reduced access to health and social services	*States Parties shall provide those health services needed by persons with disabilities specifically because of their disabilities, including early identification and intervention as appropriate, and services designed to minimize and prevent further disabilities….* —Article 25, United Nations Convention on the Rights of Persons with Disabilities
Reduced access to emergency relief services	*States Parties shall take… all necessary measures to ensure the protection and safety of persons with disabilities in situations of risk, including situations of armed conflict, humanitarian emergencies and the occurrence of natural disasters.* —Article 11, United Nations Convention on the Rights of Persons with Disabilities
Lack of educational opportunities	*States Parties shall ensure that persons with disabilities are not excluded from the general education system on the basis of disability, and that children with disabilities are not excluded from free and compulsory primary education, or from secondary education, on the basis of disability.* —Article 24, United Nations Convention on the Rights of Persons with Disabilities
Exclusion from income generation and employment opportunities	*States Parties recognize the right of persons with disabilities to work on an equal basis with others…* —Article 27, United Nations Convention on the Rights of Persons with Disabilities

The concept of "human development" arose out of growing dissatisfaction with the development approach that presumed an automatic link between economic growth and human advancement, a concept not supported by observations such as the persistence of poverty even in the midst of economic growth, the many social problems that emerge in tandem with economic growth, and the sometimes severe and widespread human costs of macroeconomic interventions aimed at securing economic growth. A broader view, a focus on "human development," encompassing critically important aspects of human flourishing beyond economic growth, was ably advanced by economist Mahbub-ul-Haq and elaborated upon in successive Human Development Reports, annual reports since 1990 commissioned by the United Nations Development Programme (UNDP).

Although there is no universally accepted definition of *human development*, it is conceived as "a process of enlarging people's choices and building human capabilities (the range of things people can be and do), enabling them to live a long and healthy life, have access to knowledge, have a decent standard of living and participate in the life of their community and the decisions that affect their lives."[78] The substance of this conception, and the necessary conceptual clarity, has been provided by Amartya Sen's work on capabilities and freedoms.[79] The Human Development Index, a composite measure of life expectancy, education, and income, has been used to establish trends and to rank and classify countries into four tiers: very high, high, medium, and low human development. The least developed nations are the most likely to experience violent conflict and the severe consequences of natural disasters, to be the least prepared to deal with natural disasters, and the least capable of effectively protecting the human rights of their citizens.

While the concepts of human development and human rights are distinct, they overlap, have much in common, and complement each another. Human rights and human development share a common vision and a common purpose, "to secure, for every human being freedom, well-being and dignity."[78]

Millennium Development Goals: The Biggest Mental Health Promotion Program Ever Implemented?

The most prominent program of work to advance human development since the establishment of the United Nations has been the Millennium Development Goals (MDGs) program. This has been a remarkably ambitious program to achieve clearly articulated global objectives in a relatively small number of priority development domains (see Panel 8.2).

Although the program has attracted some skepticism about the possibility of success, and periods in the past decade when progress appeared to stall, the 2012 report on progress documents some remarkable achievements (Panel 2). The UN Secretary-General rightly emphasized the importance of Millennium Development Goal 8 (MDG-8), the establishment of a vibrant partnership for development. Bilateral development agencies have been prominent partners for development, taking the MDGs as a core part of their development mission.[80] They have become increasingly focused on the issue of development effectiveness and the efficient and effective use of development assistance funds and expertise.[65]

"Mental health" is not specifically included in the MDGs. While it is common to hear mental health advocates refer to this fact as "a lost opportunity for mental health," the reality is quite different. Everything we know about social determinants of mental health and illness (see Chapter 7 in this volume) suggests that the MDG program is the biggest mental health promotion program ever implemented. There is no question that progress towards achievement of a number of the goals will make a positive and very substantial contribution to mental health and to prevention of mental disorder.

Panel 8.2 Millennium Development Goals

http://www.undp.org/content/undp/en/home/mdgoverview.html

(The following text is quoted from the Foreword to the *Millennium Development Goals Report 2012*.[105])

1. Eradicate extreme hunger and poverty
2. Achieve universal primary education
3. Promote gender equality and empower women
4. Reduce child mortality
5. Improve maternal health
6. Combat HIV/AIDS, malaria and other diseases
7. Ensure environmental sustainability
8. Develop a global partnership for development

This year's report on progress towards the Millennium Development Goals (MDGs) highlights several milestones. The target of reducing extreme poverty by half has been reached five years ahead of the 2015 deadline, as has the target of halving the proportion of people who lack dependable access to improved sources of drinking water. Conditions for more than 200 million people living in slums have been ameliorated— double the 2020 target. Primary school enrolment of girls equaled that of boys, and we have seen accelerating progress in reducing child and maternal mortality.

These results represent a tremendous reduction in human suffering and are a clear validation of the approach embodied in the MDGs. But, they are not a reason to relax. Projections indicate that in 2015 more than 600 million people worldwide will still be using unimproved water sources, almost one billion will be living on an income of less than $1.25 per day, mothers will continue to die needlessly in childbirth, and children will suffer and die from preventable diseases. Hunger remains a global challenge, and ensuring that all children are able to complete primary education remains a fundamental, but unfulfilled, target that has an impact on all the other Goals. Lack of safe sanitation is hampering progress in health and nutrition, biodiversity loss continues apace, and greenhouse gas emissions continue to pose a major threat to people and ecosystems.

The goal of gender equality also remains unfulfilled, again with broad negative consequences, given that achieving the MDGs depends so much on women's empowerment and equal access by women to education, work, health care and decision-making. We must also recognize the unevenness of progress within countries and regions, and the severe inequalities that exist among populations, especially between rural and urban areas.

Achieving the MDGs by 2015 is challenging but possible. Much depends on the fulfillment of MDG-8—the global partnership for development. The current economic crises besetting much of the developed world must not be allowed to decelerate or reverse the progress that has been made. Let us build on the successes we have achieved so far, and let us not relent until all the MDGs have been attained.

Ban Ki-moon
Secretary-General, United Nations

Mental health is crucial to the overall well-being of individuals, societies, and countries. The importance of mental health has been recognized by WHO since its origin, and is reflected by the definition of health in the WHO constitution as *not merely the absence of disease or infirmity*, but rather, *a state of complete physical, mental, and social well-being*. Mental health is related to the development of societies and countries. Poverty and its associated psychosocial stressors (e.g., violence, unemployment, social exclusion, and insecurity) are correlated with mental disorders. Relative poverty, low education, and inequality within communities are associated with increased risk of mental health problems. Community and economic development can also be used to restore and enhance mental health. Community development programs that aim to reduce poverty, achieve economic independence and empowerment for women, reduce malnutrition, increase literacy and education, and empower the underprivileged contribute to the prevention of mental and substance use disorders and promote mental health. (WHO mhGAP 2008[40])

A major issue, and opportunity, for the global mental health community over the next few years is to ensure that mental health, particularly the need to focus on the development of effective and accessible mental health systems as part of the broader development agenda, is an explicit component of the emerging post-MDG development landscape.

COMPLEX ADAPTIVE SYSTEMS

It will be clear from this brief outline that threats, risks, and vulnerabilities are highly complex, fluid, and interdependent. Causality is not linear, and seeking to deal with one problem requires attention to many others in as integrated a fashion as possible. The mental health dimensions of these human security and development issues are similarly inseparable in reality, while we still need to have simplified conceptual frameworks and language that will guide action in the face of seemingly impossible complexity.

Mental health systems are complex adaptive systems (CAS).[62] They are composed of subsystems and are part of supra-systems, and are the product of the social, economic, cultural, and political contexts in which they are developed. In human systems these sub- and supra-systems range from activity at the molecular level, through physiological and organ systems, to the individual, inter-individual, and group interactivity, to social and cultural systems of which the mental health system is a part. Regardless of the composition of complex adaptive systems (e.g., physical, biological, ecological, social/cultural systems) they share key properties[81–84]—multiple levels of organization, open boundaries, rule sets, or control parameters that determine the state of the system at any point in time, adaptation and structural coupling, self-organization, emergence, and nonlinear causality. Table 8.4 outlines the core characteristics of complex adaptive systems and gives some examples of each feature in mental health systems.[62]

Complex adaptive systems may exist in three broad regimes—an ordered regime, a chaotic regime (or a phase transition between these two), or a complex regime. Kauffman[85] has suggested a number of features of networks that will determine in which of these regimes the network will operate, thereby identifying in a preliminary fashion some possible sources of order in complex adaptive systems. An important finding from Kauffman's work is that the region just near the phase transition from an orderly to a chaotic regime is where the most complex behaviors can occur, sufficiently orderly to ensure stability, yet "full of flexibility and surprise. Indeed, this is what we mean by complexity."[85] A living system must "strike an internal compromise between malleability and stability. To survive in a variable environment, it must be stable but not so stable that it remains forever static."[86] Nor can it be so unstable that slight internal or external perturbations can cause the whole structure to collapse.

Where the system is stable, with high certainty and agreement, technical solutions to problems and the exercise of competence are appropriate. Leadership for change in complex systems occurs in the zone of complexity.[62] In this zone, there is a relatively low degree of certainty and degree of agreement concerning what needs to be changed and how this is to be achieved. The emerging environment or context for the change is unfamiliar, and the tasks that will be necessary are also unfamiliar. Here competence is

Table 8.4 Core Features of Complex Adaptive Systems

Core Features	Brief description	Mental health systems
Multiple levels of organization	Multiple levels of organization with subsystems and supra-systems. Simultaneous membership of multiple systems is common.	This is a key feature of mental health systems everywhere. There are different forms of organization at international, national, state/provincial, area/district, service agency, team, and individual mental health practitioner levels. This applies also to civil society organizations and groupings, families and people with mental disorders.
Open boundaries	Complex adaptive systems have open or fuzzy rather than fixed boundaries. They are open to the flow of matter, energy, information (depending on the nature of the system). Membership of the system can change and agents can be simultaneously members of several systems simultaneously.	Individuals move into and out of the mental health system at a great rate, and between agencies in the system. Particular organizations appear and disappear. Team structures and functions emerge, evolve and are modified, and disappear. The boundaries between different elements of the system are more or less open, with this changing over time. A key requirement for effective global mental health system development is to further open boundaries (for example between ministries of health and social affairs, between professional and civil society organizations, and between local and international development agencies) and to encourage and enable exchange and collaboration. The key flows in mental health systems are people, information and money, and these move across elements and levels of the system. Increasing or reducing the flows of information and money through various elements of the system will have major impacts on the shape and organization of the system.
Rule sets	The actions or behavior of agents are governed by rule sets. The settings or values of these rules are the system's control parameters. In human systems the actions of agents are governed by laws and regulations, and cultural values, beliefs and commitments.	In the global mental health field international legal instruments and international polices ("rule sets") are influential in LAMICs. The agents in the mental health system are individuals (clinicians, managers, clerical and other support staff) and organizations (hospitals, community mental health centers, NGOs, academic departments, mental health branches of health departments.) Whiteford[97] suggests that there are "only five main levers available" to government to implement policy. They are: information collection and publication; the financing system; the payment system; the distribution of services and how they respond to consumer demands; and the regulatory system. These levers may be thought of also as those key system parameters in which government has the ability to reset settings or values in order to bring about change.

Adaptive	The agents and the system are adaptive. Both the agents and the rule sets within a system change over time. The nature and extent of interaction of the system with its environment or context also characteristically changes over time. CASs are frequently structurally coupled, that is they co-evolve, with other systems as they adapt to each other. As systems change they change each other's environment, resulting in changes in the structure and organization of each other and of the environment. A structurally coupled system is also a developing (self-organizing) system.	The rule sets change over time in response to changing economic social and policy contexts. They also change as the prevailing conceptions of what should constitute a functioning mental health system, for example the move from institution-based to community-focused systems of treatment and care. Particularly important is the increasing and legitimate demands of consumers and carers for safer, more responsive services, and for participation in decision-making. Mental health services everywhere are adapting to the demands of the recovery movement and, as they develop coherent responses in terms of service values, structures and practices, are contributing to the further development of the recovery construct. This is a clear example (there are very many others) of structural coupling.
Self-organization	Self-organization, based on internal interaction rules and external constraints. More or less stable patterns—with capacity for massive change—based on the interaction of the component parts of the system.	The specific organizational arrangements and functions and activities of various multidisciplinary teams, for example crisis assessment teams, vary in metropolitan and rural settings because of available resources, local needs, distances that have to be traveled and so on. In some inner city locations local needs give rise to specific teams, such as those focusing on mental ill people who are homeless. An injection of funds can give rise to new teams, such as early psychosis teams, where they did not exist before. A reduction in funds, as is now happening in the context of the global financial crisis, is also forcing different forms of self-organization in mental health systems in order to ensure survival of critically important elements or components of systems.

(continued)

Table 8.4 Continued

Core Features	Brief description	Mental health systems
Emergence	The behavior of a system emerges as a result of the rich interaction over time of multiple component agents and of the system with its context.	International cultures (such as that of the World Health Organization) and local social, cultural, economic and political contexts will influence the types of systems that will emerge, even following very similar development efforts. It is important to be aware of the relative power of different agents in the system, since this will have a clear impact on the pattern that emerges from the interactions of the agents in the system.
Non-linear causality	Complex adaptive systems are characterized by non-linear causality, with multiple positive and negative feedback loops, the influence of external constraints, and exquisite sensitivity to initial conditions. Because of this non-linearity and sensitivity to initial conditions, the details of the emergent behavior are inherently unpredictable.	A change introduced into any level of the mental health system, e.g., new policy, may have little impact because of the inherent stability of key elements of the system (e.g., the attitudes of senior clinical staff to the change). "The environment of political decision making is complex. Factors such as the relative power of each player in the political landscape, the positions taken by them and the intensity of commitment for or against the policy all come into play."[97] Similarly, relatively small changes, for example the appointment of a consumer consultant to the management structure of the service, can result in large and essentially unpredictable changes in the functioning of a system. The implementation of policy virtually never goes as planned. Flexibility in responding and adapting to emerging issues, which can create barriers and opportunities, is essential.

insufficient. There is a need for capability—the ability to generate creative adaptive solutions to new and emerging problems.

CURRENT GLOBAL MENTAL HEALTH SITUATION

Mental, neurological, and substance use (MNS) disorders are prevalent in all regions of the world and are major contributors to morbidity and premature mortality. Worldwide, community-based epidemiological studies have estimated that lifetime prevalence rates of mental disorders in adults are 12.2%–48.6%, and 12-month prevalence rates are 8.4%–29.1%. Fourteen percent of the global burden of disease, measured in disability-adjusted life years (DALYs), can be attributed to MNS disorders. About 30% of the total burden of non-communicable diseases is due to these disorders. Almost three quarters of the global burden of neuropsychiatric disorders is in countries with low and lower middle incomes. The stigma and violations of human rights directed towards people with these disorders compounds the problem, increasing their vulnerability; accelerating and reinforcing their decline into poverty; and hindering care and rehabilitation. Restoration of mental health is not only essential for individual well-being, but is also necessary for economic growth and reduction of poverty in societies and countries. Mental health and health security interact closely. Conditions of conflict create many challenges for mental health. (WHO, 2008[40])

The current global mental health situation, particularly in low- and middle-income countries, is considered in detail in the other chapters of this book. Some particular features are worthy of note here, and are summarized in Table 8.5. Mental health has been a low priority for governments and for other key decision-makers. This is the product of many factors, including limited understanding of mental health as an important public health and development issue; little understanding that effective treatments and social interventions are available, affordable, and feasible, even in low-resource environments; low population mental health literacy, with a consequent low demand for services; and a low demand for action on improving mental health systems. Governance arrangements for mental health programs and services in LAMICs have been poorly developed, with low levels of capability in important places, particularly in Ministries of Health, Social Affairs, Education, and Science. There has therefore been little incentive to invest, and little development of skills in clinical and social services, mental health service development and management, and mental health research, particularly mental health systems research. Mental health information systems are either poor or virtually nonexistent, making planning, monitoring, and evaluation difficult, and keeping the mental health needs of the population invisible. As a consequence of these and no doubt many other factors, investment in mental health has been pitifully low. The poorest countries invest the lowest proportion of already very small health budgets in mental health.[40] One of the major and continuing deficiencies is human resources for mental health.[23] (See Chapter 10.)

The outcomes of these deficiencies include poorly developed and poorly integrated mental health service systems, a focus on institution-based service delivery in poorly resourced and often dysfunctional mental hospitals,[86,87] extremely limited community-based services, and little capacity for rehabilitation and social support. The frequent lack of income and social protection arrangements in LAMICs often means that people with mental disorders are among the most destitute of the poor. Stigma and discrimination are prominent and human rights abuses frequent and widespread.[37,54–56,68] (See Chapter 18.)

In response to this unsatisfactory state of affairs, there has been increasing attention to and calls for scaling up what we already know.[15,22] However, the task before us is considerably greater and more complex than "scaling up." It is an issue of development; the need to build functioning, integrated systems, informed by human security and complexity

Table 8.5 Mental Health Systems in Low- and Middle-Income Countries

Context	System elements	Outcomes
• Little understanding of mental health as an important public health and social and economic development issue • Little understanding that effective and affordable interventions and service models are available • Mental health is a low political and social priority • Weak investment • Weak drive for mental health system reform and development • Low levels of skill in policy development and implementation • Weak governance and management arrangements • Low population "mental health literacy"	• Inadequate infrastructure, facilities, equipment, drug distribution systems. • Shortage of skilled mental health workers • Geographic maldistribution of available workforce • Disciplinary imbalance—doctor and nurse dominated • Hospital-centered • Undeveloped information systems, with lack of high-quality local information to support planning • Poorly developed mental health systems research capacity • No culture of evaluation and continuous quality improvement • Poorly organized and marginalized consumers, carers, civil society	• Narrow population coverage—wide "treatment gap" • Very wide gap between best (usually in major urban centers) and worst (usually in poor rural areas) mental health services • Low and inequitable access (geographic, economic, linguistic, cultural) to mental health services • Stigma, discrimination, social and economic exclusion • Mental health training is unattractive for most disciplines • Inadequate protection of rights, with widespread human rights abuses • Lack of locally relevant evidence for policy and practice • Poorly developed advocacy by civil society and groups

Source: Minas. *Harv Rev Psychiatry*, p. 38. Used with permission from Lippincott Williams & Wilkins.

perspectives. There is also a need to translate international and national policy aspirations into practical, culturally appropriate local realities.

Discussions about global mental health tend to be focused on low- and middle-income countries in contrast with high-income countries. While overall level of resources is of course important, it is essential not to forget that in every country there is wide variation in the distribution of resources, threats, and capabilities by geographic region and by population subgroup. Figure 8.1, showing within-country regional differences in poverty in Kenya, graphically illustrates this point. High-income countries invariably have population subgroups that experience a pattern of social determinants of mental disorders that put them at high risk, often associated with socioeconomic circumstances that limit their capability to respond effectively to such risks, included reduced access to mental health and social services. (This is of course also true in low- and middle-income countries.) As an example, such groups in Australia include indigenous populations, asylum seekers and refugees, prison populations, illicit drug users, and people who are extremely poor and homeless. A nuanced approach to global mental health must go beyond national populations and concern itself with particularly vulnerable subpopulations. The approach to development, the application of human security interventions, and the development of mental health systems would, for example, need to vary considerably from Nairobi and Central Rural districts to North-Eastern Rural districts of Kenya.

The analysis by Alkire and Santos[88] (Figure 8.1) focuses on the geographic distribution of multidimensional poverty. Analyses of a similar kind that focus on geographic distribution of other threats and risks would be just as informative in terms of planning and implementing mental health promotion programs and design of mental health services. Similar distributional analyses also need to be developed by population subgroups rather than by geographic region.

In May 2012, the World Health Assembly (WHA), having considered the report of the secretariat,[38] requested the director-general of the World Health Organization to develop a comprehensive mental health action plan in collaboration with WHO member states.[89] WHO recommended four broad strategies for consideration by the WHA: (a) improve the provision of good-quality treatment and care for mental health conditions; (b) improve access for people with or at risk of mental disorders to social welfare services and opportunities for education and employment; (c) introduce human rights protection for people with mental health conditions; and (d) protect and promote mental health. In August 2012, WHO released the Zero Draft of a proposed Global Mental Health Action Plan 2013–2020, for consultation with member states.[39] The draft vision for the plan is:

A world in which mental health is valued, mental disorders are effectively prevented and in which persons affected by these disorders are able to access evidence-based health and social care and exercise the full range of human rights to attain the highest possible level of health and functioning free from stigma and discrimination.

MENTAL HEALTH SYSTEM DEVELOPMENT

Mental health organizations, and the mental health system overall, are complex, adaptive, nonlinear, dynamic systems. Where one draws the boundary of a system is arbitrary, depending on the purposes for which the boundary is drawn. There is structural coupling between mental health agencies, the general health system, consumer and carer groups, professional organizations, health departments, etc. They are in constant interaction with each other, and, over time, each reciprocally shapes the structure of the others.[90] Moving from one level of the system to another is associated with emergent phenomena that could not be predicted from knowledge of the lower-order subsystem, and that transcend the properties of the lower-order system. Each level requires different forms of investigation and of understanding.

Whole System Performance

It is now recognized that "improving quality of care involves improving whole systems around the doctor or clinician–patient interaction," and that a key task for quality improvement is the creation of an "environment in which excellence in clinical care will flourish."[91] This need to focus on whole system performance is consistent with the human security perspective that often requires multiple interventions in different domains to bring about desirable outcomes. The interactions within a complex adaptive system are more important than the discrete actions of the component parts. Mental health system development requires collaboration across sectors and disciplines, partnerships, and cooperative working practices. Productive or generative relationships occur when interactions produce new and valuable capabilities that are not possible through individual action of the parts.[83] Leaders and managers need to look increasingly across the parts of the system and to have a system-wide perspective.

Minimum Specifications

Progress towards goals that are desirable but difficult to achieve can occur through applying to the system a few simple, flexible rules, sometime referred to as *minimum specifications*. The tendency in policy implementation and management is to do the opposite, to specify in great detail what is to be done at all levels of the system. Minimum specifications leave room for creativity and innovation. They encourage discussion about how they are to be achieved locally, thereby increasing connectedness and facilitating shared views of what is to be done. If minimum specifications focus on system-wide targets they encourage generative relationships and the emergence of solutions that are relevant to local conditions. The setting of minimum specifications (e.g., principles, values, outcomes), without trying to specify everything in detail, and the task of securing the commitment of all players to the achievement of these minimum specification, may be a critical leadership function. The task of moving towards these goals in a way where everyone is clear about their individual roles, the tasks that need to be accomplished, the accountabilities that have to be established and monitored, the information systems that need to be in place, are management responsibilities.

Understanding Attraction for Change Rather Than Battling Resistance

Although it is common to read in the global mental health literature about "barriers to change," this may be an unhelpful framing of what needs to be done to bring about change. If resistance or barriers are seen as the reason that change is difficult to achieve, then the solution is to battle against and to overcome resistance, wherever it is to be found. However, in complex adaptive systems, behavior follows "attractors" in the system. Understanding where the attractors in the system are is part of the art of leadership and management. Understanding how a change in system parameter settings can shift the system from one attractor pattern to a more desirable one is a key task of leadership for change. An example of such a control parameter change is attending to payment systems, such as creating financial incentives for desirable outcomes, and changing the regulatory arrangements that will push behaviors and system structures in desirable directions.

Variation and Diversity

Standards and guidelines encourage uniformity. This is desirable when we are thinking of minimum standards and guidelines that encourage evidence-based practice. However, in a system that is far from perfect and looking to continually improve, there is merit also in encouraging diversity, in fostering creativity and accepting locally relevant structures and processes rather than seeking to impose a stifling uniformity. Variation and diversity are core features of any complex evolving system. The importance of biodiversity to the health of the biosphere is now well understood. The importance of cultural diversity in social systems is less well understood and less accepted. Diversity in service systems, such as the mental health system, and to a certain extent in clinical practice, tends to be regarded with suspicion. This is a critical error, one that can have a very negative impact on the continuing evolution of the service system.

Learning for Capability

Professional education currently focuses on competence—what individuals know and are able to do, expressed in terms of attitudes, knowledge, and skills. In dealing with complex adaptive systems we need to shift to thinking about educating for capability—the extent to which individuals can adapt to change, generate new knowledge, and continue to improve their, and their organization's, performance.[92] This involves a commitment to issues such as lifelong learning, learning networks, evidence-based practice, quality improvement, and inter-disciplinary and cross-sectoral connectedness. This is a further example of co-evolution, or structural coupling, of different elements of the system and the system with its context. Reflective learners transform as the world changes around them, and transform the world around them.

Values and Leadership

A key component of any minimum specifications approach to leadership for mental health system development is the clear and explicit articulation of the values that will underpin everything else that occurs in the system. It is also critically important that, as far as possible, values are shared by all who are involved in the change agenda. The values that should guide mental health system development are those enunciated in the human security agenda and the many instruments that seek to guarantee protection of human rights, and a commitment to evidence-informed development and practice.[93]

CONCLUSION

Bringing about positive change in complex systems requires skilled, sustained, and distributed leadership.[94] In seeking to develop more effective mental health systems globally we do not yet have a sufficiently good understanding of the relevant control parameters, and can generally not predict with any certainty the impact of changing those control parameters that we can change. There is a clear need for strengthening capability in implementation science and mental health systems research (see Chapter 19), understanding of effective leadership, and understanding of the most effective strategies for securing political commitment (see Chapter 20).

It is clear that, in thinking of mental health systems as complex adaptive systems, and of leadership for change in such systems, command and control styles of leadership are dead. An analogy for the changes that are occurring in our mental health systems can be found in economics. We are moving from a command economy to a market economy. There are many remnants of the command economy style of thinking in development programs broadly and the management of mental health systems particularly.

It is uncertain whether the insights and methods of complexity theory can be directly applied to the task of global mental health system development. The presence in such systems of intentionality, planning, control, and direction may require substantial modification of the concepts that have been developed in physical and biological systems. However, for our purposes, the concepts of complexity (emergence, structural coupling, etc.) may offer a powerful metaphor for thinking creatively about leadership for, and management of, change. We need to develop research programs that will allow us to investigate and to better understand mental health systems as complex adaptive systems. While the traditional research disciplines such as epidemiology and randomized trials will continue to be important, it will be necessary also to develop research and analytical methods that will enable the rigorous study of qualities and patterns. Whether a complexity perspective is anything more than simply a useful and engaging metaphor will become clearer as research programs on complexity in sociocultural systems are developed.

The consumer-initiated recovery movement that is having such a profound impact on mental health policy and practice globally is fully consistent with both the human security and the complexity perspectives outlined in this chapter. Deegan, one of the founders and most influential proponents of recovery-oriented policy and practice, and a psychologist who is in recovery from schizophrenia, has written:

Recovery is not a linear process marked by successive accomplishments. The recovery process is more accurately described as a series of small beginnings and very small steps. Professionals cannot manufacture the spirit of recovery and give it to consumers. Recovery cannot be forced or willed. However, environments can be created in which the recovery process can be nurtured like a tender and precious seedling. To recover, psychiatrically disabled persons must be willing to try and fail, and try again. (Deegan 1988, p. 11; cited in ref. 96)

The phrase "environments can be created" highlights the fact that the task of system-building, from the perspective of complex adaptive systems, is to create environments in which desirable and intended configurations can emerge. Here the emergent phenomenon is *recovery*. The global mental health enterprise is seeking the development (emergence) of mental health systems that are effective, equitably distributed, affordable, and appropriate to local social and cultural context.

REFERENCES

1. Commission on Human Security. *Human security now.* New York: Commission on Human Security; 2003.
2. United Nations General Assembly. *General Assembly Resolution A/RES/60/1: 2005 World Summit Outcome.* New York: United Nations, 2005.
3. Kessler RC, Angermeyer M, Anthony JC, et al. Lifetime prevalence and age-of-onset distributions of mental disorders in the World Health Organization's World Mental Health Survey Initiative. *World Psychiatry.* 2007;6(3):168–76. Epub 12/1/2008.
4. Levi F, La Vecchia C, Saraceno B. Global suicide rates. *Eur J Public Health.* 2003;13(2):97–8. Epub 2003/06/14.
5. Mathers CD, Ezzati M, Lopez AD. Measuring the burden of neglected tropical diseases: the global burden of disease framework. *PLoS Negl Trop Dis.* 2007;1(2):e114. Epub 2007/12/07.
6. Elwan A. Poverty and disability: a survey of the literature 1999. Available from: http://siteresources.worldbank.org/SOCIALPROTECTION/Resources/SP-Discussion-papers/Disability-DP/9932.pdf.
7. Patel V, Kleinman A. Poverty and common mental disorders in developing countries. *Bull WHO.* 2003;81(8):609–15. Epub 2003/10/25.
8. Patel V, Pereira J, Coutinho L, Fernandes R, Fernandes J, Mann A. Poverty, psychological disorder and disability in primary care attenders in Goa, India. *Br J Psychiatry.* 1998;172:533–6. Epub 1998/11/26.
9. Patel V, Rodrigues M, DeSouza N. Gender, poverty, and postnatal depression: a study of mothers in Goa, India. *Am J Psychiatry.* 2002;159(1):43–7. Epub 2002/01/05.
10. Saraceno B, Barbui C. Poverty and mental illness. *Can J Psychiatry.* 1997;42(3):285–90. Epub 1997/04/01.
11. Bhugra D, Minas IH. Mental health and global movement of people. *Lancet.* 2007;370(9593):1109–11. Epub 2007/09/07.
12. Chisholm D, Flisher AJ, Lund C, et al. Scale up services for mental disorders: a call for action. *Lancet.* 2007;370(9594):1241–52.
13. Horton R. Launching a new movement for mental health. *Lancet.* 2007;370(9590):806.
14. Jacob KS, Sharan P, Mirza I, et al. Mental health systems in countries: where are we now? *Lancet.* 2007;370(9592):1061–77.

15. Lancet Global Mental Health Group. Scale up services for mental disorders: a call for action. *Lancet.* 2007;370(9594):1241–52.

16. Patel V, Araya R, Chatterjee S, et al. Treatment and prevention of mental disorders in low-income and middle-income countries. *Lancet.* 2007;370(9591):991–1005.

17. Patel V, Flisher AJ, Hetrick S, McGorry P. Mental health of young people: a global public-health challenge. *Lancet.* 2007;369(9569):1302–13. Epub 2007/04/17.

18. Prince M, Patel V, Saxena S, et al. No health without mental health. *Lancet.* 2007;370(9590):859–77.

19. Saraceno B, van Ommeren M, Batniji R, et al. Barriers to improvement of mental health services in low-income and middle-income countries. *Lancet.* 2007;370(9593):1164–74.

20. Saxena S, Thornicroft G, Knapp M, Whiteford H. Resources for mental health: scarcity, inequity, and inefficiency. *Lancet.* 2007;370(9590):878–89.

21. Drew N, Funk M, Tang S, et al. Human rights violations of people with mental and psychosocial disabilities: an unresolved global crisis. *Lancet.* 2011;378(9803):1664–75. Epub 2011/10/20.

22. Eaton J, McCay L, Semrau M, et al. Scale up of services for mental health in low-income and middle-income countries. *Lancet.* 2011;378(9802):1592–603. Epub 2011/10/20.

23. Kakuma R, Minas H, van Ginneken N, et al. Human resources for mental health care: current situation and strategies for action. *Lancet.* 2011;378(9803):1654–63. Epub 2011/10/20.

24. Kieling C, Baker-Henningham H, Belfer M, et al. Child and adolescent mental health worldwide: evidence for action. *Lancet.* 2011;378(9801):1515–25. Epub 2011/10/20.

25. Lund C, De Silva M, Plagerson S, et al. Poverty and mental disorders: breaking the cycle in low-income and middle-income countries. *Lancet.* 2011;378(9801):1502–14. Epub 2011/10/20.

26. Benegal V, Chand PK, Obot IS. Packages of care for alcohol use disorders in low- and middle-income countries. *PLoS Med.* 2009;6(10):e1000170. Epub 2009/10/28.

27. de Jesus MJ, Razzouk D, Thara R, Eaton J, Thornicroft G. Packages of care for schizophrenia in low- and middle-income countries. *PLoS Med.* 2009;6(10):e1000165. Epub 2009/10/21.

28. Mbuba CK, Newton CR. Packages of care for epilepsy in low- and middle-income countries. *PLoS Med.* 2009;6(10):e1000162. Epub 2009/10/14.

29. Patel V, Simon G, Chowdhary N, Kaaya S, Araya R. Packages of care for depression in low- and middle-income countries. *PLoS Med.* 2009;6(10):e1000159. Epub 2009/10/07.

30. Patel V, Thornicroft G. Packages of care for mental, neurological, and substance use disorders in low- and middle-income countries: PLoS Med Series. *PLoS Med.* 2009;6(10):e1000160. Epub 2009/10/07.

31. Prince MJ, Acosta D, Castro-Costa E, Jackson J, Shaji KS. Packages of care for dementia in low- and middle-income countries. *PLoS Med.* 2009;6(11):e1000176. Epub 2009/11/06.

32. Flisher AJ, Sorsdahl K, Hatherill S, Chehil S. Packages of care for attention-deficit hyperactivity disorder in low- and middle-income countries. *PLoS Med.* 2010;7(2):e1000235. Epub 2010/02/27.

33. Editorial. A movement for global mental health is launched. *Lancet.* 2008;372(October 11):1274.

34. Patel V, Garrison P, de Jesus Mari J, Minas H, Prince M, Saxena S. The *Lancet's* series on global mental health: 1 year on. *Lancet.* 2008;372(9646):1354–7. Epub 2008/10/22.

35. Patel V, Boyce N, Collins PY, Saxena S, Horton R. A renewed agenda for global mental health. *Lancet.* 2011;378(9801):1441–2. Epub 2011/10/20.

36. Funk M, Drew N, Freeman M, Faydi E. *Mental health and development: Targeting people with mental health conditions as a vulnerable group.* Geneva: World Health Organization; 2010.

37. Minas H. Mental health and human rights: never waste a serious crisis. *Int J Ment Health Syst.* 2009;3(1):12. Epub 2009/06/18.

38. World Health Organization. *Global burden of mental disorders and the need for a comprehensive, coordinated response from health and social sectors at the country level.* A/65/10. Geneva: World Health Organization; 2012.

39. World Health Organization. *Global Mental Health Action Plan 2013–2020.* Zero Draft, August 27, 2012. Geneva: World Health Organization; 2012. http://www.who.int/mental_health/mhgap/mental_health_action_plan_EN_27_08_12.pdf

40. World Health Organization. *mhGAP: Mental health Gap Action Programme: Scaling up care mental, neurological, and substance use disorders.* Geneva: World Health Organization; 2008.

41. UK Department for International Development. *DFID research.* London 2010; Available from: http://www.dfid.gov.uk/Working-with-DFID/Research/.

42. Grand challenges in global mental health. http://grandchallengesgmh.nimh.nih.gov/.

43. Minas H. International observatory on mental health systems: a mental health research and development network. *Int J Ment Health Syst.* 2009;3(1):2. Epub 24/1/2009.

44. Minas H. International observatory on mental health systems: structure and operation. *Int J Ment Health Syst.* 2009;3(1):8. Epub 2009/04/07.

45. Minas H. *National taskforce on community mental health system development in Vietnam.* Melbourne: Centre for International Mental Health; 2010; Available from: http://blogs.unimelb.edu.au/internationalmentalhealth/2010/03/08/national-taskforce-on-community-mental-health-system-development-in-vietnam/.

46. The Royal Commission into Institutional Responses to Child Sexual Abuse. 2012; Available from: http://www.childabuseroyalcommission.gov.au/Pages/default.aspx.

47. United Nations Secretary-General. *In larger freedom: Towards development, security and human rights for all.* A/59/2005. New York: United Nations; 2005.

48. United Nations Development Programme. *Human development report, 1994.* New York: UN Development Programme; 1994.

49. United Nations General Assembly. *Resolution A/RES/33/53. Human rights and scientific and technological developments.* New York: United Nations; 1978.

50. United Nations General Assembly. *Principles for the protection of persons with mental illness and the improvement of mental health care.* Resolution 46/119. New York: United Nations; 1991.

51. United Nations. *The Universal Declaration of Human Rights.* 1948; Available from: http://www.un.org/en/documents/udhr/index.shtml.

52. United Nations. *International Covenant on Economic, Social and Cultural Rights.* 1966; Available from: http://www2.ohchr.org/english/law/cescr.htm.

53. United Nations. *International Covenant on Civil and Political Rights.* 1966; Available from: http://www2.ohchr.org/english/law/ccpr.htm.

54. Minas H, Diatri H. Pasung: Physical restraint and confinement of the mentally ill in the community. *Int J Ment Health Syst.* 2008;2(1):8. Epub 2008/06/17.

55. Puteh I, Marthoenis M, Minas H. Aceh Free Pasung: Releasing the mentally ill from physical restraint. *Int J Ment Health Syst.* 2011;5:10. Epub 17/5/2011.

56. Irmansyah I, Prasetyo YA, Minas H. Human rights of persons with mental illness in Indonesia: more than legislation is needed. *Int J Ment Health Syst.* 2009;3(1):14. Epub 24/6/2009.

57. Tol WA, Barbui C, Galappatti A, et al. Mental health and psychosocial support in humanitarian settings: linking practice and research. *Lancet.* 2011;378(9802):1581–91. Epub 20/10/2011.

58. Tol W, Bastin P, Jordans M, et al. Mental health and psychosocial support in humanitarian settings. In: Patel V, Minas H, Cohen A, Prince M, editors. *Global Mental Health: Principles and Practice.* New York: Oxford University Press; 2014.

59. *Natural disasters: coping with the health impact.* Disease Control Priorities project, 2007. Available at http://www.dcp2.org/file/121/.

60. Shoaf K, Rottman S. Public health impact of disasters. *Aust J Emerg Manag.* 2000;15:58–63.

61. Irmansyah I, Dharmono S, Maramis A, Minas H. Determinants of psychological morbidity in survivors of the earthquake and tsunami in Aceh and Nias. *Int J Ment Health Syst.* 2010;4(1):8. Epub 2010/04/29.

62. Minas H. Leadership for change in complex systems. *Australas Psychiatry.* 2005;13(1):33–9. Epub 2005/03/22.

63. Ogata S, Sen A. Foreword. *Human security now.* New York: Commission on Human Security; 2003.

64. Lund C. Social determinants of mental disorders. In: Patel V, Minas H, Cohen A, Prince M, editors. *Global Mental Health: Principles and Practice.* New York: Oxford University Press; 2014.

65. AusAID. *An effective aid program for Australia: Making a real difference—delivering real results.* Canberra: Australian Agency for International Development; 2012.

66. AusAID. *Development for all: Towards a disability-inclusive Australian aid program 2009–2014.* Canberra: Australian Agency for International Development; 2008.

67. Minas H. Mentally ill patients dying in social shelters in Indonesia. *Lancet.* 2009;374(9690):-592–3. Epub 2009/08/25.

68. Regional Office for Europe. *Impact of economic crises on mental health.* Copenhagen: World Health Organization; 2011.

69. WHO Secretariat. *The financial crisis and global health: Report of a high-level consultation.* Geneva: World Health Organization; 2009.

70. Fast-moving fire takes properties in central Victoria as New South Wales battles 135 blazes. [January 8, 2012]; Available from: http://www.theaustralian.com.au/news/fast-moving-fire-takes-properties-in-central-victoria-as-nsw-battles-135-blazes/story-e6frg6n6-1226549351466.

71. Karoly D, England M, Steffen W. *Off the charts: Extreme Australian summer heat.* Canberra: Climate Commission, 2013.

72. Minas H. The problem is detention, not asylum seekers. *Sydney Morning Herald.* September 22, 2010. Available at http://www.smh.com.au/opinion/politics/the-problem-is-detention-not-asylum-seekers-20100921-15l9l.html.

73. Organization for Economic Co-operation and Development. *Paris Declaration and Accra Agenda for Action, 2005/2008.* Available at http://www.oecd.org/dac/effectiveness/34428351.pdf.

74. AusAID. *An Effective Aid Program for Australia.* Canberra: Australian Agency for International Development; 2012.

75. United Nations General Assembly. *Convention on the Rights of Persons with Disabilities and the Optional Protocol thereto.* A/RES/65/154. New York: United Nations; 2010.

76. Alkire S. *Human development: Definitions, critiques, and related concepts*: United Nations Development Programme; 2010. Available at dr.undp.org/en/reports/global/hdr2010/papers/HDRP_2010_01.pdf.

77. United Nations Development Programme. *Human development report, 1990.* New York: UN Development Programme; 1990.

78. United Nations Development Programme. Human development: Concept. Nd; Available from: http://hdr.undp.org/en/media/SupportPackage_eng.pdf.

79. Sen A. *Development as freedom.* Oxford, UK: Oxford University Press; 2001.

80. Australian Agency for International Development. *Millennium Development Goals: The fight against global poverty and inequality.* Available from: http://www.ausaid.gov.au/aidissues/mdg/Pages/home.aspx.

81. Waldrop MM. *Complexity: The emerging science at the edge of order and chaos.* London: Penguin Books; 1994.

82. Plsek P, Greenhalgh T. Complexity science: the challenge of complexity in health care. *BMJ.* 2001;323(7314):625–8.

83. Plsek PE, Wilson T. Complexity science: complexity, leadership, and management in health care organizations. *BMJ.* 2001;323(7314):746–9.

84. Wilson T, Holt T, Greenhalgh T. Complexity and clinical care. *BMJ.* 2001;323(7314):685–8.

85. Kauffman S. *At home in the universe: The search for laws of self-organization and complexity.* London: Penguin Books; 1996.

86. World Health Organization. *Mental health atlas.* Geneva: World Health Organization; 2005.

87. Saraceno B, Saxena S. Mental health resources in the world: results from Project Atlas of the WHO. *World Psychiatry.* 2002;1(1):40–4. Epub 2006/09/02.

88. Alkira S, Santos E. *Multidimensional poverty index.* Oxford, UK: Oxford Poverty and Human Development Initiative, University of Oxford, 2010.

89. World Health Assembly. *The global burden of mental disorders and the need for a comprehensive, coordinated response from health and social sectors at the country level.* WHA A65/R4. Geneva: World Health Organization; 2912.

90. Butler M. *Partners in recovery: new, practical support for people living with severe mental illness.* New Paradigm: *Aust J Psychosoc Rehabil.* 2012(Spring/Summer):6–8.

91. Callaly T, Arya D, Minas H. Quality, risk management and governance in mental health: an overview. *Australas Psychiatry.* 2005;13(1):16–20. Epub 2005/03/22.

92. Fraser SW, Greenjalgh T. Coping with complexity: Educating for capability. *BMJ.* 2001;323:799–803.

93. Movement for Global Mental Health. Available from: http://www.globalmentalhealth.org/articles.html.

94. Minas H. The Centre for International Mental Health approach to mental health system development. *Harv Rev Psychiatry.* 2012;20(1):37–46. Epub 2012/02/18.

95. Craze L. *National Recovery-Oriented Mental Health Practice Framework Project: Discussion paper.* Glen Alpine NSW: Craze Lateral Solutions; 2012.

96. World Health Organization. *Risks to mental health: An overview of vulnerabilities and risk factors.* Geneva: World Health Organization; 2012.

97. Whiteford H. Leadership in mental health policy: the national context. *Australas Psychiatry.* 2005;13(1):21–6. Epub 2005/03/22.

98. Fritze JG, Blashki GA, Burke S, Wiseman J. Hope, despair and transformation: Climate change and the promotion of mental health and wellbeing. *Int J Ment Health Syst.* 2008;2(1):13. Epub 2008/09/19.

99. Intergovernmental Panel on Climate Change. http://www.ipcc.ch/.

100. Parmesan C, Yohe G. A globally coherent fingerprint of climate change impacts across natural systems. *Nature.* 2003;421(6918):37–42. Epub 2003/01/04.

101. Patz JA, Campbell-Lendrum D, Holloway T, Foley JA. Impact of regional climate change on human health. *Nature.* 2005;438(7066):310-7. Epub 2005/11/18.

102. Narayan SM, Stein MB. Do depression or antidepressants increase cardiovascular mortality? The absence of proof might be more important than the proof of absence. *J Am Coll Cardiol.* 2009;53(11):959–61. Epub 2009/03/14.

103. Costello A, Abbas M, Allen A, et al. Managing the health effects of climate change: Lancet and University College London Institute for Global Health Commission. *Lancet.* 2009;373(9676):1693–733. Epub 2009/05/19.

104. Patz JA, Kovats RS. Hotspots in climate change and human health. *BMJ.* 2002;325(7372):1094–8. Epub 2002/11/09.

105. United Nations. *The Millennium Development Goals Report 2012.* New York: United Nations; 2012.

9 Global Mental Health Resources

Pallab K. Maulik, Amy M. Daniels,
Ryan McBain, and Jodi Morris

INTRODUCTION

Recent trends have seen an increase in the prevalence of non-communicable disorders and injuries, especially in low- and middle-income countries.[1] Not only are cardiovascular disorders, stroke, cancer, diabetes and respiratory diseases on the rise, but mental health conditions such as alcohol use disorders have also shown an increasing trend in recent years. Furthermore, many non-communicable disorders like cardiovascular diseases, cancers, and stroke, and communicable diseases, such as HIV/AIDS, are associated with an increased risk of mental disorders, which add to the increasing numbers of people affected with mental disorders.[2] The World Mental Health Survey estimated that the 12-month prevalence of any mental disorder varies between 4.3% to 26.4% across different countries.[3] More recently, analyses from Europe suggests that almost 38% Europeans suffer from mental disorders in any given year, which corresponds to almost 168 million people.[4]

The number of people suffering from mental illnesses of different types and severity is large and growing. Factors contributing to the increased diagnosed prevalence of mental disorders include improved identification, increased awareness among the general population and care providers, increased stress, the growing prevalence of other chronic health conditions including conditions like HIV-AIDS, alcohol and substance use disorders, and an aging population.[5] Over the past half century, developments in the areas of neurobiology and pharmacology have led to a better understanding of many mental disorders and their treatments. However, the complexities of mental disorders do not have a unique solution that fits all, and numerous resources are required to tackle the problem. Such resources vary from the easily understood need for infrastructure and suitably trained health personnel who can deliver good care, to more complex issues related to community-based support facilities and legislative and policy initiatives that can provide the necessary governance and oversight to implementing evidence-based care.[5,6] However, it is the lack of many such factors and their inequitable distribution that contributes to a large treatment gap and causes increased disability due to mental illnesses. While true of low- and middle-income countries,[7] the treatment gap—i.e., the difference between the number of people in need of mental health care and those actually receiving it—is large even in high-income countries.[8] Even when mental health care is received, it can be inadequate or inappropriate due to the lack of health professionals trained to manage mental illness.

Patel and Prince[9] defined global mental health in the context of global health as an "area of study, research and practice that places a priority on improving [mental] health and achieving equity in [mental] health for all people worldwide."[10] Global mental health resources can mean many things to many people and encompass a large array of specific components that help reduce the burden of mental disorders, improve mental health, and promote positive mental health across the world. In 2001, World Health Organization (WHO) launched Project Atlas,[11] which defined and outlined key mental health resources. The areas that Atlas included were: mental health policies and programs; legislation; availability of mental health services for the general population; availability of services for specific populations such as children and adolescents, women, the elderly, persons with disabilities, refugees, and persons with alcohol and substance use disorders; primary care and community care services; number of mental health personnel and mental health care facilities; mental health financing; facilities for training and education in mental health; monitoring and surveillance and research facilities; and availability of essential psychotropic medicines. While this list is not exhaustive, this chapter on global mental health resources will focus on these key resources.

Several important questions arise while discussing global mental health resources. What is known about existing mental health resources, and where are the gaps? How are the gaps to be closed? What works best, and in which settings? Is research sufficiently advanced to address such concerns? Who should be responsible for developing mental health resources, and in which areas should government and non-governmental organizations (NGOs) collaborate? While not all such questions have an easy answer, some can be answered and will be discussed in the following sections of this chapter.

KNOWLEDGE ABOUT GLOBAL MENTAL HEALTH RESOURCES AND THE RELEVANCE OF DATA COLLECTED BY THE WORLD HEALTH ORGANIZATION

The concept of global mental health has been around for some years, but it is only in the past decade that there has been a renewed focus in the area. Some factors that have regenerated interest are the availability of new, cross-culturally relevant epidemiological studies that highlighted the burden of mental illness, awareness about treatment modalities that can be delivered using non-specialist health workers,[9] and global leadership provided by WHO and other international organizations. As the realization about global mental health needs increased, so did a felt need to gather information about available resources to manage mental illness. In the latter half of 2000, there was a sudden impetus to gather such information when WHO decided to focus on mental health in their World Health Report of 2001. Project Atlas[11] originated out of that need and has continued to develop many editions and variants.[12–18] Project Atlas remains the only source of data about global mental health resources that uses similar definitions to gather data across all countries of the world. While Atlas collects only macro-level data, and the accuracy of such data can be questioned, it provides a broad overview of global mental health resources that can be compared across countries.

Project Atlas

Since 2001, the primary objective of Project Atlas has been to "raise public and professional awareness of the inadequacies of existing [mental health] resources and services and the large inequities in their distribution at national and global level."[18] To this end, Project Atlas has published updated reports roughly every five years—in 2001, 2005, and 2011—with particular attention to process indicators on various components of countries' mental health systems. The 2011 edition of the Mental Health Atlas represents the most up-to-date, internationally representative compilation of resources for mental health currently available, comprising data on 184 of 193 United Nations member states and covering 95% of the world population.

WHO Assessment Instrument for Mental Health Systems (WHO-AIMS)

Alongside the WHO Mental Health Atlas, a number of other initiatives and instruments such as WHO-AIMS[19] and the World Mental Health (WMH) Surveys have made substantial contributions to the global mental health resource database. The chief goal of WHO-AIMS is to provide a comprehensive assessment of a country's mental health system, as well as the services and support offered to people with mental disorders outside of the psychiatric service sector. Through WHO-AIMS, countries are able to develop information-based mental health policy and plans with clear baseline information and targets. Moreover, through regular assessments, countries are able to monitor progress in implementing reform policies, providing community services, and involving consumers, families, and other stakeholders in mental health promotion, prevention, care, and rehabilitation.

Project Atlas and WHO-AIMS Comparisons

The overlap between Project Atlas and WHO-AIMS deserves particular attention, as commonalities across indicators have allowed for a contextualized and comparative representation of many countries' mental health systems. Unlike other available indicator schemes, WHO-AIMS was specifically designed with the needs of low- and middle-income countries in mind.[20] In comparison to the Mental Health Atlas, the methodology of data collection involved in the WHO-AIMS is more rigorous, covers a wider range of indicators, and involves several rounds of review. This reflects the different primary objectives of the two projects. Whereas the primary purpose of WHO-AIMS is to provide countries with a tool that allows them to gather in-depth information that can be used for mental health planning and policy development, information collected through Atlas is primarily used for advocacy and research. Though the methodologies and primary goals of these projects differ, both projects provide a comprehensive picture of existing mental health resources. An accurate and up-to-date picture along these lines is important for several reasons. It provides statistical evidence of successes and shortcomings in terms of resource provisions at national levels as well as disparities across global regions and income levels. This in turn has the capacity to draw attention to current needs in mental health and to identify priorities and strategies to improve services and patient protections.[21] Coupled with epidemiological data and information on the global burden of mental illness—estimated at 13.5% of the global burden of disease—these data can also raise awareness of the existing "resources gap" between current resource levels and those needed to adequately treat patients. Beyond this, data generated from assessments such as the WHO-AIMS and Mental Health Atlas provide a lens through which countries can view their own resource levels and distribution in order to identify areas for strengthening. Ultimately, it is likely that efforts in this direction will be modest given the resource constraints of many countries, and realistic goals must be bolstered by actionable mental health plans.

EXISTING GLOBAL MENTAL HEALTH RESOURCES: FINDINGS FROM PROJECT ATLAS AND OTHER GLOBAL INITIATIVES

Detailed country-level statistics on mental health resources may be available from some countries; however, to provide an overview of the global perspective, this chapter highlights updated findings from the Mental Health Atlas 2011[18] and outlines key initiatives in the area of global mental health resources across the world, including the WHO-AIMS.[19] In addition to the Mental Health Atlas and WHO-AIMS, information on global mental health services, training, and public health priorities have been compiled in specialized atlases—*Atlas: Psychiatric Education and Training across the World 2005*,[12] *Atlas: Child and Adolescent Mental Health Resources*,[13] and *Atlas: Nurses in Mental Health 2007*[15]—and have been incorporated into the discussion of findings below. Examples from other individual initiatives and country-specific data have also been included to highlight specific gaps.

Governance

At a conceptual level, governance can be thought of in terms of the existence and content of a mental health legislative and policy framework—including a national mental health policy, a national mental health plan or strategy, and ratified laws pertaining to mental health—as well as in terms of the enforcement of existing legislation and the implementation of policy.

Mental Health Policies

"Mental health policies" may be broadly defined as official statements of governments which convey an organized set of values, principles, objectives, and areas for action to improve the mental health of a population. While the content areas of a policy may vary from country to country, good-practice principles can ensure that the most important processes have been addressed and key content issues have been included.[22] According to Mental Health Atlas 2011,[18] mental health policies exist in 60% of countries and cover approximately three-quarters (72%) of the world's population. However, as indicated in Figure 9.1, this statistic masks considerable heterogeneity by World Bank income group classifications[7]: over three-quarters (77%) of high-income countries maintain policies, compared with half (49%) of low-income countries. Importantly, there has been little change in the percentage of countries reporting mental health policies from *Atlas 2001* to *Atlas 2011*: at all three time points, approximately two-thirds of countries have reported the presence of a mental health policy.

Mental Health Plans

In conjunction with mental health policies, mental health plans serve to delineate strategies and activities that will be implemented to realize the objectives of a policy, and typically specify elements such as the budget and timeframe for implementation. Mental health plans have a unique implementation orientation. They play a critical role in translating policy into practice.[23] In comparison to national mental health policies, plans exist in approximately three-quarters (72%) of countries and cover 95% of the world's population; this compares with 70% of countries in 2005, signifying that there has been limited progress over the past six years. As shown in Figure 9.1, level of coverage today ranges from 62% of low-income countries to 88% of high-income countries.

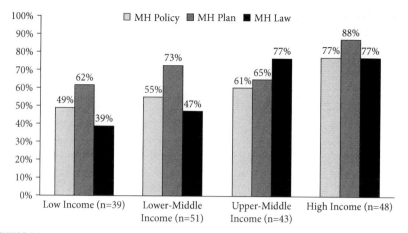

FIGURE 9.1

Percent of countries with mental health policies, plans, and laws, by World Bank Income Group.

Among countries with mental health plans, over 80% have approved or revised their plan since 2005, while only 6% have continued with plans created or adapted before 2000. This evolution may be seen, in part, as a greater prioritization of mental health within the global health arena over the past ten years, as embodied in seminal publications such as the *2001 World Health Report*.[5] In 2009, the health ministers of Latin American and Caribbean countries formulated the Strategy and Plan of Action on Mental Health, which for the first time outlined a vision and direction for development of mental health services and capacity building over a 10-year period in the region, for taking better care of patients with mental disorders and promoting positive mental health.[24] Other WHO regions have adopted similar initiatives.

Mental Health Laws

Although national mental health policies and plans provide a strong foundation for a functional mental health system, mental health laws are particularly important for securing the rights and protections of persons suffering from mental illness. In a diversity of contexts, those with mental illness are formally and informally discriminated against in terms of employment, voting, and a variety of personal freedoms.[17] Given this reality, mental health laws provide legal recourse for guarding individuals' autonomy in pursuing meaningful lives. Such laws can cover a broad array of issues, including access to mental health care; consent to treatment; freedom from cruel, inhuman, and degrading treatment; freedom from discrimination; and protection of a full range of civil, cultural, economic, political, and social rights. A dedicated mental health law refers more narrowly to legislation which covers *all* issues of relevance to persons with mental disorders.

Worldwide, approximately 60% of countries have dedicated mental health laws, with global coverage also representing approximately 60% of the world's population. Figure 9.1 illustrates that there is more variability in the existence of these laws than of national policies or plans: roughly four in ten (39%) low-income countries—as compared to eight in ten (77%) high-income countries—have mental health laws. Among countries with mental health legislation, less than half (42%) of these laws were enacted or revised in 2005 or later, and 15% have continued with legislation enacted before 1970.

In addition to disparities in the legislative frameworks between low- and high-income countries, a number of critical knowledge gaps remain in the evaluation of global mental health governance. Chief among these is the quality of mental health policies, plans, and laws.[25] Ideally, mental health legislation forms a foundation for a well-functioning mental health system; however, in many instances legislation remains inchoate and ineffectual as a positive force for change.[26] For example, Cooper and colleagues,[27] while reporting on Uganda's mental health policy, found that though a draft policy exists that is in line with international norms, it is stigmatizing and does not adequately protect the human rights of people with mental illness. In Ghana, the existence of the Mental Health Act was not widely known, and the policy was not effective.[28] Uganda or Ghana are only two of many countries where mental health laws or policies do not adequately address human rights concerns of people with mental illness, and there is a need to develop strategies that correct that situation. This inadequacy of existing laws also extends to laws related to persons with disabilities, including intellectual disability.[29] Often, existing laws lack adequate executive processes in place that can implement such laws and do not have any clauses stating that failure to implement them would lead to prosecution. At times, such mental health laws can be impediments to delivery of human rights-based care, and are worse than having no laws. This in turn raises the question whether mental health legislation is reflective of a country's prioritization of mental health care and an intention to take concrete steps moving forward, or whether policy formation remains an exercise of abstraction simply meant to convey a country's normative principles.

Financing and Payment Systems

Financing represents a critical component of mental health resources. In particular, mental health expenditures per capita provide an overall picture of the amount of funding dedicated to mental health facilities, training and employment of mental health professionals, and the purchase of medicines for the treatment of mental illness. In addition, financing provides a general picture of resource allocation, as one can view both the percentage of government expenditures allocated to mental health and the percentage of the mental health budget allocated to various systems components, such as mental hospitals and research and training facilities.[30]

One major finding from the 2011 edition of the *Mental Health Atlas* shows that the level of country expenditures on mental health is a function of country income as measured by gross national income (GNI) per capita.[7] As indicated in Figure 9.2A, over 60% of the variability in countries' mental health expenditures per capita is explained by country GNI. For example, in Bangladesh, a low-income country with a GNI of US$580 per capita, US$0.03 is spent per person on mental health. In contrast, Singapore—a high-income country with a GNI of US$37,220—spends US$26.05 per capita on mental health. Nonetheless, even countries with similar income levels have substantially different levels of mental health expenditures: for instance, while Brazil and Lebanon have comparable GNIs, Brazil spends 2.6 times more on mental health per capita.

Overall, the global median expenditure on mental health is estimated at US$1.63 per capita per year. As illustrated in Figure 9.2B, this figure varies substantially by income per capita and income group classification. While median mental health expenditure in low-income countries is more than 200 times below that of high-income countries, median GNI in low-income countries is only 76 times lower than that of high-income countries, indicating that income level does not fully account for funding differences. One additional factor liable to contribute to such income-based disparities is differential rates of infectious diseases like HIV/AIDS, tuberculosis, and malaria: given higher rates of such diseases in poorer countries, such countries tend to allocate a larger proportion of their health budget towards communicable than towards non-communicable diseases.[16]

The percentage of total government health expenditures dedicated to mental health is an indication of the priority given to mental health within the government's health

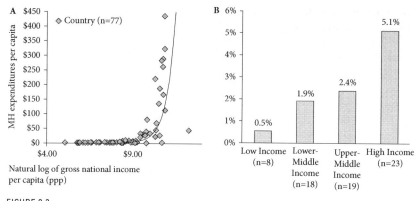

FIGURE 9.2

A: Association between GNI and financing. **B:** Percent of health expenditures dedicated to mental health, by World Bank Income Group.

sector. On this measure, the global median percentage of health expenditures dedicated to mental health is 2.8%. As shown in Figure 9.2B, lower-income countries tend to spend a smaller percentage of their health budget on mental health: in low-income countries, a median of 0.5% of health expenditures is dedicated to mental health, compared to 1.9% in lower-middle-income countries, 2.4% in upper-middle-income countries, and 5.1% in high-income countries.

Globally, the three commonest methods of financing mental health care are through government-levied taxation (63%), followed by out-of-pocket payments (17%), and social insurance (15%).[31] However, in some of the poorest and most populous countries, such as India, Pakistan, and Nigeria, taxes and social insurance form a smaller component. In most of these countries, individuals often spend more out-of-pocket in order to receive better treatment.

One of the principles operationalized by WHO's mental health Gap Action Programme (mhGAP) project has been the decentralization of mental health resources by shifting treatment from institutionalized care in mental hospitals to a more integrated approach that emphasizes the role of the primary care sector.[32] Along these lines, the proportion of mental health expenditures allocated to mental hospitals serves as a proxy for the concentration and priority of institutionalized care in a country. According to *Atlas 2011*, almost three-quarters (73%) of mental health expenditures are spent at mental hospitals in low- and middle-income countries, compared to roughly half of expenditures (54%) in high-income countries. Andreoli and colleagues[33] reported that, in Brazil, mental health expenditure as a proportion of total health expenditure fell from 5.8% in 1995 to 2.3% in 2005, mainly due to a significant drop in the budget allocated to mental hospitals, which fell from almost 96% to 50% of the mental health budget. However, the same period also saw an increase in the budget for community services, from less than 1% to 15%. India's mental health budget increased from a little more than US $6 million in the period from 1997 to 2002 to a proposed US $210 million in 2008 to 2012.[34] However, reality suggests that this increase is insufficient to support all the mental health needs of the population, and even the allocated amounts are often not utilized efficiently or equitably.

Stepping back, it is apparent that even basic data on countries' mental health financing are lacking. Only slightly more than one-third of countries included in Project Atlas were able to provide a dollar amount allocated to mental health expenditures. This raises questions about the representativeness of the existing sample. In addition to facile indicators such as mental health expenditures per capita, it also behooves countries to document their financing and payment systems, if one has been established. For example, information on a country's payment system provides critical knowledge on existing incentives and disincentives for health care workers, which are liable to have an impact on the level and quality of patient care.[35] In China, for instance,doctors receive greater compensation for prescribing more medicines at higher costs, leading to significant over-prescription and over-consumption, especially in private sector healthcare facilites where profit margins are important metrics for success.[36] Since psychiatric care can be expensive due to longer durations of treatment, it is important to reduce out-of-pocket expenses to a minimum, and governments should cover mental disorders as part of social insurance packages. However, social insurance is dependent on government funds, so a poor country will have limited resources to fund such initiatives. In other countries where social insurance is not compulsory and universal, such facilities are available to only those who are employed or in urban settings. Private insurance also has its own risks, as is evident by the managed care provided by private insurers in United States that may limit psychiatric care to specific modalities and for specified periods of time.[37] Thus methods of financing mental health care across countries are not ideal, and more efforts should be made by individual governments to reduce the financial burden on their citizens.

Mental Health Services

Mental health services provide interventions for mental disorders. Most countries provide mental health care within primary health care systems and through dedicated mental health facilities such as mental hospitals and mental health outpatient facilities. Outpatient facilities, psychiatric wards within general hospitals, community residential facilities, and mental hospitals have their own roles in care of patients with mental illnesses. For example, mental hospitals and psychiatric wards in general hospitals typically provide treatment for acute psychiatric episodes or long-term care for those with severe mental disorders. In comparison, outpatient facilities, and community-residential facilities provide community-based support for those seeking follow-up care or who are in recovery. Mental hospitals are not an efficient use of resources, and the shift should be for primary care and community care. However, in many countries where community care is not developed mental hospitals may be the only care available and in this context may be considered a resource. Ideally, the distribution of and funding for different types of facilities accurately reflect patterns of access to care as well as the function for which facilities are designed.[22]

Primary Health Care

Primary health care (PHC) encompasses health clinics offering a first point of entry into the health system, and typically provides initial assessment and treatment for common health conditions while referring those requiring specialized care. In many instances, mental disorders can be managed effectively at the PHC level if adequate resources are available. Furthermore, an emphasis on community-based care can improve early detection and treatment, minimize stigma from treatment-seeking, and improve the cost-effectiveness of interventions.[31] Availability of protocols for treatment and diagnosis, and official referral procedures exemplify vital components of countries' mental health systems. Globally, only 36% of countries have approved manuals for treatment and diagnosis of mental disorders at the PHC level, with little variability by income-group classification. The existence of formal referral procedures is more frequent, although poorer countries are less likely to have procedures in place: while 82% of high-income countries have referral procedures from primary to secondary and tertiary care, only 72% of low-income countries have these procedures formalized.

Outpatient Facilities

Outpatient facilities specifically focus on the management of mental disorders and related clinical problems on an outpatient basis. Worldwide, there is a median of 0.6 outpatient facilities per 100,000 population. However, this value ranges from 0.04 facilities per 100,000 population in low-income countries to 2.32 facilities in high-income countries (Table 9.1). In Mexico, for example, there is approximately one outpatient facility for every four million people, whereas in Croatia there is one facility for every 30,000 people.

Psychiatric Wards Within General Hospitals

Psychiatric wards within general hospitals are those reserved for care of persons with mental disorders within general hospitals. Such wards are present in 85% of countries. While the global median number of beds in these wards is 1.4 per 100,000 population, the median ranges from 0.4 per 100,000 population in lower-middle-income countries to 13.6 per 100,000 population in high-income countries. In comparison with declining rates of psychiatric beds in mental hospitals, globally there has been no change in the rate of general hospital psychiatric beds. Only in low-income countries was the median rate of change negative, indicating that more than half of low-income countries saw a decrease in their rate of general hospital beds reserved for psychiatric patients.

Community Residential Facilities

Another form of decentralized care is embodied in community residential facilities, which are community-based mental health facilities that provide overnight residence for people with mental disorders. Community residential facilities are present in 54% of countries. While the global median rate of community residential facilities is 0.008 per 100,000 population (or 8 per 100 million population), there is presently a median of zero facilities per 100,000 in low- and middle-income countries, as compared to 10 facilities per 100,000 population in high-income countries.

Mental Hospitals

Mental hospitals are inpatient facilities that typically provide care and long-stay residential services for people with severe mental disorders. Mental hospitals are present in 80% of countries. The global median prevalence of mental hospitals is 0.03 hospitals per 100,000 population and ranges from 0.01 in low-income countries to 0.10 in high-income countries. A greater contrast can be found in terms of the number of beds in

Table 9.1 Number of Outpatient Facilities and Psychiatric Beds in General and Mental Hospitals per 100,000 Population, by World Bank Income Group Classification

Income Group (n = no. of respondent countries)	Outpatient Facilities	Psychiatric Beds in General Hospitals	Psychiatric Beds in Mental Hospitals
Low-income (n = 30–35)	0.04	0.6	1.3
Lower-middle-income (n = 40–47)	0.29	0.4	4.5
Upper-middle-income (n = 35–43)	1.05	2.7	21.0
High-income (n = 40–47)	2.32	13.6	30.9

mental hospitals, which varies from 1.3 per 100,000 population in low-income countries to 30.9 per 100,000 population in high-income countries (Table 9.1). Yet, even within income groups, differences persist. For example, while Pakistan has approximately one psychiatric bed per 100,000 population, India, Nigeria, and Viet Nam—three additional lower-middle-income countries with equivalent GNIs—have 1.5, 2.5, and 18.0 psychiatric beds per 100,000 population, respectively.

Interestingly, when comparing rates of psychiatric beds in mental hospitals reported in *Atlas 2005* and *Atlas 2011*, one finds a clear trend indicating a reduction. Globally, there is a median decrease of approximately 0.1 mental hospital beds per 100,000 population, with the greatest declines in upper-middle (0.9 per 100,000 population) and high-income countries (0.4 per 100,000 population). It is likely that this trend reflects a global shift from institutionalized to community-based care in outpatient and primary care facilities; however, additional research is needed to confirm this.

Across all types of facilities, availability of appropriate psychotropic medications for treating mental disorders is important. Studies have shown that pharmacological interventions are beneficial and cost-effective in treating a range of mental disorders, such as schizophrenia, major depressive disorder, and so forth.[38] Based on data from 50 respondent countries, median expenditures on medicines is US$6.81 per capita. However, it should be noted that the majority of respondents were high-income countries, and that the actual global median is liable to be considerably lower than this. By income, a median of US$0.02 per capita is dedicated to medicines for mental health in low-income countries, as compared to US$0.17 in lower-middle-income countries, US$0.83 in upper-middle-income countries, and US$26.31 in high-income countries.

There are two key concerns about available mental health care facilities, globally— inadequate number of facilities, and inequitable distribution of those even when available. Data from Atlas and WHO-AIMS show that the availability of community-based services and primary care facilities for mental health is very limited. Where available, the services are often not comprehensive. Community-based support services for people with mental illnesses are especially poor in low- and middle-income countries, and people in such settings are often left to fulfill their own needs even when they need support for daily household chores, shopping, transport services, education, or work-based needs, acute or long-term, etc. Often community-based care is provided through a mix of governmental and non-governmental organizations that involve consumers and families. In countries like Brazil, which have shown significant improvement in providing care to those with mental illness, it has been largely due to the advocacy of families and consumers. Also, in many low- and middle-income countries, families are responsible for provision of a considerable amount of care since formally trained human resources are scarce. Furthermore, even when such services exist, they are often not organized properly and exist within "silos."[37] Inpatient or outpatient care specific to mental illnesses varies across and within countries. There are huge differences in the availability and quality of care provided. Within a country, available services are mostly located in urban centers, leaving large parts of the country without any access to mental health care. India, a country with a large, diverse population, is an example of one country that suffers from similar problems. Even when services are available, they vary considerably in quality. Inadequate numbers of mental health professionals, unavailability of inpatient beds, and poor supplies of essential psychotropic medications are only a few of the factors that undermine existing services.[37]

Human Resources

Human resources for mental health comprise the most versatile input in countries' mental health systems. While the human resources in global mental health will be elaborated upon in the next chapter, for now it will suffice to say that they serve a variety of functions, including making diagnoses and referrals, providing treatment in the form of psychotherapy and prescription of medicines, training future generations of human resources, and advocating for greater resources as well as patient rights and protections.[39,40] The WHO *Mental Health Atlas* provides an overview of both human resource training, which is predictive of future human resource levels, and the numbers of human resources presently working in mental health. In addition, the specialized *Atlas of Psychiatric Education and Training*[12] provides more comprehensive information on training.

Training

Globally, there are more nursing graduates (a median of 5.2 per 100,000 population) than all other health professionals combined—which includes a median of 0.04 psychiatrists, 0.09 psychologists, and 3.34 other medical doctors (not specialized in psychiatry) per 100,000 population. Additionally, in all categories of professional graduates, there are many more who completed training in high as compared to low-income countries.

The *Mental Health Atlas* also provides basic information about training at the primary health care level. As of 2011, less than one-third (28%) of countries reported a majority of PHC doctors with official in-service training on mental health within the past five years; this figure was even lower for PHC nurses—22%. Percentages did not vary substantially by income level, indicating that the existing knowledge gap is not primarily reflective of a country's inability to pay for training.

According to the *Atlas of Psychiatric Education and Training*, which covered 73 countries, roughly 70% of countries had psychiatric training programs in place—slightly more than half (55%) of low-income countries, and approximately three-quarters (77%) of high-income countries.[12] Half of respondent countries reported having an accredited diploma or master's degree in psychiatry. Each country has specific criteria to determine psychiatric training programs; approximately 45 countries reported using availability of a minimum number of beds as the predetermined criterion, and the average number of beds used for establishing a program was 136. Outpatient attendance was also a training criterion in 33 countries. Furthermore, teaching and research skills were evaluated during some point of training in about 55% and 70% of countries, respectively.

Current Human Resources

Consistent with the number of graduates from different health professions, globally there are more nurses working in the mental health sector—a median of 5.8 per 100,000 population—than all other health professionals combined. In 2007, the specialized *Atlas on Nurses in Mental Health* found a median of 0.3 nurses per 100,000 population working in the mental health sector of low-income countries, 2.1 in lower-middle-income countries, 6.4 in upper-middle-income countries, and 29.8 in high-income countries.[15] In both Atlases, the principal message is clear: while the proportion of nurses is lower in poor countries, nurses play a central role in providing care for patients with mental disorders.

Across all professions, the global median prevalence of human resources working in the mental health sector is 10.7 per 100,000 population (Table 9.2). While data on human resources levels were also collected by Project Atlas in 2001 and 2005, modifications in operational definitions preclude comparisons of earlier editions and 2011 rates, with the exception of rates of psychiatrists. On this particular measure, it was found that— between 2005 and 2011—rates of psychiatrists increased by 0.65 per 100,000 population in high-income countries, by 0.31 per 100,000 population in upper-middle-income countries, by 0.03 in lower-middle-income countries, and *decreased by* 0.01 per 100,000

Table 9.2 Current Level of Health Professionals Working in the Mental Health Sector per 100,000 Population, by World Bank Income Group Classification

Income Group (n = no. of respondent countries)	Psychiatrists	Other medical doctors	Nurses	Psychologists	Social workers	Occupational therapists
Low-income (n = 25–38)	0.05	0.06	0.42	0.02	0.01	0.00
Lower-middle-income (n = 31–52)	0.54	0.21	2.93	0.14	0.13	0.01
Upper-middle-income (n = 26–42)	2.03	0.87	9.72	1.47	0.76	0.23
High-income (n = 26–47)	8.41	1.49	29.15	3.79	2.16	1.51

population in low-income countries. This decrease reflects both "brain drain," in terms of the number of psychiatrists emigrating to higher-income countries, as well as a failure to train new psychiatrists at a rate commensurate with population growth rates.[41]

In addition to health professionals, family and user associations may be considered informal human resources that play vital roles in patient advocacy and support. Globally, family and user associations are present in 64% and 62% of countries, respectively, with much greater representation in high-income countries. Among countries in which user and family associations are present, over three-quarters of the time, these associations participate in the formulation and implementation of mental health policies, plans, and legislation. While such findings are promising, greater research is needed with respect to the magnitude and impact these associations have in resource-limited settings.

The quality of psychiatric education and training of mental health professionals is not uniform across countries. Even within countries, the training standards vary considerably. For example, in India, while the basic curriculum is similar across medical institutions, the focus on psychiatric training at both the under- and post-graduate levels varies across them. At the post-graduate level, the quality of psychiatric training also varies. Often the differences are not due to a lack of initiative but to inadequate infrastructure or the unavailability of adequately trained teaching staff. Mental health professionals, including psychiatrists, should receive both clinical and research training that tunes them in to issues like cultural differences, human rights, ethics, research methodologies, and so forth, which would not only help them in their clinical practice but also guide their research principles and help them to function more effectively globally.[42] Due to inadequate training facilities, it is not surprising to find inadequate numbers of trained mental health personnel across countries. Not only is the distribution skewed across countries, with poorer countries having fewer trained personnel, but it also varies within different regions of a given country, with most trained personnel located in urban centers. The lack of adequate resources is also apparent in other areas of mental illness, such as addictions. For example, one-third of countries lack a government unit or official responsible for treatment services for substance use disorders, and less than half of countries report a specific budget allocated to the treatment of substance use disorders.[17] This is despite the fact that, globally, some 39 deaths per 100 000 population are attributable to alcohol and illicit drug use, out of which 35 are attributable to alcohol use.

Given the lack of resources, it is time to acknowledge that responsibilities to manage mental health problems need to be shared across other health disciplines and systems of medicine, including traditional healers, especially in low- and middle-income countries.[43]

The governments of such countries should take effective measures to develop an integrated policy of care that factors in inadequate resources and the need to involve other health practitioners.

Information Systems: Surveillance and Monitoring

Information systems provide a critical framework for evaluating the structure and delivery of mental health resources within a country's health system. Information gathering through an organized data collection system allows for an overview of system *inputs*— i.e., the level and distribution of various resources, which is critical to identifying shortcomings and areas for strengthening. Data collection and analysis also allows for an overview of system *outputs*, including the number and demographic distribution of individuals seeking treatment at different types of facilities, the availability of various types of services to individuals, and whether the same or different individuals are seeking treatment at facilities over time.[44]

A majority of *Atlas 2011* respondent countries reported collecting data on numbers of admissions to mental hospitals (80%), general hospitals (73%), outpatient facilities (68%), and day treatment facilities (63%). In contrast, fewer countries report collecting data on patient levels at primary health care facilities (56%) and community residential facilities (34%). Data on diagnosis and service users' age and gender are also collected less frequently than information on admissions. Beyond these basic estimates outlined in Project Atlas, it remains unclear whether and to what extent countries collect mental health care data at local, district, and regional levels. Moreover, countries do not offer details on information system infrastructure, including whether medical records are stored on hardcopy or in electronic form, or whether health care providers are required to document patient information in a systematic and uniform manner. Given these realities, the level of quality and reliability of estimates (e.g., on admissions rates) provided to WHO are liable to vary dramatically from one country to the next.

Mental Health Resources for Special Populations

Inequity of access to care for certain groups, such as children, women, people in rural or remote settings, and the poor, is a serious issue in many countries, as resources for mental health are often not evenly distributed among the population.[22,45] For example, facilities and human resources are often concentrated in urban centers, thereby limiting access to appropriate services for rural populations. Data from WHO-AIMS indicate that, controlling for population density, the availability of beds, psychiatrists, and nurses is approximately three times greater in urban areas.[19] Moreover, services in many low- and middle-income countries are also concentrated in the private sector, therefore limiting access for the poor, especially those of ethnic and linguistic minority groups.[22]

In addition, vulnerable populations often have unique needs and require treatment by professionals with specific training, which is unavailable in many countries. For example, most health facilities in low- and middle-income countries are staffed by health workers who have not received training for child mental health and are therefore unable to distinguish the differing mental health needs of infants, children, and adolescents.[46] Lack of training can result in the misidentification or over-diagnosis of disorders in children and adolescents, which, in turn, may perpetuate stigma; for example, mental health conditions may be mislabeled as discipline problems, laziness, or even witchcraft.[47,48] Developing awareness about child and adolescent mental health problems amongst different stakeholders in the community was identified as a key first step in increasing the willingness to discuss emotional issues in a study conducted across nine low- and middle-income countries.[49] Moreover, research on global child mental health suggests that resources for children and adolescents greatly lag behind those available for adults.[13,50] For instance, a recent study of the treated prevalence in mental health services for children and adolescents in 42 low- and middle-income countries found that children comprise only 12% of the patient population in mental health outpatient facilities and less than 6% in all other types of mental health facilities, and that less than 1% of beds in inpatient facilities is reserved for this population.[50] The creation of national mental health policies for children, the promotion of international legislation on children's rights, and other global initiatives can be instrumental in addressing treatment disparities and in improving availability of and access to services for children and adolescents with mental health needs.[51]

Other vulnerable populations, such as women,[52] refugees,[53] and the elderly[18,54] may have less access to general health services, including mental health services than the rest of the population. Given that women in resource-poor countries are more likely to be poor and less educated and to experience trauma, such as intimate-partner violence,[55] and that these factors put individuals at greater risk for experiencing psychological and emotional distress, efforts to close the gender treatment gap are urgently needed.

While the mental health needs of refugees and internally displaced populations and those affected by war, for instance, may be greater than those of the general population,[56] these groups encounter multiple barriers to accessing needed care. Barriers to care can be both structural and cultural in nature, and include language, high cost, general distrust, lack of knowledge, and low social acceptability of psychiatric care.[53,57]

Resources to address the mental health needs of older adults, particularly those suffering from dementia, are especially lacking in low- and middle-income countries.[2] In general, health systems of resource-poor countries are not equipped to address the growing physical health needs of the elderly, let alone the mental health needs. As such, cost-effective programs, such as education campaigns and supporting family caregivers, will need to be considered.[2] Thus, while mental health resources in general need to be strengthened, special attention needs to be paid to particular populations and current inequities in access to services.

In addition to the 2011 *Mental Health Atlas,* special atlases have also been released on substance use,[17] and on neurological disorders such as multiple sclerosis[58] and epilepsy.[14] The findings in these reports are broadly similar to those reported in the 2011 *Mental Health Atlas*—namely, that resources are very limited.

THE ROLE OF INTERNATIONAL ORGANIZATIONS AND INITIATIVES IN DEVELOPING GLOBAL MENTAL HEALTH RESOURCES

In the previous section, we highlighted Project Atlas and WHO-AIMS as examples of global initiatives spearheaded by the WHO to map resources for mental health. Results show that resources for mental health remain scarce, inequitably distributed globally, and inefficiently utilized. Though there is little evidence of substantial changes in the level of available resources over the past decade, there have been numerous initiatives led by various stakeholders—including national governments, other groups such as nonprofit organizations, research centers, advocacy groups, and professional associations—that have been instrumental in the development of resources for mental health. For instance, over the last few years, international organizations, and the global initiatives that formed as a result of collaborations among them, have played increasing roles in enhancing global mental health resources, particularly in the areas of research, advocacy, and capacity building. This section describes some of the international initiatives and organizations that have been instrumental in such efforts.

A brief description of global and regional mental health initiatives is provided in Table 9.3. Here we define an "initiative" as a distinct program or strategy that was created to document or address gaps in global mental health. These may include initiatives that focus on specific populations or on a particular topic, such as policies or services. A list of organizations that exclusively focus on mental health is provided in Table 9.4. It is important to note that, while the lists of initiatives and organizations are convenience samples and are not intended to be exhaustive, they highlight the range of programs and groups from around the globe that have been established in response to global mental health resource gaps. While many organizations and initiatives have existed for decades, others have formed in response to calls for action following publication of the 2001 *World Health Report* and the 2007 *Lancet* series on global mental health.[5,21] Common among those listed, however, is their scope—all focus specifically on global mental health, and all play leading roles in mental health research, advocacy, and capacity building. The following section features some of the initiatives and organizations in the context of their roles in each of these areas.

Table 9.3 Global and Regional Mental Health Initiatives

Initiative	Scope	Primary role(s)	Website
Global Consortium for the Advancement of Promotion and Prevention in Mental Health	Global	Research, advocacy, capacity building	www.gcappmentalhealth.org
Grand Challenges in Global Mental Health	Global	Research	http://grandchallengesgmh.nimh.nih.gov/
International Alliance for Child and Adolescent Mental Health and Schools	Global	Research, advocacy	www.intercamhs.org
International Mental Health Policy and Services Project: Mental Health Country Profile	Global	Capacity building (policy)	–
Mental Health Gap Action Program	Global	Capacity building (services)	www.who.int/mental_health/mhGAP/en/
Mental Health and Poverty Project	Regional (Ghana, South Africa, Uganda, Zambia)	Capacity building (policy)	www.who.int/mental_health/policy/development/mhapp/en/
Movement for Global Mental Health	Global	Research, advocacy, capacity Building	www.globalmentalhealth.org
Program for Improving Mental Health Care	Regional (Ethiopia, India, Nepal, South Africa, Uganda)	Research, capacity building	http://www.prime.uct.ac.za/
The World Mental Health Survey Initiative	Global	Research	www.hcp.med.harvard.edu/wmh/

Table 9.4 Organizations With a Global Mental Health Focus

Initiative	Organization type	Primary role(s)	Website
Basic Needs	Charitable/ non-profit	Capacity building	www.basicneeds.org
Cittadinanza	Charitable/ non-profit	Advocacy, capacity building	http://en.cittadinanza. org/
Global Alliance of Mental Illness Advocacy Networks–Europe*	User/ professional association	Advocacy	www.gamian.eu
Global Initiative on Psychiatry	Charitable/- Non-profit	Advocacy, capacity building	www.gip-global.org
Global Network for Research in Mental and Neurological Health	Non-profit	Research, capacity building	www.mental- neurological-health. net
International Association for Child and Adolescent Psychiatry and Allied Professions	Professional society	Research, advocacy, capacity building	www.iacapap.org
Mental Health and Psychosocial Support Network	Non-profit	Advocacy	http://mhpss.net/
World Federation for Mental Health*	Non-profit	Advocacy	www.wfmh.org
World Psychiatric Association	Professional society	Advocacy, capacity building	www.wpanet.org

* European region only.

Research

In recent years there have been a number of global research initiatives that have developed to advance the understanding of the burden of mental illness, to evaluate the evidence base for treatment of the most common and debilitating mental disorders, and to reduce the treatment gap. The World Mental Health Survey, first launched in 1998,[59] is an example of an initiative that has been instrumental in advancing the global mental health research agenda.[60] Coordinated by the Assessment, Classification, and Epidemiology Group of the World Health Organization, the World Mental Health Survey is a multistage, 28-country study on the prevalence and correlates of mental and substance use disorders. The World Mental Health Survey is a valuable resource insofar as it provides national and global prevalence estimates, and its findings have been a catalyst for accelerating global mental health research beyond psychiatric epidemiology to include mental health services and implementation research. In 2011, another study reviewed existing literature from the European Union and estimated the burden of mental illness in Europe.[4]

The Movement for Global Mental Health (MGMH) and the Grand Challenges in Global Mental Health (GCGMH) are examples of initiatives that were created to advance mental health research from estimating disease to identifying both the major challenges of and potential solutions to reducing the treatment gap and improving health outcomes. Launched in 2007, the MGMH comprises individuals and institutions dedicated to improving services for people with mental disorders worldwide. In addition to its advocacy and capacity-building roles, the MGMH established a number of research priorities based on the "Call for Action" of the *Lancet* series on global mental health.[61,62] These include clinical, cost-effectiveness, and large-scale implementation trials on multiple behavioral health conditions in a variety of settings (e.g., school, primary care), the findings of which will be used to inform mental health system and policy changes. In October 2011, the *Lancet* published the second global mental health series, an update to its 2007 series, which highlighted global efforts over 2007–11 in closing the treatment gap and improving the rights of persons with mental disorders in low-resource settings.[62]

The Grand Challenges in Global Mental Health initiative, coordinated by the U.S. National Institute for Mental Health (NIMH) and the Global Alliance for Chronic Diseases (GACD), is an initiative to bring psychiatric, neurological, and substance use disorders to the forefront of global attention and the research agenda.[63] Established in 2010, the GCGMH comprises researchers, clinicians, and advocates from around the world with a common goal of identifying challenges and research priorities that, over the next 10 years, will lead to improvements in the lives of people with neuropsychiatric illnesses. In response to the top 25 global mental health "challenges,"[64] the group identified research priorities in the areas of disease etiology, early intervention, treatment improvement and care access, increasing awareness, building human resource capacity, and improving health systems and policy. Findings from research on these areas are intended to help inform improvements to mental health systems and the lives of those with neuropsychiatric illness.

The Program for Improving Mental Health Care (PRIME) (C. Lund, personal communication) is another example of an initiative to develop a research base on the implementation and scaling up of treatment programs for alcohol use disorders, depression, and psychosis in primary care settings of resource-poor countries. Participant countries include Ethiopia, India, Nepal, South Africa, and Uganda. Research focuses on the feasibility and effectiveness of implementing the mental health Gap Action Program, or mhGAP, for the treatment of the aforementioned disorders in primary care. It is anticipated that the lessons learned from the studies conducted across five countries will contribute to a broader understanding of how mental health services can be implemented in resource-poor settings and provide the framework for future services development in primary care cross the globe.

Advocacy

While there is no question that stigma against individuals with mental illness remains pervasive in low and high-income countries alike,[65] international organizations have played a valuable role in reducing stigma by promoting greater awareness of and advocating for individuals affected by mental illness. One of the earliest advocates for the rights and proper treatment of individuals with mental illness throughout the globe is the World Federation of Mental Health (WFMH). WFMH members are mental health professionals and consumers and their families from over 100 countries. Since 1948, the WFMH has worked to prevent mental disorders, advocate for the appropriate treatment of individuals with mental illness, and promote mental health.[66]

Over the decades since WFMH was founded, a number of other regional and global organizations have been formed to promote mental health and to advocate for those affected by mental illness. This includes organizations such as the International Association for Child and Adolescent Psychiatry and the Allied Professions, and the Global Initiative on Psychiatry and initiatives like the Global Consortium for the Advancement of Promotion and Prevention in Mental Health. Regional organizations such as the Global Alliance of Mental Illness Advocacy Networks–Europe[67] have also played instrumental roles. Formed in 1997, GAMIAN-Europe is a primarily user-driven, European organization that represents the interests of individuals affected by mental illness and advocates for their rights. The organization's focal areas include advocacy, information and education, anti-stigma and discrimination, patients' rights, and capacity building. Examples of some of the organization's activities include a stigma survey to understand discrimination experienced by individuals with mental illness and training for consumers interested in starting their own self-help groups.[67]

Capacity Building

Several new initiatives have been developed to build the capacity of (primarily low- and middle-income) countries to form and implement mental health policy and to develop and scaled-up evidence-based services for mental health. While the World Health Organization and their university partners have taken leading roles in the creation of a number of initiatives, such as the Mental Health and Poverty Project (MHaPP) and the Mental Health Gap Action Plan, others have been spearheaded by charitable nonprofit organizations, such as Basic Needs. The following sections highlight a few examples of the efforts of international organizations in the areas of mental health policy and services development. Two projects carried out by the Institute of Psychiatry, London, have undertaken a detailed study of the gaps and needs of Kenya and Tanzania over the last decade. In both countries, the methods included stakeholder analysis, epidemiological assessments, and the development of suitable tools for integrating mental health in all levels of care, especially primary care, across the country. The eventual objective was to develop a suitable mental health policy based on the needs of each country and integrate mental health into the overall health system using a multi-sectoral approach.[68,69]

Policy

The underlying premise of the MHaPP is that mental illness and poverty are inextricably linked, and by developing strong mental health policy, the cycle of poverty and mental illness can be broken.[70,71] The goal of MHaPP is to assist poor countries in the development, implementation, and evaluation of mental health policies. The MHaPP began in 2005 and is a partnership among the University of Cape Town, South Africa; the Human Sciences Research Council; the University of KwaZulu-Natal; the University of Leeds, England; and the World Health Organization. In Ghana, South Africa, Uganda, and Zambia, MHaPP uses the WHO framework for policy, plan, and legislation development to identify strategies for strengthening mental health systems. Since its inception, the program has been successful in a number of key areas. In Ghana, for instance, research among various stakeholders has elucidated the primary barriers to mental health policy implementation.[72] In turn, this information will be used to develop a mental health policy with the primary goal of reducing the burden of mental illness.

Services

The mental health Gap Action Plan (mhGAP) was launched in 2002 by the WHO to scale up services with a known evidence-base for individuals with mental, neurological, and substance use disorders living in resource-poor countries.[32,73] Conditions targeted by mhGAP were identified on the basis of their high prevalence, high economic costs, and associations with human rights violations, and include depression, schizophrenia spectrum disorders, dementia, and substance use disorders. The mhGAP Intervention Guide (mhGAP-IG) consists of interventions for the prevention and management of each priority condition; each intervention was identified on the basis of the evidence for its effectiveness and feasibility of implementation.[32] The program is being implemented in Ethiopia, Jordan, Nigeria, and Panama. As most participating countries are only just completing training on selected interventions, both short- and long-term results of the mhGAP program are forthcoming. However, all of the mhGAP countries have made a strong commitment to increasing resources for mental health. For example, Ethiopia, a country with 85 million people and only 36 psychiatrists, has recognized the need to scale up mental health services and strengthen human resources. Work has already begun on adaptation of mhGAP-IG for the local situation and on developing the training material. It is also proposed that mhGAP become part of the undergraduate medical training in universities across Ethiopia. Though this program is in the early stages, it is anticipated that mhGAP will substantially increase access to mental health and substance use treatment and improve mental health outcomes for individuals in resource-poor countries.

Basic Needs is an international development organization, based primarily in Africa and Asia, dedicated to improving the lives of individuals with mental illness (http://www.basicneeds.org/). Specifically, the organization empowers individuals with mental illness who are living in the community to function independently and earn a living and provides regular access to community-based mental health and substance-use treatment services. Since its inception in 1999, over 45,000 individuals with mental illnesses have benefited from the organization's services.

Other Initiatives

The initiatives and organizations presented in this chapter highlight some of the current global efforts to address mental health resource gaps, particularly in the areas of research, policy, and capacity building. The lists provided in Tables 9.3 and 9.4 are not exhaustive, nor do they cover all areas of behavioral health. For instance, substance use disorders were not a focus of this review; however, there are several efforts, such as the United Nations Office on Drugs and Crime/WHO Global Initiative on Primary Prevention of Substance Abuse,[74] and programs led by non-governmental organizations, like those of the Open Society Foundations (Open Society Foundations 2011), that were initiated to reduce the global burden of substance use disorders through the development of effective policies and services.

In addition, there are a number of other international initiatives and organizations that do not exclusively focus on mental health but nonetheless have helped narrow the global mental health resources gap. An example of such an initiative is the Global Burden of Disease Study.[75,76] Findings from this study highlighted mental illness as constituting a significant proportion of the global disease burden and have helped stimulate international efforts in the areas of research, advocacy, and capacity building. With respect to organizations, WHO collaborating centers, such as the Schizophrenia Research Foundation (SCARF), research centers at universities in both low- and high-income countries, and non-governmental organizations, such as the Carter Center, the St. Camille de Lellis Foundation, and HealthNet TPO, and many others not listed here, play crucial roles in global mental health, particularly in the areas of research and provision of mental health services for underserved and vulnerable populations.

IMPACT OF MENTAL HEALTH INITIATIVES ON GLOBAL MENTAL HEALTH RESOURCES AND IMPLICATIONS FOR THE FUTURE

The year 2001 marked an important transition in global mental health in general, and specifically in global mental health resources.[6] The *World Health Report* of that year was on mental health and refocused the world's attention to global mental health and related issues.[5] The same year, WHO also published results of the global survey on mental health resources called Project Atlas.[11] Prior to 2001, information about mental health resources was primarily available from some high-income countries like the United States, United Kingdom, Australia, etc., but following Project Atlas, such data are available across all countries of the world. Since then, there have been other updates and variants on Atlas and also related projects like WHO-AIMS,[19] which have gathered more in-depth information about mental health resources from selected low- and middle-income countries. Other international projects have also contributed to information on mental health resources and capacity development.[77,78] Epidemiological projects have also been undertaken to ascertain the burden of mental illness.[4,59]

Epidemiological studies to estimate the burden of mental disorders have been undertaken across many countries for some decades now, but without the knowledge about existing mental health resources, it was difficult to assess the gaps in developing appropriate mental health services and related factors, whether in infrastructure; primary or community-based human resources, programs, and legislations; or services focused on special populations like children and women. Countries also were unable to understand deficiencies in their own mental health resources, as comparative data from other countries with similar economic and human development were lacking. For example, a low-income sub-Saharan country had no way of understanding where they were ranked using data from the United States, as the needs and capacity to develop mental health resources were vastly different. However, with the development of initiatives that have plotted mental health resources, such comparison is possible using data across countries of similar development levels or within the same geographic regions.[79] Researchers and policymakers across countries also have some common indicators to measure development and report program or policy outcomes. The Mental Health Action Plan, a survey of mental health resources across 42 European countries, identified major differences in resources across the countries in the region and also gaps in knowledge that could be used to inform better mental health policy development across the region.[80]

Since 2001, there has also been a realization that specific mental health terms such as mental health law, intellectual disability related legislation, mental health policy or plan, and mental health financing had been ill-defined in the past. Even concepts of psychiatric nurses, social workers specific to mental health, and clinical psychologists were defined quite variably across countries. This led to confusion about the magnitude of available mental health resources and an inability to compare data. With Project Atlas, clearer definitions started to emerge and continue to be refined, allowing a uniform understanding of those concepts across countries. The Mental Health Action Plan from Europe also identified differences in definitions of different resources among the countries of Europe.[80]

Chisholm and colleagues[61] estimated current and projected per capita expenses for delivering a set of core mental health packages for conditions like schizophrenia, depression, bipolar disorder, and alcohol use disorder across 12 low- and middle-income countries. They used a few key indicators that covered the areas of sufficient planning and investment for mental health care; sufficient workforce to provide mental health services; consistency of mental health care inputs and processes with best practice and human-rights protection; and improved outcomes for people with mental disorders, to guide their estimates. They estimated that US$2/person-year was needed in low-income countries and US$3–$4/person-year in middle-income countries. Based on current estimates, expenditure would have to increase tenfold in low-income countries and almost fourfold in middle-income countries to achieve the expenditure target by 2015 (see Figure 9.3). Based on their finding, a series of steps were suggested as part of the "Call for Action" that the Lancet Mental Health Series proposed. The key strategies were to place mental health on

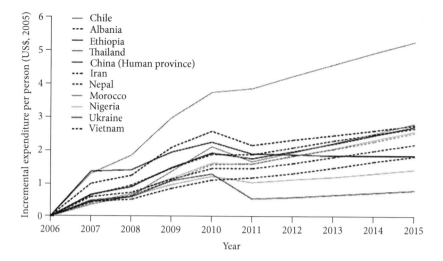

FIGURE 9.3

Incremental expenditure for a core package of mental health interventions, 2006–2015. *Source:* Chisholm et al., 2007. Used with permission from Elsevier.[61]

the public-health priority agenda, improve organization of mental health services, integrate the availability of mental health in general health care; develop human resources for mental health, and strengthen public mental health leadership. The *World Health Report* of 2001 had suggested similar steps for improving mental health resources in countries based upon their existing capacity.[5] With the increased focus on global mental health, international organizations and many institutional and non-governmental organizations have over the past decade played a more active role in highlighting mental health issues through their activities and have put pressure on their respective governments to prioritize mental health, but a lot still remains to be done.[34,77,81,82]

While mental health in low- and middle-income countries has been particularly under-served, developed countries also have their own issues. Mental health care for special populations like children and adolescents, the elderly, women, those in correctional facilities, refugees, and populations affected by migration and conflict affect all countries. Knowledge about appropriate mental health services prior to the recent shift in focus towards global mental health was in separate silos, and the flow of knowledge was mostly from developed to developing countries. However, with greater awareness about global mental health, there is a need to develop expertise that can flow both ways.[9] Both sides can and should learn from each other's experiences and apply what is appropriate to their settings. Cultural considerations play a big role in managing mental health care, and lessons can be drawn from each other.

Prior to Atlas, it was common knowledge that mental health facilities and resources across the world were lacking, but it was with projects that quantified the resources across numerous countries that these poor conditions was underlined even more.[31] While macro-level data have their limitations in scope and accuracy, more accurate and detailed data are now being generated. Emerging data have also highlighted the need for good governance,[81] conducting evidence-based research in areas of mental health policies and services,[68,69,83,84] and increasing budgets for developing adequate mental health resources.[61] While such research and oversight were present to varying extents in more developed countries, resource-poor countries neither had the knowledge nor the expertise to concentrate on such issues or to develop a level of governance that was focused on mental health care. It is with the renewed emphasis on global mental health that the international community of experts is focusing more on the situation in low- and middle-income countries. There is a host of initiatives that focus on different aspects of mental health resource development. However, there is a need to develop a coordinated effort such that limited resources can be used as efficiently as possible. There is also a need to be mindful about the needs of marginalized populations across countries—rural/tribal, women/children/elderly, or people with disabilities/refugees—and to develop mental health services that are more equitable and culturally appropriate.

Even with the recent initiatives, many issues remain. As described in the previous sections, the quantitative data obtained through global projects fail to provide a complete picture about resources. Questions about the quality of policies and legislation, the distribution of psychiatric beds and human resources, the quality of available primary and community care facilities are only some of the key questions that remain unanswered from most countries. Future projects should focus more on gathering qualitative information about these and other resources. Data-gathering should be complemented by developing strategies to overcome any shortcomings. From all the data available about the burden of mental illness globally and available resources and budget, it is evident that mental disorders need to be managed with other health conditions in most countries, especially low- and middle-income countries, where resources are extremely limited. Given the complexities involved in managing mental illness, experts from other sectors like urban planning, poverty alleviation programs, rural and tribal development, social services, labor, finance, etc., should also be involved as and when necessary. It becomes the responsibility of mental health professionals in all countries to make every effort to involve their colleagues from other health and non-health sectors. As in any multisectoral approach of this magnitude, it is always useful to have the government on board. Both government and non-governmental organizations need to develop a cooperative association built on transparency. Finally, all these should be backed with adequate finances—be it grants to fund individual research, or government or private funding that supports service and program development at local, regional, or national levels. The recent call for increasing funding for mental health research is welcome,[64] but it also is the responsibility of individual governments to support large-scale mental health policies and programs that can use research findings to take effective programs to scale.

CONCLUSION

Overall, global mental health resources are inadequate in most countries, and in low- and middle-income countries there is an acute need to develop infrastructure and human resources and to support these efforts with appropriate mental health policies and legislation. There should be a substantial increase in investment in the mental health sector. An oft-quoted comment is that there is not enough research from countries to estimate the burden of mental disorders or the needs of the society. International and national funding agencies should take note of this and develop strategies to correct this problem. Efforts have started in this area and need to develop further. Finally, with this increased focus on global mental health, there is a need to develop adequate stewardship of programs and outline coordinated strategies that are inclusive of all countries and use each other's strengths.

REFERENCES

1. Beaglehole R, Bonita R, Horton R, Adams C, Alleyne G, Asaria P, et al. Priority actions for the non-communicable disease crisis. *Lancet.* 2011;377(9775):1438–47.
2. Prince M, Patel V, Saxena S, Maj M, Maselko J, Phillips MR, et al. No health without mental health. *Lancet.* 2007;370(9590):859–77.

3. Demyttenaere K, Bruffaerts R, Posada-Villa J, Gasquet I, Kovess V, Lepine JP, et al. Prevalence, severity, and unmet need for treatment of mental disorders in the World Health Organization World Mental Health Surveys. *JAMA*. 2004;291(21):2581–90.

4. Wittchen HU, Jacobi F, Rehm J, Gustavsson A, Svensson M, Jönsson B, et al. The size and burden of mental disorders and other disorders of the brain in Europe 2010. *Eur Neuropsychopharmacol.* 2011;21:655–79.

5. World Health Organization. *The World Health Report 2001—Mental health: new understanding, new hope.* Geneva, Switzerland: WHO; 2001.

6. Saraceno B. Mental health: scarce resources need new paradigms. *World Psychiatry.* 2004;3(1):3–5.

7. World Bank. *Country and lending groups.* Washington, DC: World Bank; 2011. Available at: http://data.worldbank.org/about/country-classifications/country-and-lending-groups. Accessed August 23, 2011.

8. Kohn R, Saxena S, Levav I, Saraceno B. The treatment gap in mental health care. *Bull WHO.* 2004;82:858–66.

9. Patel V, Prince M. Global mental health: a new global health field comes of age. *JAMA.* 2010;303(19):1976–7.

10. Koplan JP, Bond TC, Merson MH, Reddy KS, Rodriguez MH, Sewankambo NK, et al. Towards a common definition of global health. *Lancet.* 2009;373(9679):1993–5.

11. World Health Organization. *Atlas: Mental health resources in the world 2001.* Geneva, Switzerland: WHO; 2001.

12. World Health Organization. *Atlas: Psychiatric education and training across the world 2005.* Geneva, Switzerland: WHO; 2005.

13. World Health Organization. *Atlas: Child and adolescent mental health resources: global concerns, implications for the future.* Geneva, Switzerland: WHO; 2005.

14. World Health Organization. *Atlas: Epilepsy care in the world 2005.* Geneva, Switzerland: WHO; 2005.

15. World Health Organization. *Atlas: Nurses in mental health 2007.* Geneva, Switzerland: WHO; 2007.

16. World Health Organization. *The global burden of disease—2004 update.* Geneva, Switzerland: WHO; 2008.

17. World Health Organization. *Atlas on substance use (2010): Resources for the prevention and treatment of substance use disorders.* Geneva, Switzerland: WHO; 2010.

18. World Health Organization. *Mental Health Atlas 2011.* Geneva, Switzerland: WHO; 2011. Available at: http://www.who.int/mental_health/evidence/atlas/en/. Accessed September 15, 2011.

19. World Health Organization. *Mental health systems in selected low- and middle-income countries: a WHO-AIMS cross-national analysis.* Geneva, Switzerland: WHO; 2009.

20. Saxena S, Lora A, van Ommeren M, Barrett T, Morris J, Saraceno B. WHO's Assessment Instrument for Mental Health Systems: collecting essential information for policy and service delivery. *Psychiatr Serv.* 2007;58:816–21.

21. The Lancet. Lancet Global Mental Health Group; Series on Global Mental Health. 2007. Available at: http://www.thelancet.com/series/global-mental-health. Accessed September 8, 2011.

22. World Health Organization. *Improving health systems and services for mental health.* Geneva, Switzerland: WHO; 2009.

23. World Health Organization. *Mental health policy, plans and programmes.* Geneva, Switzerland: WHO; 2004.

24. Pan American Health Organization. *Strategy and plan of action on Mental Health/Resolution of the PAHO Directing Council (CD49.R17).* Washington, DC: Pan American Health Organization; 2009. Available at: http://new.paho.org/hq/dmdocuments/2009/CD49.R17%20(Eng.).pdf. Accessed September 20, 2011.

25. Faydi E, Funk M, Kleintjes S, Ofori-Atta A, Ssbunnya J, Mwanza J, et al. An assessment of mental health policy in Ghana, South Africa, Ghana and Zambia. *Health Res Policies Syst.* 2011;9:17

26. Omar MA, Green AT, Bird PK, Mirzoev T, Flisher AJ, Kigozi F, et al. Mental health policy process: a comparative study of Ghana, South Africa, Uganda and Zambia. *Int J Ment Health Syst.* 2010;4:24.

27. Cooper S, Ssebunnya J, Kigozi F, Lund C, Flisher A, The MHaPP Research Programme Consortium. Viewing Uganda's mental health system through a human rights lens. *Int Rev Psychiatry.* 2010;22(6):578–88.

28. Bhana A, Petersen I, Baillie KL, Flisher AJ, The MHaPP Research Programme Consortium. Implementing the World Health Report 2001 recommendations for integrating mental health into primary health care: a situation analysis of three African countries: Ghana, South Africa and Uganda. *Int Rev Psychiatry*. 2010;22(6):599–610.

29. Dhanda A, Narayan T. Mental health and human rights. *Lancet*. 2007;370(9594):1197–8.

30. Saxena S, Sharan P, Saraceno B. Budget and financing of mental health services: baseline information on 89 countries from WHO's Project Atlas. *J Ment Health Policy Econ*. 2003;6:135–43.

31. Saxena S., Sharan P, Garrido M, Saraceno B. World Health Organization's Mental Health Atlas 2005: implications for policy development. *World Psychiatry*. 2006;5:179–84.

32. World Health Organization. *mhGAP Mental Health Action Programme: Scaling up care for mental, neurological and substance abuse disorders*. Geneva, Switzerland: WHO; 2008.

33. Andreoli SB, Almeida-Filho N, Martin D, Mateus MDL, Mari JJ. Is psychiatric reform a move for reducing the mental health budget? The case of Brazil. *Rev Bras Psiquiatr*. 2007;1:43–6.

34. Jacob KS, Sharan P, Mirza I, Garrido-Cumbrera M, Seedat S, Mari JJ, et al. Mental health systems in countries: where are we now? *Lancet*. 2007;370(9592):1061–77.

35. Roberts MJ, Hsiao W, Berman P, Reich MR. *Getting health reform right: a guide to improving performance and equity*. New York: Oxford University Press; 2004.

36. Liu Y. China's public health-care system: facing the challenges. *Bull World Health Organ* 2004;82:532–8.

37. Saxena S, Thornicroft G, Knapp M, Whiteford H. Resources for mental health: scarcity, inequity, and inefficiency. *Lancet*. 2007;370:878–89.

38. Patel V, Araya R, Chatterjee S, Chisholm D, Cohen A, De Silva M, et al. Treatment and prevention of mental disorders in low-income and middle-income countries. *Lancet*. 2007;370(9591):991–1005.

39. Barrett T, Boeck R, Fusco C, Ghebrehiwet T, Yan J, Saxena S. Nurses are the key to improving mental health services in low- and middle-income countries. *Int Nurs Rev*. 2009;56:138–41.

40. Patel V. The future of psychiatry in low- and middle-income countries. *Psychol Med*. 2009;39(11):1759–62.

41. Patel V. 2003. Recruiting doctors from poor countries: the great brain robbery? *BMJ*. 2003;327:926–8.

42. Fahrer R, Jorge MR, Ruiz P. Addressing psychiatric education in Latin America: challenges and opportunities. *Int Rev Psychiatry*. 2010;22(4):378–81.

43. Patel V. Mental health in low- and middle-income countries. *Br Med Bull*. 2007;81–82:81–96.

44. World Health Organization. *The World Health Report 2000—Health systems: Improving performance*. Geneva, Switzerland: WHO; 2000.

45. Ngui EM, Khasakhala L, Ndetei D, Roberts LW. Mental disorders, health inequalities and ethics: a global perspective. *Int Rev Psychiatr*. 2010;22(3):235–44.

46. Tyano S, Keren M. Some reflections on the development of child and adolescent psychiatry. *World Psychiatry*. 2005;4(3):154–5.

47. Rahman A, Mubbashar M, Harrington R, Gater R. Developing child mental health services in developing countries. *J Child Psychol Psychiatry*. 2000;41(5):539–46.

48. Robertson B, Mandlhate C, Seif El-Din A, et al. Systems of care in Africa. In: Remschmidt H, Belfer M, Goodyer I, editors. *Facilitating pathways: Care, treatment and prevention in child and adolescent mental health*. Berlin: Springer; 2004:71–88.

49. Hoven CW, Doan T, Musa GJ, Jaliashvili T, Duarte CS, Ovuga E, et al. Worldwide child and adolescent mental health begins with awareness: a preliminary assessment in nine countries. *Int Rev Psychiatry*. 2008;20(3):261–70.

50. Morris J, Belfer M, Daniels A, Flisher A, Villé L, Lora A, et al. Treated prevalence of and mental health services received by children and adolescents in 42 low-and-middle-income countries. *J Child Psychol Psychiatry*. 2011;52(12):1239–46.

51. Vostanis P. Mental health services for children in public care and other vulnerable groups: implications for international collaboration. *Clin Child Psychol Psychiatry*. 2010;15(4):555–71.

52. Buvinić M, Medici A, Fernández E, Torres AC. Gender differentials in health. In: Jamison DT, Breman JG, Measham AR, et al., editors. *Disease control priorities in developing countries*. 2nd edition. Washington, DC: World Bank; 2006: 195–210.

53. Wong EC, Marshall GN, Schell TL, Elliott MN, Hambarsoomians K, Chun C, et al. Barriers to mental health care utilization for U.S. Cambodian refugees. *J Consult Clin Psychol*. 2006;74(6):1116–20.

54. Prince M, Livingston G, Katona C. Mental health care for the elderly in low-income countries: a health systems approach. *World Psychiatry.* 2006;6:5–13.

55. Ellsberg M, Jansen H, Heise L, Watts CH, Garcia-Moreno C, and on behalf of the WHO Multi-Country Study on Women's Health and Domestic Violence against Women Study Team. Intimate partner violence and women's physical and mental health in the WHO multi-country study on women's health and domestic violence: an observational study. *Lancet.* 2008;371(9619):1165–72.

56. Onyut LP, Neuner F, Ertl V, Schauer E, Odenwaldm M, Elbert T. Trauma, poverty and mental health among Somali and Rwandese refugees living in an African refugee settlement—an epidemiological study. *Confl Health.* 2009;3(6):1–16.

57. Sheikh-Mohammed M, MacIntyre CR, Wood NJ, Leask J, Isaacs D. Barriers to access to health care for newly resettled sub-Saharan refugees in Australia. *Med J Aust.* 2006;185:594–7.

58. World Health Organization. *Atlas: Multiple sclerosis resources in the world 2008.* Geneva, Switzerland: WHO; 2008.

59. Kessler RC, Ustun BT. The World Mental Health (WMH) Survey Initiative version of the World Health Organization (WHO) Composite International Diagnostic Interview (CIDI). *Int J Methods Psychiatr Res.* 2004;13(2):93–121.

60. The World Mental Health Survey Initiative. The World Mental Health Survey Initiative. 2005. Available at: http://www.hcp.med.harvard.edu/wmh/. Accessed September 8, 2011.

61. Chisholm D, Flisher AJ, Lund C, Patel V, Saxena S, Thornicroft G, et al. Scale up services for mental disorders: a call for action. *Lancet* 2007;370(9594):1241–52.

62. *The Lancet.* Lancet Global Mental Health Group; Series on Global Mental Health. 2011. Available at: http://www.thelancet.com/series/global-mental-health-2011. Accessed May 10, 2013.

63. Grand challenges in global mental health. Grand Challenges in Global Mental Health. 2011. Available at: http://grandchallengesgmh.nimh.nih.gov/. Accessed September 8, 2011.

64. Collins PY, Patel V, Joestl SS, March D, Insel TR, Daar AS, et al. Grand challenges in global mental health. *Nature.* 2011;475:27–30.

65. Thornicroft G, Brohan E, Rose D, Sartorius N, Leese M, for the INDIGO Study Group. Global pattern of experienced and anticipated discrimination against people with schizophrenia: a cross-sectional survey. *Lancet.* 2009;373:408–15.

66. World Federation for Mental Health. WFMH: World Federation for Mental Health; Making mental health a global priority. 2007. Available at: http://www.wfmh.org/. Accessed September 8, 2011.

67. GAMIAN-Europe. Global Alliance of Mental Illness Advocacy Networks–Europe, 2010. Available at: http://www.gamian.eu/. Accessed September 8, 2011.

68. Kiima D, Jenkins R. Mental health policy in Kenya—an integrated approach to scaling up equitable care for poor populations. *Int J Ment Health Syst.* 2010;4:19.

69. Mbatia J, Jenkins R. Development of a mental health policy and system in Tanzania: an integrated approach to achieve equity. *Psychiatr Serv.* 2010;61(10):1028–31.

70. Department for International Development. *Policy Brief 1. Breaking the vicious cycle of mental ill-health and poverty: Mental Health and Poverty Project.* London: Department for International Development, United Kingdom; 2008. Available at: http://www.dfid.gov.uk/r4d/PDF/Outputs/MentalHealth_RPC/MHPB1.pdf. Accessed on September 30, 2011.

71. World Health Organization. *Mental health and development: Targeting people with mental health conditions as a vulnerable group.* Geneva, Switzerland: WHO; 2010.

72. Awenva AD, Read UM, Ofori-Attah AL, Doku VC, Akpalu B, Osei AO, et al. From mental health policy development in Ghana to implementation: what are the barriers? *Afr J Psychiatry.* 2010;13(3):184–91.

73. World Health Organization. *WHO mental health Gap Action Programme (mhGAP).* Geneva, Switzerland: WHO; 2011. Available at: http://www.who.int/mental_health/mhgap/en/index.html. Accessed September 8, 2011.

74. World Health Organization. *UNODC/WHO global initiative on primary prevention of substance abuse.* Geneva, Switzerland: WHO; 2011. Available at: http://www.who.int/substance_abuse/activities/global_initiative/en/. Accessed September 8, 2011.

75. Institute for Health Metrics and Evaluation. *The Global Burden of Disease study.* The Global Burden of Disease Study, Seattle. 2011. Available at: http://www.globalburden.org/. Accessed September 9, 2011.

76. Murray C, Lopez A. *The global burden of disease.* Boston, MA: Harvard School of Public Health, World Health Organization, and World Bank; 1996.

77. Lund C. Mental health in Africa: findings from the Mental Health and Poverty Project. *Int Rev Psychiatry.* 2010;22(6):547–9.

78. Jenkins R, Gulbinat W, Manderscheid R, Baingana F, Whiteford H, Khandelwal S, et al. The mental health country profile: background, design and use of a systematic method of appraisal. *Int Rev Psychiatry.* 2004;16(1–2):31–47.

79. Saxena S, Maulik PK. Mental health services in low- and middle-income countries—an overview. *Curr Opin Psychiatry.* 2003;16(4):437–42.

80. World Health Organization. *Policies and practices for mental health in Europe—meeting the challenges.* Copenhagen, Denmark: WHO Regional Office for Europe; 2008.

81. Saraceno B, Dua T. Global mental health: the role of psychiatry. *Eur Arch Psychiatry Clin Neurosci.* 2009;259(Suppl 2):S109–17.

82. Rodriguez JJ. Mental health care systems in Latin America and the Caribbean. *Int Rev Psychiatry.* 2010;22(4):317–24.

83. Khandelwal S, Avode G, Baingana F, Conde B, Cruz M, Deva P, et al. Mental and neurological health research priorities setting in developing countries. *Soc Psychiatry Psychiatr Epidemiol.* 2010;45(4):487–95.

84. Razzouk D, Sharan P, Gallo C, Gureje O, Lamberte EE, de Jesus Mari J, et al. Scarcity and inequity of mental health research resources in low- and middle-income countries: a global survey. *Health Policy.* 2010;94(3):211–20.

10 Strategies for Strengthening Human Resources for Mental Health

Ritsuko Kakuma, Harry Minas, and
Mario R. Dal Poz

INTRODUCTION

At the heart of each and every health system, the workforce is central to advancing health.
—World Health Organization, 2006[1]

The 2006 World Health Report[1] focused global attention on the shortage of health workers. Many low- and middle-income countries (LMICs) face a health workforce crisis, and the shortage of human resources and training is similarly overwhelming for mental health.[2-5] Reports such as the World Health Report 2001[6] and the Atlases for Mental Health Resources,[3,7,8] Neurological Disorders,[9] and Nurses in Mental Health[10] have clearly shown the minimal supply of HRMH in LMICs (particularly compared to high-income countries (HICs)) and the urgency with which this must be addressed.

According to the 2011 Mental Health Atlas,[8] nurses were the largest workforce category in the mental health system, with a global median number of 5 nurses per 100,000 population, followed by psychiatrists, with 1.3 per 100,000 population. While numbers of psychologists and social workers were much smaller, occupational therapists were particularly rare, with not a single occupational therapist working in the mental health system in at least 50% of low-income countries (LICs). Psychiatrists were far more numerous in HICs, with the median number 748 times greater than in LICs. Figure 10.1 and Table 10.1 show the changes in HRMH between 2005 and 2010. The increase in psychiatrists was greatest in HICs, with a median change rate of 0.65 psychiatrists per 100,000 population, whereas in LICs there was a decrease by 0.005 per 100,000 population.

Only recently have empirical data on the extent of the HRMH *shortage* and *needs* become available. Findings of a large study to estimate the needs and shortages of psychiatrists, psychosocial care providers, and nurses in mental health settings in 58 LMICs using 2005 Mental Health Atlas data were published by the World Health Organization

193

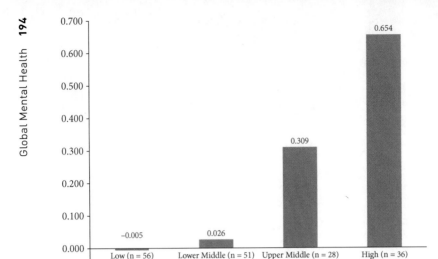

FIGURE 10.1

Median change in number of psychiatrists per 100,000 population for countries by income group (World Bank, 2004). *Source:* Kakuma et al., 2011, p. 1656. Used with permission from Elsevier.[12]

(WHO).[11] The estimated total number of mental health care workers needed in 2005 was 362,000, representing 22.3 workers per 100,000 population in LICs and 26.7 workers per 100,000 in middle-income countries (MICs): 6% psychiatrists, 54% nurses in mental health settings, and 41% psychosocial care providers (Table 10.2). These data reflect an overall shortage of 190,300 mental health workers (17.3 workers in LICs and 14.9 in MICs). With the exception of Latvia, all LMICs are faced with mental health workforce shortages in at least one of the three categories of workers. Figure 10.2 shows regional variations in the magnitude of the mental health workforce shortages.

The largest shortages were seen in Vietnam, with 1.7 psychiatrists and 11.52 psychosocial health providers per 100,000; and in Uruguay, with 22.20 nurses per 100,000. All

Table 10.1 Median Number of Health Professionals for Mental Disorders (per 100,000 population) in 2001, 2005, and 2010 By Income Categories. Source: Kakuma et al., 2011, p. 1656[12]

	Psychiatrists			*Nurses†*			*Psychologists*			*Social Workers*			*Occupational Therapists*		
	2001	*2005*	*2010*	*2001*	*2005*	*2010*	*2001*	*2005*	*2010*	*2001*	*2005*	*2010*	*2001*	*2005*	*2010*
Low	0.06	0.05	0.05	0.16	0.16	0.42	0.04	0.04	0.02	0.03	0.04	0.01	UN	UN	0.00
Lower middle	0.9	1.05	0.54	1.0	1.05	2.93	0.6	0.60	0.14	0.3	0.28	0.13	UN	UN	0.01
Higher middle	2.4	2.70	2.03	5.7	5.35	9.72	0.7	1.80	1.47	1.42	1.50	0.76	UN	UN	0.23
High	9.0	10.50	8.41	33.5	32.95	29.94	26.7	14.0	3.79	25.5	15.70	2.16	UN	UN	1.51
World	1.0	1.2	1.27	2.0	2.00	4.95	0.4	0.60	0.33	0.3	0.40	0.24	UN	UN	0.06
N=	182	183	177	164	172	158	164	173	147	147	157	129	UN	UN	119

† The 2005 Atlas defined nurses as "psychiatric nurses"; 2011 Atlas defined nurses as "nurses in mental health setting" (broader definition). UN =Unknown.

Table 10.2 Supply and Shortage of Mental Health Workers per 100,000 Population, and Total Scale-up Cost (Wage Bill) Estimate to Eliminate Shortage of Mental Health Workers (Thousands $US, 2005) in 58 LMICs By Income Category for 2005. Source: Kakuma et al., 2011, p. 1656.[12]

	Psychiatrists			Nurses			Psychosocial Health Providers			Total FTE Staff		
	Supply	Shortage	Wage bill	Supply	Shortage	Wage bill	Supply	Shortage	Wage bill	Supply	Shortage	Wage bill
Low	0.26	1.04	$48,588	5.15	7.90	$136,652	1.35	8.40	$162,523	6.76	17.34	$347,764
Middle	2.15	0.46	$31,845	5.70	9.37	$282,871	11.43	5.05	$151,423	19.28	14.88	$466,139
All LMICs	1.18	0.76	$80,433	5.42	8.61	$419,523	6.25	6.77	$313,947	12.85	16.14	$813,903

FTE=Full-Tiem Equivalent

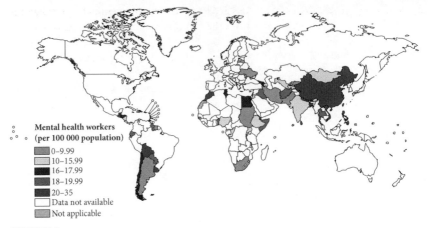

Mental health workers
(per 100 000 population)
0–9.99
10–15.99
16–17.99
18–19.99
20–35
Data not available
Not applicable

FIGURE 10.2

Shortage of mental health workers in 58 LMIC, 2005. *Source:* Kakuma et al., 2011. Used with permission from the World Health Organization.

LICs and approximately two-thirds of MICs had far fewer mental health workers than needed to deliver a required core set of mental health interventions. Countries with greater shortages of psychiatrists per 100,000 population reported a greater proportion of other medical doctors working in mental health settings.

HRMH continue to be grossly inadequate in most LMICs, and those available are concentrated in urban settings. The very small increase in the number of psychiatrists in the majority of MICs and an actual decrease in LICs raises concerns and has serious implications for HRMH.[8] The shortage and distribution difficulties are likely to worsen unless significant investments are made to train a wider range of specialist and non-specialist mental health care providers in substantially higher numbers, and strategies are in place to address underserved areas.[12] Practical guidelines to assist policymakers, health planners, and educators to address shortages of HRMH are now available,[13–15] and evidence on new and feasible models of mental health services from LMICs is emerging.[12]

An essential response to scaling up of HRMH and to develop a sustainable and comprehensive mental health system in LMICs includes *task shifting*, defined as "delegating tasks to existing or new cadres with either less training or narrowly tailored training."[16] This is particularly important for three reasons: (1) Most countries simply do not have sufficient numbers of mental health specialists to meet the population needs for mental health care; (2) there are particular tasks of mental health care that can be delivered by non-specialist health workers with sufficient training and supervision (see Task-Shifting section, below); and (3) the increasing shift towards a comprehensive and recovery-based system of care necessitates an increasingly multidisciplinary and multi-sectoral approach to mental health reform (see Policy section, below).

Also critically important is implementation of a systemic approach, such as the Human Resources for Health Action Framework (HRH Action Framework) developed by the World Health Organization. This includes six interconnected components: policy, health workforce management, finance, education, partnership, and leadership.[12,17] The current scarcity of evidence on interventions to strengthen HRMH poses challenges in developing evidence-informed HRMH strategy.

STRATEGIES FOR STRENGTHENING HRMH

Accurate HRMH Data

Access to accurate, up-to-date information on HRMH through research and effective monitoring and evaluation is essential in order to ensure appropriate mental health policy, planning, and evaluation.[18] An effective monitoring and evaluation strategy and mental health information system enable the availability of reliable and timely information on the existing mental health system, and facilitates appropriate implementation of mental health services. The need for a mental health information system has been and continues to be a priority area.[19–21]

The critical role of research in improving health, equity and development is indisputable[22–24] yet in a recent review, only 45 studies were found that evaluated the impact of task-shifting interventions on patient outcomes, and just 27 studies evaluated training programs on staff performance in LMICs.[12] Of these, 23 studies were from South Asia, 13 from Africa, ten from Latin America and the Caribbean, five from the Middle East, five from China, four from Turkey, two from East Asia, and one from Russia. There is an urgent need for mental health research evidence, such as health policy and systems research and delivery of cost-effective interventions in low-resource contexts, which can inform policymakers and planners in developing the most appropriate mental health care package in resource-poor settings.[25–27]

Effectiveness of Task Shifting

Task shifting, defined as "delegating tasks to existing or new cadres with either less training or narrowly tailored training"[16] is an essential response for the HRMH shortages. It can include mental health care providers employed in different sectors; and inter-sectoral collaborations with other professionals (such as teachers and prison staff) to strengthen mental health awareness, mental health promotion, prevention, early detection, referrals, treatment, and recovery. A summary of the evidence on task shifting in mental health care is provided below.

Specialist Mental Health Professionals and Psychosocial Workers

Even if task shifting is extensively implemented, mental health specialists will continue to be essential in providing clinical care with an emphasis on complex psychiatric cases and training and supervising non-specialist health workers (NSHWs) to manage less complex cases.[28] Mid-level mental health workers (e.g., medical officers for mental health) have also helped reach rural areas where psychiatrists are often unavailable.

Psychosocial workers also play an important role. Social workers have facilitated support groups for service users and caregivers as part of a multidisciplinary mental health team in India[29] and provided psycho-education and monitoring in Chile.[30] Psychologists have also been effective in providing psycho-education intervention in reducing caregiver burdens and improving attitudes in Chile.[31,32]

In the majority of studies, psychiatrists, neurologists, non-specialist medical doctors, nurses, and psychosocial workers have effectively provided short-term training, supervision, and monitoring for NSHWs for detection, referral, treatment, psycho-education, and follow-up care, with positive patient outcomes.[30,33–35]

Non-Specialist Health Workers (NSHWs)

There is growing evidence from LMICs that NSHWs can effectively deliver mental health care. They have contributed in various services such as clinics, halfway homes, and community outreach services. They have been involved in a variety of activities, including detecting, diagnosing, treating and preventing common and severe mental disorders, epilepsy, mental retardation and dementia as part of a complex stepped-care intervention[30,33,36,37] or single intervention such as group interpersonal therapy (IPT),[38] cognitive behavioral therapy (CBT)[39] and psycho-educational programs for caregivers.[40]

Their roles differ according to their level of training. For example, trained nurses, social workers, and lay workers take on follow-up and educational and promotional roles.[30,41,42] Primary care doctors with mental health training have been involved in the identification, diagnosis, treatment, and referral of complex cases.[2,42,43] In addition, lay health workers have been involved in supporting caregivers, befriending, ensuring adherence, and in detection of mental health problems.[36,39,41,44]

Most studies showed significant improvements in patient outcomes: better recovery, and reduced dysfunction and severity. Infants of mothers with maternal depression have also benefited from improvement in symptom severity.[39,44] While training community health workers to screen for dementia was not found to be effective in one study,[45] other NSHW interventions have been effective in reducing burden on caregivers of patient with dementia.[36] Although results are promising, these approaches need to be studied further in routine service settings.

Mental Health Users and Caregivers for Mental Health Care Delivery

The involvement of mental health care users and caregivers as providers of mental health care is relatively recent worldwide, and existing evidence on its impact on patient outcomes is primarily based in HICs,[46–49] also, many of the studies have methodological weaknesses. Nonetheless, they demonstrate the beneficial roles users and caregivers can play in supporting caregivers and providing mental health care.

Family caregivers contribute to detection, treatment seeking, and support of a person with a mental disorder, and evidence on educational programs for caregivers, particularly for patients with neurological conditions in LMICs, is increasing.[50,51] In Iran, parents of inpatients with chronic schizophrenia were better equipped to manage their children's behaviors and provide a supportive role in producing better patient outcomes after a one-month training program.[52] In a more recent study in Iran, eight weekly educational sessions were effective in reducing caregiver distress and challenging behaviors of patients with dementia.[53] An RCT examining the impact of a psycho-education program for caregivers of patients with schizophrenia in India found that caregivers who received monthly sessions for nine months showed better outcomes in psychopathology and disability levels among patients as well as caregiver support and caregiver satisfaction.[54]

Users of mental health services can provide support to others, share personal experiences, and participate in self-help and mutual aid initiatives.[35,55] Although some mental health user organizations provide psycho-education and skills-building sessions to users and families for home-based care, self-help, and entrepreneurship,[56] no rigorous evaluations have been done to examine their impact in LMICs. The role of users and caregivers needs to be better explored and evaluated, and possibly expanded.

The existing evidence, though limited, demonstrates that non-specialist health workers, including users and caregivers, can and should play a role as members of the mental health workforce. The role of community resources such as indigenous, traditional, or alternative care providers must also be better examined. More context-appropriate research evidence is urgently needed to inform decision makers and health planners in developing innovative strategies for strengthening the mental health workforce.

Human Resources for Health Action Framework

The worldwide need to address the human resources for health (HRH) shortage has led to efforts by diverse stakeholders to develop a technical framework to assist governments and health managers to develop and implement a comprehensive strategy to achieve an effective and sustainable health workforce.[1] The Human Resources for Health Action

Framework (HRH Action Framework) consists of six components that are interconnected and necessary in human resource development: policy, health workforce management, finance, education, partnerships, and leadership (Figure 10.3).[17]

- *Policy*: Rules, regulations, and legislation for conditions of employment, work standards, and development of the health workforce. Key subcomponents include professional standards, licensing, and accreditations; authorization of scopes of practice of health workforce cadres; political, social, and financial decisions related to health workforce; and employment law and rules for civil service.
- *Health workforce management*: Integrated use of data, policy, and practice to plan for necessary staff, recruit, hire, deploy, and develop health workers. Key subcomponents include personnel systems (e.g., workforce planning, recruitment, hiring, and deployment); work environment and conditions (e.g., employee relations, workplace safety, job satisfaction, career development); human resource information system; performance management (e.g., performance appraisal, supervision); and staff retention.
- *Finance*: Obtaining, allocating, and dispersing adequate funding for human resources. Key subcomponents include salaries and allowances; budget for human resources for health; and mobilizing financial resources.
- *Education*: Production and continuous development of an appropriately skilled workforce. Key subcomponents include pre-service education; in-service training; capacity of training institutions; and training of community health workers and non-formal care providers. An emerging issue in delivery of education is the use of technology—handheld devices, web-based material, and simulated learning environments—to improve the efficiency and effectiveness of learning.
- *Partnerships*: Formal and informal linkages aligning key stakeholders; e.g., service providers, sectors, donors, to maximize use of human resources. Key subcomponents include community mobilization; public–private sector agreements; and mechanisms and processes for multi-stakeholder cooperation.
- *Leadership*: Capacity to provide direction, to align people, to mobilize resources, and to reach goals. Key subcomponents include identification and support for health workforce champions; leadership development for health workforce managers; and capacity for multi-sector and sector-wide collaboration; and modernization and strengthening of associations.

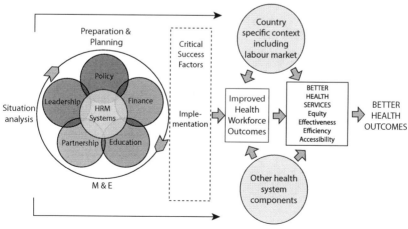

FIGURE 10.3
HRH action framework.[17]

The comprehensive approach of the HRH Action Framework helps address challenges such as staff shortages, uneven staff distribution, gaps in skills and competencies, low retention, and poor motivation. Effective HRH management is central in integrating all of the components. The guiding process-related principles in applying the framework are that the strategy is country-led, government-supported, multi-sectoral, multi-stakeholder, donor-aligned, and gender sensitive. The content-related principles are that the strategy be results-focused, system-linked, knowledge-based, learning-oriented and innovation-prone.[17]

The World Health Report 2006[1] proposed the "working lifespan" approach to systematically address the dynamics of the HRH, by focusing on strategies related to the stage when people enter the workforce, the period of their lives when they are part of the workforce, and the point at which they make their exit from it (Figure 10.4). At each stage, specific policy interventions can be designed and implemented.

This framework clearly illustrates the need for a systemic approach to strengthening HRMH, which in turn is part of a systemic approach to health system development (Figure 10.5). A systems approach enables the development of a strategy that can handle the complexities of a health system to maximize the sustainability of services.[57]

The HRH Action Framework also demonstrates the need for collaboration with a wide range of relevant stakeholders (e.g., decision makers, specialist and non-specialist health professionals, community health workers, researchers, non-government organizations, civil society organizations, faith-based organizations, user and caregivers, media, etc.) and institutional and infrastructural capacity building. Although the shortages in HRH are evident across all health areas in LMICs, the crisis is particularly significant for mental disorders. Existing evidence on health and mental health policies, plans, and services demonstrates that the need for, and importance of, mental health services is not yet recognized in many LMICs.

An example of HRMH strategies consistent with the HRH Action Framework is presented in Box 10.1.

Policy

To effectively develop HRMH, a clear policy (at national, provincial, and district levels) is necessary to define the overall values and goals; provide a coherent framework within

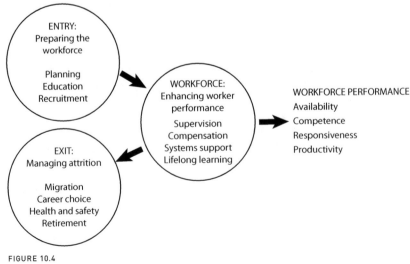

FIGURE 10.4
Working lifespan strategies.[1]

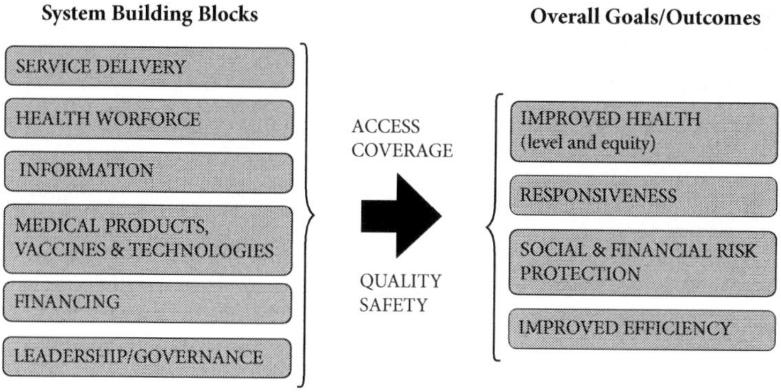

FIGURE 10.5

Building blocks of a health system: The WHO health system framework[57]

which the country can plan, train, and develop their HRMH; provide a means of account-ability; and encourage continuous improvement in the quality of care. The types, members, and distributions of human resources required will depend on the mental health services that will be delivered in the particular setting. This can be a stand-alone HRMH develop-ment policy or be integrated into the overall mental health policy.

Box 10.1 HRMH Development in Aceh, Indonesia

The approach taken to strengthening HRMH in Aceh, Indonesia, has been consis-tent with the HRH Action Framework. There is a provincial mental health policy, and a number of the districts have developed a district mental health policy. Information on the mental health workforce has improved steadily, although there is a good deal more work to do to develop a workforce data system that would be adequate for planning, recruitment, deployment, and further skill development for mental health workers. Thirteen of the 23 districts have an identified mental health budget, and all 23 districts employ community mental health nurses through the core district health budget, and provide support for the extensive village volunteers program. Education and training has been a major part of the provincial strategy for develop-ing the provincial mental health system. In partnership with Gadjah Mada University (Yogyakarta), the Syah Kuala University in Banda Aceh has established a psychology training program and is attracting large numbers of Acehnese students. Training and support for village mental health volunteers has seen rapid growth in the number of these essential community-level workers. A key area of continuing deficiency is the lack of an Aceh-based training program for psychiatrists. The provincial and district governments of Aceh, continuously supported by the Indonesian Ministry of Health, have shown exemplary leadership in their sustained commitment to the development of the most comprehensive community-based mental health system in Indonesia. Many of the key people involved in the development of the Acehnese mental health system have received training in the Melbourne-based International Mental Health Leadership Program. Finally, the whole enterprise of building a community-based mental health system, and a community mental health workforce, has been a series of partnerships involving the provincial and district governments of Aceh; the Indonesian Ministry of Health; Acehnese, other Indonesian, and interna-tional universities; UN agencies, including WHO, UNICEF, and IOM; and local and international NGOs.

In terms of global initiatives, the Sixty-Fifth Session of the World Health Assembly in May 2012 adopted resolution WHA-65.4—*The global burden of mental disorders and the need for a comprehensive, coordinated responds from health and social sectors at the country level*, and called on WHO to develop a comprehensive global mental health action plan.[19,20] *Zero Draft: Global Mental Health Action Plan 2013–2020* was released in 2012, inviting WHO member states, intergovernmental organizations, WHO Collaborating Centers, NGOs, and other organizations and associations to submit comments. *Zero Draft* presents a transformative agenda that aims to support member states, international partners, and the WHO Secretariat in developing focused, aligned, and country-owned strategies and guiding investments to deliver maximum returns for people in need.[21]

Defining mental disorders WHO adopts a broad spectrum of conditions to define mental disorders, including neurological and substance use disorders. It includes depression and anxiety disorders, alcohol and other substance use and misuse, severe and disabling conditions such as schizophrenia and bipolar disorder, as well as neurological problems such as epilepsy and dementia.[19]

Defining mental health services One of the most important changes in mental health care in the last few decades has been the shift from institution-based treatment to community-based care. Implications of this shift for HRMH include the need for (1) redeployment of staff from hospital to community-based service settings; (2) the development of new competencies for work among staff in community-based settings with a new emphasis on recovery and rehabilitation in both hospital and community-based settings; (3) training of a wider range of HRMH (such as informal community care and primary care); and (4) reform of associated training models in keeping with the new service delivery models.[13]

Integration of mental health into general health care, primary care in particular, has also been one of the most feasible approaches to address the significant treatment gap.[58] This has also had significant HRMH implications, such as the need for appropriate training in mental health competencies to detect mental illnesses, provide basic care, and refer complex cases to specialist services, and mental health specialists must work collaboratively with general health workers to provide support and supervision.

The WHO proposes the WHO Service Organization Pyramid for an Optimal Mix of Services for Mental Health in which integration of mental health services into primary care is a fundamental component and is supported by other levels of care, including community-based and hospital services.[59] This pyramid, however, will require significant modification if we are to incorporate the increasingly multidisciplinary and multi-sectoral contexts in which mental health services are being delivered (health, education, labor, housing, criminal justice, and social services). The *A65/10 Report*,[19] *Resolution WHA-65.4*, and[20] *Zero Draft: Global Mental Health Action Plan 2013–2020*[21] call for a comprehensive, community-based, integrated, and responsive mental heath and social care services. It highlights the need for community-based services to go beyond the provision of clinical care and to adopt a recovery-based approach that includes support services for individuals to achieve their own goals and aspirations, such as employment, housing, educational opportunities, and community engagement. Efforts to develop coordinated, comprehensive, community-based mental health and social services for people with mental disorders are currently underway in Vietnam, and this program's description is presented in Box 10.2.

An effective mental health care system also requires paying adequate attention to mental health promotion and prevention of mental disorders across the life course. Strategies for mental health promotion and prevention of mental disorders may include interventions to nurture core individual attributes during childhood and adolescents; early detection

Box 10.2 Vietnam

Vietnam has had a community mental health program, delivered through primary care, since 1998. Although the program has been rolled out across most of the country, it focuses only on schizophrenia and epilepsy, and services for people with common mental disorders remain limited. Staffing at the primary care level is as good as in any comparable country in the world. However, there are significant shortages in mental health workers at all levels (i.e., psychiatrists, psychologists, occupational therapists, psychiatric social workers, and psychiatric nurses), and Vietnam has the most severe shortage of psychiatrists worldwide.[11] The government of Vietnam has devoted increased attention to the mental health of the population and to developing an integrated hospital and community mental health system that has the capacity to respond to the mental health service needs of the population. The National Action Plan for Mental Health for 2011–2015 aims to develop community teams for all 63 provinces. The initial composition of the teams will include psychiatrists, at least 10 nurses, and 5 psychosocial workers. This composition is expected to change, once training programs in psychology, psychiatric social work, occupational therapy, and community psychiatric nursing are developed and launched over the coming four years.

In terms of the role of social workers, the government of Vietnam approved Decision 32/2010/QD-TTg on March 25, 2010, which announced the development of social work as a profession and commits to training 60,000 social workers by 2020. Furthermore, Decision 1215/QD-TTg to approve the proposal to develop community-based social support and rehabilitation for people with mental disorder was announced on July 22, 2011. Decision 1215 aims to mobilize community and family members in providing resource support, psychological support, and rehabilitation for people with mental disorders for the purposes of assisting with care and community integration of people with mental disorders, prevention of mental disorders, and ensuring social security. Accordingly, the Ministry of Labor, Invalids and Social Affairs, in collaboration with the Ministries of Health, Education and Training, Finance, Planning and Investment, and Information and Communications, will develop community-based human resources on social assistance and rehabilitation for people with mental disorders by (1) organizing training for staff and collaborators working in the field of mental health care; (2) supporting training institutions to develop training curricula and training programs on social work in the field of mental health care, and to improve the teaching capacity of staff; and (3) training families of people with mental disorders with skills in caring and rehabilitation.

and prevention of emotional problems and behavioral problems; provision of healthy living and working conditions; social protection for the poor; anti-discrimination laws; community education about mental health and mental illnesses; promotion of human rights; and harm-reduction initiatives.[21]

The shifts in the scope of mental health services pose further challenges in defining, coordinating, and managing roles and functions. Depending on the extent to which mental health services include mental health promotion, prevention, detection, treatment, rehabilitation, and social support, the breadth of HRMH and the need for inter-sectoral collaboration and coordination will vary. Furthermore, the variability in the roles of different mental health workers across settings highlights the importance of focusing on a skills-mix rather than a staff-mix approach in increasing HRMH.[16]

An example of how a mental health care structure might incorporate the various services and human resources is depicted in Figure 10.6.

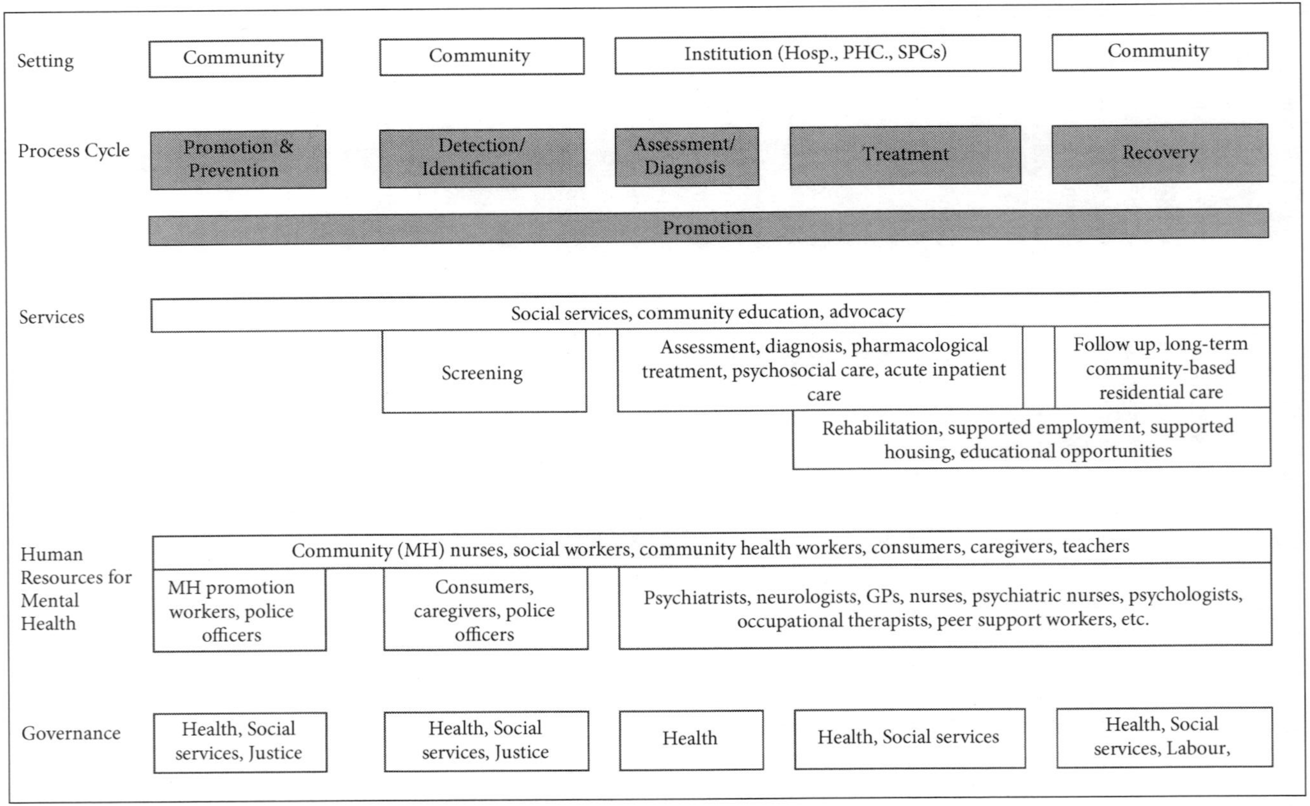

Setting	Community	Community	Institution (Hosp., PHC., SPCs)	Community
Process Cycle	Promotion & Prevention	Detection/Identification	Assessment/Diagnosis	Treatment	Recovery
			Promotion		
Services	Social services, community education, advocacy				
		Screening	Assessment, diagnosis, pharmacological treatment, psychosocial care, acute inpatient care	Rehabilitation, supported employment, supported housing, educational opportunities	Follow up, long-term community-based residential care
Human Resources for Mental Health	Community (MH) nurses, social workers, community health workers, consumers, caregivers, teachers				
	MH promotion workers, police officers	Consumers, caregivers, police officers	Psychiatrists, neurologists, GPs, nurses, psychiatric nurses, psychologists, occupational therapists, peer support workers, etc.		
Governance	Health, Social services, Justice	Health, Social services, Justice	Health	Health, Social services	Health, Social services, Labour,

FIGURE 10.6

Example of mental health care system structure

In the context of task shifting and varying levels of services, HRMH can include (1) specialist workers, such as psychiatrists, neurologists, psychiatric nurses, psychologists, mental health social workers, and occupational therapists; (2) non-specialist health workers (NSHWs) such as doctors, nurses and lay health workers, mental health care users, and caregivers; and (3) other professionals such as teachers, police officers, and community-level workers. They can work in different settings (hospital, clinic, community, etc.) and different sectors (education, labor, correctional, etc.).

Defining the different types of scale-up Once a mental health service package and an optimal mix of human resources are determined, a strategy to increase HRMH is required. There are different interpretations of "scaling up" across the health context, and its definition has direct implications for HRMH planning. Scaling up typically includes several common components: an increase in the number of people receiving services that have been shown to be effective in similar contexts; increase in the range of such services; and services made sustainable through policy formulation, implementation, and financing.[60]

Scaling up can also refer to a process that includes mobilization of political will, human resource development, increase in the availability of essential medicines, and monitoring and evaluation.[61] WHO describes scaling up as "deliberate efforts to increase the impact of health service innovations successfully tested in pilot or experimental projects so as to benefit more people and to foster policy and program development on a lasting basis."[62] The different types of scale-up which are relevant for HRMH are:

- *Horizontal scale-up* (also called *expansion* or *replication*) is when services are replicated in different geographical sites or are extended to serve larger or new population groups.
- *Vertical scale-up* (also called *policy/political/legal/institutional scale-up*) is when formal government decisions are made to adopt an innovation on a national or sub-national level and to institutionalize it through national planning mechanisms, policy changes, or legal action. Systems and structures are adapted and resources distributed to build the institutional mechanisms that can ensure sustainability.
- *Functional scale-up* (also called *diversification* or *grafting*) involves testing and adding interventions to an existing package.

All three types of scale-up will be required to effectively develop appropriate, adequate, and sustainable human resources to close the treatment gap for mental health care, and policies need to be in place to enable scale-up activities.

Mobilizing political will is one of the most common and most significant challenges in mental health system development and requires organized actions to effectively respond to the mental health needs of the population (see Chapter 20). These actions include reforming legal, policy, and regulatory frameworks; increasing investment in mental health; modifying existing programs or establishing new mental health programs; strengthening human resources for mental health; generating research evidence; and effectively using evidence to inform policy and practice.[63]

Evidence to inform appropriate rules, regulations, and legislation for employment conditions, work standards, and workforce development are scarce. In many contexts, mental health services are provided by workers with limited competencies and knowledge of professional standards, and in contexts where there are inadequate licensing or accreditation arrangements, and where there is a lack of clarity about scope of practice to guide the work of various health workers. In essence, many health workers are providing mental health services that they are legally not authorized to provide, most often because there is no other option. Not only are policies necessary to provide the framework for mental health services, they are also essential to protect and enable the health workers to provide the services that they are trained to provide.[64]

Education and Training

Ongoing development of an appropriately skilled workforce is essential for strengthening HRMH. Training should be relevant to the mental health needs of the population, and include in-service training (e.g., continuing education) and institutional capacity-strengthening to implement training programs effectively.

However, psychiatric training programs are present in only 55% of LICs and 69% of lower MICs and 60% of upper MICs,[5] and approaches to psychiatric education vary across countries.[65–68] In Nigeria, a specialist training program in psychiatry has been in place for over 25 years, yet only half of the country's tertiary mental health facilities have enough psychiatrists to provide accredited training.[5]

Training of NSHWs also needs scaling up. Evidence on training in mental health among primary health care providers as well as other health providers has consistently shown positive results for detection and treatment of mental disorders.[58,69] Overall, short-term training by specialist mental health professionals with ongoing supervision can effectively improve confidence, detection, treatment, and treatment compliance of individuals with mental disorders and reduce caregiver burden. Training of community health workers and non-formal care providers is also a critical component of the health workforce to meet treatment needs.[34,52–54,66,68,70–81] Training programs must also be strengthened, or developed, to train non-specialist workers and psychosocial workers. Many countries are still lacking training programs in areas such as psychology, social work, and occupational therapy. As service models increasingly shift towards a multidisciplinary skills mix to promote mental health, prevent mental illness, detect and treat mental illness, and support recovery, the needs of psychosocial workers will also increase, and training programs will be needed to meet the demand.

Health Workforce Management

Skilled health managers are essential in developing a successful health workforce. Health managers oversee the strategic direction of mental health service development, manage resource allocation, and monitor policy targets and outcomes. Health managers are responsible for planning and implementing health personnel systems, managing work environments and conditions, HRH information systems, workforce performance, and staff retention. Inequitable resources for mental health training and inequitable salaries for psychiatrists and other mental health care providers relative to other health professions make a career in mental health less appealing. These are important issues that health managers must be able to address to improve mental health services, yet capacity-building of policymakers and health planners and managers is often neglected when developing HRH development plans.

Information on health managers in developing countries is lacking. The managerial function is rarely included in HRH plans. A survey of health managers in Ethiopia, Ghana, and the United Republic of Tanzania[82] demonstrated that managers are primarily clinicians with additional management roles and responsibilities. They included doctors, nurses, assistant medical officers, health administrators, pharmacists, health officers, and clinical officers, with the largest proportion being doctors. Furthermore, training in management is not a requirement to assume a managerial role. The findings highlight the major lack of recognition for the role of skilled health mangers in scaling up service delivery.

Recruitment Negative attitudes of health professionals towards mental disorders still remain a significant challenge. Even when training programs are available, very few students are choosing a career in psychiatry.[83,84] Ignorance, stigma, and discrimination contribute to the lack of willingness in many medical trainees to undertake specialist training in mental health. In Kenya, medical students enrolled at University of Nairobi were surveyed on their attitudes towards psychiatry.[77] Although almost 75% of respondents held overall favorable attitudes towards psychiatry, only 14% would consider psychiatry as a career choice. In Brazil, focus group discussions with primary health care providers found that, although they accept their role in detecting the mental health problems of their clientele, they still believe that diagnosis and treatment should remain the responsibility of the mental health specialists.[71,85] Misconceptions about mental disorders, fear, perceived low status of mental health professionals, and inadequate training contribute to the reluctance of many health professionals to provide mental health care in Ghana, South Africa, Uganda, and Zambia.[86–89]

However, educational interventions in mental health for primary care professionals have been shown to improve attitudes towards mental illness.[70–73, 75, 76, 90–92] Similar interventions during medical training may improve recruitment of mental health specialists, but this needs further exploration.[93]

Managing distribution, migration, and attrition Migration of health workers from LMICs to HICs, and from rural to urban settings, significantly constrains human resource development,[94–98] and mental health is no exception.[99–101] Professional isolation and better training and career opportunities are key reasons for emigrating to HICs and to urban settings.[102] Factors such as salaries and working conditions (e.g., inadequate facilities and supplies), lack of training and continuing education opportunities become push factors to leave LMICs, and pull factors for HICs to use as strategies to recruit health professionals to their own countries.[103] Professional isolation and better training opportunities were identified as key reasons for emigrating by the World Psychiatric Association (WPA) Taskforce on "brain drain."[102]

Salaries and working conditions in LMICs are even worse in mental health than in general health settings, because of the lack of priority for mental health care in many countries, with consequent lack of resources to develop training programs, facilities, and services for mental health care. Jenkins and colleagues examined the international migration of psychiatrists in LMICs by examining the professional databases of the four leading recipient countries in 2008 to determine the number of psychiatrists with specialist qualifications from their own countries.[104] The authors found that collectively, the United Kingdom, United States, New Zealand, and Australia had 4,687 psychiatrists from India, 1,593 from the Philippines, 1,158 from Pakistan, 149 from Bangladesh, 384 from Nigeria, 484 from Egypt, and 142 from Sri Lanka (a total of almost 9,000 psychiatrists).[99] The detrimental impact on donor countries was that, without this migration, many of the countries would have more than double (in some cases five to eight times) the number of psychiatrists per 100,000 population. These results clearly demonstrate the urgent need to develop innovative strategies to deal effectively with the issue of professional migration.

Establishing local training programs where none exist, strengthening existing programs, and addressing incentives to foster rewarding career pathways are particularly important in reducing the likelihood of out-migration. International collaborations have been an important strategy in scaling up HRMH.[105] Psychiatric training was conducted in Ethiopia through a partnership between the University of Toronto and the University of Addis Ababa (TAAP), and the number of psychiatrists in Ethiopia increased from 11 to 34 between 2003 and 2009.[106] The success of the program has led to its expansion to cover 14 different health programs.[107]

Working conditions also play a role in HRMH retention. In a cross-sectional study in Kenya, 95% of respondents working at a psychiatric hospital reported low to high levels of emotional exhaustion, and 88% reported depersonalization. Almost 40% of respondents reported having low levels of accomplishment.[108] In Brazil, 62% of mental health professionals from four mental health services in Rio de Janeiro reported only moderate levels of job satisfaction.[109]

Retention and equitable distribution of HRMH remain a challenge. Financial incentive strategies, institutional capacity-building that promotes career development, opportunities to receive and provide mentorship, and favorable workplace conditions are areas that need to be strengthened to minimize attrition.

Monitoring and evaluation, information systems Evaluation of strategies to scale up HRMH remains a challenge. The lack of agreed-upon indicators for monitoring and evaluating HRH development strategies is a key impediment. To date, indicators of HRMH have focused primarily on the number of mental health specialists, availability of training programs, number of health workers who received specialist training, and number of non-specialists with mental health training. Brain drain has mainly been assessed through international studies that look at mental health specialists working in high-income countries who were trained in LMICs.

Despite the emerging evidence on mental health systems in LMICs, applying the evidence to develop and evaluate HRMH is a difficult and complex task that will continue to pose challenges in the coming years. It requires a systemic approach with interdisciplinary and multi-sectoral collaborations and strong partnerships between ministries, researchers, NGOs, health professionals, service users/caregivers, and communities if significant long-term gains are to be made. Adequate attention to these aspects is essential to achieve the objective of scaling up care for mental disorders.

The HRH Action Framework and the monitoring and evaluation framework have not yet been applied in the mental health context. Strategies to scale up HRMH should be aligned with the evidence and framework on developing human resources for health.

Finance

Mobilizing financial resources to develop HRH is one of most significant obstacles in mental health. The efficient use of existing funds is also challenging.[110] Existing data from the Mental Health Atlas 2005 showed the inadequate allocation of health expenditure for mental health in all LMICs.[3] Cost-effectiveness studies for scaling up NSHWs are few,[111] and further studies are necessary to inform HRMH planning.

Scheffler and colleagues addressed this gap by estimating the annual wage bill required to fill the mental health workforce shortages for all LMICs.[11] Mental health workforce needs were subtracted from the 2005 supply of mental health workers to calculate shortages (or surplus). The wage bill was determined by multiplying the shortages by annual wages in 58 LMICs based on 2005 data. Annual wage bill costs estimated to eliminate the mental health workforce shortages are approximately US$814 million in 2005: US$80 million for psychiatrists, US$420 million for nurses in mental health settings, and US$315 million for psychosocial care providers. The estimates vary from country to country. Nigeria was found to have the highest estimated cost to eliminate workforce shortages for all workforce categories: US$14.8 million for psychiatrists, US$49.6 million for nurses, US$53.7 million for psychosocial health providers, for a total of US$118.2 million.

A needs-based approach was also used to determine costs for scaling up child and adolescent mental health care in South Africa.[112] It was found that, per child or adolescent, per annum, nationally, it would cost US$21.50 to provide full coverage and US$5.00 to provide minimum coverage.

Strategic changes in payment systems are as important as financing in bringing about system change.[113] For example, increasing the role of psychiatrists as supervisors and trainers, and increasing the number of other mental health workers, will need payment arrangements that recognize these changed roles. These changes will also be important in shifting practice from institutions to community services.

Partnerships

Effective partnerships play a crucial role in establishing appropriate and adequate human resources to deliver a comprehensive, integrated, and sustainable health system. In Burma, a partnership between a local health department and internally displaced villagers enabled the training of villagers so that they could perform an increasingly comprehensive set of interventions for a malaria control program. This partnership resulted in a significant increase in the number of villagers trained, from 3,000 to 40,000 over the course of five years.[114]

In Somaliland, a public–academic partnership between Kings College London, THET (Tropical Health and Education Trust), and their Somaliland partners includes work in Somaliland with four nurse-training institutions, two medical schools, two professional associations, an emerging health professionals council, some of the public hospitals and regional health boards, and the Ministry of Health and Labor.[115] Mental health is incorporated into this program, which includes equipment and training aids, books, and some funding. Through this program, all 62 final-year medical students and interns in 2008 and 2009 received intensive mental health training and rigorous examinations. Mental health has become an intrinsic part of medical training.

Research evidence on the impact of partnerships on HRMH development is scarce, but described here are current collaborative initiatives to strengthen mental health systems, including HRMH.

ASEAN Mental Health Taskforce The Assocation of Southeast Asian Nations (ASEAN) Strategic Framework for Health Development (2010–2015) was endorsed in 2010. Mental heath is included under B4: Promote ASEAN Health Lifestyle. This serves as the operational guideline for the implementation of the ASEAN Socio-Cultural Community Blueprint on health development and provides direction for relevant technical working groups to further develop their respective work plans and have ownership for its implementation. An ASEAN Meeting held in Bangkok in June 2011 established the ASEAN Mental Health Taskforce (AMT) and developed a work plan, allocating responsibility to individual member states for different elements of the work plan, the overall objective of which is to ensure access to adequate and affordable mental health treatment and care and psychosocial services, and to promote healthy lifestyles for the people of ASEAN member states. The World Health Organization and the Centre for International Mental Health at the Univesity of Melbourhe have been invited by the ASEAN Secretariat to provide technical assistance to the AMT since its inception. The AMT provides a unique policy-relevant and policy-led opportunity to engage actively and share experiences to develop and evaluate current programs, develop strategies to integrate mental health into general health care, and to strengthen the capacity of researchers and decision makers at individual and organizational levels.

Mental Health Consortium in Vietnam The government of Vietnam, although committed to mental health, faces many challenges in mental health service provision. The existing primary care–based community mental health program is limited to treatment of psychotic and very severe affective disorders and epilepsy. People suffering from depression and other common mental disorders have very limited access to treatment or care. Capacity to provide non-pharmacological treatments is extremely limited, and there is extremely limited access to community-based rehabilitation and psychosocial support services. Massive under-recognition of mental disorders as a national public health problem results in significant under-investment in mental health,[116] almost total reliance on mental hospitals, and a serious shortage of skilled mental health professionals at all levels.[8] Existing mental health policies and plans require development and implementation, and mental health legislation is lacking.[*,**] Inter-sectoral collaboration and coordination between Ministry of Health-managed services and other sectors (e.g., social, education, criminal justice, etc.) is inadequate. Neglect and abuse of the human rights of people with mental disorders (PWMDs) must also be urgently addressed.

Services for PWMDs are implemented through the Ministry of Health (MoH) and the Ministry of Labour, Invalids, and Social Affairs (MoLISA). MoLISA provides care for PWMDs through their social protection services. The network of 17 Social Protection Centers in 16 cities and provinces has limited technical and financial support and is unable to provide the full range of necessary services.

Lack of collaboration between the two key ministries poses significant complexities. No mechanism and guidelines exist to facilitate collaboration between the two sectors. There is an urgent need to establish an inter-ministerial mechanism to develop and implement a comprehensive and integrated system of care for PWMDs through a national action framework on mental health that maximizes the capacity, efficiency, and effectiveness of the mental health system.

Current barriers to developing and implementing such a framework include: (1) lack of collaboration and coordination of services by MoH and MoLISA; (2) lack of an effective monitoring and evaluation system (both MoH and MoLISA) to track quality of care and policy implementation, and to identify determinants of success in achieving national mental health objectives; (3) insufficient capacity of provincial and district-level managers in leadership for integrated mental health system development and implementation; (4) lack of accurate and up-to-date information on workforce needs; (5) no comprehensive workforce development plan; and (6) minimal access to existing evidence, practical experiences, and best practices in community mental health.

Adequate documentation and dissemination of local evidence on effective mental health care is essential for planning, implementation, and evaluation. The Centre for International Mental Health, the University of Melbourne (CIMH), has been working in Vietnam since 1994,[117,118] and has collaborated closely with MoH since 2010 to establish the National Taskforce on Community Mental Health System Development in Vietnam through funding from Atlantic Philanthropies (2010–2014). The goal of the National Taskforce Project is to develop community mental health services in Vietnam by strengthening the capacity of MoH, in cooperation with key stakeholders, including other relevant ministries (such as MoLISA, and ministries of finance and education), to plan, design, and deliver effective, accessible, and affordable community mental health services to the population of Vietnam. The key components of the National Taskforce Project are to establish and manage the National Taskforce and secretariat; policy and research support; training and human resource development; and demonstration projects. The National Taskforce Project has five key areas of work: (1) mental heath legislation, policy, and financing; (2) human resources for mental health; (3) community

---

[*] Ha Mai Luan: Project on planning of network of nursing, rehabilitation centers for psychiatric people, Son La. In: *Workshop on taking care of mental patients*. Hanoi: Social Protection Bureau, Ministry of Labour, Invalids and Social Affairs; 2009:58–66.

[**] Le Van Thach: Project on planning of network of nursing, rehabilitation centers for psychiatric people, Son La. In: *Workshop on taking care of mental patients*. Hanoi: Social Protection Bureau, Ministry of Labour, Invalids and Social Affairs; 2009:47–57.

mental health services; (4) women and children's mental health; and (5) mental health advocacy and human rights.

In 2010, Prime Ministerial Decision 32/2010/QD-TTg was announced, to develop social work as a profession and to train 60,000 social work staff, including social workers and officials, by 2020. In 2011, Prime Ministerial Decision 1215/QD-Ttg Project, Community-Based Assistance and Functional Rehabilitation for Mental Ill and Mentally Disordered Project, 2011–2020 was announced. This project set out an ambitious program of national reform and development of community-based functional rehabilitation and social support services[119] for PWMDs in Vietnam, and has made available substantial funds from the state budget to implement this reform.

The National Taskforce Project and the two new MoLISA-managed programs enable MoH and MoLISA to collaboratively develop and implement an integrated mental health system.[119] If done well, Vietnam is well positioned to become a global leader in successfully designing and implementing a truly inter-sectoral mental health care system that is led in partnership by the two key ministries. Establishing such a process involves considerable complexity, coordination, and sensitivities and a Mental Health Consortium Program (funded by Atlantic Philanthropies, Jan. 2013–Dec. 2015) was established to support this initiative. This Consortium of local and international partners (UNICEF-Vietnam, CIMH, Vietnam Veterans of America Foundation, and Research and Training Center for Community Development), share their experience, expertise, and resources to provide coordinated technical assistance to MoH and MoLISA to implement the three programs. The work of the Mental Health Consortium will support the two ministries to maximize their capacity to achieve national mental health objectives, examples of which include: (1) development of a National Action Framework on Mental Health; (2) development of an integrated monitoring and evaluation system to track implementation of the National Action Framework on Mental Health; (3) a needs assessment and development of a human resource development plan; (4) building capacity for managers on leadership in integrated mental health system development and implementation; and (5) review and dissemination of evidence, practical experiences, and best practices in community mental health care.

PRIME: Program for Improving Mental Health Care The Program for Improving Mental Health Care (PRIME; funded by the U.K. Department for International Development, 2011–2017) aims to generate evidence on the implementation and scaling up of integrated packages of care for priority mental disorders in primary and maternal health care settings in Ethiopia, India, Nepal, South Africa, and Uganda.[120] PRIME has three objectives:

1. Develop draft mental health care plans, comprising packages of mental health care for delivery in primary health care and maternal health care;
2. Evaluate the feasibility, acceptability, and impact of the packages of care in primary health care and maternal health care in one low-resource district (or sub-district) in each country; and
3. Evaluate the scaling up of these packages of care to other districts.

One of the guiding principles of PRIME is to work in partnerships. It seeks to address the knowledge gap through partnerships between academic researchers, Ministry of Health members responsible for the national mental health program in the participating study countries, international NGOs with experience in mental health interventions in primary care and community settings, and WHO. Through these partnerships, each of the five countries has developed a draft mental health action plan that is informed by local needs and resources (e.g., human resource cadres delivering service packages components that vary across study countries) and are continuing to produce research evidence to inform HRMH development that is applicable to many countries. The mental health care plan for Ethiopia is now available.[121]

Leadership

Effective leadership is essential in scaling up HRMH,[122] yet little evidence exists that addresses this issue adequately. Studies on leadership training for human resources development for general health services clearly demonstrate its importance.[123] In six provinces in the Republic of Kenya, health teams receiving six-month leadership and management training had significantly better improvements in health care coverage and number of client visits at the facility level than those not receiving the training intervention.[124] A 13- to 16-week Virtual Leadership Training Program delivered using a web-based platform that combines face-to-face and distance learning methods has also been found to be effective in improving leadership skills. Participants of this training program involved in the Developing Human Resources for Health Project in Uganda were better able to improve the learning environment and opportunities for laboratory skills among medical and nursing students.[125]

The University of Melbourne has been running an International Mental Health Leadership Program since 2001.[126] This four-week intensive course provides training in mental health policy and systems, mental health workforce, and mental health and human rights for researchers, psychiatrists, mental health professionals, and decision makers. Shorter two-week leadership courses have subsequently been developed in Indonesia, India, and Nigeria. Anecdotal evidence suggests that the courses and ongoing support for alumni make an impact in their home countries. An international diploma in mental health law and human rights has also been launched by the Indian Law Society and the World Health Organization. The number of applications to these courses clearly demonstrates the need for such courses, and anecdotal evidence demonstrates their success in inspiring and supporting participants to become leaders in mental health in their own countries. Unfortunately, systematic evaluations of such initiatives have not yet been carried out.

In addition to organized training programs, initiatives such as the Movement for Global Mental Health provide opportunities for a variety of stakeholders to take leadership in a variety of activities to carry this movement forward. Another initiative, called the EMPOWER project (funded by WellcomeTrust, 2010–2011), provided opportunities for mental health–user organizations from India, Kenya, Nepal, and Zambia to collaborate with researchers to lead mental health advocacy projects in these countries to develop communication tools to reduce stigma and discrimination and advocate for change. Such experiences must be captured and shared in the global mental health community so that others can learn and benefit to develop innovative strategies to strengthen HRMH (see Box 10.3).

CONCLUSION

HRMH continue to be grossly inadequate in most LMICs. The shortage is likely to worsen unless significant investments are made to train a wider range of mental health workers in substantially higher numbers. Task shifting seems to be an effective and feasible approach for this, but this, too, will involve significant investment, innovative thinking, and effective leadership.

Examples of innovative and effective strategies to expand services to primary care settings and into the community are emerging. The variability in the roles of different mental health workers across settings highlights the importance of focusing on a skills-mix rather than a staff-mix approach in increasing HRMH.[16] Training programs

Box 10.3 Relevant Guides and Tools to Strengthen HRMH

The following list of tools and resources aims to help readers in contributing towards HRMH development (NB: this list is not meant to be comprehensive or exhaustive):

HRH policy-impact assessment tools:

- WHO Human Resources for Health Tools and Guidelines:http://www.who.int/hrh/tools/situation_analysis/en/index.html
- Incorporating the Right to Health into Health Workforce Plans: Key Considerations: https://s3.amazonaws.com/PHR_other/incorporating-right-to-health.pdf
- Walt G, Gilson L. Reforming the health sector in developing countries: the central role of policy analysis. *Health Policy and Planning*. 1994;9:353–70: http://info.worldbank.org/etools/docs/library/122031/bangkokCD/BangkokMarch05/Week2/4Thursday/S2EngagingStakeholders/ReformingtheHealthSector.pdf
- WHO. WHO-AIMS Mental health systems in selected low- and middle-income countries: a WHO-AIMS cross-national analysis. [Online]. Geneva, WHO; 2009. Available from: http://whqlibdoc.who.int/publications/2009/9789241547741_eng.pdf.
- Aaron Tjoa, Margaret Kapihya, Miriam Libetwa, Kate Schroder, Callie Scott, Joanne Lee, and Elizabeth McCarthy (2010). Meeting human resources for health staffing goals by 2018: a quantitative analysis of policy options in Zambia. *BioMed Central Ltd. Hum Resour Health.* 2010;8:15: http://www.human-resources-health.com/content/8/1/15.
- World Health Organization (2008). *WHO Human resources for health minimum data set.* Geneva, World Health Organization. http://www.who.int/hrh/documents/hrh_minimum_data_set.pdf

HRH toolkits:

- The WHO Service Availability Mapping tool: www.who.int/healthinfo/systems/serviceavailabilitymapping
- Assessment for human resources for health: Survey instruments and guide to administration. (2002) World Health Organization: http://www.who.int/entity/hrh/tools/hrh_assessment_guide.pdf
- A guide to rapid assessment of human resources for health. (2004). World Health Organization: http://www.who.int/hrh/tools/en/Rapid_Assessment_guide.pdf
- Gupta, N. and M. R. Dal Poz (2009). Assessment of human resources for health using cross-national comparison of facility surveys in six countries. *Hum Resour Health.* 7:22: http://www.human-resources-health.com/content/7/1/22
- The Service Provision Assessment by Macro International: www.measuredhs.com/aboutsurveys/spa/start.cfm
- The PHRplus survey tool by Partners for Health Reformplus: www.healthsystems2020.org/content/resources/detail1704/
- The Facility Audit of Service Quality rapid monitoring tool by MEASURE Evaluation: http://ihfan.org/home/docs/attachments/wp-09-111_Comparative_analysis.pdf.

(continued)

Box 10.3 Continued

- iHRIS Software Suite by Capacityplus including: iHRIS Quality, iHRIS Manage, iHRIS Plan, iHRIS Appliance: www.capacityplus.org/hris/suite/
- Incorporating the Right to Health into Health Workforce Plans: Key Considerations by Health Workforce Advocacy Initiative (HWAI): https://s3.amazonaws.com/PHR_other/incorporating-right-to-health.pdf
- The Right to Health and Health Workforce Planning: A Guide for Government Officials, NGOs, Health Workers and Development Partners by Physicians for Human Rights: https://s3.amazonaws.com/PHR_other/health-workforce-planning-guide-2.pdf. And also in French: https://s3.amazonaws.com/PHR_other/health-workforce-planning-guide-2-french.pdf).
- Guiding Principles on National Health Workforce Strategies by HWAI: English: http://www.healthworkforce.info/advocacy/HWAI_Principles.pdf. French: http://www.healthworkforce.info/advocacy/HWAI_Principles_FR.pdf. Spanish: http://www.healthworkforce.info/advocacy/HWAI_Principles_ES.pdf.
- Addressing the Health Workforce Crisis: A Toolkit for Health Professional Advocates by HWAI: http://www.healthworkforce.info/advocacy/HWAI_advocacy_toolkit.pdf.
- Dal Poz M, Gupta N, Quain E, Soucat ALB, editors. Handbook on monitoring and evaluation of human resources for health with special applications for low- and middle-income countries. [Online]. Geneva, WHO; 2009. Available from: http://whqlibdoc.who.int/publications/2009/9789241547703_eng.pdf
- Bruckner TA, Scheffler RM, Shen G, Yoon J, Chisholm D, Morris J, et al. The mental health workforce gap in low- and middle-income countries: a needs-based approach. *Bull WHO* [Online] 2011; 89:84–194. Available from: http://www.who.int/bulletin/volumes/89/3/10-082784.pdf
- Tjoa A, Kapihya M, Libetwa M, Lee J, Pattinson C, McCarthy E, et al. Doubling the number of health graduates in Zambia: estimating feasibility and costs. *BioMed Central Ltd. Hum Resour Health*. 2010;8:22. http://www.human-resources-health.com/content/8/1/22.
- Varpilah ST, Safer M, Frenkel E, Baba D, Massaquoi M, Barrow G. Rebuilding human resources for health: a case study from Liberia. *BioMed Central Ltd. Hum Resour Health*. 2011;9:11. http://www.human-resources-health.com/content/9/1/11.
- WHO. Workload Indicators of Staffing Need: http://www.who.int/hrh/tools/workload_indicators.pdf
- Paphassarang C, Theppanya K, Rotem A. Improving availability and retention of health workers in remote and underserved areas: The Lao PDR experience. Paper presented at the Joint AAAH-WHO conference. "Getting committed health workers to the underserved areas: a challenge for the health systems" November 23–25, 2009, in Hanoi, Vietnam. Department of Organization and Personnel, Ministry of Health, Lao PDR. http://www.aaahrh.org/4th_conf_2009/Chantakhath_LAOS.pdf
- Beaudoin O, Forest L, et al. (2006). Working together towards recovery: consumers, families, caregivers and providers. A toolkit for consumers, families and caregivers. Canadian Collaborative Mental Health Initiative: http://www.ccmhi.ca/en/products/toolkits.html

Box 10.3 Continued

- World Health Organization (2008). Toolkit on monitoring health systems strengthening: human resources for health. Geneva, World Health Organization: http://www.who.int/healthinfo/statistics/toolkit_hss/EN_PDF_Toolkit_HSS_HumanResources_oct08.pdf
- WWPT: WPRO Workforce Projection Tool, version 1.0: User's Manual. by World Health Organization: http://www.healthworkforce.info/aaah/workshop/gf_hss/05-04-2008/AAAH%20TRAINING%20WORKSHOP/Session%209/WPRO%20Workforce%20Projection%20Tool-%20description.PDF
- Pacque-Margolis S, Ng C, et al. (2011). Human resources for health (HRH) indicator compendium. USAID and CapacityPlus http://capacityplus.org/human-resources-health-indicator-compendium
- Lorenzo FME, Ronquillo K, et al. Development of regional HRH indicators and monitoring template: profess report submitted to Asian Alliance for HRH Development. Asia Pacific Action Alliance on Human Resources for Health: http://www.who.int/workforcealliance/knowledge/resources/aaah_indicators/en/index.html

Training Manuals

- An introduction to mental health: facilitator's manual for training community health workers in India (2009). http://www.basicneeds.org/html/Publications_BasicNeeds_Manuals.htm
- Learning for Performance: A Guide and Toolkit for Health Worker Training and Education Programs (2007). IntraHealth International, Inc. http://www.intrahealth.org/page/learning-for-performance
- Eisenman D, Weine S, et al. (2006). The ISTSS/Rand guidelines on mental health training of primary healthcare providers for trauma-exposed populations in conflict-affected countries. *J Trauma Stress*. 19(1):5–17.
- Weine S, Danieli Y, et al. (2002). Guidelines for international training in mental health and psychosocial interventions for trauma exposed populations in clinical and community settings. *Psychiatry*. 65(2):156–64. http://www.who.int/mental_health/resources/training_guidelines_for_trauma_interventions.pdf
- World Health Organization (1998). A WHO Educational Package: Mental Disorders in Primary Care. Geneva, World Health Organization: http://whqlibdoc.who.int/hq/1998/WHO_MSA_MNHIEAC_98.1.pdf

Guidelines

- World Health Organization (2010). mhGAP Intervention Guide for mental, neurological and substance use disorders in non-specialized health settings: http://www.who.int/mental_health/publications/mhGAP_intervention_guide/en/index.html
- World Health Organization (2005). Mental Health Policy and Service Guidance Package—Module 11: Human resources and training in mental health. Geneva, World Health Organization: http://www.who.int/mental_health/policy/essentialpackage1/en/index.html
- World Health Organization (2012). WHO QualityRights Tool Kit: Assessing and improving quality and human rights in mental health and social care facilities. Geneva, World Health Organization: http://whqlibdoc.who.int/publications/2012/9789241548410_eng.pdf

will need to be accompanied by effective supervision to maintain and to continue to develop skills, and ongoing career development opportunities will be critical in minimizing attrition.

Involvement of workers from a broad range of workforce categories is likely to facilitate scaling up of mental health care in LMICs. The specific composition of the mental health workforce will vary across settings and will need to be aligned with existing delivery system and resource structures.

Despite the growing evidence on mental health systems in LMICs, HRMH is a neglected area in the scientific literature. It is a field that requires urgent attention if we are to develop effective strategies to scale up services for mental health. It is a complex task that requires a systemic approach with interdisciplinary and multi-sectoral collaborations and strong partnerships between ministries, researchers, NGOs, health professionals, service users/caregivers, and communities if we are to make significant gains.

Skilled health management and support workers, who compose up to a third of the health workforce, are critical in overseeing the implementation of strategic directions, while policymakers manage resource allocation and monitor policy targets and outcomes. They are responsible for planning and implementing HRH, managing the work environment and conditions, HRH information systems, workforce performance, and staff retention. Greater investments in strengthening health management capacity for mental health will be an important component in increasing HRMH. A systemic approach to capacity building is necessary to addressing human resources management with strong emphasis on country-led initiatives with multi-sectoral and multi-stakeholder collaborations (including community engagement), community-based services, evidence-based with appropriate monitoring and evaluation strategies.[127]

Need for More Research in HRMH and for More Skilled Researchers

Evidence for cost-effective and comprehensive community-based mental health care in LMICs is scarce. Only 10% of the world's health research addresses 90% of the global population living in LMICs, and furthermore, only 3%–6% of the mental health research in high-impact medical journals is from LMICs.[128,129] There is an urgent need for research to generate relevant scientific evidence to address HRMH.[129–133] Twenty-two priority areas for research in HRH were identified through stakeholder interviews from 25 LMICs, review of the literature, and an international workshop.[134] A similar exercise is needed to identify priority research areas for HRMH. Based on our review, examples of key areas to be addressed include:

- Adequacy and impact of mental health policies on HRMH;
- Adequacy and impact of HRH policies on mental health;
- Cost of non-specialist health workers (e.g., expansion of Scheffler et al. model to incorporate different mental health care providers in the wage bill);
- Development and validation of HRMH toolkits in different contexts, etc.;
- Evidence on the effectiveness of user/caregiver involvement in service delivery;
- Better understanding of push and pull factors for migration;
- Systematic evaluation of training programs.

Additional evidence is needed on the effectiveness and cost-effectiveness of task shifting in identification and management of mental disorders by NSHWs. Information and evidence is also needed on training requirements and application of newly acquired knowledge and skills in everyday practice. Evidence on the effectiveness of user/caregiver involvement in service delivery and better understanding of push and pull factors for migration of mental health specialists is also needed for effective HRMH planning.

Stronger inter-sectoral collaborations will also contribute to reducing the HRMH shortage and must be explored further.[135] We found only one study that examined the impact of trained schoolteachers for raising mental health awareness.[64] Teachers were effective in raising awareness about mental disorders among school children, parents, and neighbors. Evaluation studies on the role of community resources such as traditional or alternative care providers were not found in our review. This issue requires careful examination, given that, in many LMICs, alternative care is often sought before care from a mental health specialist or primary care practitioner.

A key challenge in increasing research evidence in many LMICs is the weak capacity to conduct high-quality research and to disseminate findings to knowledge-users effectively. Although this is not specific to mental health research, the general lack of recognition of mental health as a priority health research area contributes to the lack of support for capacity-building initiatives. The Global Forum for Health Research, in collaboration with the World Health Organization, carried out a project in 2004 to map research capacity in LMICs with the aim to raise awareness of the need for research capacity strengthening for mental health in LMICs.[136] Evaluation of research outputs from 114 LMICs found significantly skewed distributions. While 57% of countries contributed fewer than five articles to an international mental health indexed literature between 1993 and 2003, countries such as Argentina, Brazil, China, India, the Republic of Korea, and South Africa published significantly more articles. Over half of the respondents had not received formal training in epidemiology, public health, or basic sciences. Financial support for training is low, and access to literature and technical support to carry out research is also limited. The three leading challenges for mental health research reported by researchers were lack of funds, trained staff, and time. Lack of a research culture and lack of collaborators were also considered important challenges.

This mapping project highlights the gap in research capacity for mental health at individual, organization, and national levels. It provides the evidence base for the urgent need for research capacity strengthening initiatives that provide skills in epidemiological or public health research methods, knowledge translation and exchange, leadership, mentorship, and advocacy. Increasing such capacity at all levels will yield a greater impact and provide a stronger infrastructure to support mental health research. A global coordinated strategy for capacity building for research on and development in mental health services and policy is warranted.[137]

Despite the emerging evidence on mental health systems in LMICs, its application to develop and evaluate HRMH is a difficult and complex task that will continue to pose substantial challenges in the coming years. It requires a systemic approach with interdisciplinary and multi-sectoral collaborations and strong partnerships between ministries, researchers, NGOs, health professionals, service users/caregivers, and communities if significant long-term gains are to be made. Adequate attention to these aspects is essential to achieve the objective of scaling up care for people with mental disorders.

REFERENCES

1. World Health Organization. *The World Health Report 2006: Working together for health.* Geneva: World Health Organization; 2006.
2. Saxena S, Thornicroft G, Knapp M, Whiteford H. Resources for mental health: scarcity, inequity, and inefficiency. *Lancet.* 2007;370(9590):878–89.
3. World Health Organization. *Mental Health Atlas 2005.* Geneva: World Health Organization; 2005.
4. World Health Organization. *Atlas: Child and adolescent mental health resources. Global concerns: Implications for the future.* Geneva: World Health Organization; 2005.

5. World Health Organization. *Atlas: Psychiatric education and training across the world 2005.* Geneva: World Health Organization; 2005.

6. World Health Organization. *The World Health Report 2001: Mental health: New understanding, new hope.* Geneva: World Health Organization; 2001.

7. World Health Organization. *Atlas: Mental health resources in the world 2001.* Geneva: World Health Organization; 2001.

8. World Health Organization. *Mental Health Atlas 2011.* Geneva: World Health Organization; 2011.

9. World Health Organization. *Atlas: Country resources for neurological disorders 2004.* Geneva: World Health Organization; 2004.

10. World Health Organization. *Atlas: Nurses in mental health 2007.* Geneva: World Health Organization; 2007.

11. Scheffler RM, Bruckner TA, Fulton BD, Yoon J, Shen G, Chisholm D, et al. *Human resources for mental health: workforce shortages in low- and middle-income countries.* Geneva: World Health Organization; 2011.

12. Kakuma R, Minas H, van Ginneken N, Dal Poz MR, Desiraju K, Morris JE, et al. Human resources for mental health care: current situation and strategies for action. *Lancet.* 2011;378(9803):1654–63. Epub 10/20/2011.

13. World Health Organization. *Mental Health Policy and Service Guidance Package—Module 11: Human resources and training in mental health.* Geneva: World Health Organization; 2005.

14. World Health Organization, World Organization of Family Doctors. *Integrating mental health into primary care.* Geneva: World Health Organization and World Organization of Family Doctors (WONCA); 2008.

15. World Health Organization. *mhGAP intervention guide for mental, neurological and substance use disorders in non-specialized health settings: mental health Gap Action Programme.* Geneva: World Health Organization; 2010.

16. Fulton BD, Scheffler RM, Sparkes SP, Auh EY, Vujicic M, Soucat A. Health workforce skill mix and task shifting in low income countries: a review of recent evidence. *Hum Resour Health.* 2011;9(1):1. Epub 01/13/2011.

17. Dal Poz MR, Quain EE, O'Neil M, McCaffery J, Elzinga G, Martineau T. Addressing the health workforce crisis: towards a common approach. *Hum Resour Health.* 2006;4:21. Epub 08/05/2006.

18. Riley PL, Zuber A, Vindigni SM, Gupta N, Verani A, Sunderland NL, et al. Information systems on human resources for health: a global review. *Hum Resour Health.* 2012;10(1):7. Epub 05/02/2012.

19. World Health Organization. A65/10—Global burden of mental disorders and the need for a comprehensive, coordinated response from health and social sectors at the country level. 2012.

20. Sixty-Fifth World Health Assembly. *A65/10 Global burden of mental disorders and the need for a comprehensive, coordinated response from health and social sectors at the country level.* Report by the Secretariat. Geneva: World Health Organization. 2012.

21. World Health Organization. *Zero Draft: Global Mental Health Action Plan 2013–2010 (version dated August 27, 2012).* Geneva: World Health Organization, 2012.

22. Nuyens Y. *No development without research: A challenge for research capacity strengthening:* Geneva: Global Forum for Health Research; 2005.

23. Hanney SR, Gonzalez Block MA. Building health research systems to achieve better health. *Health Res Policy Syst.* 2006;4:10.

24. Hanney SR, Gonzalez-Block MA, Buxton MJ, Kogan M. The utilisation of health research in policy-making: concepts, examples and methods of assessment. *Health Res Policy & Syst/ BioMed Central.* 2003;1(1):2.

25. Lund C, Stein DJ, Corrigall J, Bradshaw D, Schneider M, Flisher AJ. Mental health is integral to public health: a call to scale up evidence-based services and develop mental health research. *S Afr Med J.* 2008;98(6):444, 6.

26. Tomlinson M, Rudan I, Saxena S, Swartz L, Tsai A, Patel V. Setting investment priorities for research in global mental health. *Bull WHO.* 2009;87(6):438–46.

27. Sharan P, Gallo C, Gureje O, Lamberte E, Mari JJ, Mazzotti G, et al. Mental health research priorities in low- and middle-income countries of Africa, Asia, Latin America and the Caribbean. *Br J Psychiatry.* 2009;195(4):354–63.

28. Patel V. The future of psychiatry in low- and middle-income countries. *Psychol Med.* 2009;39(11):1759.

29. Srinivasa Murthy R, Kishore Kumar KV, Chisholm D, Thomas T, Sekar K, Chandrashekar CR. Community outreach for untreated schizophrenia in rural India: a follow-up study of symptoms, disability, family burden and costs. *Psychol Med.* 2005;35(3):341–51.

30. Araya R, Rojas G, Fritsch R, Gaete J, Rojas M, Simon G, et al. Treating depression in primary care in low-income women in Santiago, Chile: a randomised controlled trial. *Lancet.* 2003;361(9362):995–1000.

31. Gutierrez-Maldonado J, Caqueo-Urizar A. Effectiveness of a psycho-educational intervention for reducing burden in Latin American families of patients with schizophrenia. *Qual Life Res.* 2007;16(5):739–47. Epub 02/09/2007.

32. Gutierrez-Maldonado J, Caqueo-Urizar A, Ferrer-Garcia M. Effects of a psychoeducational intervention program on the attitudes and health perceptions of relatives of patients with schizophrenia. *Soc Psychiatry & Psychiatr Epidemiol.* 2009;44(5):343–8. Epub 11/05/2008.

33. Rojas G, Fritsch R, Solis J, Jadresic E, Castillo C, González M, et al. Treatment of postnatal depression in low-income mothers in primary-care clinics in Santiago, Chile: a randomised controlled trial. *Lancet.* 2007;370(9599):1629–37.

34. Ran MS, Xiang MZ, Chan CL, Leff J, Simpson P, Huang MS, et al. Effectiveness of psychoeducational intervention for rural Chinese families experiencing schizophrenia—a randomised controlled trial. *Soc Psychiatry & Psychiatr Epidemiol.* 2003;38(2):69–75. Epub 02/04/2003.

35. Chatterjee S, Pillai A, Jain S, Cohen A, Patel V. Outcomes of people with psychotic disorders in a community-based rehabilitation programme in rural India. *Br J Psychiatry.* 2009;195(5):-433–9. Epub 11/03/2009.

36. Dias A, Dewey ME, D'Souza J, Dhume R, Motghare DD, Shaji KS, et al. The effectiveness of a home care program for supporting caregivers of persons with dementia in developing countries: a randomised controlled trial from Goa, India. *PloS One.* 2008;3(6):e2333. Epub 06/05/2008.

37. Patel V, Weiss HA, Chowdhary N, Naik S, Pednekar S, Chatterjee S, et al. Effectiveness of an intervention led by lay health counsellors for depressive and anxiety disorders in primary care in Goa, India (MANAS): a cluster randomised controlled trial. *Lancet.* 2010;376(9758):2086–95. Epub 12/17/2010.

38. Bolton P, Bass J, Neugebauer R, Verdeli H, Clougherty KF, Wickramaratne P, et al. Group interpersonal psychotherapy for depression in rural Uganda: a randomized controlled trial. *JAMA.* 2003;289(23):3117–24.

39. Rahman A, Malik A, Sikander S, Roberts C, Creed F. Cognitive behaviour therapy-based intervention by community health workers for mothers with depression and their infants in rural Pakistan: a cluster-randomised controlled trial. *Lancet.* 2008;372(9642):902–9.

40. Xiang M, Ran M, Li S. A controlled evaluation of psychoeducational family intervention in a rural Chinese community. *Br J Psychiatry.* 1994;165(4):544–8.

41. Chatterjee S, Patel V, Chatterjee A, Weiss HA. Evaluation of a community-based rehabilitation model for chronic schizophrenia in rural India. *Br J Psychiatry.* 2003;182:57–62.

42. Patel VH, Kirkwood BR, Pednekar S, Araya R, King M, Chisholm D, et al. Improving the outcomes of primary care attenders with common mental disorders in developing countries: a cluster randomized controlled trial of a collaborative stepped care intervention in Goa, India. *Trials.* 2008;9:4. Epub 01/29/2008.

43. Murthy RS. *Integration of mental health with primary health care—Indian experience.* Bangalore: National Institute of Mental Health and Neurosciences, 1987.

44. Tripathy P, Nair N, Barnett S, Mahapatra R, Borghi J, Rath S, et al. Effect of a participatory intervention with women's groups on birth outcomes and maternal depression in Jharkhand and Orissa, India: a cluster-randomised controlled trial. *Lancet.* 2010;375:1182–92.

45. Jacob KS, Senthil Kumar P, Gayathri K, Abraham S, Prince MJ. Can health workers diagnose dementia in the community? *Acta Psychiatr Scand.* 2007;116(2):125–8. Epub 07/26/2007.

46. Simpson EL, House AO. Involving users in the delivery and evaluation of mental health services: systematic review. *BMJ.* 2002;325(7375):1265. Epub 11/30/2002.

47. Simpson EL, House AO. User and carer involvement in mental health services: from rhetoric to science. *Br J Psychiatry.* 2003;183:89–91.

48. Goodwin V, Happell B. Consumer and carer participation in mental health care: the carer's perspective: part 1—the importance of respect and collaboration. *Issues Ment Health Nurs.* 2007;28(6):607–23.

49. Goodwin V, Happell B. Consumer and carer participation in mental health care: the carer's perspective: part 2—barriers to effective and genuine participation. *Issues Ment Health Nurs.* 2007;28(6):625–38.

50. Ghanizadeh A, Shahrivar FZ. The effect of parent management training on children with attention deficit hyperactivity disorder. *J Child & Adolesc Ment Health.* 2005;17(1):31–4.

51. Gavrilova SI, Ferri CP, Mikhaylova N, Sokolova O, Banerjee S, Prince M. Helping carers to care—the 10/66 dementia research group's randomized control trial of a caregiver intervention in Russia. *Int J Geriatr Psychiatry.* 2009;24(4):347–54. Epub 09/25/2008.

52. Assadollahi GA, Ghassemi GR, Mehrabi T. Training families to better manage schizophrenics' behaviour. *East Mediterr Health J.* 2000;6(1):118–27.

53. Javadpour A, Ahmadzadeh L, Bahredar MJ. An educative support group for female family caregivers: impact on caregivers psychological distress and patient's neuropsychiatry symptoms. *Int J Geriatr Psychiatry.* 2009;24(5):469–71. Epub 10/22/2008.

54. Kulhara P, Chakrabarti S, Avasthi A, Sharma A, Sharma S. Psychoeducational intervention for caregivers of Indian patients with schizophrenia: a randomised-controlled trial. *Acta Psychiatr Scand.* 2009;119(6):472–83. Epub 11/27/2008.

55. Saraceno B, van Ommeren M, Batniji R, Cohen A, Gureje O, Mahoney J, et al. Barriers to improvement of mental health services in low-income and middle-income countries. *Lancet.* 2007;370(9593):1164–74.

56. Kleintjes S, Lund C, Swartz L. Organising for self-advocacy in mental health: experiences from 6 African countries (Submitted, *Transcultural Psychiatry*). 2011.

57. de Sevigny D, Adam T. *Systems thinking for health system strengthening*: Geneva: World Health Organization, Alliance for Health Policy and Systems Research; 2009.

58. World Health Organization. *Integrating mental health into primary care: A global perspective.* Geneva: World Health Organization and World Organization of Family Doctors (WONCA); 2008.

59. World Health Organization. *Improving health systems and services for mental health.* Geneva: World Health Organization; 2009.

60. Eaton J, McCay L, Semrau M, Chatterjee S, Baingana F, Araya R, et al. Scale up of services for mental health in low-income and middle-income countries. *Lancet.* 2011;378(9802):1592–603. Epub 2011/10/20.

61. Mangham LJ, Hanson K. Scaling up in international health: what are the key issues? *Health Policy Plan.* 2010;25(2):85–96. Epub 2010/01/15.

62. Simmons R, Fajans P, Ghiron L, editors. *Scaling up health service delivery from pilot innovations to policies and programmes.* Geneva: World Health Organization & ExpandNet; 2007.

63. Caldas de Almeida JM, Minas H. Generating political commitment for mental health system development. In: Patel V, Prince M, Cohen A, Minas H, editors. *Global mental health: Principles and practice*: Oxford University Press.

64. Minas H, Mahoney J, Kakuma R. Health for the South Community Mental Health Project: evaluation report. Prepared for World Vision Australia. 2011.

65. Singh B, Ng CH. Psychiatric education and training in Asia. *Int Rev Psychiatry.* 2008;20(5):413–8. Epub 2008/11/18.

66. Savin D. Developing psychiatric training and services in Cambodia. *Psychiatr Serv.* 2000;51(7):935.

67. Das M, Gupta N, Dutta K. Psychiatric training in India. *Psychiatr Bull.* 2002;26:70–2.

68. Gao X, Jackson T, Chen H, Liu Y, Wang R, Qian M, et al. There is a long way to go: a nationwide survey of professional training for mental health practitioners in China. *Health Policy.* 2010;95(1):74–81. Epub 2009/12/08.

69. Patel V, Cohen A. Mental health services in primary care in "developing" countries. *World Psychiatry.* 2003;2(3):163–4.

70. Al-Faris E, Al-Subaie A, Khoja T, Al-Ansary L, Abdul-Raheem F, Al-Hamdan N, et al. Training primary health care physicians in Saudi Arabia to recognize psychiatric illness. *Acta Psychiatr Scand.* 1997;96(6):439–44. Epub 1998/01/08.

71. Ballester DA, Filippon AP, Braga C, Andreoli SB. The general practitioner and mental health problems: challenges and strategies for medical education. *Sao Paulo Med J.* 2005;123(2):72–6.

72. Budosan B, Jones L. Evaluation of effectiveness of mental health training program for primary health care staff in Hambantota District, Sri Lanka post-tsunami. *J Humanitarian Assistance.* 2009. Available at http://sites.tufts.edu/jha/archives/509

73. Chinnayya HP, Chandrashekar CR, Moily S, Puttamma test, Raghuram A, Subramanya KR, et al. Training primary care health workers in mental health care: evaluation of attitudes towards mental illness before and after training. *Int J Soc Psychiatry*. 1990;36(4):300–7.

74. Duran-Gonzalez LI, Hernandez-Rincon M, Becerra-Aponte J. [Education of psychologists and their role in primary health care]. *Salud Publica de Mexico*. 1995;37(5):462–71.

75. Engin E, Cam O. Effect of self-awareness education on the self-efficacy and sociotropy-autonomy characteristics of nurses in a psychiatry clinic. *Arch Psychiatr Nurs*. 2009;23(2):148–56. Epub 03/31/2009.

76. Mohit A, Saeed K, Shahmohammadi D, Bolhari J, Bina M, Gater R, et al. Mental health manpower development in Afghanistan: a report on a training course for primary health care physicians. *East Mediterr Health J*. 1999;5(2):373–7. Epub 05/04/2000.

77. Ndetei DM, Khasakhala L, Ongecha-Owuor F, Kuria M, Mutiso V, Syanda J, et al. Attitudes toward psychiatry: a survey of medical students at the University of Nairobi, Kenya. *Acad Psychiatry*. 2008;32(2):154–9.

78. Park YS, Kim KS, Song KJ, Kang J. [A preliminary survey of nurses' understanding of delirium and their need for delirium education—in a university hospital]. *Taehan Kanho Hakhoe Chi*. 2006;36(7):1183–92.

79. Shukla GD. Undergraduate education in mental health in UP and MP: a need for redemption. *J Indian Med Assoc*. 1996;94(2):62–3, 5.

80. Sidorov PI, Solov'ev AG, Tevlina VV. [Factors of social workers' training in a medical school for work in psychiatric and substance abuse rehabilitation clinics]. *Zhurnal nevrologii i psikhiatrii imeni SS Korsakova / Ministerstvo zdravookhraneniia i meditsinskoi promyshlennosti Rossiiskoi Federatsii, Vserossiiskoe obshchestvo nevrologov [i] Vserossiiskoe obshchestvo psikhiat*. 1999;99(5):41–3.

81. Uçok A, Soygür H, Atakli C, Kuşcu K, Sartorius N, Duman ZC, et al. The impact of anti-stigma education on the attitudes of general practitioners regarding schizophrenia. *Psychiatry & Clin Neurosci*. 2006;60(4):439–43.

82. World Health Organization. *Who are health managers? Case studies from three African countries*. Geneva: World Health Organization; 2009.

83. Adewuya AO, Oguntade AA. Doctors' attitude towards people with mental illness in Western Nigeria. *Soc Psychiatry & Psychiatr Epidemiol*. 2007;42(11):931–6. Epub 08/28/2007.

84. Minas H, Zamzam R, Midin M, Cohen A. Attitudes of Malaysian general hospital staff towards patients with mental illness and diabetes. *BMC Public Health*. 2011;11:317. Epub 05/17/2011.

85. Farooq S, Akhter J, Anwar E, Hussain I, Khan SA. The attitude and perception of hospital doctors about the management of psychiatric disorders. *J Coll Phys Surg Pak*. 2005;15(9):552–5.

86. Doku V, Ofori-Atta A, Akpalu B, Osei A, Ae-Ngibise K, Read U, et al. *Country report of mental health policy development and implementation in Ghana*. Accra: Mental Health and Poverty Project: 2008.

87. Kigozi F, Ssebunnya J, Kizza D, Green A, Omar M, Bird P, et al. *Phase 1 Country Report: A situation analysis of the menal health system in Uganda*. Kampala: Mental Health and Poverty Project. 2008.

88. Lund C, Kleintjies S, Campbell-Hall V, Mjadu S, Petersen I, Bhana A, et al. *Mental health policy development and implementation in South Africa: a situation analysis. Phase 1. Country report*. Cape Town: Mental Health and Poverty Project. 2008.

89. Mwanza J, Sikwese A, ayeya J, Lund C, Bird P, Drew N, et al. *Phase 1 Country Report: Mental health policy development and implementation in Zambia: a situation analysis*. Lusaka: Mental Health and Poverty Project. 2008.

90. Budosan B. Mental health training of primary health care workers: case reports from Sri Lanka, Pakistan and Jordan. *Intervention*. 2011;9(2):125–36.

91. Henderson DC, Mollica RF, Tor S, Lavelle J, Culhane MA, Hayden D. Building primary care practitioners' attitudes and confidence in mental health skills in a post-conflict society: a Cambodian example. *J Nerv Ment Dis*. 2005;193(8):551–9. Epub 08/06/2005.

92. Ganatra HA, Bhurgri H, Channa R, Bawany FA, Zafar SN, Chaudhry RI, et al. Educating and informing patients receiving psychopharmacological medications: are family physicians in Pakistan up to the task? *PloS One*. 2009;4(2):e4620. Epub 02/28/2009.

93. Reddy JP, Tan SM, Azmi MT, Shaharom MH, Rosdinom R, Maniam T, et al. The effect of a clinical posting in psychiatry on the attitudes of medical students towards psychiatry and mental illness in a Malaysian medical school. *Ann Acad Med Singapore*. 2005;34(8):505–10. Epub 10/06/2005.

94. Awofeso N. Improving health workforce recruitment and retention in rural and remote regions of Nigeria. *Rural & Remote Health.* 2010;10(1):1319.

95. Kanchanachitra C, Lindelow M, Johnston T, Hanvoravongchai P, Lorenzo FM, Huong NL, et al. Human resources for health in southeast Asia: shortages, distributional challenges, and international trade in health services. *Lancet.* 2011;377(9767):769–81. Epub 01/29/2011.

96. Sherr K, Mussa A, Chilundo B, Gimbel S, Pfeiffer J, Hagopian A, et al. Brain drain and health workforce distortions in Mozambique. *PloS One.* 2012;7(4):e35840. Epub 05/05/2012.

97. Kirigia JM, Gbary AR, Muthuri LK, Nyoni J, Seddoh A. The cost of health professionals' brain drain in Kenya. *BMC Health Serv Res.* 2006;6:89. Epub 07/19/2006.

98. Ferrinho P, Siziya S, Goma F, Dussault G. The human resource for health situation in Zambia: deficit and maldistribution. *Hum Resour Health.* 2011;9(1):30. Epub 12/21/2011.

99. Jenkins R, Kydd R, Mullen P, Thomson K, Sculley J, Kuper S, et al. International migration of doctors, and its impact on availability of psychiatrists in low and middle income countries. *PloS One.* 2010;5(2):e9049. Epub 02/09/2010.

100. Awenva AD, Read UM, Ofori-Atta AL, Doku VCK, Akpalu B, Osei AO, et al. From mental health policy development in Ghana to implementation: what are the barriers? *Afr J Psychiatry.* 2010;13:184–91.

101. Araya M, Mussie M, Jacobson L. Decentralized psychiatric nursing service in Ethiopia—a model for low income countries. *Ethiop Med J.* 2009;47(1):61–4.

102. Gureje O, Hollins S, Botbol M, Javed A, Jorge M, Okech V, et al. Report of the WPA task force on brain drain. *World Psychiatry.* 2009;8(2):115–8.

103. Huicho L, Canseco FD, Lema C, Miranda JJ, Lescano AG. [Incentives to attract and retain the health workforce in rural areas of Peru: a qualitative study][Spanish]. *Cadernos de Saude Publica [Reports in Public Health].* 2012;28(4):729–39. Epub 04/11/2012..

104. Mullan F. The metrics of the physician brain drain. *N Engl J Med.* 2005;353(17):1810–8.

105. Hauff E. The Cambodian Mental Health Training Programme. *Australas Psychiatry.* 1996;4:187–8.

106. Alem A, Pain C, Araya M, Hodges BD. Co-creating a psychiatric resident program with Ethiopians, for Ethiopians, in Ethiopia: the Toronto Addis Ababa Psychiatry Project (TAAPP). *Acad Psychiatry.* 2010;34(6):424–32.

107. Toronto Addis Ababa Academic Collaboration. 2011 (http://www.taaac.com), (accessed 10 Nov 2012).

108. Ndetei DM, Pizzo M, Maru H, Ongecha F, Khasakhala LI, Mutiso V, et al. Burnout in staff working at the Mathari psychiatric hospital. *Afr J Psychiatry.* 2008;11(3):199–203.

109. Reboucas D, Abelha L, Legay LF, Lovisi GM. [Work in mental health: a job satisfaction and work impact study]. *Cadernos de Saude Publica.* 2008;24(3):624–32.

110. Saxena S, Sharan P, Saraceno B. Budget and financing of mental health services: baseline information on 89 countries from WHO's Project Atlas. *J Ment Health Policy & Econ.* 2003;6(3):135–43.

111. Chisholm D, Lund C, Saxena S. Cost of scaling up mental healthcare in low- and middle-income countries. *Br J Psychiatry.* 2007;191:528–35. Epub 12/07/2007.

112. Lund C, Boyce G, Flisher AJ, Kafaar Z, Dawes A. Scaling up child and adolescent mental health services in South Africa: human resource requirements and costs. *J Child Psychol Psychiatry.* 2009;50(9):1121–30. Epub 02/27/2009.

113. Chisholm D. Mental health system financing in developing countries: policy questions and research responses. *Epidemiol Psychiatr Soc.* 2007;16(4):282–8.

114. Lee CI, Smith LS, Shwe Oo EK, Scharschmidt BC, Whichard E, Kler T, et al. Internally displaced human resources for health: villager-health worker partnerships to scale up a malaria control programme in active conflict areas of eastern Burma. *Glob Public Health.* 2009;4(3):229–41.

115. Syed Sheriff RJ, Baraco AF, Nour A, Warsame AM, Peachey K, Haibe F, et al. Public-academic partnerships: Improving human resource provision for mental health in Somaliland. *Psychiatric Serv.* 2010;61(3):225–7.

116. Lancet Global Mental Health Group. Scale up services for mental disorders: a call for action. *Lancet.* 2007;370(9594):1241–52.

117. Minas H. Vietnam. *Australas Psychiatry.* 1994;2(6):280–4.

118. Hung P, Minas I, Liu Y, Dahlgren G, Hsiao W, Duong H, et al., editors. *Cham Soc Suc Khoe Nhan Dan Theo Dinh Huong Cong Bang Va Hieu Qua [Efficient, equity-oriented strategies*

for health: international perspectives, focus on Vietnam]. Hanoi: Hanoi Medical Publishing Company; 2001.

119. Minas H. *Technical assistance to restructure system of Centres for care of mental health patients run by MOLISA: Report to WHO Vietnam*. Melbourne: Centre for International Mental Health, 2009.

120. Lund C, Tomlinson M, De Silva M, Fekadu A, Shidhaye R, Jordans M, et al. PRIME: a programme to reduce the treatment gap for mental disorders in five low- and middle-income countries. *PLoS Med.* 2012;9(12):e1001359. Epub 01/10/2013.

121. Federal Democratic Republic of Ethiopia Ministry of Health. National Mental Health Strategy 2012/13—2015/16. Addis Ababa, Federal Democratic Republic of Ethiopia Ministry of Health. 2012.

122. Minas H. Leadership for change in complex systems. *Australas Psychiatry.* 2005;13(1):33–9. Epub 03/22/2005.

123. Schiffbauer J, O'Brien JB, Timmons BK, Kiarie WN. The role of leadership in HRH development in challenging public health settings. *Hum Resour Health.* 2008;6:23. Epub 11/06/2008.

124. Seims LR, Alegre JC, Murei L, Bragar J, Thatte N, Kibunga P, et al. Strengthening management and leadership practices to increase health-service delivery in Kenya: an evidence-based approach. *Hum Resour Health.* 2012;10(1):25. Epub 08/31/2012.

125. Sherk KE, Nauseda F, Johnson S, Liston D. An experience of virtual leadership development for human resource managers. *Hum Resour Health.* 2009;7:1. Epub 01/10/2009.

126. Beinecke RH, Minas H, Goldsack S, Peters J. Global mental health leadership training programmes. *Int J Leadersh Public Serv.* 2010;6(supplement):63–72.

127. Potter C, Brough R. Systemic capacity building: a hierarchy of needs. *Health Policy Plan.* 2004;19(5):336–45.

128. Saxena S, Paraje G, Sharan P, Karam G, Sadana R. The 10/90 divide in mental health research: trends over a 10-year period. *Br J Psychiatry.* 2006;188:81–2.

129. Patel V, Sumathipala A. International representation in psychiatric literature: survey of six leading journals. *Br J Psychiatry.* 2001;178:406–9.

130. White J, Patel V, Herrman H. Mental health research in low and middle-income countries: role of research institutions. *ANZ J Psychiatry.* 2005;39(3):202.

131. de Jesus MJ, Patel V, Kieling C, Anders M, Jakovljevi M, Lam LC, et al. The 5/95 Gap on the dissemination of mental health research: The World Psychiatric Association (WPA) task force report on project with editors of low and middle income (LAMI) countries. *Afr J Psychiatry.* 2009;12(1):33–9.

132. Patel V. Closing the 10/90 divide in global mental health research. *Acta Psychiatr Scand.* 2007;115(4):257–9. Epub 03/16/2007.

133. Sumathipala A, Siribaddana S, Patel V. Under-representation of developing countries in the research literature: ethical issues arising from a survey of five leading medical journals. *BMC Med Ethics.* 2004;5:E5. Epub 10/06/2004.

134. Ranson MK, Chopra M, Atkins S, Dal Poz MR, Bennett S. Priorities for research into human resources for health in low- and middle-income countries. *Bull WHO.* 2010;88(6):435–43. Epub 06/12/2010.

135. Skeen S, Kleintjes S, Lund C, Petersen I, Bhana A, Flisher AJ, et al. "Mental health is everybody's business": roles for an intersectoral approach in South Africa. *Int Rev Psychiatry.* 2010;22(6):611–23. Epub 01/14/2011.

136. Sharan P, Levav I, Olifson S, de Francisco A, Saxena S, editors. *Research capacity for mental health in low- and middle-income countries: Results of a mapping project*. Geneva: World Health Organization & Global Forum for Health Research; 2007.

137. Collins PY, Tomlinson M, Awuba J, Kakuma R, Minas H. Research priorities, capacity and networks in global mental health. In: Patel V, Prince M, Cohen A, Minas H, editors. *Global mental health: Principles and practice*: Oxford University Press.

11 Mental Health Promotion and the Prevention of Mental Disorders

Inge Petersen, Margaret Barry,
Crick Lund, and Arvin Bhana

INTRODUCTION

Scaling up treatment efforts is imperative to reduce the substantial global burden of mental disorders (see Chapter 6). However, scaling up treatment cannot substantively reduce the prevalence of mental disorders, for two major reasons. Firstly, there are limitations to existing treatment methods. Using epidemiological data on depression from Australia, Andrews and colleagues[1] calculated that current psychological and pharmacological treatment methods are unable to halve the burden of depression, even with maximum coverage, clinician competence, and patient compliance. Secondly, the increasing burden posed by mental disorders, notably depression[2] (see Chapter 6), raises concern about the sustainability of the escalating cost of treating mental illness.[3] The prevention of mental disorders is thus important to reducing the burden of mental disorders and containing the escalating cost of treatment. In addition, there is a moral imperative to promote mental health and well-being of populations. Acknowledgement of this need is reflected in a number of key international publications, which advocate a comprehensive public health approach to improving mental health at a population level.[4–8]

DEFINITION OF MENTAL HEALTH, MENTAL HEALTH PROMOTION, AND PREVENTION OF MENTAL DISORDERS

Mental health is fundamental to good health and contributes to the functioning of individuals, families, communities, and society. It is more than the absence of mental illness. The World Health Organization (WHO) describes it as "a state of well-being in which the individual realizes his or her own abilities, can cope with the normal stresses of life, can work productively and fruitfully, and is able to make a contribution to his or her community."[4] Positive mental health is a multidimensional concept, encompassing a subjective sense of one's own self-worth and the worth of others; affective balance; and the capacity to think, perceive, and interpret adequately, as well as to cope in the face of normal adversities. Positive mental health is thus a resource for living, contributing to the effective functioning of individuals, families, communities, and societies.[9] Other definitions also include a spiritual dimension. For example, in African and Aboriginal societies, personal well-being is explicitly connected with the spiritual world.[10] In addition, in these societies, a person's well-being is also connected to the well-being of his or her community. This resonates with materialist or critical perspectives that embed well-being in the social, economic, and cultural life of the individual and community.

Mental health promotion is concerned with promoting positive mental health, and employs strategies for strengthening protective factors to enhance the social and emotional well-being and quality of life of the general population. It brings a shift from the clinical and treatment focus of current mental health service delivery to the promotion of protective and competence enhancing factors that keep individuals and populations mentally healthy. Within the mental health promotion framework, recognition of the broader social determinants of mental health has led to a growing emphasis on policy interventions to remove the structural barriers to mental health through initiatives to reduce poverty, discrimination, and inequalities as well as programmatic interventions to strengthen the mental health of individuals, groups, and communities.[9,11]

Prevention of mental disorders, on the other hand, is specifically concerned with reducing the incidence, prevalence, duration, and recurrence of mental disorders.[8] Adopting Caplan's [12] public health approach to preventive psychiatry, mental disorder prevention occurs at three levels; namely, primary, secondary, and tertiary. *Primary prevention* aims to reduce the onset of mental ill-health, thus reducing the incidence of mental disorders. Secondary and tertiary prevention do not reduce the incidence of mental disorders, but seek to lower the prevalence of established cases. *Secondary prevention* is concerned with early detection and treatment of a mental disorder, and *tertiary prevention* aims to reduce relapse and disability as well as enhance rehabilitation, reduce morbidity, and support recovery.

Primary prevention interventions can be universal, selective, or indicated. *Universal* interventions target a whole population; *selective* interventions target individuals or groups whose risk of developing a mental disorder is elevated as a result of biological, social, or psychological risk factors; and *indicated* prevention programs target individuals having symptoms of mental disorders, which do not meet the criteria for diagnosis of a mental disorder. It has been suggested that indicated prevention is actually early intervention, as symptoms could be part of the prodromal phase of a disorder. Nevertheless, the importance of indicated prevention is underscored by the finding that the longer the duration of a disorder, the more difficult it is to treat.[13] Thus, even if it is considered early intervention, indicated prevention is likely to lead to better outcomes.

Mental health promotion thus focuses on positive mental health, and its main aim is the building of psychosocial strengths, competencies, and access to resources. Prevention of mental disorders is concerned with reducing the risk for mental disorders. The scope of this chapter is limited to *mental health promotion* and *primary prevention* of mental disorders, given the overlap that primary prevention has with mental health promotion, as well as the overlap that secondary and tertiary prevention have with treatment and ameliorative care (see Chapter 16). Mental health promotion and primary prevention of mental disorders (hereafter referred to as mental health promotion and prevention) use similar strategies, reducing risk and strengthening protective factors that have the dual outcomes of promoting mental health and reducing risk for a range of mental disorders. The two concepts are interrelated. Promoting mental health may reduce the incidence of mental disorders, as positive mental health is protective against mental disorders; and interventions to prevent the onset of mental disorders can promote mental health. Both concepts may be present in the same intervention and use similar strategies, but they have different and complementary outcomes.[8]

MENTAL HEALTH PROMOTION AND PREVENTION OF MENTAL DISORDERS: A PUBLIC HEALTH AND SOCIOECONOMIC DEVELOPMENT PRIORITY

As discussed in Chapter 8, mental health is inextricably linked to the UN Millennium Development Goals (MDGs), with the social determinants of mental disorders now well established.[14] From our current knowledge, it is reasonable to expect that the achievement of the MDGs will, thus, contribute to promoting the mental health and well-being of the poorest people across the globe. Multifaceted, comprehensive policies and intersectoral actions are required, both globally and at a country level (see Chapter 8). Global solutions to climate change and addressing global shortages of food, energy, land, and water, which disproportionately impact poor people and poor countries, are vital to this project.[15] Furthermore, mental well-being also demands the removal of oppressive regimes in order to promote equality and democratic participation and to ensure that people worldwide have the independence, capacity, and freedom to pursue a life that they view as good and is coterminous with their social and cultural identities.[15]

On the other hand, mental health promotion and prevention interventions can also contribute to the achievement of the MDGs. The social determinants of poor mental health diminish people's likelihood of reaching their potential, reducing the human capabilities or human capital available for socioeconomic development across the globe. Individual and proximal mental health promotion and prevention interventions can support the realization of people's potential, promoting positive mental health outcomes in contexts that increase vulnerability to poor mental health outcomes described in Chapter 7. This can ultimately contribute to human capital development and the achievement of a number of MDGs. For example, mental health promotion interventions to improve maternal responsiveness can contribute to the achievement of the MDGs that relate to maternal and child health. Poor maternal responsiveness, which is associated with maternal depression, impacts negatively on a range of child outcomes, including stunting, poor socio-emotional development, and cognitive deficits.[16] Interventions to improve maternal responsiveness can promote better child health outcomes, breaking the intergenerational cycle of poverty and poor mental health, and ultimately contributing to socioeconomic development in vulnerable populations (see section on prenatal development and infancy in this chapter).

CONCEPTUAL MODELS FOR MENTAL HEALTH PROMOTION AND THE PRIMARY PREVENTION OF MENTAL DISORDERS

The Ottawa Charter[17] views mental health as being embedded in, and influenced by, a wider social, economic, and cultural ecology. This charter emerged from the first International Conference on Health Promotion, held in Ottawa in 1986, and mapped out public health actions to achieve health for all by 2000 and beyond. The inextricable link between people and their environments was thus acknowledged, with mental health being embedded within this wider ecology and influenced by the interplay of multiple "risk" and "protective" factors. These include biological and genetic factors, interpersonal factors, and environmental factors, as well as wider political, economic, social, and cultural factors.

The impact of these risk and protective factors on mental health and development varies across the lifespan and is dependent on developmental vulnerabilities and challenges associated with different developmental phases. There is an emerging body of evidence from developmental neuroscience, as well as epidemiological and life-course development studies, that highlights specific opportunities for strengthening protective factors and reducing risk factors at critical developmental stages when the effect of such interventions are likely to be most beneficial.

Bronfenbrenner[18] provides an ecological systems theory that understands human development to be shaped by a series of nested interactive systems, with the individual existing within layers of social relationships, from immediate to more remote, which vary in their impact depending on developmental vulnerabilities across the lifespan. "Immediate" systems encompass a person's microsystems where a person's immediate experience and personal interactions occur; for example, family and peer relationships. "Mesosystems" refer to a person's accumulated microsystems, with Bronfenbrenner[18] suggesting that development will be enhanced if there is synergy in the value systems of different microsystems. It follows that mental health promotion and prevention interventions within these proximal systems strive to strengthen health-enhancing microsystems; for example, parent–child microsystems.

The "exosystem" refers to community-environmental contexts that influence the micro- and mesosystems, such as the school or neighborhood, which are influenced by organizations such as community development boards or school governing bodies and which do not necessarily involve the person directly. The "macrosystem" is more remote and refers to societal influences such as culture and structural influences. Examples include patriarchal culture that promotes gender inequities, and global and national socioeconomic policies that promote wealth inequalities. The macrosystem ultimately accounts for many of the social determinants of poor mental health described in (see Chapter 7), such as gender inequities and unemployment, which have an impact on the micro-, meso-, and exosystems and ultimately a person's mental health. It follows that mental health promotion and prevention interventions within the macrosystem would emphasize interventions to address the cultural and structural barriers to mental health through initiatives to reduce poverty, discrimination, and inequalities.

Amartya Sen's concept of *capability*,[19] which refers to a person's ability to achieve a given functioning of "doing" or "being" with a given set of commodities, was originally conceived as a framework for thinking about poverty and has also been used as a conceptual model for understanding inequality, human development, well-being, health, and disability. Applying Sen's concept of capability to mental health provides a complementary conceptual model to Bronfenbrenner's ecological developmental theory. It illuminates how developmentally appropriate capabilities are achieved across the lifespan with the necessary environmental support and highlights the interaction of innate personal factors with social factors in the development of capabilities across the lifespan. Nussbaum's extension of Sen's concept of capability[20] clearly distinguishes between *basic, internal,* and *combined* capabilities. *Basic capabilities* are the innate or genetic *potential* of an individual for optimal neurocognitive and socio-emotional development. During prenatal development and infancy, basic capabilities are transformed into *internal capabilities*, or *actual* optimal cognitive and socio-emotional development with support from the environment and life experiences. Recent evidence from developmental neuroscience provides empirical support for this, with developmental outcomes being determined by the interaction of multiple interacting genetic and environmental factors and experiences.[21] Given heightened neural plasticity during prenatal development and infancy, exposure to negative environmental factors and experiences can compromise the development of optimal cognitive and socio-emotional development during this early developmental phase.

During childhood and adolescence, although neural plasticity declines, malleable external conditions, such as adequate parenting and schooling, are necessary to facilitate the development of *combined* or *functional capabilities*, such as socio-emotional regulation and numeracy and literacy, which emerge when internal capabilities are combined with suitable external conditions. In scarce-resource contexts, inappropriate or inadequate parenting and poor schooling can compromise the development of these combined capabilities, trapping vulnerable children in a negative cycle of poor social-relatedness and self-regulation and low educational achievement, resulting in greater vulnerability to poor mental health and reduced wage-earning potential as adults. It should be noted, however, that vulnerabilities to negative health outcomes that emerge early in life do not necessarily have a linear trajectory. There are opportunities later on in childhood, adolescence, and adulthood for health-promoting interventions that can lead to the amelioration of earlier vulnerabilities towards healthy outcomes.[22]

A PRACTICE FRAMEWORK FOR MENTAL HEALTH PROMOTION AND PREVENTION

In the process of engaging in mental health promotion and prevention efforts, a *competency enhancement* approach is central. The competency enhancement model focuses on the process of enabling and achieving positive mental health and enhancing the well-being of individuals, communities, and society through an empowering, participative, and collaborative process, which enables people to increase control over their mental health and its determinants.[23] In keeping with the fundamental principles of health promotion as articulated in the Ottawa Charter,[17] adopting a competency enhancement approach to mental health promotion includes strategies for strengthening individuals, relationships, and communities together with "upstream" policy interventions across multiple sectors in order to reduce structural barriers to mental health.

With regard to the actual activities of mental health promotion and prevention practice, in keeping with the fundamental principles of health promotion as articulated in the Ottawa Charter[17] as well as Bronfenbrenner's and Sen's conceptual models described previously, both of which acknowledge the inextricable link between people and their environments, a socio-ecological perspective (depicted in Figure 11.1) provides a conceptual framework for practice. This framework embraces a systems approach to mental health promotion, spanning individual, social, and environmental factors, and underlines the importance of multisectoral involvement and synergistic action from the micro to the macro level, to bringing about tangible and enduring change.[11,24] The importance of enhancing resourcefulness and life skills, developing supportive environments, reorienting existing services, and advocating for the development of healthy public policy designed to promote and protect positive mental health at a population level is underscored.

A version of the socio-ecological perspective is presented in Figure 11.1 and distinguishes between three broad nested and interactive levels of risk and protective factors. These levels encompass: *intrapersonal* factors, such as genetic makeup, physical health, cognitions, emotions, skills, and behavior; *proximal* factors, referring to interpersonal and immediate factors related to family, peer, school, and community; and *distal* factors, which refer to macro structural factors, both at country level and globally, such as cultural influences and socioeconomic and environmental policies. This framework can be applied to understanding risk and protective factors across the lifespan.

At a *distal level*, the development of health enabling public policies is important in order to address the negative impact of wider structural factors on mental health, such as poverty, poor education, gender inequity, unemployment, and income inequality. These actions are, however, not unique to mental health promotion and primary prevention,

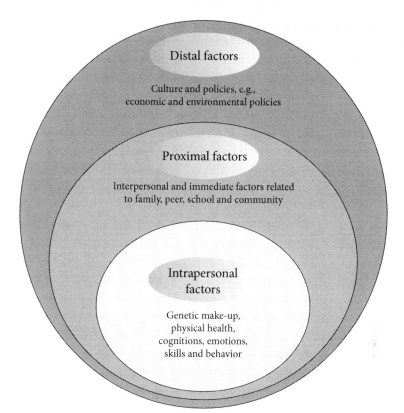

FIGURE 11.1
Socio-ecological framework.

and they overlap with many other initiatives, such as the MDGs, aimed at promoting human and socioeconomic development at country level and globally (see Chapter 8).

Interventions at the *intrapersonal* and *proximal levels* aim to build resilience through strengthening protective factors to moderate or mediate the impact of risk factors. Moderation and mediation are distinguished in the following way. With moderation, protective factors *interact* with risk factors to reduce the impact of risk factors. An existing supportive relationship with a significant other, such as a parent, can, for example, moderate the impact of exposure to a traumatic event. On the other hand, mediation occurs with the introduction of protective factors that account *directly* and *independently* for an improved outcome.[21] An example would be the introduction of a family support program to improve child functioning and parent–child interaction following exposure to a traumatic event. It plays a compensatory role and operates independently from the risk factor.

Common *intrapersonal* interventions to promote mental health include building the capacity of people through positive thinking, knowledge, and social skills. *Proximal* interventions commonly involve building supportive environments in the home, schools, workplaces, and communities, with these contexts also providing key settings for promoting positive mental health.[9]

PLANNING MENTAL HEALTH PROMOTION AND PREVENTION INTERVENTIONS

In planning mental health promotion and primary prevention, five distinct stages have been identified that should occur at each ecological level.[25,26] The first stage involves selecting appropriate theories for informing interventions. The second stage entails developing an understanding of the socio-cultural context and specific risk and protective factors influencing the mental health of the target group in order to promote cultural congruence of interventions. The third stage involves developing and implementing theoretically and contextually informed interventions using an empowering competency enhancement approach. The fourth stage involves assessing the intervention effects in relation to the identified measurable variables. The final stage is concerned with dissemination of the intervention more broadly in a manner that ensures that fidelity is maintained. These stages are elaborated in greater detail below.

Theories for Informing Interventions

Theories underpin the content or elements of mental health promotion and prevention programs. Within the overarching socio-ecological perspective, mental health promotion and primary prevention interventions draw on theories from a number of disciplines, including lifespan developmental theories, community and health psychology, and social and organizational theories. We review a selection of these (see Table 11.1).

Intrapersonal and proximal level theories generally strive to strengthen protective factors for positive mental health through moderating or mediating the impact of risk factors, building resilience in the face of exposure to risk. At the *intrapersonal* level, cognitive behavioral models have been successfully used with adolescents and adults to moderate and mediate the impact of risk exposure through changing a person's response to risk exposure, promoting mental health and preventing the onset of depression and anxiety disorders.[13,26] The most commonly used cognitive behavioral health promotion theory to facilitate behavioral change at this level is the "theory of planned behavior," which understands behavior change to occur when there is a change in: attitude or beliefs about the outcome of a behavior; subjective norms or perceived social expectations of a behavior and motivation to comply with these expectations; and perceived behavioral control, which refers to people's subjective belief that they can perform a particular behavior. Also at this level, the "challenge model" is an example of a human development model successfully used for building self-efficacy and coping skills in children and adolescents. It underpins many life skills training programs and understands a moderate amount of stress as being useful to enhance resilience and capacity to deal with stressors later in life.[26]

Table 11.1 Examples of Theoretical Models Underpinning Mental Health Promotion and Prevention Interventions

Ecological Level	Theories
Intrapersonal level	Cognitive behavioral therapy Cognitive behavioral health promotion models; e.g., Theory of Planned Behavior, Challenge model
Proximal level	Social Support theory Authoritative Parenting model Compensatory and Protective Factor models Community Development and Social Action models
Distal level	Outside Initiative model (using social action and advocacy) Inside Initiative model (using advocacy)

At the *proximal* level, common theories for strengthening interpersonal systems include models for strengthening health-enhancing social support, with social support having been shown to bolster mental and physical health through helping to buffer the negative effects of stress on health, as well as providing access to resources to help cope with stressors;[26] the "authoritative parenting" model, which encompasses promoting high parental involvement and support and control found to promote more effective parenting;[26] as well as the "compensatory" and "protective factor" models for building resilience in children and adolescents,[27] both of which may adopt strategies to promote greater social support or authoritative parenting and are distinguished by whether the intervention has a mediating effect (compensatory model) or moderating effect (protective factor model).

A number of community level theories have their roots in "social capital theory." Social capital denotes the benefits derived from belonging to social networks. Besides the individual health-promoting benefits of bonding and bridging social capital, which provide access to emotional support and resources, respectively,[28] social capital forms the basis for promoting collective empowerment of community members to address the social determinants of poor mental health as well. Social capital theory thus provides a model not only for promoting resilience in the face of risk but also for empowering community members to gain control over their mental health and its determinants.[29] Two common models that draw on social capital for informing interventions at the community level include the "community development" and "social action" models. In the former, community members are encouraged to increase their collective capacity to address common problems within their communities through participation in support groups, self-help groups, or action-oriented groups. Empowerment, which is understood to be a process whereby individuals and communities assume control over their lives and environment, is central. The social action model uses the same community-organizing principles, but has an activist agenda, promoting collective action to promote structural level change through peaceful protest action such as boycotts and demonstrations.[29]

At a *distal* level, policy change can be initiated from the outside (outside initiative model) using social action and advocacy; as well as from inside governments and governing bodies (inside initiative model).[30] Advocacy work is central to both approaches. The outside initiative model utilizes advocacy and activist groups to highlight policy issues. With the inside initiative model, health advocates may form relationships with policymakers to influence the policy change process through the provision of timely and accurate information. Legitimacy or public acceptance of the policy, feasibility, public support, and timing all influence how much attention is paid to a policy issue.[30] (For a more detailed description of these theories and others, please consult Petersen et al.[29])

Understanding the Local Context—Responding to Local Needs and Ensuring Cultural Congruence

Understanding the local cultural context, social realities, and needs of the beneficiaries of an intended program is essential for ensuring cultural congruence and ecological fit with the needs of a population. Cultural congruence is understood as a process of working within the cultural framework of the beneficiaries of a program, using culturally appropriate skills and interventions[31] (see Chapter 12). Interventions can be newly developed, drawing on local practices and strategies; or existing evidence-based interventions can be adapted and modified to be contextually appropriate. For both types, community members should be involved in the development or adaptation of the intended program, providing meaningful insight and local knowledge on interventions that may mediate or moderate pathways to health.

Implementation

The implementation of theoretically and contextually informed interventions needs to be guided by a competency enhancement or empowerment approach. This demands that interventions be delivered in a democratic participatory way, drawing on existing strengths, competencies, and knowledge to strengthen or develop new capacities and capabilities. Furthermore, capacitating local resources to deliver the interventions wherever possible is important in order to promote community control over mental health. Moreover, from a critical empowerment perspective, interventions should strive to promote a critical awareness or questioning of the assumed social order of things, such as gender inequities or other structural roots of poor mental health. According to Paulo Freire, this entails an exploration of the root causes of social problems, and leads to the development of a critical consciousness and empowerment of people to take action to address the structural roots of their problems.[32] This should lead to improved community control over the social determinants of mental health.

Evaluating Interventions

Establishing the evidence base of interventions is important to ensuring optimal outcomes for beneficiaries as well as best use of scarce resources. While randomized controlled trials (RCTs) are the gold standard for establishing the effectiveness of interventions, they are not always possible to implement, particularly in community-based trials, because of cost, ethical, practical, and political reasons. In these instances, various non-randomized designs can be effectively used for evaluating the effects of interventions. Examples include a matched-control before-and-after study in which observations are made before and after implementation, both in a group that receives the intervention and in a control group that does not; or an interrupted time series study where multiple observations occur before and after in a single group that receives the intervention.[33]

Other constraints to assessing the effects of mental health promotion and prevention interventions include the fact that distal interventions often involve multiple public health efforts and socioeconomic development initiatives, making it difficult to distinguish the impact of any specific intervention on mental health outcomes. In addition, the majority of primary prevention trials measure changes in protective factors or severity of symptoms as opposed to a reduction in the incidence of new cases.[13]

Economic-evaluation studies are also important to undertake in order to demonstrate the value of investing resources in mental health promotion and prevention interventions to policymakers. Such studies are able to model the savings that may be retrieved from interventions. Challenges in doing economic evaluation studies include the multi-sectoral and long-term nature of mental health promotion and primary prevention programming, with benefits often experienced much later in another sector from the sector where the program was administered.[3] For example, prevention of the development of disruptive disorders typically occurs through home-based and school-based programs, but the long-term impact is experienced in the criminal justice system as a reduction in arrests and incarceration costs.

Dissemination

Dissemination and scaling up of mental health promotion and primary prevention interventions requires advocacy efforts both globally and at a country level, with the World Health Organization (WHO) and other international bodies such as the United Nations Children's Fund (UNICEF) and the World Bank playing a crucial role in ensuring distal global policies that are health-promoting. The role of national governments in the development of health-promoting policies at country level is also key.

Successful strategies for the scaling up of effective intrapersonal and proximal-level interventions draw on diffusion of innovation theory,[34] and lessons from successes and failures of dissemination attempts globally. Applying diffusion of innovation theory to program dissemination and uptake essentially comprises three stages: (a) Adoption of the program by the uptake body, which involves awareness of the need for the program; (b) implementing the program with fidelity, which refers to the degree to which all the elements of the original program are retained in the implemented program; and (c) institutionalizing or incorporating the program into the routine activities of the uptake organization.

Ensuring contextual compatibility and involving key stakeholders, particularly institutions and government partners responsible for service delivery systems, from the outset is central to providing opportunities for integration of mental health promotion and prevention interventions into existing service delivery systems. In the context of scarce resources, task sharing (see Chapter 1) is equally applicable to mental health promotion and prevention, with emerging evidence of the efficacy of task shifted interventions for mental health promotion from low- and middle-income countries (LMICs).[35]

MENTAL HEALTH PROMOTION AND PREVENTION ACROSS THE LIFESPAN

The following section introduces each developmental phase with a description of the particular developmental challenges associated with the different developmental phases across the life span. Using the socio-ecological framework described previously, risk and protective factors for each developmental phase are described. This is followed by an overview of distal policy interventions needed, as well as more specific mental health promotion programs and primary prevention interventions for each developmental stage.

PRENATAL DEVELOPMENT AND INFANCY (0–2 YEARS)

Prenatal development and infancy are crucial periods for sensorimotor, neurocognitive, and socio-emotional development, and are a particularly vulnerable period for the development of a wide range of neurocognitive and socio-emotional deficits.[36] Developmental neural plasticity is most prominent during this period. The brain develops rapidly, and environmental influences can affect basic neurodevelopmental processes such as neuronal migration, synaptogenesis, synaptic pruning, and myelination.[21]

During this period, the developing child is particularly vulnerable to an array of environmental assaults that originate from distal "upstream" poverty-related factors. Chronic and severe malnutrition prenatally and during infancy can result in deprivation of essential micronutrients and is associated with neurocognitive deficits, resulting in poor school performance and poor socio-emotional development.[37] Iodine deficiency is particularly hazardous for mental health, and can cause irreversible mental retardation.[38] Prenatal exposure to influenza, rubella, and toxoplasmosis, as well as prenatal, perinatal, and postnatal exposure to the human immunodeficiency virus (HIV) can also result in cognitive impairment, as can postnatal exposure to cerebral malaria, meningitis, and encephalitis during early childhood. Birth trauma, still prevalent in LMICs, is associated with cerebral insults that can also lead to brain malfunction and a range of mental and physical disabilities.[22] Prenatal and postnatal exposure to environmental toxins such as high levels of lead, arsenic, pesticides, tobacco smoke, and alcohol also negatively affects the developing brain, exposing the developing fetus and infant to risk for neurocognitive deficits.[37] Exposure to alcohol in the unborn fetus can cause fetal alcohol syndrome (FAS), which can result in facial anomalies, growth retardation, and abnormalities in the central nervous system, resulting in neurocognitive and social deficits in exposed children.[39]

Postnatally, the development of a secure attachment relationship between an infant and his or her caregiver is essential for healthy socio-emotional development. Caregiver sensitivity and responsiveness are influenced by caregiver emotional and motivational states. Maternal depression can impair parent–child interactions and fragment the attention a caregiver gives a young child.[16] This can result in disturbances in social and emotional development as well as interpersonal attachments later in life. Given that development of the synapses peaks during infancy, lack of psychosocial stimulation as a result of poor maternal responsiveness can also impede optimal cognitive development.[21]

Distal policy interventions during this developmental phase overlap with many other public health actions. These include: strengthening of health systems to improve the provision of obstetric care; immunization; increasing the general public's knowledge of the dangers of alcohol use and other narcotics during pregnancy; promoting child safety such as wearing of seatbelts to prevent head injuries; and increasing access to micronutrients for vulnerable populations such as salt iodization programs (see Box 11.1); folic acid food fortification; and selective protein nutrition supplementation programs.

Specific Mental Health Promotion Programs

Home Visitation Programs and Clinic Care

A combination of home visits and clinic care for at-risk families has the greatest success for promoting healthy socio-emotional and cognitive development in infants.[41] One of the most successful and emulated programs demonstrating long-term health-enhancing effects of a mental health–promoting program during infancy is the Prenatal and Infancy Home Visiting Program in the United States of America. The program was multifaceted, involving both improved prenatal clinic care to produce better pregnancy outcomes and home visits to promote, *inter alia*, more responsive and sensitive maternal care. In addition to improved developmental outcomes in the short term, child participants demonstrated better social and behavioral outcomes in the long term. (see Box 11.2.)

While there have been fewer studies to enhance responsive parenting in LMICs, the evidence base is growing, with emerging evidence suggesting that the promotion of more responsive parenting and psychosocial stimulation through parenting interventions can promote better health and improved infant attachment in exposed infants. In LMICs, the value of home-based visitation programs that encourage maternal responsiveness is demonstrated by at least two trials. In Jamaica, trained community workers were tasked to improve mother–infant interactions through play during weekly home visits over two years in stunted children. The study involved a control group, a stimulation-only group, a nutritional supplementation–only group, and a combined stimulation and supplementation group. During the first two years of infancy, children in receipt of both interventions showed higher levels of cognitive development than children in receipt of a single intervention. At 22 years, participants who received the psychosocial stimulation intervention had higher adult intelligent quotient (IQ) scores, obtained higher educational attainment, displayed fewer depressive symptoms, and reported less involvement in fights or serious violent behaviors than those who did not.[42] Cooper and colleagues[43] have recently implemented a psychosocial stimulation program for deprived women in South Africa to improve maternal sensitivity and mother–infant attachment using trained community workers. An RCT found that the program improved maternal sensitivity and reduced intrusiveness at 12 months post-intervention. At 18 months, exposed children also were more securely attached than controls.[43] Unfortunately, no long-term data on this intervention is available.

Specific Primary Prevention Interventions

Primary prevention interventions during prenatal development and infancy are focused largely on the prevention of *mental retardation* and *developmental disabilities*.

Primary prevention of mental retardation and developmental disabilities involves distal interventions described previously; specifically, the prevention of iodine deficiency through salt iodization and iodine supplementation for "at risk" women and children (see Box 11.1), with the greatest impact on child IQ being shown to occur with supplementation beginning in the first two trimesters of pregnancy.[38] Other interventions include folic acid and protein nutrition supplementation; immunization and treatment programs to prevent diseases that can have an impact on brain development; reducing exposure to toxins; ensuring adequate obstetrical care to prevent birth trauma; and the prevention of head injuries such as the promotion of the use of seatbelts.

Intrapersonal and proximal interventions include genetic counseling where there is a risk of genetic or chromosomal defects that may be responsible for mental retardation. The prevention of FAS, which increases risk for mental retardation and other developmental disabilities in utero, is also possible. In this regard, the integration of screening and brief interventions using motivational interviewing into maternal health care has been shown to help reduce alcohol intake during pregnancy.[39]

CHILDHOOD AND ADOLESCENCE

There is still a high degree of neural plasticity in preschool children who begin to regulate their attention, emotions, motor behavior, and cognitions, developing a sense of a

---

Box 11.1 China's Iodine Deficiency Eradication Program

Iodine is a trace element that occurs in low concentrations in water and soil and is ingested by plants and animals. It is essential for the synthesis of thyroid hormones, which help regulate the metabolic activities of cells, as well as for cell replication. Given that replication of cells during brain development occurs mainly during prenatal development and the first two years of life, iodine during this developmental phase is critical for optimal brain development. Iodine deficiency is the most common cause of preventable mental retardation. While only a very small amount of iodine is required to ensure optimal brain development, it is not uniformly found in the soil and is often deficient in mountainous regions. Fortification of food with iodine, especially iodized salt, has been shown to be the most effective mechanism for combating iodine deficiency. In addition, iodized oil capsules distributed to select populations such as pregnant women and children 0–2 years of age and even entire populations at risk of iodine deficiency can play a complementary role to iodized salt.

China embarked on a national iodine deficiency disorder elimination program after 1990 with the support of the World Bank, which assisted with upgrading of facilities for the production of iodized salt as well ensuring quality control and effective distribution in China. Coverage of salt with the necessary iodine content to prevent iodine deficiency disorder increased from 30% in 1995 to 81% in 1999. Iodine oil capsules were also distributed to "at-risk" populations but discontinued in 1998. The success of China's iodized salt program has been attributed to the central role played by the state in controlling the production and distribution of iodized salt to ensure easy access to iodized salt and prevent the fraudulent sale of non-iodized salt as edible iodized salt.[40]

Box 11.2 The Prenatal and Infancy Home Visiting Program

The **Prenatal and Infancy Home Visiting Program** in the United States of America involved pre- and postnatal nurse home visits to vulnerable low-income women with no previous live births over two years. The goals of the program were to improve prenatal health to produce better pregnancy outcomes, encourage sensitive and competent care by parents to improve child health and developmental outcomes, and improve the future prospects of mothers so as to facilitate better planning of future pregnancies as well as improved education and employment prospects. Three separate large-scale RCTs spanning 27 years all found improvements in child care reflected in fewer injuries and ingestions of harmful substances such as poisons; reductions in child abuse and neglect, and better infant emotional and language development; improved reproductive and sexual health, as shown in fewer subsequent pregnancies; greater participation in the workforce; and a reduction in dependency on public assistance and food stamps. Long-term follow-up of children of the first trial found that, at 15 years, child beneficiaries evidenced fewer arrests, convictions, substance abuse, or promiscuous sexual behavior than control participants.[44] These positive outcomes were estimated to result in cost savings four times the original program investment.[45]

distinct self-identity. This also marks a period of greater exposure to influences beyond the family, and the development of social relatedness and self-regulatory control, which are important for healthy cognitive and social competence.[22]

Middle childhood is generally considered as the period from six to 12 years, marked by the commencement of formal schooling. Failure to accomplish self-regulatory control and social relatedness during the preschool years, as well as preexisting neurocognitive deficits, can jeopardize children's chances of succeeding in the school environment and establishing healthy peer relations. In the absence of supportive school environments which cater for their special needs, these children may experience social rejection, academic failure, and conflict with teachers, and consequently withdraw from successful peers and school activities. This can impede the development of healthy self-esteem and competence, which are important developmental milestones during middle childhood. As they grow older, these children may also be more vulnerable to gravitating towards deviant peer groups, which increases the risk of engaging in anti-social behavior.[46]

Adolescence is defined as commencing with the onset of puberty and can range from as early as 10 years to as late as 20 years. The concept of "youth" includes young adults up to 24 years old, who may be vulnerable to many of the risk influences associated with adolescence.[26] In addition to further cognitive development, including the acquisition of abstract thought processes, key developmental challenges include developing psychological autonomy, establishing intimate friendships, and developing a sense of identity.[26] There is still a fair amount of neural plasticity, and adolescents are particularly vulnerable to environmental factors that interact with genetic factors to influence their risk of developing mental disorders. In addition, while rational decision-making is present, this may be compromised by emotional arousal to which adolescents are prone, leading to impulsive decision-making and a consequent increase in risk-taking that can have a negative impact on the mental health and life course of a person.[47]

Fundamental to mental health promotion and primary prevention efforts in children and adolescents is the need to understand the factors influencing healthy cognitive, social, and emotional development, and the role of stressful life experiences on the development of internalizing disorders such as anxiety and depression and externalizing behavioral disorders, such as conduct disorder and attention-deficit/hyperactivity disorder (ADHD). Exposure to harsh, inconsistent, or abusive parenting can interfere with the development of self-regulatory processes in preschool children, impeding their capacity to function effectively in a school environment and to establish healthy peer relationships. In older children, continued exposure to harsh, punitive, or abusive parenting can result in increased aggression, violence, and conduct disorders. Aggressive social behavior is a key risk factor for progression to externalizing disorders, as well as being a predictor of internalizing disorders.[26]

Exposure to traumatic events also negatively affects socio-emotional development in children. Children and adolescents of divorced parents or whose parents have died have an elevated risk of developing multiple cognitive, emotional, and behavioral problems, such as depression, anxiety, and higher rates of post-traumatic stress disorder (PTSD).[48,49] Early exposure to violence such as direct physical, sexual, or emotional abuse; parental intimate-partner abuse; and exposure to community violence, including bullying, have also been associated with elevated risk for PTSD, depression, anxiety, and behavioral disorders in children.[50,51]

Distal interventions to promote mental health in children and adolescents include policies to improve contextual and environmental factors, such as upgrading neighborhoods to ensure safe recreational spaces, as well as adequate health care, educational, and social welfare and development services.

At the intrapersonal and proximal levels, a consistent finding is that caregiver warmth and support, as well as developmentally appropriate monitoring and control, associated with authoritative parenting, can moderate or mediate the relationship between stressors and mental distress in children. The school environment and school-based programs that promote academic and socio-emotional coping and interpersonal skills can also help build positive social and emotional development in children and adolescents. There are numerous specific mental health promotion programs and primary prevention interventions that have been shown to reduce risks and strengthen protective factors. We briefly review some of these.

Specific Mental Health Promotion Programs

Preschool Cognitive Stimulation Programs

Given that heightened neural plasticity continues during the preschool years, poor cognitive stimulation during these crucial years can retard optimal cognitive development. Reviews of child-focused programs such as day care and preschool programs in HICs indicate that exposure to structured social interactions and cognitive stimulation have a positive impact on academic and social outcomes of "at risk" children from disadvantaged backgrounds. These programs can promote early cognitive gain, reduce the likelihood of being placed in special educational classes or having to repeat grades, and increase the likelihood of graduating from high school.[52]

Early childhood programs that combine early education with family support and parenting programs to foster nurturing parent–child relationships also demonstrate promising outcomes in HICs for promoting healthy socio-emotional outcomes and reducing risk for delinquent and antisocial behavior in later years.[53] The Perry Preschool Project (see Box 11.3) developed in the United States of America, provides an example of an excellent program that combines high-quality early childhood education, as well as an extensive home visitation and parent-support program for disadvantaged children. In addition to academic gains, long-term follow-up also found social gains for program participants who had fewer out-of-wedlock births, relied less on social services, and had higher average earnings and reduced rates of criminal behavior than control participants.[50]

> **Box 11.3** The Perry Preschool Project: A Cognitive Stimulation Intervention
>
> **The Perry Preschool Project** in the United States is a community-based preschool education intervention designed to promote intellectual and social development in children aged three and four years from disadvantaged backgrounds. This project uses an active learning approach, imparting cognitive and learning skills and encouraging independent and intuitive thinking that support children's development through school and into young adulthood. Findings from a randomized control trial that followed 123 disadvantaged African-American children over 40 years found that this high-quality, early childhood program led to improved school performance, higher employment rates, better jobs, higher earnings, more likelihood of being married, of owning a home, of having significantly fewer arrests, and less likelihood of being in receipt of social service benefits.[50] The program improves the academic success of low-income children and assists parents in providing the necessary supports for their children to develop intellectually, socially, and mentally. The program reduces the risk of underprivileged children becoming delinquent and continuing a life of poverty, by improving their chances of finishing school and thus attaining greater economic and social wealth.
>
> A cost-benefit analysis of the program by Barnett[52] indicated that there was a seven- to eightfold return on the initial investment, due to decreased schooling costs, welfare and justice costs, and higher earnings due to improved academic and social outcomes of the program participants.

In addition, a review of mental health promotion interventions in LMICs[32] reports promising findings, albeit from a limited number of studies, on the positive impact of preschool interventions on children's social and emotional well-being in low-resource settings. An example is a seventeen-year follow-up study of a Turkish early enrichment program,[51] which found immediate and long term benefits of preschool and parent training on child development, school attainment, and occupational status, which mirrors the findings from the Perry Preschool Project.[51]

Caregiver-Strengthening Interventions

Programs that promote disciplinary consistency using mild and consistent negative consequences for undesirable behavior (e.g., "time out" or loss of privileges); positive involvement of parents with their children (e.g., playing and reading); as well as emotional communication, through *in vivo* practice of these skills with their children, have been found to promote healthy socio-emotional development and adaptive behavior.[54]

In addition to developing greater school readiness, the success of the Perry Preschool Project (see Box 11.2) in promoting better social adjustment is thought to be as a result of building more effective home–school linkages and more supportive home environments.[55]

Examples of mental health promoting caregiver-strengthening programs following exposure to specific stressors include programs for divorce and violence exposure. The New Beginnings Program is an example of the former and has been shown to have positive effects of enhancing parent–child relationships, reducing inter-parental conflict, and strengthening coping skills in the child affected by divorce.[56]

With regard to the impact of violence exposure, children's socio-emotional coping is moderated by caregiver responses and exacerbated in the context of disrupted families and poor caregiver mental health.[51] There is emerging evidence from LMICs such as Bosnia and Herzegovina of the efficacy of using nonspecialists to provide both psycho-education to caregivers on the impact of trauma exposure on preschool children as well as support to engage in sensitive, emotionally expressive communication and stimulating interaction with their children. Outcomes of this program demonstrated a positive impact on children's emotional well-being.[57]

School-Based Programs

Schools provide ideal settings for mental health promotion programs for children and adolescents. As indicated in the introduction to this section, the development of social and emotional competencies and healthy self-esteem are important developmental tasks during middle childhood. These competencies are important to assist adolescents, in particular, to negotiate emotional arousal in social situations. There is robust evidence from HICs and emerging evidence from LMICs of the mental health promoting impact of *school-based social and emotional learning programs*, which have been shown to help to improve academic performance and develop children's socio-emotional competencies to manage emotions, set and achieve goals, develop an appreciation of others' perspectives, develop and maintain positive relationships, and handle interpersonal conflict constructively. Life skills training is the most commonly used strategy to build socio-emotional competencies within school settings and is typically delivered using interactive teaching methods that involve demonstration, practice, and feedback using structured activities such as role-plays and games.[58]

The concept of "health-promoting schools" applies the eco-holistic principles of the Ottawa Charter[17] to school settings. Central to this approach is a comprehensive program that strengthens the school system through health-enabling school policies to promote the health and well-being of students; e.g., policies that discourage bullying; physical environments that are conducive to good health and well-being, such as recreational facilities; health-enabling social environments, such as good teacher–student relationships and parent–school relationships and community linkages; formal and informal curricula that promote health-enhancing skills and competencies; and access to appropriate adolescent-friendly health services. The rationale behind the whole-school approach is that there is considerable interaction between environment, risky behaviors, and mental health that demands a comprehensive systems intervention.[58] Systematic reviews show that such system-level comprehensive programs implemented continuously for more than one year are an effective strategy for promoting socio-emotional well-being and school adjustment.[59]

Whole-school programs have been found to be particularly successful in reducing bullying and are based on the assumption that bullying is a systemic problem requiring a systemic response. Such programs typically include anti-bullying school policies, which include non-physical consequences of bullying; sensitization of the whole school community, including staff, students, and parents, about what constitutes bullying, its impact on the bully and the bully-victim, and appropriate responses; life skills programs to instill anti-bullying attitudes and pro-social conflict resolution skills; and counseling interventions for students at risk of becoming bullies or bully-victims.[60]

A review of school-based interventions in LMICs also indicates emerging evidence that school programs implemented across diverse LMIC contexts demonstrate significant positive effects on students' emotional and social well-being and on students' school adjustment.[35] These findings are particularly encouraging in relation to interventions for children living in areas of war and conflict, where the school provides an accessible forum for reaching out to young people and their families coping with the negative impacts of war. There is also some emerging evidence that multi-component interventions that combine life-skills with reproductive and sexual health education and substance-abuse education can have a significant positive effect on students' risk-taking behavior.[35]

Specific Interventions for the Prevention of Mental Disorders in Children and Adolescents

Given the overlap between mental health promotion and primary prevention strategies, it is not surprising that many prevention interventions shown to be effective use strategies similar to those described in the above mental health promotion programs.

Disruptive Disorders

In addition to promoting mental health, school-based programs promoting socio-emotional competencies and improving academic capacities, as well as parent-training programs, have also been shown to prevent the development of disruptive disorders.[61,62] (See Box 11.4 for an example of an evidence-based primary prevention program for the prevention of disruptive disorders.)

Substance-Use Disorders

Systematic reviews indicate that a variety of mental health promoting school and family interventions are also effective in preventing substance-use disorders in children and adolescents. Effective school-based programs include specific skills-training interventions, such as harm reduction, decision making, and social skills to resist peer pressure. Effective family interventions include parent skills-training in effective communication and monitoring and control.[64]

Depression

Interventions that have been shown to reduce the incidence of depression in children and adolescents have been largely selective or indicated and based on cognitive behavioral therapy (CBT).[65] Specifically, the Clarke Cognitive-Behavioral Prevention intervention for adolescents has proved effective for preventing future depression in several randomized trials.[21]

Psychosis

Schizophrenia and other psychotic disorders typically begin during adolescence and early adulthood and are preceded by a prodromal phase wherein a person

---

Box 11.4 *The Fast Track Prevention Program*

The *Fast Track Prevention Program* provides long-term evidence of the effectiveness of a multi-component program in preventing lifetime prevalence of all externalizing disorders. This was a selective program targeting vulnerable children from Grades 1–10 and focused on addressing a set of risk factors for the development of antisocial behavior, including poor parental monitoring and control of behavior, deficient child cognitive and socio-emotional coping skills, poor peer relations, weak academic skills, and disruptive and rejecting classroom environments. An RCT using multiple assessments over ten years, including two years after the intervention, found significant reductions in psychiatric diagnoses of conduct disorder, oppositional defiant disorder, ADHD, and any other externalizing disorder in those rated as being at highest initial risk in the intervention arm compared to the control arm.[63]

presents with non-psychotic symptoms, thus providing an opportunity for targeted primary-prevention interventions. Interventions with people with prodromal symptoms involve phase-specific treatment that includes medication regimes specifically developed for people with prodromal symptoms and/or psychological treatment, typically CBT and/or case-management involving individual and family psychosocial support. A systematic review of six randomized control trials in HICs spanning age ranges from 12 to 36 years suggests, however, that while such interventions may delay the onset of psychosis, the evidence as to whether phase-specific treatment can prevent the development of psychosis in the long term in people with prodromal symptoms is inconclusive.[66]

ADULTS

The impact of the interaction of risk and protective factors on the development of positive mental health and mental disorders in adults is cumulative but not necessarily linear. Twenty-five percent of mental disorders in adulthood begin before the age of eight years, and 50% by adolescence.[67] Prevention of many adult mental disorders thus requires interventions earlier in the lifespan.

There are, however, also many social risk factors that may operate independently or interact with preexisting vulnerabilities to impede mental health and promote the onset of mental disorders during adulthood. A recent review of the social determinants of depression, which contributes the highest disease burden of neuropsychiatric disorders and is more prevalent in young adults and females, indicates that there is convincing evidence of the association of depression with stressful life events and violence, strong evidence of an association with crime, conflict, disasters, and stressful working environments; and reasonable evidence associating depression with stigma and discrimination and poverty-related factors such as food insecurity, poor housing, and unemployment or underemployment.[14]

"Poverty" includes a number of domains of social and economic deprivation, and there is ongoing debate over its definition and how it is to be measured. From the data that are currently available, there are some indications that low levels of income *per se* do not increase the risk of common mental disorders, but that relative poverty, sudden changes in income, income insecurity, adverse life events, and the stressors of living in poverty are more predictive of poor mental health status than is absolute poverty (as measured by a fixed level of income).[68]

Common stressful life events that have been associated with depression include loss and bereavement, interpersonal disputes, role transitions such as becoming chronically ill, and social isolation.[69] Exposure to traumatic events such as violence, conflict, and disasters is also associated with PTSD and other common mental disorders (CMDs), especially in women following exposure to assaultive violence.[70]

Just as schools provide a setting wherein specific risk factors operate for children (for example, bullying), workplace settings are similarly beset with specific risk factors for poor mental health in adults. Research from HICs suggests that job strain resulting from high demand and low control increases the risk for depression.[71] There is also evidence to suggest that effort–reward imbalance, organizational injustice, undesirable work events, and bullying are also associated with increased risk for CMD symptoms.[71] The impact of job loss and unemployment on CMDs is also well established.[72] While there is a paucity of data on the impact of work strain on mental health in LMICs, there are numerous factors that render employees in LMICs more vulnerable to exploitation, which is likely to have a negative impact on their mental health. These include a large informal sector that is uncontrolled by labor legislation, as well as pressure to keep wages low as many LMICs strive to enter the global economy.

In addition to distal policy interventions that overlap with many public health and poverty-alleviation strategies, gender-equity initiatives, and actions to reduce oppression and exploitative practices globally (see Chapter 7), there are many specific mental health promotion programs and prevention interventions that can help promote more positive mental health outcomes in adults.

Specific Mental Health Promotion Programs

Building Social Capital and Economic Empowerment

Social capital provides people with access to emotional support as well as the resources to deal with stressful life events. Promising programs combine building social capital with community development and economic empowerment initiatives, with the latter helping to provide resources to address poverty-related social determinants of poor mental health. Examples of such programs include the Comprehensive Rural Health Project (CRHP) in India, where the mental health of women was reported to improve through participation in the program,[73] as well as the Microfinance for AIDS and Gender Equity (IMAGE) program in South Africa, which promoted both gender and economic empowerment, although microfinance interventions in other contexts have not shown such positive outcomes[74] (see Box 11.5).

In addition, women in armed-conflict situations in LMICs, who are often exposed to extreme assaultive trauma, have been found to benefit from mental health promotion strategies that encourage community social capital and solidarity, and build on traditional methods of support.[75] Strategies that have been found to promote resilience and coping amongst genocide rape survivors in Rwanda, for example, include the development of post-conflict women's associations that provide social support and a safe space for survivors to share their experiences without the threat of stigma and discrimination.[76]

Box 11.5 Empowerment Programs to Combat Intimate-Partner Violence and Poverty

The **Intervention with Microfinance for AIDS and Gender Equity (IMAGE)** program targeted deprived women in South Africa and combined a microfinance intervention with a participatory learning program that included HIV prevention, communication skills, gender roles, power relations, and domestic violence to promote critical thinking, confidence, and communication skills. Wider community mobilization also engaged men and youth in the intervention. An RCT found that two years after completing the program, participants reported 55% fewer acts of violence by their intimate partners in the previous 12 months than did control participants. The inclusion of men in the program was deemed important, given findings from other microfinance programs that the economic empowerment of women can increase friction with their male partners.[74]

The **Comprehensive Rural Health Project (CRHP)** targeted mainly women in India. The project adopted an empowerment community-development approach and engaged people through farmer's clubs, women's groups, and adolescent girls' groups. Interventions were delivered by village health workers (VHWs) in the main, and included income-generation projects, agricultural and environment programs, education, and health care, including primary health care and hospital services as well as rehabilitation services for disabilities. Qualitative evaluation of the impact of the program on women's mental health suggests that economic empowerment afforded them increased psychological empowerment, with women suggesting that they had greater participation in decision-making, increasing their sense of control over their lives and their mental health.[73]

Alternative Therapies: Yoga and Exercise

There is increasing evidence that yoga and as well as high-energy exercise can improve one's mood and help reduce symptoms of anxiety and depression. Yoga, in particular, helps people regulate their response to stress through reducing physiological arousal, such as reducing the heart rate.[77]

Work-Based Programs

Just as schools provide a convenient setting for the delivery of mental health promotion interventions for children, workplace settings provide a similarly convenient setting for the delivery of mental health promotion interventions for adults. Both individual and organizational change is needed to promote mental health in the workplace.[9] Mental health promotion interventions shown to be effective in reducing CMD symptoms in the workplace in HICs have been selective and include stress management and CBT programs.[78] Participatory interventions at an organizational level to provide less stressful work environments are also a promising strategy.[79]

Interventions for the Primary Prevention of Specific Mental Disorders in Adults

Depression

Interventions that have been shown to be effective in preventing the onset of depression in selected and indicated groups include the use of CBT or interpersonal therapy (IPT) techniques.[13] CBT as a prevention strategy helps promote more adaptive coping strategies for stressful life events. IPT helps through strengthening social support and problem management strategies.[13]

Alcohol-Use Disorders

The importance of preventing the development of alcohol use disorders is highlighted by the biopsychosocial and economic consequences of these disorders, which have been associated with decreased productivity, increased unintentional injuries, and aggression and violence, including child and spouse abuse. In addition to distal interventions to increase awareness of the dangers of alcohol misuse and restricting access to alcohol, specific prevention programs found to be effective in reducing hazardous drinking and the onset of alcohol-use disorders include screening and brief interventions (SBIs) for adults and pregnant women in primary care settings, emergency departments, and college student health centers. However, the evidence for SBIs reducing alcohol consumption among adolescents and heavy alcohol users in hospitals and primary care settings is inconclusive.[80]

Suicide Prevention

Globally, suicide rates have increased by 60% in the last 45 years, and suicide is in the top three leading causes of death in people between the ages of 15 and 44. Rates amongst young people have increased rapidly, with suicide being the second leading cause of death in the 10- to 24-year age group.[81] Although the population's attributable risk of suicide associated with mental disorders, particularly mood disorders and alcohol-use disorders, does vary across countries, they are the most important health-related risk factor. Other contributory factors include extreme social difficulties, interpersonal violence, access to lethal means to commit suicide, and attitudes towards suicide.

It follows that suicide prevention requires a multifaceted response. While reported under this section for adults, the following strategies for the prevention of suicide are equally applicable to adolescents and older people. Strategies that have been found to assist in the reduction of suicide risk include:

(a) Improved identification and treatment of depression and substance-use disorders by primary care workers. Studies indicate that the majority of persons with completed suicides had contact with a primary care physician within a year of their death;

(b) Restricting access to common lethal means for committing suicide, such as pesticides and firearms;

(c) Follow-up care of people who have engaged in non-fatal suicide attempts, to prevent future attempts;

(d) School, work, and community gatekeeper training is a promising strategy and involves training key people such as teachers, clergy, etc., to identify and refer people at risk of suicide.[82]

OLDER PEOPLE

Risk factors for dementia in older adults include factors associated with vascular disease, such as hypertension, type II diabetes, hypercholesterolemia, obesity, and smoking; all of which relate to adult lifestyles that may persist in older people. The need for general health promotion programs to promote healthy lifestyles amongst adults and older people is thus highlighted. Such programs in LMICs are particularly important, given their greater use of tobacco products.[83] Deficiencies of folate and vitamin B_{12} have also been identified as risk factors.[83] In relation to protective factors, complex cognitive activity across the lifespan has been found to be protective against dementia risk.[84]

Increased risk for late-life depression in HICs is associated with female gender, disability and functional impairment, prior depression, bereavement, sleep disturbance, and social isolation. As people get older, their social networks shrink, and social engagement, such as visiting friends, may also be impaired in those with disabilities.[83]

At a distal level, mental health promotion and prevention interventions for older people should include policy-level interventions to reduce tobacco and alcohol consumption within the general population, as well as to ensure the provision of adequate social protection, adequate nutrition, and health care services to facilitate the early detection and treatment of chronic conditions in older people.[83] Policies to support the provision of micronutrient supplementation with folic acid and vitamin B_{12} in healthy adults to prevent dementia is a promising intervention, although more evidence is required.[85]

Evidence of the effectiveness of intrapersonal and proximal mental health promotion and prevention programs for older people across HICs and LMICs is sparse. Promising approaches for promoting older people's mental health focus on improving their overall quality of life; engagement to strengthen supportive social networks, including befriending, peer, and group support; volunteering and intergenerational projects; work with carers of older people to promote greater uptake of education, sports, and leisure; and targeted outreach with those who are most isolated and vulnerable.[83,86] With regard to the prevention of dementia specifically, training in memory strategies and cognitive exercises is also a promising intervention for at-risk individuals.[87]

CHALLENGES AND RECOMMENDATIONS FOR SCALING UP MENTAL HEALTH PROMOTION AND PRIMARY PREVENTION OF MENTAL DISORDERS GLOBALLY

Distal interventions generally overlap with other public health efforts and socioeconomic development initiatives. Specific evidence of the impact of such efforts on the promotion of mental health and the prevention of mental disorders is difficult to ascertain, given the lack of controlled trials and lack of measurement of mental health outcomes. Evidence of risk factors for mental disorders do, however, indicate that the following interventions will promote mental health and have an impact on preventing the onset of mental disorders (see Tables 11.2 and 11.3).

During prenatal development and infancy, reducing exposure to environmental risk factors such as toxins and micronutrient deficiencies, especially iodine deficiency, and improving public health services to prevent and treat communicable diseases, improve obstetrical care, and prevent birth complications and head injuries are indicated.

From childhood through to adulthood, many social and environmental risk factors aggregate in poorer communities. Achieving the MDGs through country and global policies would assist in addressing many of the social determinants of poor mental health. These include global policies to address global shortages in food, water, land, and energy, as well as global efforts to eradicate oppressive regimes and armed conflict. At the country level, legislation to limit and regulate access to alcohol and other narcotics; economic policies that promote greater socioeconomic equality; labor policies promoting employment security and improved working conditions; and welfare policies that provide social protection to the sick, disabled, and unemployed are some examples of policies that, if implemented, should have a positive impact on mental health across the lifespan.[14]

With regard to *intrapersonal and proximal interventions*, economic evaluation studies suggest that early interventions with children and adolescents offer the greatest cost savings to societies via reduced health and social spending later in life.[88] Furthermore, while universal interventions are ideal to support healthy development for all, in scarce-resource contexts, selective and indicated interventions show greater effects and may be more efficient.[21]

During prenatal development and infancy, home-visitation programs are most effective for selected vulnerable groups. These can be delivered as part of primary health care programs to improve, *inter alia*, maternal mental health, parental responsiveness, and attachment. These programs have largely been delivered by professional nurses in HICs. Given the scarcity of professional resources in LMICs, training community care workers to deliver similar interventions should be considered in these contexts, and evidence attests to the efficacy of this approach.

During childhood and adolescence, parenting skills training and socio-emotional learning programs, especially life skills programs, have been shown to reap good returns for investment in the long term.[3,88] Multifaceted preschool and school-based programs to enhance, *inter alia*, child academic achievement and social relatedness as well as parental involvement and monitoring and control, are most successful in promoting mental health and preventing disruptive behavioral disorders and substance-use disorders. CBT has been shown to be an effective strategy for preventing depression in "at risk" adolescents. Phase-specific intervention during adolescence and early adulthood for the prevention of psychosis has emerged as a promising strategy, although the long-term effectiveness of such interventions is currently not clearly established (see Table 11.2).

In adults, CBT and IPT for selected and indicated groups at risk for depression can promote more adaptive functioning and prevent or delay the onset of clinical depression (see Table 11.3). Yoga and high-energy exercise can improve mood and also help reduce

Table 11.2 Suggestions for Mental Health Promotion Interventions Across the Lifespan

Life Phase	Programs	Distal interventions
Prenatal development and infancy	Home visitation and clinic programs to promote maternal mental health, maternal responsiveness, and psychosocial stimulation of infants.	Policies to reduce poverty and promote greater socioeconomic equality, eradicate oppressive regimes and armed conflict; improve contextual and environmental factors; as well as ensure adequate health care, educational and social welfare/development services
Childhood and adolescence	Parenting skills training programs School-based life skills and socio-emotional learning programs Whole-school programs	
Adults and older people	Gender and economic empowerment programs Building supportive social networks in adults and older people Organizational change to promote less stressful working environments Yoga and other exercise	

Table 11.3 Suggested Interventions for Prevention of Mental Disorders

Disorder	Suggested Interventions
Mental retardation and developmental disabilities	Iodine, folic acid, and protein nutrition supplementation Immunization and treatment programs to prevent diseases that negatively impact brain development Reducing exposure to toxins that negatively impact brain development Ensuring adequate obstetrical care to prevent birth trauma Prevention of head injuries through programs to promote child safety; e.g., use of seatbelts Genetic counseling Brief screening interventions to reduce alcohol use during pregnancy to prevent FAS
Disruptive disorders	Comprehensive interventions for children and adolescents, including building socio-emotional competencies, improving academic capacities, and parent training programs
Substance use disorders	Comprehensive interventions involving specific skills training interventions for children and adolescents, such as harm reduction, decision making, and social skills to resist peer pressure, as well as parent training programs. Policy interventions to reduce consumption of narcotics and alcohol. Brief screening interventions for hazardous drinking in adults.
Depression	Cognitive behavioral therapy for selected and indicated groups of adolescents and adults with sub-clinical symptoms of depression, as well as interpersonal therapy for adults.

Table 11.3 Continued

Disorder	Suggested Interventions
Psychosis	Phase-specific treatment for psychosis in indicated groups of adolescents and young adults in the prodromal phase of psychosis.
Suicide	Improved identification and treatment of depression and substance-use disorders by primary care workers. Restricting access to common lethal means for committing suicide, such as pesticides and firearms. Follow-up care of people who have engaged in non-fatal suicide attempts to prevent future attempts. Training of gatekeepers to identify and refer people at risk of suicide.
Dementia	Cognitive stimulation exercises in older people. Policies to reduce tobacco and alcohol consumption across the lifespan. Micronutrient supplementation in older people.

symptoms of anxiety and depression. Promising initiatives in poor-resourced contexts for addressing the stressors associated with poverty as well as differential exposure to stressful life events include programs that combine strengthening social capital with gender and economic empowerment to promote greater gender equity and sustainable livelihoods. Promising strategies in older adults include building supportive social networks to prevent social isolation, which can contribute to late-life depression, as well as folic acid and vitamin B supplementation and cognitive exercises to prevent dementia.

Settings such as primary health care, preschool, school, and the workplace provide opportunities for both screening and interventions. These multiple settings demand a multi-sectoral response with diverse disciplines such as medicine, education, psychology, social work, and public health being involved in service delivery. Given the shortage of professionals across disciplines in LMICs, engaging local community resources is essential. There is emerging evidence of the efficacy of task-shifted mental health promotion interventions delivered by trained community members in LMICs.[35] Engaging community members in the development and delivery of mental health services also holds potential for empowering community members through increased awareness and capacities to act on the social determinants of poor mental health, thereby engendering greater community control over their mental health. Task shifting requires, however, the development of technical support materials as well as the diversification of professional roles to ensure ongoing support and supervision. This poses a challenge in both HICs and LMICs, given that few training curricula across the relevant disciplines include the science of mental health promotion and prevention of mental disorders.[21]

Scaling up mental health promotion and the primary prevention of mental disorders requires advocacy and education of policymakers, civil society, and service providers across multiple sectors about the need for mental health promotion and prevention efforts, and the wider health and social benefits that can accrue therefrom. To this end, highlighting returns on investment is an important strategy. It has been suggested that nearly 90% of the costs associated with poor mental health are incurred in sectors outside of health and social care.[89] Highlighting the importance of mental health to the achievement of the MDGs is a further strategy for LMICs in particular. Renewed global interest in primary health care, which embraces prevention and health promotion, also provides a window of opportunity for placing mental health promotion and the prevention of mental disorders on the agendas of national governments, international donor agencies, and global bodies that influence global development policies. These advocacy efforts should be promoted alongside investments to generate further evidence of the role and cost-effectiveness of mental health promotion and prevention interventions in promoting human capital and social economic development globally, and in LMICs especially.

ACKNOWLEDGMENTS

We acknowledge and thank Tasneem Kathree for assisting with literature searches for the chapter.

REFERENCES

1. Andrews G, Sanderson K, Corry J, Lapsley HM. Using epidemiological data to model efficiency in reducing the burden of depression. *J Ment Health Policy Econ.* 2000;3(4):175–86.
2. World Health Organization. *The global burden of disease: 2004 update.* Geneva: World Health Organization; 2008.
3. Knapp M, McDaid D, Parsonage M. *Mental health promotion and mental illness prevention: The economic case.* London; 2011.
4. World Health Organization. *Strengthening mental health promotion.* (Fact sheet no. 220). Geneva: World Health Organization; 2001.
5. World Health Organization. *Mental health: New understanding, new hope. The World Health Report.* Geneva: World Health Organization; 2001.
6. World Health Organization. *Prevention and promotion in mental health.* Geneva: World Health Organization; 2002.
7. World Health Organization. *Promoting mental health. Concepts, emerging evidence, practice. Summary Report.* Geneva: World Health Organization; 2004.
8. World Health Organization. *Prevention of mental disorders: Effective interventions and policy options. Summary Report.* Geneva: World Health Organization; 2004.
9. Barry MM, Jenkins R. *Implementing mental health promotion.* Oxford, UK: Churchill Livingstone Elsevier; 2007.
10. Ypinazar VA, Margolis SA, Haswell-Elkins M, Tsey K. Indigenous Australians' understandings regarding mental health and disorders. *Aust N Z J Psychiatry.* 2007;41(6):467–78.
11. Barry MM. Addressing the determinants of positive mental health: concepts, evidence and practice. *Int J Ment Health Promot.* 2009;11(3):4–17.
12. Caplan G. *Principles of preventive psychiatry.* New York: Basic Books; 1964.
13. Cuijpers P, van Straten A, Smit F, Mihalopoulos C, Beekman A. Preventing the onset of depressive disorders: a meta-analytic review of psychological interventions. *Am J Psychiatry.* 2008;165(10):1272–80.
14. Patel V, Lund C, Hatherill S, Plagerson S, Corrigall J, Funk M, et al. Mental disorders: equity and social determinants. In: Blas E, Kurup AS, editors. *Equity, social determinants and public health programmes.* Geneva: World Health Organization; 2010:115–34.
15. Evans A, Evans J. *Resource scarcity, wellbeing and development.* London: Bellagio Initiative; 2011.
16. Richter LM. *The importance of care-giver child interactions for the survival and healthy development of young children: A review.* Geneva: World Health Organization; 2004.
17. World Health Organization. Ottawa Charter for Health Promotion. 1986 [cited October 25, 2011]. Available from: http://www.who.int/hpr/NPH/docs/ottawa_charter_hp.pdf
18. Bronfenbrenner U. *The ecology of human development: Experiments by nature and design.* Cambridge, MA: Harvard University Press; 1979.
19. Sen A. *Development as freedom.* Oxford, UK: Oxford University Press; 1999.
20. Nussbaum MC. *Women and human development: the capabilities approach.* Cambridge, UK: Cambridge University Press; 2000.
21. O'Connell ME, Boat T, Warner KE, editors. *Preventing mental, emotional, and behavioral disorders among young people: Progress and possibilities.* Washington, DC: National Academies Press; 2009.
22. Richter L, Dawes A, de Kadt J. Early childhood. In: Petersen I, Bhana A, Flisher AJ, Swartz L, Richter L, editors. *Promoting mental health in scarce-resource contexts.* Cape Town, SA: Human Sciences Research Council Press; 2010:99–123.

23. Barry MM. Researching the implementation of community mental health promotion programs. *Health Promot J Austr.* 2007;18(3):240–6.

24. Barry MM. Generic principles of effective mental health promotion. *Int J Ment Health Promot.* 2007;9(2):4–16.

25. Petersen I. At the heart of development: an introduction to mental health promotion and the prevention of mental disorders in scarce-resource contexts. In: Petersen I, Bhana A, Flisher AJ, Swartz L, Richter L, editors. *Promoting mental health in scarce-resource contexts.* Cape Town, SA: Human Sciences Research Council Press; 2010:3–20.

26. Breinbauer C, Maddaleno M. *Youth: Choices and change: Promoting healthy behaviors in adolescents.* Washington DC: Pan American Health Organization; 2005.

27. Fergus S, Zimmerman MA. Adolescent resilience: a framework for understanding healthy development in the face of risk. *Annu Rev Public Health.* 2005;26:399–419.

28. Putnam R. *Bowling alone: The collapse and revival of American community.* New York: Simon and Schuster; 2000.

29. Petersen I, Govender K. Theoretical considerations. From understanding to intervening. In: Petersen I, Bhana A, Flisher A, Swartz L, Richter L, editors. *Promoting mental health in scarce-resource contexts: Emerging evidence and practice.* Cape Town, SA: HSRC Press; 2010:21–48.

30. Hall P, Land H, Parker A. *Change, choice and conflict in social policy.* London: Heineman; 1975.

31. Wilson DW. Culturally competent psychiatric nursing care. *J Psychiatr Ment Health Nurs.* 2010;17(8):715–24.

32. Freire P. *Education for critical consciousness.* Continuum: New York; 1993.

33. Bhana A, Govender A. Evaluating interventions. In: Petersen I, Bhana A, Flisher AJ, Swartz L, Richter L, editors. *Promoting mental health in scarce-resource contexts Emerging evidence and practice.* Cape Town, SA: HSRC Press; 2010:60–81.

34. Rogers E. *Diffusion of innovations,* 4th ed. New York: Free Press; 1995.

35. Barry MM, Clarke AM, Jenkins R, Patel V. *Rapid review of the evidence on the effectiveness of mental health promotion in low and middle income countries. Mainstreaming health promotion: Reviewing the health promotion actions on priority public health conditions.* Geneva: World Health Organization; 2012.

36. Grantham-McGregor S, Cheung YB, Cueto S, Glewwe P, Richter L, Strupp B. Developmental potential in the first 5 years for children in developing countries. *Lancet.* 2007;369(9555):60–70.

37. Walker SP, Wachs TD, Gardner JM, Lozoff B, Wasserman GA, Pollitt E, et al. Child development: risk factors for adverse outcomes in developing countries. *Lancet.* 2007;369(9556):145–57.

38. Engle PL, Grantham-McGregor S, Black M, Walker SP, Wachs TD. How to avoid the loss of potential in over 200 million young children in the developing world. *Child Health & Educ.* 2009;1(2):58–72.

39. Hankin JR. Fetal alcohol syndrome prevention research. *Alcohol Res Health.* 2002;26(1):58–65.

40. Goh G. *An analysis of combating iodine deficiency: Case studies of China, Indonesia, and Madagascar.* Washington, DC: The World Bank; 2001.

41. Eshel N, Daelmans B, de Mello MC, Martines J. Responsive parenting: interventions and outcomes. *Bull WHO.* 2006;84(12):991–8.

42. Walker SP, Chang SM, Vera-Hernández M, Grantham-McGregor S. Early childhood stimulation benefits adult competence and reduces violent behavior. *Pediatrics.* 2011;127(5):849–57.

43. Cooper PJ, Tomlinson M, Swartz L, Landman M, Molteno C, Stein A, et al. Improving quality of mother–infant relationship and infant attachment in socio-economically deprived community in South Africa: randomised controlled trial. *BMJ.* 2009;338:b974.

44. Olds DL. The nurse–family partnership: An evidence-based preventive intervention. *Infant Ment Health J.* 2006;27(1):5–25.

45. Karoly LA, Greenwood PW, Everingham SS, Houbé J, Kilburn MR, P. RC, et al. *Investing in our children: What we know and don't know about the costs and benefits of early childhood interventions.* Santa Monica, CA: Rand Publishers; 1998.

46. Dodge KA, Greenberg MT, Malone PS. Testing an idealized dynamic cascade model of the development of serious violence in adolescence. *Child Dev.* 2008;79(6):1907–27.

47. Spear LP. Rewards, aversions and affect in adolescence: emerging convergences across laboratory animal and human data. *Dev Cogn Neurosci.* 2011;1(4):390–403.

48. Cluver L, Gardner F, Operario D. Psychological distress amongst AIDS-orphaned children in urban South Africa. *J Child Psychol Psychiatry.* 2007;48(8):755–63.

49. Amato PR. Children of divorce in the 1990s: an update of the Amato and Keith (1991) meta-analysis. *J Fam Psychol.* 2001;15(3):355–70.

50. Briggs-Gowan MJ, Carter AS, Clark R, Augustyn M, McCarthy KJ, Ford JD. Exposure to potentially traumatic events in early childhood: differential links to emergent psychopathology. *J Child Psychol Psychiatry.* 2010;51(10):1132–40.

51. Barbarin OA, Richter L, deWet T. Exposure to violence, coping resources, and psychological adjustment of South African children. *Am J Orthopsychiatry.* 2001;71(1):16–25.

52. Nelson G, Westhues A, MacLeod J. A meta-analysis of longitudinal research on preschool prevention programs for children. *Prev & Treat.* 2003;6(31). doi: 10.1037/1522-3736.6.1.631a

53. Barnett WS. Long-term effects of early childhood programs on cognitive and school outcomes. *Future of Children.* 1995;5(3):25–50.

54. Kaminski JW, Valle LA, Filene JH, Boyle CL. A meta-analytic review of components associated with parent training program effectiveness. *J Abnorm Child Psychol.* 2008;36(4):567–89.

55. Schweinhart LJ, Montie J, Xiang Zea. *Lifetime effects: The High/Scope Perry Preschool Study through age 40.* Michigan: High/Scope Press; 2005.

56. Wolchik SA, Sandler IN, Weiss L, Winslow EB. New beginnings: an empirically based program to help divorced mothers promote resilience in their children. In: Breismeister JM, Schaefer CE, editors. *Handbook of parent training: Helping parents prevent and solve problem behaviors.* New York: Wiley; 2007:25–62.

57. Dybdahl R. Children and mothers in war: an outcome study of a psychosocial intervention program. *Child Dev.* 2001;72(4):1214–30.

58. Patel V, Flisher AJ, Nikapota A, Malhotra S. Promoting child and adolescent mental health in low and middle income countries. *J Child Psychol Psychiatry.* 2008;49(3):313–34.

59. Wells J, Barlow J, Stewart-Brown S. A systematic review of universal approaches to mental health promotion in schools. *Health Educ.* 2003;103(4):197–220.

60. Smith JD, Schneider BH, Smith PK, Ananiadou K. The effectiveness of whole-school anti-bullying programs: a synthesis of evaluation research. *School Psychol Rev.* 2004;33(4):547–60.

61. MacMillan HL. New insights into prevention of depression and disruptive behaviour disorders in childhood: where do we go from here? *Can J Psychiatry.* 2009;54(4):209–11.

62. Bayer J, Hiscock H, Scalzo K, Mathers M, McDonald M, Morris A, et al. Systematic review of preventive interventions for children's mental health: what would work in Australian contexts? *Aust N Z J Psychiatry.* 2009;43(8):695–710.

63. Conduct Problems Prevention Research Group. The effects of the fast track preventive intervention on the development of conduct disorder across childhood. *Child Dev.* 2011;82(1):331–45.

64. Schwartz C, Harrison E, Garland O, Waddell C. *Preventing substance use disorders in children and youth.* Vancouver: Children's Health Policy Centre, Faculty of Health Sciences, Simon Fraser University; 2007.

65. Calear AL, Christensen H. Systematic review of school-based prevention and early intervention programs for depression. *J Adolesc.* 2010;33(3):429–38.

66. Marshall M, Rathbone J. Early intervention for psychosis. *Cochrane Database Syst Rev.* 2011; (6): CD004718.

67. Swartz L, Herrman H. Adults. In: Petersen I, Bhana A, Flisher A, Swartz L, Richter L, editors. *Promoting mental health in scarce resource contexts: Emerging evidence and practice.* Cape Town, SA: HSRC Press; 2010:167–79.

68. Lund C, Breen A, Flisher AJ, Kakuma R, Corrigall J, Joska JA, et al. Poverty and common mental disorders in low and middle income countries: A systematic review. *Soc Sci Med.* 2010;71(3):517–28.

69. Klerman GL, Weissman MM, Rounsaville BJ, Chevron ES. *Interpersonal psychotherapy of depression:* New York: Basic Books; 1984.

70. Breslau N. Epidemiologic studies of trauma, posttraumatic stress disorder, and other psychiatric disorders. *Can J Psychiatry.* 2002;47(10):923–9.

71. Bonde JP. Psychosocial factors at work and risk of depression: a systematic review of the epidemiological evidence. *Occup Environ Med.* 2008;65(7):438–45.

72. Dooley D, Catalano R, Wilson G. Depression and unemployment: panel findings from the Epidemiologic Catchment Area study. *Am J Community Psychol.* 1994;22(6):745–65.

73. Kermode M, Herrman H, Arole R, White J, Premkumar R, Patel V. Empowerment of women and mental health promotion: a qualitative study in rural Maharashtra, India. *BMC Public Health.* 2007;7:225.

74. World Health Organization. *Preventing intimate partner and sexual violence against women: Taking action and generating evidence.* Geneva: World Health Organization; 2010.

75. Ghosh N, Mohit A, Murthy RS. Mental health promotion in post-conflict countries. *J R Soc Promot Health.* 2004;124(6):268–70.

76. Zraly M, Nyirazinyoye L. Don't let the suffering make you fade away: an ethnographic study of resilience among survivors of genocide-rape in southern Rwanda. *Soc Sci Med.* 2010;70(10):1656–64.

77. Saeed SA, Antonacci DJ, Bloch RM. Exercise, yoga, and meditation for depressive and anxiety disorders. *Am Fam Physician.* 2010;81(8):981–6.

78. Martin A, Sanderson K, Cocker F. Meta-analysis of the effects of health promotion intervention in the workplace on depression and anxiety symptoms. *Scand J Work Environ Health.* 2009;35(1):7–18.

79. Graveling RA, Crawford JO, Cowie H, Amati C, Vohra S. *A review of workplace interventions that promote mental well-being in the workplace.* Edinburgh, UK: Institute of Occupational Medicine; 2008.

80. Botelho R, Engle B, Mora JC, Holder C. Brief interventions for alcohol misuse. *Primary Care.* 2011;38(1):105–23, vii.

81. World Health Organization. *Suicide prevention.* [Cited January 20, 2012]; available from: http//:www.who.int/mental_health/prevention/suicide/suicideprevent/en/.

82. Mann JJ, Apter A, Bertolote J, Beautrais A, Currier D, Haas A, et al. Suicide prevention strategies: a systematic review. *JAMA.* 2005;294(16):2064–74.

83. Prince M. Older people. In: Petersen I, Bhana A, Flisher AJ, Swartz L, Richter L, editors. *Promoting mental health in scarce-resource contexts.* Cape Town, SA: Human sciences Research Council Press; 2010:180–207.

84. Valenzuela MJ, Matthews FE, Brayne C, Ince P, Halliday G, Kril JJ, et al. Multiple biological pathways link cognitive lifestyle to protection from dementia. *Biol Psychiatry.* 2011; 71:783–91.

85. Malouf R, Grimley Evans J. Folic acid with or without vitamin B_{12} for the prevention and treatment of healthy elderly and demented people. *Cochrane Database Syst Rev.* 2008;(4):CD004514.

86. Wheeler FA, Gore KM, Greenblatt B. The beneficial effects of volunteering for older volunteers and the people they service: A meta-analysis. *Int J Aging & Hum Dev.* 1998;47(1):69–79.

87. Gates NJ, Sachdev PS, Fiatarone Singh MA, Valenzuela M. Cognitive and memory training in adults at risk of dementia: a systematic review. *BMC Geriatrics.* 2011;11:55.

88. Zechmeister I, Kilian R, McDaid D. Is it worth investing in mental health promotion and prevention of mental illness? A systematic review of the evidence from economic evaluations. *BMC Public Health.* 2008;8:20.

89. Roberts G, Grimes K. *Return on investment. Mental health promotion and mental illness prevention.* London and Canada: Canadian Policy Network at the University of Western Ontario: Canadian Institute for Health Information; 2011.

12 Interventions for Mental Disorders

Charlotte Hanlon, Abebaw Fekadu, and
Vikram Patel

INTRODUCTION

Therapeutic nihilism about mental, neurological, and substance use (MNS) disorders
has been a potent factor perpetuating the treatment gap worldwide. The notion that
MNS disorders are untreatable or too complicated and difficult to treat, especially in
resource-poor settings, has been challenged for many years;[1] however, recently there has
been substantial progress in increasing awareness of the robust, global evidence for effective treatments for MNS disorders.[2–4]

It is important to take a broad view of interventions to alleviate MNS disorders,
recognizing that the majority of people suffering from these disorders will rely upon
self-care or the informal care sector; for example, through religious institutions, traditional or alternative healers, or the advice of friends and families.[5] In this chapter, we shall focus on specific interventions for MNS disorders, usually delivered by
health professionals, as this is where the evidence base is best-developed. We will
start by outlining some of the key principles that should underpin any intervention
for MNS disorders and will argue for the value of an evidence-based approach. This
will be followed by an in-depth focus on the ground-breaking work of the World
Health Organization's (WHO) mental health Gap Action Programme (mhGAP)[6]
in synthesizing the global evidence base and producing evidence-based guidelines
(mhGAP-Implementation Guide; MIG) for a set of "priority" MNS disorders; namely,
depression, alcohol and drug use disorders; suicide and self-harm; psychosis, bipolar
disorder, epilepsy, dementia, and child developmental and behavioral disorders.[4] The
inclusion of epilepsy, a neurological disorder, in the MIG (and in this textbook on
global mental health) arises because epilepsy is commonly managed by mental health
professionals in low- and middle-income country (LAMIC) settings.

Moving from evidence-based guidelines to the development and implementation of packages of care is the next step required for scale-up of mental health care (see Chapter 14), and the current state of the art will be discussed. While noting the success of these approaches, areas requiring further attention will be highlighted.

PRINCIPLES OF INTERVENTION

The usefulness of an intervention for any disorder needs to be considered in terms of its effectiveness, feasibility, equity, acceptability and affordability. Each of these principles will now be considered in turn.

Effectiveness

In order to evaluate whether or not an intervention has helped a person who is suffering from a disorder, relying on anecdotal evidence from the person, their caregivers, or their treating clinician will not give us the information we need. It does not tell us whether the person would have got well without the intervention, or whether they have actually improved in objective terms. In order to gain such information, a methodologically rigorous scientific study needs to be conducted. You have already been introduced to different types of epidemiological study design (see Chapter 4). When it comes to the evaluation of interventions there is a hierarchy of evidence produced by different study designs, based on the relative susceptibility of each study design to bias, confounding, and reverse causality (see Figure 12.1).

In this hierarchy of evidence, meta-analyses or systematic reviews of well-conducted randomized controlled trials (RCTs) are located at the top; from a scientific perspective, they offer the best evidence. The defining advantage of an RCT compared to other study designs is that the intervention is allocated randomly to eligible participants. As a consequence, selection bias is minimized, and any potential confounding variables will not interfere with the result, because both known and unknown confounders are distributed randomly between the two groups. RCTs can still, however, be susceptible to bias, chance, and confounding, depending on how they are carried out in practice. The key methodological features of RCTs that need to be adhered to in order to generate high-quality evidence are set out in the Consolidated Standards of Reporting Trials (CONSORT) guidelines.[7] These guidelines were developed from an expert consensus of reporting requirements to enable evaluation of the quality of any published RCT. An important distinction is made between efficacy and effectiveness trials[8] (see Box 12.1); the latter also sometimes called pragmatic trials.[9]

Despite the large treatment gaps that exist in LAMICs,[10] the evidence base for effective interventions comes predominantly from high-income countries (HICs).[2] Out of 11,501 RCTs of mental health interventions for schizophrenia, depression, alcohol use disorders or child developmental disorders conducted worldwide, fewer than 1% had been carried out in low-income countries.[2] Apart from this imbalance in the global distribution of intervention evidence, the findings from individual RCTs are not usually sufficient in themselves to be able to guide clinical practice. Hence the importance of systematic reviews of the evidence base in order to identify good-quality RCTs, the results of which can then be combined statistically in a "meta-analysis" or summarized in a narrative overview. (See Box 12.2 for useful sources of evidence-based clinical guidance.) Criteria for evaluating the quality of a meta-analysis are available.[11]

Although they are the gold standard for evaluation of an intervention, RCTs are not always ethical or feasible. Ethical constraints to carrying out an RCT may arise when the client group is extremely vulnerable: for example, those who are imprisoned or

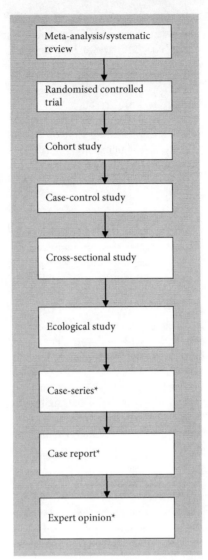

FIGURE 12.1

Hierarchy of study designs for best evidence. (*Examples of methods for "practice-based evidence.")

homeless, or located in any setting where there is risk of coercion. In the global mental health context, this is particularly pertinent to RCTs carried out in poor populations within LAMICs where participation in the study may provide access to medications or care that would otherwise be unavailable, thus potentially undermining voluntary consent. RCTs of medications in pregnant women are rarely considered ethical, due to possible risks to the unborn child, so that the evidence base on teratogenicity of medications is limited to observational or laboratory-based studies. In terms of feasibility, trials of antidepressant therapy for postnatal depression may struggle to recruit women because of their reluctance to take medications while breastfeeding.[12] Another example would be when mental health service reforms are implemented throughout a population, making it difficult to identify a control group. A range of "quasi-experimental" study designs are gaining credibility[13] and may constitute the "best available" evidence when an RCT is not possible.

Box 12.1 Efficacy vs. Effectiveness Trials

Efficacy trials

Defined as *"the extent to which a specific intervention […], produces a beneficial result under ideal conditions."*[8] Most published trials are efficacy rather than effectiveness trials. Efficacy trials are often required before proceeding to the relatively greater complexity and expense of effectiveness trials.

Effectiveness trials

Defined as *"a measure of the extent to which a specific intervention […], when deployed in the field in the usual circumstances, does what it is intended to do for a specified population."*[8]

Compared to efficacy trials, effectiveness studies are usually set in routine health care or community settings, with broader eligibility criteria for participation, outcome measures more closely tied to the priorities of patients and healthcare providers, and longer periods of follow-up that more closely reflect usual clinical practice.[68] Effectiveness trials have greater generalizability, although this can compromise their internal validity.

Box 12.2 Evidence-Based and Best Evidence Guidelines

The Cochrane Database of Systematic Reviews:
   http://www.thecochranelibrary.com/view/0/index.html
   The National Institute for Health and Clinical Excellence guidance for mental health and behavioral conditions:
   http://www.nice.org.uk/guidance/index.jsp?action=byTopic&o=7281#/search/?reload
   The World Health Organization's (WHO) Mental Health Gap Action Programme Evidence Resource Center:
   http://www.who.int/mental_health/mhgap/evidence/en/index.html

---

Where the existing evidence base is lacking, either due to an absence of studies or to studies of a poor quality, it may still be possible, and indeed necessary, to make recommendations based on the best available evidence. Rigorous and systematic methods of dealing with such an evidence gap do exist; for example, the Grading of Recommendations Assessment, Development and Evaluation (GRADE) approach used recently by the WHO[14] (see Box 12.3).

The hierarchy of evidence (Figure 12.1) has been criticised as too narrow a formulation of what constitutes evidence.[15] A complementary form of evidence has been proposed; that is, "practice-based evidence," which draws on the experience of service users, caregivers, and health workers who have accumulated expertise in managing health conditions in real-life settings.[15] Generation of practice-based evidence makes use of participatory methods involving the key stakeholders. The practice-based-evidence approach ensures that research is closely tied to local realities and addresses the pertinent research questions for the setting, thus increasing the potential for uptake of research findings. However, practice-based evidence is more susceptible to bias than evidence derived from RCTs, and this needs to be taken into account when interpreting findings from this study type.

Box 12.3 Applying GRADE to WHO's mental health Gap Action Programme Implementation Guide (MIG)[14]

The Grading of Recommendations Assessment, Development, and Evaluation (GRADE) methodology for developing MIG involved the following steps:

1. Establishing a Guideline Development Group that was multi-disciplinary, representative of different country settings, appropriately gender balanced, and checked for potential conflicts of interest.
2. Developing scoping questions to guide searches for systematic reviews and relevant primary studies, and defining the relevant outcomes.
3. Conducting systematic reviews according to established protocols.
4. Aggregating and evaluating the evidence from these systematic reviews, with explicit criteria for grading the study's quality and the strength of recommendation.
5. Systematically and transparently applying criteria to include consideration of values, preferences, and feasibility in formulating the final guidelines.

Limitations of the GRADE approach included the exclusion of evidence from non-randomized studies, concern about the reliability of application of quality-evaluation criteria, and possible bias in selecting acceptable measures of predefined outcomes.

The main advantage of the GRADE approach was to maximize applicability of the existing evidence base and identify the best available evidence for low- and middle-income country settings, despite the dearth of studies actually conducted in these settings.

Feasibility

It is critically important that an intervention be not just efficacious, but also feasible to implement. In LAMICs in particular, but also in high-income countries, there is a shortage of mental health professionals to deliver specialized interventions.[16] Therefore, interventions delivered by, for example, psychiatrists, may be of limited applicability in LAMIC settings. Task-sharing between specialists and general health workers can enable some MNS disorder interventions to be delivered in primary or general health care settings, but the feasibility of this approach needs rigorous evaluation (see Chapter 10). Sustainability also challenges the implementation of interventions. Account needs to be taken of the burden on health workers, both in terms of the time available to deliver an intervention and the emotional burden that can lead to burnout.[17,18] High staff turnover in health facilities can also undermine implementation.[19] Certain interventions are only feasible where appropriate laboratory services are readily available and affordable. For example, the mood-stabilizer lithium is a highly effective treatment for bipolar disorder, but it can only be used safely when it is possible to carry out regular blood tests to monitor the plasma level of the medication.

Equity

The principle of equity needs to be considered in relation to the population groups who can benefit from a given intervention for an MNS disorder. Population groups who are already disadvantaged, often those most burdened by MNS disorders, are frequently excluded from effective interventions because of difficulties in accessing care.[20] Particularly vulnerable groups may include, depending on the context, the poor, those with low levels of education, the elderly, young people, women, the homeless, refugees, prisoners and those in rural communities. Barriers to care are manifold, relating in part to a lack of supply of appropriate and acceptable care, and in part to difficulty with access or a lack of demand for care.

Supply side issues arise because of an inequitable distribution of mental health services and trained professionals, seen starkly when comparing high-income countries and LAMICs, but also when comparing rural and urban areas within countries.[16] Integration of mental health care into primary and general health care services is one way to overcome the chronic shortage of mental health professionals and improve access by bringing care closer to home; thus reducing the financial burden of transportation and lost working time, and facilitating access for the poor.[6] However, this strategy requires that interventions for MNS disorders be developed for delivery by these kinds of non-specialist professionals or lay health workers. Examples of this approach to treatment development are emerging,[21–23] but more needs to be done.[24]

Lack of demand for biomedical MNS interventions relates to factors such as stigma, low levels of service-user empowerment and incompatible sociocultural beliefs. Poorly developed services and unreliable supplies of drugs are key deterrents of the use of biomedical services. When interventions are developed and evaluated, the impact of these factors on equitable access needs to be addressed.

The critical role of social determinants of health, and indeed mental health, in propagating health inequalities has been emphasized.[25] In terms of global mental health, this broadens our focus from purely medical interventions for MNS disorders to considering the critical role of wider social environments. The WHO's 2010 publication emphasizing the need for persons with MNS disorders to be prioritized for inclusion in development activities (for example, livelihood schemes) illustrates this much-needed focus on social interventions.[26] However, although social inclusion and equitable access to community resources for persons with MNS disorders are desirable goals in and of themselves, there is a need for formal evaluation and adaptation of such programs in order to maximize the beneficial impact.[27]

Acceptability

Another key consideration that goes beyond the evidence base for an intervention is its acceptability. Two important aspects of acceptability relate to the sociocultural acceptability of the intervention and the contextual relevance of what the intervention is able to achieve.

Sociocultural Acceptability

There is understandable concern about the uncritical extrapolation of evidence obtained in a high-income, Western country setting to a non-Western LAMIC setting.[28] The sociocultural context affects the way in which MNS disorders are conceptualized, the preferred patterns of help-seeking behavior, the means of communication of disorder to others and detection of symptoms, the intervention delivery mechanisms, and, potentially, the effectiveness of interventions for MNS disorders. In many LAMICs, the presumed causes of psychosis, bipolar disorder and epilepsy are located within the supernatural realm, including, for example, spirit or demon possession, bewitchment, the work of an evil eye or ancestral spirits.[29] Partly as a consequence, help-seeking tends to be directed to non-health settings, such as religious or traditional healers. The persistent popularity of traditional and religious healing approaches to mental disorders attests to their sociocultural acceptability;[30] however, some healing practices have been considered abusive and may not be so acceptable to persons with mental disorders who are the recipients of such interventions.[31] Furthermore, illness attributions are not the only drivers of help-seeking behavior,[32] and it is important to recognize the non-availability of alternative therapeutic options in many LAMIC settings. Provision of biomedical interventions for psychosis and epilepsy in rural Ethiopia has stimulated demand and reduced stigma, even without extensive awareness-raising activities, due to the perceived effectiveness of the intervention within the population.[33]

Therefore, neither acceptability nor non-acceptability of an intervention can be assumed, whether biomedical or based on traditional healing practices, and this needs to be assessed carefully as part of pre-evaluation exploratory work within the community.

Individuals may accept greater deviance of interventions from their illness attribution models for severe mental disorders (for example, psychosis and bipolar disorder) compared to common mental disorders, such as depression. Indeed, often the symptoms of common mental disorders are not considered to constitute a disorder or illness, instead being attributed to psychosocial stressors,[34] in which case a medical model of intervention may be unacceptable. Although this pattern is observable in high-income countries[35] as well as LAMIC settings,[34,36] individualization of pathology and intervention may be less acceptable in traditional, non-industrialized societies that are characterized by strong social interconnectedness.[34] The largely Western theoretical models of psychological dysfunction underlying therapeutic interventions cannot be assumed to be transferable to non-Western settings. However, adaptation of these effective interventions to other cultural contexts may be possible: for example, by identifying the thinking styles and problem-solving approaches used by rural women in Pakistan, cognitive behavioral therapy principles were adapted successfully for that setting.[37]

Initial development and adaptation work for three trials of psychological interventions for common mental disorders in LAMIC settings found that the acceptability of the intervention was influenced by several factors: (a) pragmatic considerations; for example, the cost and inconvenience of repeated attendance at a health facility;[38] (b) the stigma of receiving a mental health-specific treatment;[37] and (c) a preference for medication when attending a health facility.[38] Other necessary adaptations common to each of the interventions including improving the clarity of language and content (being careful to avoid jargon terms), using visual guides for therapists and patients, using contextually appropriate ways of conveying the model of psychotherapy (for example, religious idioms), and more actively involving family members or other supports of importance to the patient's social world.[39]

Contextually Acceptable Outcomes

Development and piloting of a psychological intervention for maternal depression in Pakistan revealed that the intervention would have greater acceptability if oriented towards improving the health of the infant rather than that of the mother.[37] Subsequent evaluation of the psychological intervention assessed its impact on the child's health, as well as maternal mental health, finding that the intervention reduced infant diarrheal episodes, increased immunization take-up, and increased use of contraception as well as reducing maternal depression.[23] Another example is a trial of group interpersonal psychotherapy for depression conducted in Uganda, in which functional and symptom outcome scales were adapted to suit the cultural context.[21] Demonstrating the effectiveness of an intervention for an MNS disorder with respect to such outcomes as public health priorities, poverty reduction, improved social and interpersonal functioning, and decreasing human rights abuses is necessary to establish the acceptability of a intervention or otherwise. However, most RCTs tend to focus on demonstrating reductions in the clinical manifestations of disorder in an individual.

Affordability

An intervention for an MNS disorder may be effective, feasible, equitable, and acceptable, but it also needs to be affordable. Affordability includes costs that are borne by the affected individuals and their caregivers, as well as costs to the broader health system. Both direct and indirect costs need to be taken into account. Direct costs—for example, the out-of-pocket costs of registering with a health facility and purchasing prescribed medication—are usually outweighed by indirect costs; for example, arising when an affected person is unable to work, or their caregiver loses income when they miss work so that they can provide care. Interventions can be compared on their cost-effectiveness; that is, the health effect gained for a given level of cost. For example, meta-analyses have shown that the newer second-generation antipsychotic medications are no more efficacious that the first-generation antipsychotic medications in treating schizophrenia[40] and have a similar tolerability, but are substantially costlier, making them a less cost-effective treatment overall, particularly in resource-poor settings.[41] As part of the Disease Control in Developing Countries Project,[40] the cost-effectiveness (cost per disability-adjusted life-year [DALY] averted per million population) of treatments for schizophrenia, bipolar disorder, depression, and panic disorder, was compared, enabling the authors to make recommendations about the most appropriate interventions for low-resource settings. This approach has since been replicated and extended to also summarize evidence for the cost-effectiveness of interventions for alcohol use disorders and child developmental disorders.[2]

INTERVENTIONS FOR PRIORITY MNS DISORDERS

The preceding discussion has examined the principles against which interventions for MNS disorders need to be measured. We will now introduce the main types of interventions used for MNS disorders in general. After this, we will present the recommended interventions for the WHO's priority MNS disorders based on the best available evidence, focusing on interventions that can be delivered by non-specialists in general health care settings.

The Biopsychosocial Approach to Intervention

The "biopsychosocial" formulation is a holistic framework that seeks to understand why a particular MNS disorder has occurred in a specific individual at a particular moment in time by looking at the likely interplay between biological, psychological and social factors [42] (see Chapter 7). This approach may be contrasted with the public health perspective that looks at reducing risk exposures across a whole population to reduce the overall incidence of a disorder, rather than focusing on the causes of disorder in affected individuals.[43] Following on from the biopsychosocial approach, interventions can also be usefully grouped into biological (for the most part pharmacological), psychological and social categories, and tailored to an individual's needs. Such an approach, combined with sensitivity to the preferences of the affected individual, allows for a "patient-centered" approach to treatment, which has been shown to be associated with better outcomes for a range of chronic conditions, including MNS disorders.[44]

A brief description of the main types of pharmacological, psychological, and social interventions now follows.

Pharmacological Interventions

One component of the treatment of MNS disorders is the use of pharmacotherapy. The main classes of medication are: antidepressants, antipsychotics, mood-stabilizers, anti-epileptics, anxiolytics, and anti-Parkinsonian medications. Medications from each of these classes are included in the WHO's model list of essential medications,[45] which provides a recommended minimum set of medications that should be available in any country. (See Box 12.4.) Even this basic set of medications may not be available reliably outside of specialist centers within LAMICs.

Psychological Interventions

First-line psychological interventions First-line psychological interventions can be delivered by non-specialists with minimal prior mental health experience. Two examples are psychological first aid and psychoeducation.

Psychological first aid is an intervention for community members that aims to improve their knowledge and understanding of mental disorders, reduce stigmatizing attitudes and equip people with simple skills to help those with mental disorders: to assess risk of suicide or self-harm, listen non-judgementally, give reassurance and information, encourage help-seeking from professionals and use self-help techniques.[46] The premise is that everybody should have these skills to use in mental health emergencies, in the same way that people learn how to apply basic first aid to medical emergencies.

Psychoeducation is an intervention for patients and caregivers designed to improve their understanding of the mental disorder, its treatment and the measures the affected person can take to maximize their chances of recovery. The aim is to effect behavioral

---

Box 12.4 WHO's Model List of Essential Medications[45]

Antidepressants

Amitriptyline and clomipramine (tricyclic antidepressants)
Fluoxetine (selective serotonin-reuptake inhibitor)

Antipsychotics

Chlorpromazine, haloperidol and fluphenazine (first-generation antipsychotics)

Anti-epileptics

Diazepam (benzodiazepine)
Phenobarbitone
Phenytoin
Sodium valproate
Carbamazepine

Mood-stabilizers

Lithium
Sodium valproate
Carbamazepine

Anxiolytic

Diazepam

Anti-Parkinsonian

Biperiden

change: for example, improved adherence to medication, which is associated with better outcome.

Structured, brief psychological therapies Structured, brief therapies are time-limited and usually manualized to ensure fidelity to the treatment model. Examples of brief, structured psychological interventions include cognitive behavioral therapy, behavioral activation, interpersonal psychotherapy, problem-solving therapy and relaxation therapy. Most of these therapies are used in the management of depressive and anxiety disorders but are also effective in bipolar disorder, reducing some of the symptoms of schizophrenia and in substance abuse.

Compared to first-line psychological interventions, these more formal psychological therapies are built on psychological theories of mental disorder, require more therapist training, and are usually delivered by mental health specialists or non-specialists with a higher level of specialist supervision.

Cognitive behavioral therapy (CBT) is based on a model of mental disorder where negative cognitions (thoughts) about self, the world and the future, and associated maladaptive behaviors, can lead to and maintain emotional distress.[47] The therapy involves helping the person identify where their thinking processes are faulty, challenge the assumptions underlying their negative thinking and change their behavior (e.g., overcome social withdrawal or avoidance of situations). Behavioral activation (BA) is one component of CBT that can also be used as an independent method of therapy. BA is focused on encouraging the person to actively structure their time, reintroduce daily routine where this has been lost and, most important, increase their exposure to potentially pleasurable experiences.[48] Studies indicate that BA is as effective as CBT, yet relatively more straightforward to deliver, making this a promising therapy for low-resource contexts.[49]

Interpersonal psychotherapy (IPT) is a structured, time-limited brief psychological intervention that focuses on the interpersonal context of depression.[50] Four types of interpersonal difficulty are thought to be of particular significance for developing depression: grief, interpersonal disputes, role transitions (for example, motherhood, retirement) and interpersonal deficits (for example, social isolation and loneliness). The therapy aims to improve interpersonal communication and decision-making in relation to the problem area and thus alleviate symptoms.[51]

Problem-solving therapy (PST) requires less training than either CBT or IPT and is briefer.[52] The aim is to help patients to mobilize their existing skills and resources to tackle psychosocial stressors that are contributing to their mental health problems. Problem solving is structured into the following stages: clarification and definition of problems, choice of achievable goals, generation of solutions, choice of preferred solutions, implementation of preferred solutions and evaluation.

Relaxation techniques include progressive muscle relaxation training,[53] autogenic training[54] (a method of inducing relaxation through repetition of set phrases and visualizations), use of relaxation imagery, biofeedback and techniques from meditation and yoga. An advantage of relaxation therapies is that, once learned, the techniques can be used by the person independently of professional supervision. Furthermore, relaxation therapy can be delivered by appropriately trained non-specialists, and even by non–health workers.

Social Interventions

Social difficulties may be a cause or consequence of mental disorder. Various forms of social adversity, including poverty, poor housing, intimate-partner violence, interpersonal conflict and social isolation, are established risk factors for development of a range of mental disorders. Social consequences of mental disorders commonly include stigma, discrimination and abuse, social exclusion, social withdrawal and loss of skills or community roles (see Chapter 7). Strong social support can increase a person's resistance to developing mental disorder and facilitate their recovery from illness.

Basic social interventions for persons with MNS disorders include providing support to address the person's social difficulties, for example, by facilitating support from non-health sector organizations (housing, employment, education); helping the person to (re)activate social support networks with family and within the community; and encouraging engagement with support groups oriented to their particular need (for example, Alcoholics Anonymous for alcohol-use disorders, or grass-roots advocacy and livelihood groups for persons recovering from severe mental disorder[55]). For longer-term MNS conditions associated with residual impairments, social skills training, supported employment and supported housing can be beneficial, if available. Social interventions to promote the human rights of persons affected by MNS disorders and to counter stigma and discrimination, are included within the remit of the health professional, often working in collaboration with other agencies; for example, to reduce child abuse through raising community awareness.

Two important social models of intervention for mental disorders are the recovery model[56,57] and community-based rehabilitation.[58] Each will now be described in detail.

The recovery model The concept of "recovery" within the recovery model goes beyond the widely understood concept of a person's getting back to normal after a period of ill health. Although the majority of persons affected by mental disorders will recover in this sense, a proportion of people, particularly those affected by psychosis, bipolar disorder and severe depression, may not experience full clinical remission. In such cases, recovery may take on a different complexion, as articulated by Deegan (1996): "The goal of recovery is not to become normal. The goal is to embrace the human vocation of becoming more deeply, more fully human." To put it another way, "recovery" is a "personal process of learning how to live, and how to live well, with enduring symptoms and vulnerabilities."[57] It has been argued that this represents a paradigm shift from a medical model of chronic illness that tends to dwell on deficits and disabilities, to a more optimistic and holistic conceptualization of well-being,[57] although the distinction may be overstated.[59] Practical consequences of a recovery approach to mental disorder may include a lesser emphasis on the clinical goal of symptom-control and more focus on enabling a person affected by severe mental disorder to find meaning and hope in their life in whatever way is meaningful to them.

Community-based rehabilitation (CBR) CBR is a form of community and multi-sectoral mobilization aimed at improving the quality of life of people with disabilities, including those arising from MNS disorders, by helping them meet their basic needs and participate fully in society.[58] WHO has developed a set of guidelines for CBR, covering the domains of health, education, livelihoods, social needs, and empowerment. Feasibility and acceptability of the CBR approach, as well as beneficial functional outcomes, have been demonstrated for persons with chronic psychosis in rural India.[60,61] International non-governmental organizations (NGOs) with a particular interest in CBR for persons with mental disorders include BasicNeeds (http://www.basicneeds.org/, accessed 02/17/2012) and CBM (http://www.cbmuk.org.uk/, accessed 02/17/2012).

BEST AVAILABLE EVIDENCE: THE WHO MIG

As described in Box 12.3, using the GRADE approach,[14] the WHO conducted a rigorous, systematic and transparent evaluation of the existing evidence base for interventions for priority MNS disorders delivered in non-specialist settings, culminating in development of a series of evidence-based guidelines.[4] These guidelines are summarized for each of the priority MNS disorders in Tables 12.1 to 12.8.

As can be seen in Tables 12.1 to 12.8, the evidence base is sufficient to be able to recommend a range of pharmacological, psychological and social interventions for each priority MNS disorder. The MIG provides a powerful tool for global efforts to reduce the treatment gap for MNS disorders.

The process of deciding on the quality of evidence to support the effectiveness, feasibility, equity, acceptability and affordability of treatment interventions for priority disorder is detailed on the WHO's website: http://www.who.int/mental_health/mhgap/evidence/en/index.html (accessed 02/17/2012).

PACKAGES OF CARE

A complementary effort to the development of the WHO MIG was the publication of a series of papers that proposed packages of care for six priority MNS disorders; namely, schizophrenia (psychosis), epilepsy, depression, alcohol use disorders, dementia, and the child behavioral disorder "attention deficit hyperactivity disorder" (ADHD).[3] A *package of care* was defined as "a combination of treatments designed to improve the recognition and management of conditions to achieve optimal outcomes," and may be distinguished from the WHO MIG by a focus on mechanisms for delivery of interventions in addition to identification of effective treatments. Well-delineated packages of care are prerequisites for scaling up care within a health service (see Chapter 14). Tables 12.9 and 12.10 provide adapted summaries of the published packages of care, dividing out generic- and disorder-specific elements to the packages. Furthermore, for each disorder, two levels of package are presented, depending on the resources available. The terms "low-resource" and "better-resourced" are not synonymous with the terms "LAMICs" and "high-income countries." Instead, we wish to draw attention to the uneven distribution of resources within both high-income countries and LAMICs, such that both sets of packages may be applicable in both HICs and LAMICs.

The generic packages of interventions for MNS disorders (Table 12.9) include a number of common service delivery factors needed to support the implementation of disorder-specific evidence-based interventions. Increasing demand for services aims to increase public awareness and mental health literacy[62] and reduce stigma. For each disorder, training and screening to improve case-finding is required, although the setting and training intensity may vary; e.g., focusing on community settings for psychosis, epilepsy, dementia, and child developmental disorders, healthcare settings for common mental disorders and alcohol use disorders, and educational establishments for child behavioral disorders. The importance of integration of delivery of MNS interventions into general health care settings has already been alluded to, helping to overcome access issues, reduce stigma and improve the physical health care of persons with MNS disorders.[5] It is proposed that chronic disease models of care provide the appropriate framework within which to deliver MNS treatments. Two key elements of chronic disease models of care are a collaborative approach and the concept of stepped care. A collaborative care model recognizes that effective care is not something "delivered to" a passive recipient (the patient) by an individual health worker, but requires the active collaboration of patient, caregivers, general and specialist health workers, and workers from non-health sector organizations, all of whom bring their own expertise to the problem. Stepped-care models of care attempt to tailor disorder-specific treatments according to the severity of disorder and response to initial treatment. For example, in a model of stepped care for common mental disorders in India,[63] everybody received first-line

Table 12.1 Depression and Other Emotional or Medical Unexplained Symptoms: Summary of WHO mhGAP Guidelines for Evidence-Based Interventions in Non-Specialist Healthcare Settings[4]

Depression

Medications	• Tricyclic antidepressants (TCAs) and selective serotonin reuptake inhibitors (SSRIs) are equally effective for moderate–severe depression
Brief, structured psychological interventions	• Cognitive behavioral therapy (CBT), interpersonal psychotherapy (IPT), problem solving therapy (PST), and behavioral activation (BA)
Other psychosocial interventions	• Relaxation therapy • Physical exercise

Medically unexplained somatic complaints

Brief, structured psychological interventions	• Cognitive behavioral therapy

Panic and anxiety

Brief, structured psychological interventions	• Cognitive behavioral therapy
Other psychosocial interventions	• Relaxation therapy

Trauma-related complaints

Structured psychological interventions	• No evidence for routine, individual debriefing • Self-graded exposure based on cognitive behavioral therapy principles
Other psychosocial interventions	• Psychological first aid

Table 12.2 Self-Harm and Suicide: Summary of WHO mhGAP Guidelines for Evidence-Based Interventions in Non-Specialist Healthcare Settings[4]

Population prevention	• Restrict access to means of self-harm; e.g. pesticides, firearms • Reduce availability of alcohol to reduce harmful use • Responsible reporting of suicide by the media
Assessment	• Screening for thoughts, plans, or acts of self-harm in persons at risk

Management	• In home and health care settings, restrict access to means of self harm or suicide, and provide close monitoring, while the individual has ideas, plans, or acts of self-harm,
	• Regular contact with health workers
	• Problem solving approach to underlying stressors
	• Facilitate social support
	• For imminent risk of serious self-harm:
	  o Urgent referral to specialist mental health services, if available,
	  o Mobilization of caregivers to ensure close monitoring
	  o Routine admission to a non-specialist inpatient unit not recommended

Table 12.3 Psychosis and Bipolar Disorder: Summary of WHO mhGAP Guidelines for Evidence-Based Interventions in Non-Specialist Healthcare Settings[4]

Medications for psychosis	

Antipsychotic medication	• Both first- (FGAs; haloperidol/chlorpromazine) and second-generation antipsychotics
	• Clozapine for treatment-resistant psychosis
	• In recurrent psychosis:
	  o Long-acting injectible antipsychotic medication (depot) if adherence is a problem
	  o Regular monitoring of symptom relief, functioning, and adverse effects

Anticholinergic medication to counteract antipsychotic side-effects	• Not for routine use: only for severe and acute extra-pyramidal side effects when dose reduction/medication change is ineffective
Medications for bipolar disorder	
Medication for mania in bipolar disorder	• Antipsychotic medication (FGA or SGA) • Mood-stabilizers lithium, valproate, or carbamazepine • (Lithium should only be started where appropriate monitoring systems are in place)
Maintenance treatment of bipolar disorder	• Lithium or valproate are the first choices • Maintenance treatment for at least two years following the last episode • Lithium and valproate to be avoided in pregnancy and breastfeeding
Antidepressants for bipolar depression	• Antidepressants for moderate–severe depression in bipolar disorder, but only when prescribed with a mood-stabilizer. SSRIs preferred to TCAs.
Psychosocial interventions for psychosis and bipolar disorder	
Psychological therapies	• Psychoeducation • Cognitive behavioral therapy (CBT) and family interventions
Psychosocial strategies to increase independence	• Multi-sectoral psychosocial interventions to improve independent living skills • Social skills training • Supported housing and other housing arrangements
Interventions to increase vocational and economic inclusion	• Linking with formal and informal sectors to promote involvement in vocational and economic opportunities • Supported employment
Strategies to improve community attitudes	• Activities to improve attitudes and reduce stigma, ensuring stakeholder involvement and direct contact with persons with mental disorder

psychological interventions (psychoeducation), but antidepressant therapy and structured psychological therapies (IPT) were reserved for those with moderate-to-severe disorders, or those not responding to first-line interventions. Involvement of a mental health specialist was indicated at any time if there was concern about suicide risk, but otherwise was restricted to patients not responding to lower levels of intervention. The

Table 12.4 Epilepsy: Summary of WHO mhGAP Guidelines for Evidence-Based Interventions in Non-Specialist Healthcare Settings[4]

Acute management of seizures	
Convulsive seizures/ status epilepticus	No intravenous (IV) access: • Rectal (not intramuscular; IM) diazepam is most effective. • Phenobarbitone (IM) only recommended when rectal diazepam not possible IV access: • IV benzodiazepines; lorazepam preferred to diazepam • If ineffective, IV phenobarbitone or phenytoin
Febrile seizures in children	Simple febrile seizures: • Can be effectively managed by non-specialists • Follow Integrated Management of Childhood Illness guidelines for fever • 24-hour observation • No evidence for prophylaxis with antipyretics or anticonvulsant medication Complex febrile seizures: • Inpatient observation and secondary level care for specialist investigations of central nervous system pathology; e.g. lumbar puncture • Prophylactic intermittent diazepam if prolonged or recurrent
First, unprovoked seizure	• No indication for routine use of anti-epileptic medications • If high risk of recurrence, specialist review before starting anti-epileptic medication
Diagnosis and non-acute management of convulsive epilepsy	
Diagnosis	• Non-specialist health workers can (and should) be trained to diagnose convulsive epilepsy • Electroencephalogram (EEG) and neuroimaging are not recommended for routine use in non-specialized settings: medication can be started on basis of clinical presentation • EEG and neuroimaging can be useful for diagnosis in specialist settings with appropriate expertise; e.g., for people with risk factors for treatable causes of epilepsy • If both are available, neuroimaging using MRI* is preferred to CT[†]
Treatment with anti-epileptic medications	• Monotherapy with any standard anti-epileptic medication (carbamazepine, phenobarbitone, phenytoin, valproate) • Carbamazepine preferred for partial onset epilepsy • Consider discontinuing after two seizure-free years
Anti-epileptic medications in women of child-bearing age	• Monotherapy using the minimum dose is recommended, avoiding valproate if possible • Folic acid should always be co-prescribed • Standard advice on breastfeeding should be followed (for carbamazepine, phenobarbitone, phenytoin and valproate)
Anti-epileptic medications in intellectual disability	• Where possible, valproate and carbamazepine are preferred due to lower adverse behavioral side-effects

Table 12.4 Continued

Psychological interventions	• Relaxation therapy, interventions based on cognitive behavioral therapy principles, psychoeducation, and family counselling as adjunctive treatments • Information and advice should be given on avoidance of high-risk activities and first-aid interventions

* MRI: magnetic resonance imaging

† CT: computerized tomography

advantages of a stepped-care approach include improved efficiency and, therefore, increased health system capacity to treat more affected persons, as well as increased responsiveness to the individual's needs.

As part of *Lancet's* first series on global mental health, costing basic packages of care for selected priority MNS disorders enabled a "call for action" to scale up mental health care to be issued.[64] It was estimated that scaling up the basic packages of mental health care would cost US$2 per person per year in low-income and US$3–$4 per person per year in lower-middle-income countries, which was relatively low compared to costs of scaling up packages of care for other public health priorities in these settings. In a recent modeling of costs for five priority disorders across 44 interventions,[65] the cost-effectiveness values ranged from $Int 100–250 to $Int 10,000–25,000 for a year of healthy life gained. For the African sub-region, the most cost-effective strategies related to population-based alcohol

Table 12.5 Alcohol Use Disorders: Summary of WHO mhGAP Guidelines for Evidence-Based Interventions in Non-Specialist Healthcare Settings[4]

Hazardous and harmful use

Screening and brief interventions	• Screening (using a brief, validated instrument if feasible) and brief interventions for hazardous or harmful alcohol use

Dependence

Withdrawal	• Supported withdrawal, in an inpatient setting if dependence is severe • 3–7 days of treatment with a reducing dose of long-acting benzodiazepines to alleviate withdrawal symptoms and prevent seizures and delirium • No evidence for antipsychotic medication alone in managing withdrawal or withdrawal-related delirium • Withdrawal-related seizures or delirium should be treated with benzodiazepines • Thiamine should be prescribed routinely; IM or IV for 3 days if at high risk of Wernicke's encephalopathy • IM or IV thiamine, twice daily, is recommended for treatment of Wernicke's encephalopathy
Preventing relapse	• Acamprosate, disulfiram, or naltrexone when part of an overall treatment program, with appropriate monitoring • Psychosocial support to both patient and caregiver • Structured psychological therapies where available (e.g., motivational enhancement therapy [MET]) • Mutual-help groups for both patients and caregivers

Table 12.6 Drug Use Disorders: Summary of WHO mhGAP Guidelines for Evidence-Based Interventions in Non-Specialist Healthcare Settings[4]

Cannabis and psychostimulant use	• Brief psychosocial interventions • Short psychological treatments, based on MET • Withdrawal in a supportive environment • Relief of withdrawal symptoms with symptomatic medication • If depression or psychosis symptoms develop, close monitoring and specialist referral are required • No indication for dexamphetamine use for psychostimulant withdrawal
Benzodiazepine dependence	• Planned withdrawal if possible. A tapering regime of long-acting benzodiazepines over a period of 8 to 12 weeks, augmented by psychosocial support • Specialist advice for inpatient care of sudden or severe withdrawal • Physical or psychiatric comorbidity is an indication for inpatient withdrawal
Injecting drug use	• Facilitate access to sterile injecting equipment • In high prevalence areas, outreach activities to provide sterile injecting equipment, information, health care, and facilitate entry into drug treatment programs

control and for the Southeast Asian sub-region it related to primary care treatment of epilepsy. The estimated cumulative cost per capita for the most cost-effective interventions for all five conditions was estimated at $Int 4.90–5.70. (See Chapter 14 for a fuller discussion on scaling up packages of care for MNS disorders.)

EVIDENCE FOR TRADITIONAL HEALING INTERVENTIONS

Descriptive reports have indicated benefits of traditional and religious healer interventions for MNS disorders, but in general there is an absence of evidence on which to judge the effectiveness of their interventions and whether or not they are associated with harm. For example, temple healing in southern India was found to be associated with a diminution of symptoms in persons with severe mental disorders,[66] but without a comparison group it is not known whether the symptoms would have remitted spontaneously. Similarly, traditional healers were trained in counseling techniques in Uganda,[55] but detail on the nature of their counseling intervention and its effectiveness compared to other treatments of known efficacy has not been reported. In Uganda, persons with severe mental disorder who were attending a traditional healer were followed up.[30] In those receiving biomedical interventions in addition to traditional healing, the outcomes were better three months, but worse at six months, compared to those receiving either traditional or biomedical interventions in isolation. Given the dearth of mental health professionals in LAMICs available to deliver biomedical interventions, and the broad acceptability of traditional and religious healing approaches to mental disorders, many have argued for collaborative models of care to be developed. However, this recommendation has rarely progressed to become a reality, and one important reason for this has been the lack of evidence to support this approach. More evidence from methodologically

Table 12.7 Dementia: Summary of WHO mhGAP Guidelines for Evidence-Based Interventions in Non-Specialist Healthcare Settings[4]

Diagnosis in non-specialist health settings	• Training in use of brief cognitive screens, informant history-taking, and detection of other causes of cognitive decline • Initial medical review, repeated six-monthly • Sensitive communication of diagnosis, where appropriate, coupled with information and commitment of ongoing care and support
Cognitive symptoms	• Cholinesterase inhibitors for mild–moderate Alzheimer's disease, with adequate supervision and support • Memantine for moderate–severe Alzheimer's disease, with adequate supervision and support • Cognitive interventions: reality orientation, cognitive stimulation, reminiscence therapy
Behavioral and psychological symptoms	• Medical review to exclude underlying medical causes • Antidepressants (SSRIs) for moderate–severe depression • Short-term use of haloperidol or second-generation antipsychotic medications when risk of imminent harm and severe, distressing symptoms • Avoid thioridazine, chlorpromazine, and trazadone
Caregiver interventions	• Psychoeducation • Training in management of behavioral symptoms • Screening and intervention for carer strain (support, counselling, cognitive behavioral therapy principles) and depression • Home-based respite care

sound studies is needed before traditional or religious approaches to treating MNS disorders can be recommended.

FUTURE DIRECTIONS

Balanced against the suffering, disability, impaired quality of life, poorer physical health, reduced survival and impoverishment of persons with undetected and untreated MNS disorders, the existing evidence base provides strong justification for advocating interventions for priority MNS disorders worldwide. This is not the same as saying that the currently recommended interventions and delivery mechanisms are fully optimal or directly applicable in all settings. In the process of developing the WHO MIG, significant gaps in the evidence base, particularly for evaluations of treatments in LAMICs, and poor quality of available evidence in other areas, meant that the consensus of experts played a role in deciding which treatments should be recommended. Three areas, in particular, stand out as requiring further concerted effort to improve the quality and applicability of the existing evidence base.

First, it is essential to ensure that interventions are contextually appropriate; for example, by incorporating medical pluralism into the health care plan and, where possible, adapting interventions to suit explanatory models of illness. Second, as this chapter has emphasized, there is extensive evidence about which interventions should be used for priority MNS disorders, but much less is known about the most effective, equitable,

Table 12.8 Child and Adolescent Developmental and Behavioral Disorders: Summary of WHO mhGAP Guidelines for Evidence-Based Interventions in Non-Specialist Healthcare Settings[4]

Child development and developmental disorders	
Improving child development	• Integrate monitoring of child development into existing maternal and child health programs • Parenting interventions promoting mother–infant interactions for at-risk children (e.g., due to under-nutrition, recurrent illness) • Detect and treat maternal depression or other mental, neurological or behavioral disorder
Management of developmental disorders	• Asses delay using brief, locally validated measures • Clinical assessment to identify common causes of intellectual disability (ID), with specialist supervision • Support and refer to community-based rehabilitation programs • Parent skills training
Child emotional disorders	
Depression	• Antidepressants should not be used in children aged 12 years or younger • For adolescents (older than 12 years), fluoxetine may be used, with monitoring of suicidal ideation and specialist supervision
Anxiety disorders	• Non-specialists should avoid pharmacological interventions
Somatoform disorders	• Non-specialists should avoid pharmacological interventions • Brief psychological treatments; e.g., cognitive behavioral therapy • Active involvement of specialists
Any emotional disorder	• Parent skills training for parents of newborn to 7-year-old children
Child behavioral disorders	
Attention-deficit hyperactivity disorder (ADHD)	• Psychosocial interventions are first-line (parent education/training, social skills training) • Second line: methylphenidate (supervision and monitoring)
Conduct disorder, disruptive behavior disorder, or oppositional defiant disorder	• Non-specialists should avoid pharmacological interventions
Psychosocial interventions	• Parent skills training for parents of newborn to 7-year-olds
Prevention and promotion	
Preventing child abuse	• Home visiting and parental education for at-risk families • Collaboration with school-based "sexual abuse prevention" programs
Promoting mental health	• Collaborate and support school-based life skills programs

Table 12.9 Cross-Cutting Packages of Interventions for Priority Disorders in Low- and High-Resource Settings (modified from PLoS Medicine series)[3]

	All settings	
Cross-cutting interventions and delivery mechanisms for all disorders	<ul><li>Increase demand for services (improve mental health literacy in community, reduce stigma in all settings)</li><li>Improve case-finding (training and screening)</li><li>Improve access (integrate in all health care settings)</li><li>Adapt model of service delivery (collaborative and stepped care)</li><li>Deliver simple psychosocial interventions (psychoeducation, psychological first aid, support adherence to treatments, facilitate access to social support)</li><li>Ensure due attention is given to physical health care</li><li>Multi-sectoral collaboration to improve functional outcomes</li><li>Advocacy for better mental health care</li></ul>	
	Low-resource settings	**Better-resourced settings**
Cross-cutting interventions for CMDs/Alcohol	<ul><li>Case-finding through improved awareness and screening in health care settings</li><li>Diagnosis by nurse or clinical officer in primary health care setting</li></ul>	<ul><li>Routine or high-risk screening linked to confirmation of diagnosis by skilled clinician</li><li>Diagnosis by trained general doctor or mental health specialist</li></ul>
Cross-cutting interventions for SMDs/epilepsy/ dementia	<ul><li>Community case-finding (house-to-house surveys, use of key informants)</li><li>Initial diagnosis by nurse or clinical officer in primary health care setting</li><li>Continuity of support coordinated by primary care case manager</li></ul>	<ul><li>Detection by professionals in a range of settings, including health, housing, social care, justice system</li><li>Diagnosis by mental health/ neurology specialist</li><li>Continuity of support coordinated by specialist case manager</li></ul>

feasible, acceptable and affordable ways in which evidence-based interventions should be delivered in different health systems and sociocultural settings. Implementation evidence is a priority research goal (see also Chapter 19). Third, even though effective (and cost-effective) treatments exist for the priority MNS disorders, for many disorders the size of effect is relatively weak. For example, even with optimal care, less than 50% of people with schizophrenia make a good recovery, in both high-income countries and LAMICs.[67] The need for further research into newer, more effective pharmacological, psychological and social interventions is pressing.[24] A global mental health perspective on interventions for MNS disorders may yield gains in this respect, by identifying risk factors (and potential interventions) associated with better or worse prognoses in different settings. Similarly, mapping the approaches of traditional healers across cultural settings could lead to novel insights, which can expand the armamentarium of evidence-based interventions relevant to global mental health.

Table 12.10 Disorder-Specific Packages of Evidence-Based Interventions, in Addition to Cross-Cutting Interventions (modified from PLoS Medicine series)[3]

	Low-resource settings	Better-resourced settings
Depression[69]	• Generic antidepressants • Problem-solving therapy • Increase social support	• Choice of antidepressants • Choice of brief psychological therapies • Befriending to prevent suicide • Electroconvulsive therapy
Alcohol use disorders[70]	• Brief advice, working up to extended brief intervention • Community-based treatment of withdrawal • Structured relapse-prevention in self-help groups • Disulfiram for relapse prevention (with family monitoring) • Population-level and selective preventive interventions	• Brief advice, working up to extended brief intervention • Treatment of withdrawal in community-based or specialized centers • Structured relapse-prevention in self-help groups • Specialized psychological and social interventions • Choice of medications for relapse prevention • Population-level and selective preventive interventions
Psychosis[71]	• First- or second-generation antipsychotics • Support for family groups • Community-based rehabilitation	• Choice of antipsychotics • Clozapine for treatment-resistant psychosis • Psychosocial family interventions • Assertive community treatment • Cognitive behavioral therapy • Supported employment • Wellness training
Epilepsy[72]	• Limited choice of cheap, generic anti-epileptic medications • Psychosocial support	• Wide choice of anti-epileptic medications • Structured, brief psychological therapies • Services for epilepsy surgery or ketogenic diet, where indicated

	Low-resource settings	Better-resourced settings
Dementia[73]	• Cautious use of antipsychotic medications for BPSD*, not as first-line treatment, preferably initiated and reviewed by specialists	• Cautious use of antipsychotic medications for BPSD, not as first-line treatment, and initiated and reviewed by specialists
	• SSRI antidepressants for moderate–severe depression, with specialist review	• SSRI antidepressants for moderate–severe depression, with specialist review
	• Caregiver support	• Caregiver support
		• Caregiver training in symptom management
		• Respite care for caregivers
		• Structured, brief psychological therapy if depression present in caregivers
		• Cholinesterase inhibitors, with specialist initiation and review
		• Structured cognitive interventions (e.g., cognitive stimulation)
Child behavioral disorder (Attention-Deficit Hyperactivity Disorder)[74]	• Methylphenidate • Behavioral interventions delivered by non-specialists	• Choice of medications • Behavioral interventions delivered by specialists and non-specialists

* BPSD: behavioral and psychological symptoms of dementia. Modified from PLoS Medicine series.[3]

REFERENCES

1. World Health Organization. *Mental health care in developing countries: A critical appraisal of research findings. Technical Report Series 698.* Geneva: WHO; 1984.
2. Patel V, Araya R, Chatterjee S, Chisholm D, Cohen A, De Silva M, et al. Global Mental Health 3: Treatment and prevention of mental disorders in low-income and middle-income countries. *Lancet.* 2007;370:991–1005.
3. Patel V, Thornicroft G. Packages of care for mental, neurological, and substance use disorders in low- and middle-income countries: PLoS Medicine Series. *PLoS Med.* 2009;6(10):e1000160.
4. World Health Organization. *Mental Health Gap Action Programme Implementation Guide (mhGAP-IG) for mental, neurological and substance use disorders in non-specialized health settings.* Geneva: WHO; 2010.
5. WHO and Wonca. *Integrating mental health into primary care. A global perspective.* Geneva: World Health Organization and World Organization of Family Doctors; 2008.
6. World Health Organization. *Mental health Gap Action Programme (mhGAP): Scaling up care for mental, neurological, and substance use disorders.* Geneva: WHO; 2008.
7. Moher D, Schulz KF, Altman DG, for the CONSORT Group. The CONSORT statement: revised recommendations for improving the quality of reports of parallel-group randomized trials. *Lancet.* 2001;357:1191–94.

8. Porta M, Last JM. *A dictionary of epidemiology*. New York: Oxford University Press; 2008.

9. Zwarenstein M, Treweek S, Gagnier JJ, Altman DG, Tunis S, Haynes B, et al. Improving the reporting of pragmatic trials: an extension of the CONSORT statement. *BMJ*. 2008;337:a2390. doi:10.1136/bmj.a2390.

10. Kohn R, Saxena S, Levav I, Saraceno B. The treatment gap in mental health care. *Bull WHO*. 2004;82:858–66.

11. Moher D, Cook DJ, Eastwood S, Olkin I, Rennie D, Stroup DF, et al. Improving the quality of reports of meta-analyses of randomized controlled trials: the QUOROM statement. *Lancet*. 1999;354:1896–900.

12. Appleby L, Warner R, Whitton A, Faragher B. A controlled study of fluoxetine and cognitive-behavioral counselling in the treatment of postnatal depression. *BMJ*. 1997;314:932–36.

13. Gilbody S, Whitty P. Improving the delivery and organisation of mental health services: beyond the conventional randomised controlled trial. *Br J Psychiatry*. 2002;180:13–8.

14. Barbui C, Dua T, van Ommeren M, Yasamy MT, Fleischmann A, Clark N, et al. Challenges in developing evidence-based recommendations using the GRADE approach: the case of mental, neurological, and substance use disorders. *PLoS Med*. 2010;7(8):e1000322.

15. Fox NJ. Practice-based evidence: towards collaborative and transgressive research. *Sociology*. 2003;37(1):81–102.

16. World Health Organization. *Mental health atlas 2011* Geneva: WHO; 2011.

17. Mateen FJ, Dorji C. Health-care worker burnout and the mental health imperative. *Lancet*. 2009;374(9690):595–97.

18. Petersen I. Comprehensive integrated primary mental health care for South Africa. Pipe dream or possibility? *Soc Sci Med*. 2000;51(3):321–34.

19. World Health Organization. *The World Health Report 2006—working together for health*. Geneva: WHO; 2006.

20. Saxena S, Thornicroft G, Knapp M, Whiteford H. Global mental health 2. Resources for mental health: scarcity, inequity, and inefficiency. *Lancet*. 2007;370:878–89.

21. Bolton P, Bass J, Neugebauer R, Verdeli H, Clougherty KF, Wickramaratne P, et al. Group interpersonal psychotherapy for depression in rural Uganda. *JAMA*. 2003;289:3117–24.

22. Patel V, Weiss HA, Chowdhary N, Naik S, Pednekar S, Chatterjee S, et al. Lay health worker led intervention for depressive and anxiety disorders in India: impact on clinical and disability outcomes over 12 months. *Br J Psychiatry*. 2011;199:459–66.

23. Rahman A, Malik A, Sikanderd S, Roberts C, Creed F. Cognitive behaviour therapy-based intervention by community health workers for mothers with depression and their infants in rural Pakistan: a cluster-randomised controlled trial. *Lancet*. 2008;372(9642):902–09.

24. Collins PY, Patel V, Joestl SS, March D, Insel TR, Daar AS, et al. Grand challenges in global mental health. *Nature*. 2011;475(7354):27–30.

25. Marmot M, Friel S, Bell R, Houweling TAJ, Taylor S. Closing the gap in a generation: health equity through action on the social determinants of health. *Lancet*. 2008;372(9650):1661–69.

26. World Health Organization, Mental Health and Poverty Project. *Mental health and development: Targeting people with mental health conditions as a vulnerable group*. Geneva: WHO; 2010.

27. Lund C, De Silva M, Plagerson S, Cooper S, Chisholm D, Das J, et al. Poverty and mental disorders: breaking the cycle in low-income and middle-income countries. *Lancet*. 2011:DOI:10.1016/S0140-6736(11)60754-X.

28. Summerfield D. How scientifically valid is the knowledge base of global mental health?. *BMJ*. 2008;336:992–94.

29. Patel V. Explanatory models of mental illness in sub-Saharan Africa. *Soc Sci Med*. 1995;40(9):1291–8.

30. Abbo C. Profiles and outcome of traditional healing practices for severe mental illnesses in two districts of Eastern Uganda. *Global Health Action*. 2011;4:DOI 10.3402/gha.v4i0.7117.

31. Freeman M, Motsei M. Planning health care in South Africa—is there a role for traditional healers? *Soc Sci Med*. 1992;32(11):1183–90.

32. Lambert H. Popular therapeutics and medical preferences in rural north India. *Lancet*. 1996;348:1706–09.

33. Shibre T, Alem A, Tekle-Haimanot R, Medhin G, Tessema A, Jacobsson L. Community attitudes towards epilepsy in a rural Ethiopian setting: a re-visit after 15 years. *Ethiopian Med J*. 2008;46(3):251–59.

34. Hanlon C, Whitley R, Wondimagegn D, Alem A, Prince M. Postnatal mental distress in relation to the sociocultural practices of childbirth: An exploratory qualitative study from Ethiopia. *Soc Sci Med.* 2009;69:1211–19.

35. Kessler D, Lloyd K, Lewis G, Gray DP. Cross sectional study of symptom attribution and recognition of depression and anxiety in primary care. *BMJ.* 1999;318:436–40.

36. Rodrigues M, Patel V, Jaswal S, de Souza N. Listening to mothers: qualitative studies on motherhood and depression from Goa, India. *Soc Sci Med.* 2003;57(10):1797–806.

37. Rahman A. Challenges and opportunities in developing a psychological intervention for perinatal depression in rural Pakistan—a multi-method study. *Arch Womens Ment Health.* 2007;10:211–19.

38. Chatterjee S, Chowdhary N, Pednekar S, Cohen A, Andrew G, Araya R, et al. Integrating evidence-based treatments for common mental disorders in routine primary care: feasibility and acceptability of the MANAS intervention in Goa, India. *World Psychiatry.* 2008;7:39–46.

39. Patel V, Chowdhary N, Rahman A, Verdeli H. Improving access to psychological treatments: lessons from developing countries. *Behav Res Ther.* 2011;49(9):523–28.

40. Geddes J, Freemantle N, Harrison P, Bebbington P, for the National Schizophrenia Guideline Development Group. Atypical antipsychotics in the treatment of schizophrenia: systematic overview and metaregression analysis. *BMJ.* 2000;321:1371–76.

41. Rosenheck RA, Leslie DL, Doshi JA. Second-generation antipsychotics: cost-effectiveness, policy options, and political decision making. *Psychiatr Serv.* 2008;59:515–20.

42. Engel GL. The need for a new medical model: A challenge for biomedicine. *Science.* 1977;196: 129–36.

43. Rose G. Sick individuals and sick populations. *Int J Epidemiol.* 1985;14(1):32–8.

44. Michie S, Miles J, Weinman J. Patient-centeredness in chronic illness: what is it and does it matter? *Patient Educ Couns.* 2003;51:197–206.

45. World Health Organization. *WHO model list of essential medications.* 17th list. Geneva: WHO,; 2011.

46. Kitchener BA, Jorm AF. Mental health first aid training for the public: evaluation of effects on knowledge, attitudes and helping behavior. *BMC Psychiatry.* 2002;2(10):doi:10.1186/471-244X-2-10.

47. Beck A, Rush AJ, Shaw BF, Emery G. *Cognitive therapy of depression.* New York: The Guilford Press; 1979.

48. Cuijpers P, van Straten A, Warmerdam L. Behavioral activation treatments of depression: A meta-analysis. *Clin Psychol Rev.* 2007;27:318–26.

49. Dimidjian S, Hollon SD, Dobson KS, Schmaling KB, Kohlenberg RJ, Addis ME, et al. Randomized trial of behavioral activation, cognitive therapy, and antidepressant medication in the acute treatment of adults with major depression. *J Consult Clin Psychol.* 2006;74(4):658–70.

50. Klerman GL, Weissman MM, Rounsaville BJ, et al. *Interpersonal psychotherapy of depression.* New York: Basic Books; 1984.

51. Verdeli H, Clougherty K, Bolton P, Speelman L, Ndogoni L, Bass J, et al. Adapting group interpersonal psychotherapy for a developing country: experience in rural Uganda. *World Psychiatry.* 2003;2(2):114–20.

52. Mynors-Wallis LM, Gath DH, Day A, Baker F. Randomised controlled trial of problem solving treatment, antidepressant medication and combined treatment for major depression in primary care. *BMJ.* 2000;320:26–30.

53. Bernstein DA, Borkovec TD. *Progressive relaxation training: a manual for the helping professions.* Champaign, IL: Research Press; 1973.

54. Schultz JH, Luthe W. *Autogenic training: A psychophysiological approach in psychotherapy.* New York: Grune and Stratton; 1959.

55. BasicNeeds. *Community mental health practice. Seven essential features for scaling up in low- and middle-income countries.* Bangalore, India: BasicNeeds; 2009.

56. Deegan P. Recovery as a journey of the heart. *Psychiatr Rehabil J.* 1996;19:91–7.

57. Roberts G, Wolfson P. New directions in rehabilitation: learning from the recovery movement. In: Roberts G, Davenport S, Holloway F, Tattan T, editors. *Enabling recovery. The principles and practice of rehabilitation psychiatry.* London: The Royal College of Psychiatrists; 2006.

58. World Health Organization. *Community-based rehabilitation: CBR guidelines.* Geneva: WHO; 2010.

59. Holloway F. Is there a science of recovery and does it matter? Invited commentary on … Recovery and the medical model. *Adv Psychiatr Treat.* 2008;14:245–47.

60. Chatterjee S, Patel V, Chatterjee A, Weiss HA. Evaluation of a community-based rehabilitation model for chronic schizophrenia in rural India. *Br J Psychiatry.* 2003;182:57–62.

61. Chatterjee S, Pillai A, Jain S, Cohen A, Patel V. Outcomes of people with psychotic disorders in a community-based rehabilitation programme in rural India. *Br J Psychiatry.* 2009;195:433–43.

62. Jorm AF. Mental health literacy: public knowledge and beliefs about mental disorders. *Br J Psychiatry.* 2000;177:396–401.

63. Patel V, Weiss HA, Chowdhary N, Naik S, Pednekar S, Chatterjee S, et al. Effectiveness of an intervention led by lay health counsellors for depressive and anxiety disorders in primary care in Goa, India (MANAS): a cluster randomised controlled trial. *Lancet.* 2010. doi:10.1016/S0140-6736(10)61508-5.

64. Lancet *Global Mental Health Group.* Global Mental Health 6. Scale up services for mental disorders: a call for action. *Lancet.* 2007;370:1241–52.

65. Chisholm D, Saxena S. Cost effectiveness of strategies to combat neuropsychiatric conditions in sub-Saharan Africa and South East Asia: mathematical modelling study. *BMJ.* 2012;344:e609 1–10.

66. Raguram R, Venkateswaran A, Ramakrishna J, Weiss MG. Traditional community resources for mental health: a report of temple healing from India. *BMJ.* 2002;325:38–40.

67. Hegarty JD, Baldessarini RJ, Tohen M, Waternaux C, Oepen G. One hundred years of schizophrenia: a meta-analysis of the outcome literature. *Am J Psychiatry.* 1994;151:1409–16.

68. Hohmann AA, Shear MK. Community-based intervention research: coping with the "noise" of real life in study design. *Am J Psychiatry.* 2002;159(2):201–97.

69. Patel V, Simon G, Chowdhary N, Kaaya S, Araya R. Packages of care for depression in low- and middle-income countries. *PLoS Med.* 2009;6(10):e1000159.

70. Benegal V, Chand PK, Obot IS. Packages of care for alcohol use disorders in low- and middle-income countries. *PLoS Med.* 2009;6(10):e1000170.

71. Mari JdJ, Razzouk D, Thara R, Eaton J, Thornicroft G. Packages of care for schizophrenia in low- and middle-income countries. *PLoS Med.* 2009;6(10):e1000165.

72. Mbuba CK, Newton CR. Packages of care for epilepsy in low- and middle-income countries. *PLoS Med.* 2009;6(10):e1000162.

73. Prince MJ, Acosta D, Castro-Costa E, Jackson J, Shaji KS. Packages of care for dementia in low- and middle-income countries. *PLoS Med.* 2009;6(11):e1000176.

74. Flisher AJ, Sorsdahl K, Hatherill S, Chehil S. Packages of care for attention-deficit hyperactivity disorder in low- and middle-income countries. *PLoS Med.* 2010;7(2):e1000235.

PART TWO
PRACTICE
OF GLOBAL
MENTAL HEALTH

13 Mental Health Policy Development and Implementation

Crick Lund, José Miguel Caldas de Almeida, Harvey Whiteford, and John Mahoney

INTRODUCTION

What Is Mental Health Policy?

Public policy represents the official commitment by a government to address a particular political, social or economic issue. Policy is usually articulated through a complex array of proclamations by politicians, policy documents, and laws. It is implemented through a number of policy "instruments," from strategic plans and budgets, to legislation that sets out the particular legal consequences of implementing, or failing to implement, a particular policy.

The World Health Organization (WHO) defines *mental health policy* as "an organized set of values, principles, and objectives for improving mental health and reducing the burden of mental disorders in a population".[1] A mental health policy therefore attempts to embrace the aspirations of a group of stakeholders (those considered to have a direct stake in mental health) regarding how the mental health of a population can be improved, while also providing realistic and achievable goals for doing so.

Classically, the process of mental health policy development and implementation has been described in terms of a cycle,[2] which begins with problem identification, moves on to policy development (through a process of stakeholder consultation, information gathering, option development, and political decision), and subsequently to implementation and evaluation (Figure 13.1).

In reality, this cycle is complicated by power struggles among a range of stakeholders, all of whom have vested interests;[3] the priority that mental health is given in relation to other policy issues;[4] the ownership of the policy by a range of stakeholders;[5] and the systems that are in place to implement that policy, including the services, information systems, and wider social and economic structures in a given society.

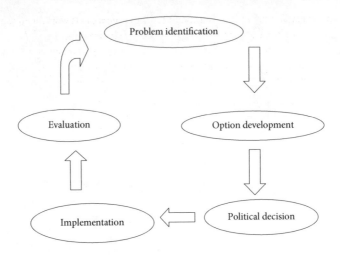

FIGURE 13.1
Generic policy cycle, as identified by Roberts et al.,[2] cited by Whiteford 2012.[23]

Why Is Mental Health Policy Important?

For those who are interested in promoting the mental health of populations and preventing or treating mental illness, policy is essential. A well-formulated mental health
policy and implementation plan provide a road map for how governments and a range
of stakeholders intend to address mental health within a given population over a specified period. It can help develop mental health services in a coordinated and systematic
manner, which is vital in settings in which services are fragmented and inconsistent. It
is a way of leveraging political commitment to the area of mental health; particularly
important in many settings where mental health is not given priority on policy agendas. And the process of developing a mental health policy is important in its own right,
as a means of building consensus among a wide range of stakeholders regarding how
mental health should be addressed and what the priorities should be.

In this chapter, we will trace the process of policy development and implementation in
global mental health. We will outline some of the principles of policy development, some
key ingredients that should be covered in the content of policies, some common challenges
in implementing such policies, and ways of building capacity for sustainable mental health
policy development and implementation. We will use examples from a range of countries to
illustrate key points throughout the chapter. In doing so, our purpose is to provide practical
assistance and lessons from the field for those who are interested in developing and implementing mental health policies, particularly in low- and middle-income countries (LMIC).

MENTAL HEALTH POLICY DEVELOPMENT

Principles

How health policy is formed is often unclear to those working in the health system and to
the general population. This can be particularly true for mental health policy, an area of
health that has traditionally been neglected and in which the policy directions have been
ad hoc or obscure. It is therefore important that the development of mental health policy
be underpinned by principles that are clear and well articulated. This certainly helps a

government when, for example, it is difficult for the professionals working in the system and the community to understand the reasons behind service reform.

Understanding the principles that underpin policy development creates the potential for greater engagement, including by those outside of government, in the services ultimately delivered in the community. This engagement can deliver greater support for the policy and its implementation. It can also provide a basis on which to critically assess whether the policy implementation deviates from the espoused principles. These principles are relevant to the whole policy cycle—problem identification, policy development, policy adoption, policy implementation, and policy evaluation (Figure 13.1), but are most important in the development of the policy.

Consult Widely

To be clear about the mental health policy a country needs, it is important to be clear about the problems the policy is intended to address. The identification of the problems needing policy attention occurs within the wider social, economic, historical, and political environment. Consultation with stakeholders and the broader community can be used to determine the position of relevant groups and individuals who are likely to hold a view on the final policy choices and the success of the implementation.[6] Consultation with mental health service users is crucial in this process—those for whom services are intended should have a central role in how the services are designed and delivered.[7]

While the policy development framework needs to be broad enough to cover the spectrum of mental health promotion, illness prevention, treatment, and rehabilitation and to cover services across the lifespan, priorities will need to be set because resources are limited. Consulting widely can help to establish and prioritize what needs attention and to assemble views on possible solutions. While there will be many commonalities in policy, each country needs to focus on areas that require specific attention; for example, enhancing the capacity of primary care services, expanding specialist community services, or dealing with the mental health consequences of conflict.

In the case of Sri Lanka after the 2004 tsunami, the WHO Country office appointed two local staff and an international consultant who was made available from the U.K. Ministry of Health. It was decided early on that the development of a new mental health policy was the most urgent priority. The finalization of the new mental health policy took six months to agree on. A wide range of stakeholders took part in the process, including the Ministry of Health, WHO, regional and district authorities, other government agencies, medical colleges, professional groups, and non-governmental organizations (NGOs).

Use the Best Available Evidence

It is vital that mental health policies are developed using the best available evidence for the population at hand. Guidelines for key elements of mental health policy and related checklists have been developed by WHO, based on country experiences of mental health policy.[1,8] In addition to these guidelines, it is essential that policy be based on the latest evidence regarding the epidemiology of mental disorders in the country and the key elements of the mental health system.

Knowledge about the distribution and determinants of mental disorders in a country is important in order to help plan services so they best meet the needs of the population. In many settings, valid and reliable local epidemiological data are not available. In such situations, it may be adequate to conduct reviews of countries or regions with similar demographic and social contexts, to develop the best estimates of population need. Thornicroft and Tansella[9] recommend a hierarchy-of-evidence approach for the use of epidemiological data in service planning: first prize is local, valid epidemiological data of psychiatric morbidity. If this is not available, then country or regional epidemiological data, weighted for local socio-demographic characteristics should be used. If this is not available, international data from comparable countries or regions adjusted for local socio-demographic characteristics should be used. If this is not available, then best estimates based on other sources of local information and opinions should be used in conjunction with an expert synthesis and interpretation of the best available data.

In delivering services, it is important that mental health clinicians have the requisite professional competencies: the knowledge, skills, and attitudes required to deliver high-quality care. Clinicians can be helped to deliver this care with clinical treatment guidelines that describe optimal treatment for individuals with a particular diagnosis. Mental health service standards describe the key attributes of a modern service and provide another mechanism for ensuring quality. However, they are seldom adequate on their own, and need to be accompanied by regulatory mechanisms such as accreditation of institutions and individuals; routine monitoring and evaluation; and "watchdog" agencies such as review boards, which are supported by legislated powers and resources. Together, these help ensure that adequately qualified clinicians use evidence-based treatments while working in appropriate service systems.

Key elements of mental health services have also been described.[10,11] More recently, core "packages of care" have been identified for priority mental, neurological, and substance use disorders.[12] WHO's mental health Gap Action Program (mhGAP) (http://www.who.int/mental_health/mhgap) provides intervention guidelines for the implementation of such core packages by non–mental health specialists, especially in LMIC, based on 93 scoping documents, using the Grades of Recommendation Assessment, Development, and Evaluation (GRADE) system.[13] Each country can adapt the available evidence for its circumstances.

Presenting evidence of the potential for targeted interventions that yield a good return on investment can be pivotal in convincing policymakers. For example, a breakthrough in policy commitment for mental health in the United Kingdom occurred through presenting evidence to health ministers that most mental illnesses (including schizophrenia) have their origins in youth. The Health Ministry subsequently agreed to a large investment in mental health (£320 million), including nationwide early intervention services for young people. In Australia, changes in mental health policy emerged when the government sought to address the high cost to the economy of lost productivity from untreated mental disorders. In 1997, the Australian mental health survey found a high number of days "out of role" (lost work days) due to common mental disorders.[14] As a result of this finding, the Australian government funded the Work Outcomes and Cost Benefit (WORC) study, which assessed the prevalence of untreated anxiety and depression of employed populations and the resulting loss of productivity (measured in absenteeism and attendance). This study found the cost to the Australian economy was 5.6 billion Australian dollars a year, much of which could be averted if treatment were provided.[15] This economic argument, along with the evidence for cost-effective treatments for anxiety and depression and the need for equity in treatment rates with other common physical disorders, was powerful in changing policy. A major and successful policy change was for the national health insurance scheme in Australia to increase access to non-pharmacological treatments for common mental disorders.[16]

While evidence is important, social attitudes also influence the policy chosen. For example, a policy of deinstitutionalization was introduced from the 1950s and 1960s in many high-income countries (HIC). This was driven by a combination of factors, including the expense of hospital care, the discovery of new and relatively effective medications that made it possible for people with chronic conditions to live in community settings, changing perspectives about the necessary loci of care, and human-rights concerns that patient abuse and neglect in institutions needed to be addressed. Societal attitudes have also changed with respect to the care of people with mental illness in the community; for example, with involuntary treatment. Involuntary treatment rates are determined by a range of legal, political, economic, and social factors, with the frequency of compulsory admissions varying greatly, even between countries such as those in the European Union (from 6 per 100,000 in Portugal to 218 per 100,000 in Finland).[17] A major social factor driving policy change has been the priority that is given to public safety (where the "protection" of the community from dangerous behavior is paramount) compared to that given to individual liberty (where the right of person with mental illness to be cared for in the least-restrictive environment is paramount). When societal focus is on individual liberty, the threshold for involuntary detention and treatment is usually higher. When the focus is on right to treatment and public safety, the threshold for involuntary detention and treatment is usually lower.[18]

Obtain High-Level Political Mandate

There are many demands made on governments. In order to obtain a political mandate, it is necessary to understand how one particular issue becomes identified as needing policy attention. The environment in which political decisions are made is complex. The interaction among politicians, their advisors, and government officials is usually in flux and not well understood by those advocating for a particular policy to be adopted. In obtaining political support for mental health, it is not only the health minister, but also other key government ministers (especially the minister responsible for finance) and the head of the government (for example, the prime minister) who are very influential. Senior government officials and advisory bodies in departments exert influence through the advice they give to the ministers. Being able to secure the support of individuals from among a range of these players will help ensure that the political mandate is delivered. Often it may be useful for mental health advocates to conduct a stakeholder analysis.

In the case of Sri Lanka's mental health policy development after the tsunami, WHO ensured that, for the first time, mental health developments became an integral part of the Country Cooperation Strategy (CCS) 2006–2011.[19] The CCS is the strategy of cooperation and agreed action between the Ministry of Health and the WHO Country Office. The Health Minister of the government of Sri Lanka had very limited knowledge of mental health systems development in 2005, but on the occasion of the launch of the national mental health policy in February 2006, the Minister of Health said the following:

We are very proud of the excellent health indicators—in a global and regional sense—that Sri Lanka has been able to achieve. However, there are many areas where we have to improve, especially in the area of mental health....I must say we are focusing very much on mental health. We have spoken to all the stakeholders and are aware of their needs. The capacity building has already started in many ways. It should go to the periphery and should not be limited only to Colombo. We are very grateful to WHO for the initiatives taken in this area. (Minister of Health Speech, February 2006)

Not all stakeholders are seen as equal in the eyes of policymakers. The health sector is well recognized as having power and influence concentrated in groups such as the medical and nursing professions. The potential beneficiaries of a policy—for example, service users—are generally less powerful and less well-organized. However, if it is possible to harness the support of professional groups and user advocacy groups, the ability to influence government is greatly enhanced. An example from outside the mental health sector is the influence of the community-based Treatment Action Campaign in South Africa in successfully advocating for the roll-out of anti-retroviral therapy.[20]

Advocates can use influential international research findings to help secure political support. For example, the publication of the Global Burden of Disease Studies showing mental disorders to be a leading cause of health-related disability in most countries,[21] and the 2007 *Lancet* series on global mental health[22] outlining the need for increased action in mental health raised the expectation that governments would act in the area of mental health.

The factors that influence governments, and therefore help shape policy, can be external as well as internal to the country. International agencies can be influential, particularly in LMIC, where development or aid funding is linked to a particular area, such as the UN Millennium Development Goals (MDGs). World Bank lending in the area of mental health has been said to be linked to areas attracting political and media attention (such as suicide and substance abuse), the need to address the mental health consequences of conflict or natural disasters, and where the reform could produce a more cost-effective use of existing resources (e.g. the reorganization of services to move resources from institutional to community care).[23]

Advocates can harness international professional organizations such as the World Psychiatric Association (http://www.wpanet.org), NGOs such as the World Federation for Mental Health (http://www.wfmh.org), and movements such as the Movement for Global Mental Health (http://www.globalmentalhealth.org) to apply external pressure on governments to address mental health issues.

Tackle Stigma Head-on

The stigma attached to mental illness, and the social exclusion of people with mental illness, have for many years meant that mental health has been a politically unattractive area for government attention. The poor living conditions, inadequate quality of care, and human-rights abuses in psychiatric hospitals have been well documented. For decades, these circumstances were not seen as warranting intervention, but a change in societal attitudes has seen the human rights of people with mental illness increasingly recognized. This has been accompanied by major efforts to reduce the stigma attached to mental illness,[24] and some international organizations such as the World Psychiatric Association and some governments have endorsed and funded anti-stigma campaigns. This has included legislative provisions to address stigma.[25] (See Chapter 18, Mental Health Stigma.)

Stigma needs to be addressed, not only in the content of mental health policy and legislation, but also in the process of developing policy. Stigma may be a major barrier to even initiating policy reforms for mental health. For example, senior policymakers in ministries of health may not regard mental health as a priority as a result of their own stigmatizing beliefs, including that people with mental disorders cannot be helped or do not deserve health services in the context of other health priorities. Thus the work of initiating and developing mental health policy reform will require addressing these issues head-on, by lobbying, providing accurate information, and facilitating interactions between policymakers and service users.

Link Policy Development to Other Health and Development Priorities

The relationship between mental illness and other health conditions is well established.[26] Opportunities for mental health policy development may therefore be enhanced by linking mental health to existing health policy priorities. An example is HIV/AIDS, which has enjoyed a high policy priority in many LMIC, but also interacts substantially with mental illness.[27] By emphasizing the importance of mental illness as a risk factor for contracting HIV, and in turn emphasizing the importance of treating mental health consequences of HIV infection, mental health advocates can make the case for more integrated care that addresses mental health and HIV needs.[28]

Successful mental health policy also requires action in areas outside the traditional scope of health, such as social services, housing, education, police, and justice. Targeted policy and service coordination in these sectors can greatly improve outcomes for people with mental illness.[29] Government officials and stakeholders from these sectors should be included when mental health policy is being developed to encourage complimentary policy developments.[30]

The response to the effects of political oppression, war, and conflict also requires mental health interventions and heightens the need for a government policy response.[31,32] The focus of governments, international agencies, and development banks on social and economic development and poverty reduction can be linked to mental health. The relationship between poverty and mental health[33] has allowed a focus on poverty reduction to incorporate a mental health dimension, through both promotion of psychosocial development at a population level and the improvement of treatment services.[5] The increasing recognition of the economic burden of mental illness, especially in terms of lost productivity, has seen the engagement of government economic agencies.[34]

Use Policy "Windows"

In their framework for the analysis of why particular health issues are given priority, Shiffman and Smith stress the importance of policy "windows."[35] These are opportunities where, due to the confluence of a range of political factors, media attention, and epidemiological changes in the population, specific health policies may be given priority. Shiffman provides the example of the way in which the Millennium Development Goals, particularly MDG4, provided such a window to foreground the issue of neonatal mortality at a global level.[36] At a national level, examples of policy windows for mental health might include the priority given to non-communicable diseases due to epidemiological transitions, increased media attention, and the political impetus created by a new minister of health or change of government. Another example is that of natural disasters, following which resources and political will may be mobilized to address mental health needs, as in the example of Sri Lanka. Mental health advocates and policymakers need to pay attention to such windows, and ensure that mental health is well aligned with the particular political opportunity that is created. For example, there may be new opportunities through the development of the next set of international development targets beyond 2015, to foreground the issue of mental health.

Steps in Mental Health Policy Development

WHO has set out specific steps that are recommended for the development of national mental health policies (Box 13.1).[1] These steps fall within the generic framework outlined in Figure 13.1, and are set out in more detail in the WHO Mental Health Policy and Service Guidance Package. This package also provides a checklist of the key processes that need to be undertaken in developing mental health policy.[8]

CONTENT OF MENTAL HEALTH POLICY

While the process of developing a mental health policy is important, equally important is the actual content of the policy document that is eventually adopted by a national or regional government. A number of comparatively recent examples have shown that

> **Box 13.1** Steps in developing a national mental health policy, adapted from the WHO Mental Health Policy and Service Guidance Package[1]
>
> 1. **Gather information on mental health needs and services:** Gather epidemiological data on mental health needs and conduct a situational analysis of current services, including public and private sectors as well as NGOs.
> 2. **Gather evidence for effective strategies:** Review the local and international literature on cost-effective interventions to promote mental health, prevent mental disorders, and detect and manage priority mental disorders.
> 3. **Consultation and negotiation:** Engage with a wide range of stakeholders throughout the process.
> 4. **Exchange with other countries:** Share experiences with other countries, particularly those with similar socioeconomic and cultural contexts.
> 5. **Set out the vision, values, principles, and objectives:** Draft a policy document that sets out the vision, values, principles, and objectives of the policy. This should be strongly informed by the data and consultation process in steps 1–4.
> 6. **Determine areas for action:** For each of the policy objectives, concrete areas for action need to be identified, with clear targets and indicators that will allow policymakers to assess the extent to which they have been implemented.
> 7. **Identify major roles and responsibilities:** Clearly identify who will be responsible for implementing the various areas for action, and what their major roles will be.
>
> *Adapted from the WHO Mental Health Policy and Service Guidance Package (WHO, 2005b).*

mental health system development is possible even in very difficult circumstances. With limited resources and where there are practically no mental health services, development of a community-focused mental health system is possible, such as in Brazil,[37] Chile,[38] and Sri Lanka.[39] In these settings, the content of a mental health policy that makes reform possible is instructive. In this section, we highlight some of the key components of a mental health policy and illustrate these with specific case examples.

Realistic Vision and Related Values, Principles, and Objectives

It is relatively easy for a mental health policy consultant to write a mental health policy, even after a short visit. What is essential, however, is to develop a realistic vision and to set this out in a policy document with locally relevant values, principles, and objectives. This requires an understanding of the local context and how decisions are made. It also requires obtaining broad ownership and incorporating the views of as many people and organizations as possible. It is vital to present a unified approach.

As an example of a vision, the South African White Paper on the Transformation of the Health System in 1997 stated:

A comprehensive and community-based mental health service (including substance abuse prevention and management) should be planned and coordinated at the national, provincial, district, and community levels, and integrated with other health services.[40]

Comprehensive Approach

In order to make a break from outdated mental health systems that concentrate their resources in large psychiatric hospitals, it is vital that policies develop a comprehensive approach that includes mental health promotion, illness prevention, and the development of a wide array of community-based treatment and rehabilitation services.

The mental health policy of Sri Lanka[41] reflects a clear consensus that community mental health system development is a high priority and that reliance on centralized mental hospitals for service delivery is not in the best interests of people with mental illness. Despite its brevity (only 10 pages), the mental health policy for Sri Lanka was able to set out the requirements for a wide range of hospital and community-based services. The policy had the following aims for a population of 20 million people:

- To open acute and rehabilitation wards in all 26 districts of Sri Lanka.
- To train and appoint additional psychiatrists and medical staff devoted to mental health, as well as ward, and community-based nurses, psychologists, occupational therapists, and social workers.
- To significantly increase staffing in the community, including 270 Medical Officers of Mental Health (MOMH) (one for every Ministry of Health (MoH) area) and 600 community nurses (two per MoH area). The approximate population of an MoH area is 60,000 people.
- To consider a new cadre of community mental health workers/community-level volunteers.
- To train and continuously supervise primary care workers.
- To develop health promotion and anti-stigma campaigns.
- Where possible, to move long-stay patients nearer their district of origin.

In most resource-poor countries, most of the categories of mental health staff needed are not available, and it could take between five and 10 years to develop curricula, train and appoint sufficient numbers of staff, during which time governments and ministers change and momentum is easily lost. It is often sensible to look for alternative solutions to such shortages in staffing. In Sri Lanka, for example, new categories of workers were created through the policy reform process. Medical Officers of Mental Health (MOMHs—medical officers with additional training in psychiatry) were posted to the areas given the highest priority (i.e. districts with no psychiatrists); and Community Support Officers (CSOs), a low paid non-professional workforce (initially created in response to the massive population need following the tsunami) were continued in a number of districts. CSOs made a substantial contribution to case finding, referral, and support for people with mental illness.[42] They have also enabled access to treatment (in local clinics or specialist treatment) of increasingly large numbers of people who previously would have received no treatment. There are problems with sustainability, but one province has created permanent CSO posts by using resources for other categories of staff, and other provinces are considering similar plans.

Primary Health Care Approach

As endorsed internationally, the primary health care approach provides the best opportunity for maximizing population coverage of mental health services,[43] and this needs to be written into the policy document. Most countries have reasonably good population coverage for general primary health care, although most staff have little knowledge or involvement with mental health, even after training. Primary care staff rarely succeed in providing a mental health service on their own without specialist (and local) backup advice and support.[44] In many countries with a reasonable primary care infrastructure, mental health policy must plan to develop services that integrate new developments within this structure. For example, in Sri Lanka, the wide availability of primary care services was considered to be a major advantage, particularly the ability to integrate the management of new mental health staff into the primary health care management systems. MOMHs (who were not hospital-based) and CSOs were managed by the district head of primary care, and technical supervision was the responsibility of psychiatrists. The mental health staff were well integrated into primary care management system and attended regular meetings of all staff (medical officers, public health midwives, public health nurses, and public health inspectors) in each Ministry of Health catchment area. They were able to discuss individual cases when necessary. In addition there were also regular meetings between the mental health staff and the Regional Director of Health Services, who also chaired regular district coordination meetings with other local government agencies and NGOs.

Promote and Protect Human Rights

Increased accessibility of community and inpatient mental health treatment and care can advance the human rights of people with mental disorders. In Sri Lanka, a great number of people with mental disorders who would previously have had no treatment and therefore continuing and largely avoidable disability are now being treated. Many people have experienced personal, social, and economic benefits that come with effective treatment of mental disorders.[45] Attention was also paid to improving the quality of care at the large hospitals with improved care-planning (including discharge planning) and incident reporting, new policies and protocols, and reviews. The level of staff violence against patients at the largest psychiatric hospital has now decreased substantially.

Attention also needs to be focused on educating the general community about mental health and illness, and on fostering the engagement of people with mental illness and their families in advocacy for mental health through the creation of consumer and family associations, as shown in work from South Africa.[7] Another important component of protection for human rights, as well as facilitating access to mental health services, is the provision of readily available and understandable information about mental health to the general population and training of non-specialist staff; for example, primary health care staff, primary and pre-school teachers, and prison officers.

The latter is a key strategy in stigma reduction, which should receive substantial attention in the content of the policy. This could include foregrounding stigma reduction as a central value of the policy, setting out strategies for stigma reduction and how these will be addressed within the health sector and more broadly across the society (see Chapter 18, Mental Health Stigma).

Promote Intersectoral Collaboration

Mental health policy development and mental health services should never be seen as the responsibility of health systems alone. For example, in Sri Lanka there are intersectoral coordinating committees that have been established at a national level (with the most senior health department staff, regional and district authorities, other government agencies, medical colleges, professional groups, and NGOs) and in each district. They constitute vitally important governance for managing and continuing the process of mental health system reform and development in Sri Lanka. They also ensure the engagement of relevant sectors outside of health in contributing to further development and to identify and solve problems. Intersectoral coordinating committees or forums operate successfully in all districts. They provide an opportunity to discuss the particular responsibilities of different government departments and agencies in relation to the needs of people in the district with mental illness.

The purpose of mental health policy should not of course be the production of a policy document, but the promotion of mental health in the population and real improvements in the quality of life of people living with mental illness. Careful attention therefore needs to be paid to the process of implementing policy, to avoid the scenario of a carefully developed mental health policy document doing little more than weighing down the shelves of Ministry of Health offices. In this next section, we provide key recommendations for this process, once again illustrating points from specific country experiences.

Link Policy to an Implementation Plan

The most valuable asset in developing mental health services is the existence of a national mental health policy with an associated *implementation plan* for every district or equivalent administrative health unit. Policy should be focused on the need for system-wide organizational change, with appropriate attention paid to governance and organizational issues, and a clear commitment and plan for implementation of the policy at the community and district levels. When work at province (or state) and district levels is closely linked with national-level frameworks, the local and national efforts support each other.

After the acceptance by the government of Sri Lanka of the new mental health policy, a detailed mental health action plan was prepared for its implementation in every district and region. Managing the service in transition and improving quality at the three large psychiatric institutions was also seen as a major challenge. The implementation plan therefore also covered plans for the main psychiatric hospitals in Colombo.[46] This document set out the actions that would be necessary for successful implementation. WHO produced a detailed concept paper and fund-raising strategy which attempted to show the scale of work across the country.[47] Yearly round-table conferences were held in Colombo to which all major donors, agencies, and partners were invited.

Allocate Adequate Resources to Implement the Policy

In most countries, all new policies need to be approved by the ministry concerned as well as the finance ministry or others responsible for the budget. The process of translating a policy into a strategic plan and budget has also been set out in the WHO Mental Health Policy and Service Guidance package.[1,48] An advantage in Sri Lanka is that once a new policy is accepted by the Cabinet, resources are automatically made available for new staff appointments. All policy proposals described above were therefore funded. Once clear plans are agreed to, supported, and developed for the longer term development of community-based services, it is much easier to approach donors. Several donors expressed an interest in supporting psychosocial and mental health activities in Sri Lanka following the tsunami: the governments of Finland, Ireland, Australia (particularly World Vision Australia and the state of Victoria), and Spain (Medecins du Monde) invested limited but vitally important resources.

In the absence of a detailed mental health policy or implementation plan, funding can easily be wasted or misspent. For example, the World Bank allocated US$2 million in 2004 to the government to reduce suicide in Sri Lanka, which was managed by the Ministry of Health. The project comprised seven major components (including detailed work on referral pathways in areas where there were no services). Over half of the allocation was later given back to the World Bank, as it was unspent. It is also difficult to make progress where capacity and expertise are weak.

Link Policy to Legislation

It is always desirable for implementation of a policy to be linked to legislation that is consistent with international human rights standards. However, the timing of this is not always optimal. For example, in the case of South Africa, legislation moved ahead of policy, through the adoption of the Mental Health Care Act (2002). But because of the lack of a national-level policy and provincial-level strategic plans that would allow the Department of Health to commit budgets to assist with the implementation of the Act, the implementation of certain key features (such as the establishment of acute care facilities in regional and district hospitals) has been mixed.[49,50] In the case of Sri Lanka, the policy framework still needs to be supported by passage of mental health legislation, which has been drafted but has not yet been passed by the national parliament. Even so, significant progress has been made, and the previous mental health legislation, which is over 100 years old, is largely ignored in favor of the policy.

Who Is Going to Implement It? (Role of Government and Other Stakeholders)

The national mental health policy and strategic plan need to clearly set out the roles and responsibilities of key stakeholders in implementing the policy, and where necessary, specify how the capacity for this implementation needs to be built.[1] There are clear and important weaknesses in most governments' capacity at national and peripheral levels to design, implement and monitor, and evaluate community-focused mental health policies. It is important not to bypass this weak capacity (or to establish a parallel approach) but to contribute to strengthening that capacity.

Leadership matters most, and leadership capacity needs to be developed at all levels. It was clear from the outset in Sri Lanka that the key issue would be the quality and distribution of leadership—in different levels and in different components of the mental health system—which needed support. A mental health leadership and development team was established at the WHO, with clear support from the WHO Country Representative. It included an experienced international mental health consultant and a talented local team. This team had excellent relations with Ministry of Health, many provincial and district Directors of Health, and with other key stakeholders such as the Sri Lankan College of Psychiatrists.

Finding the Right Mix of National and International Cooperation

It is vital that national mental health policies be driven and "owned" by the local country stakeholders. Nevertheless, there may be particular circumstances in which international cooperation and support can be extremely useful. The precise "mix" of local and international contributions will vary according to the setting and local needs. This can be illustrated by two cases; namely, Uganda and Sri Lanka.

In the case of Ugandan mental health policy reform during 2008–2011, the local Ministry of Health and research collaborators had substantial experience in mental health policy and were able to drive this process.[51] The reform process was linked to an international research program consortium, the Mental Health and Poverty Project (MHaPP), which was a collaboration between four African countries: Ghana, South Africa, Uganda, and Zambia, with support from WHO and the University of Leeds in the United Kingdom.[5] In this context, there was no need for an international consultant to provide support to the Uganda team, as they already had strong leadership, good local political support, and the capacity to develop policy through a thorough consultation process. Nevertheless, having the team linked to an international network (MHaPP) strengthened the process and provided added momentum, along with technical support for evaluation of the policy process.

In Sri Lanka, a great number of both senior and junior staff of the Ministry of Health at national, provincial, and district levels have been supported and mentored by a WHO international advisor during the process of developing policy, managing the implementation of the policy, improving the quality of care in the existing institutions, and other health development projects. Most of the team at the WHO Country Office have now left, including the international consultant, and progress is continuing to be made. Experience shows, however, that support and cooperation need to be made available over a period of time (ideally over a few years, but not necessarily full-time). Short-term support and visits are rarely successful.

Having projects managed by the WHO mental health team in Sri Lanka meant that the program could be very well connected to government at a national level, which is a great benefit in that problems could be resolved at a high level, and implementation of the project could continue with minimal hold-ups and delays. This method of governance and management of a development project is a crucially important consideration, and choosing established lines of communication to the government at national and peripheral levels is an important component of project design.

For international collaborators, familiarity with, and being able to work within, the local sociocultural context is critically important. This includes being able to recognize and negotiate local coalitions and enmities and being able to work with a sometimes factionalized environment. Consultants need to engage sensitively and show humility in their dealings with staff at all levels. This is an obvious but (in development) a too frequently ignored lesson.

Monitor and Evaluate Policy Implementation

It is vital that the implementation of policy be carefully monitored and evaluated. This requires that the design of policy and plans needs to include a clear set of targets and indicators that can be used to assess the extent to which the policy has been implemented. The WHO Evaluating Mental Health Policy and Plans module[8] provides a useful step-by-step framework for how policy implementation should be monitored and evaluated:

- Step 1. Clarify the purpose and scope of the monitoring and evaluation: this should include identifying which aspects of the policy implementation need to be evaluated, and over what time period.
- Step 2. Identify the evaluators and funding for the evaluation: evaluation can be built into routine monitoring of services or can be contracted out to agencies to conduct independent non-routine evaluations.
- Step 3. Assess and manage ethical issues: the ethical implications of evaluations need to be carefully considered; e.g. informed consent needs to be obtained and confidential information protected.
- Step 4. Prepare and manage the operational plan for the evaluation: this should include the type of evaluation design, the methods to be used, the time frame, and the data to be collected. It is important to ensure that a team is employed with the requisite research skills, including collection, analysis, and dissemination of good quality data.

In addition to this, the WHO Mental Health Information Systems module[52] provides a framework for developing and evaluating information systems that can be integrated into routine health-management information systems. In South Africa, as part of the MHaPP, a pilot mental health information system was established and evaluated in five districts across two diverse provinces. This system integrated a set of simple input and process indicators into the routine district health-management information system in a partnership between researchers and local mental health and information-management staff. Although the system did not include outcome indicators, it was able to clearly monitor staffing and service utilization patterns in the districts, which had not been previously possible.

BUILDING CAPACITY FOR MENTAL HEALTH POLICY

One of the lessons learnt from mental health policy development in LMICs is that capacity building is one of the key components of strategies to support policy implementation in these countries. Mental health policy implementation is a complex process, including many different political, financial, and technical issues. It requires not only strong political support and financial and human resources, but also leaders with the capacity to conduct the implementation process, workers with the knowledge and skills to deliver services and interventions, and a wide range of stakeholders prepared to collaborate in this process. In many LMICs, there is a lack of adequately trained leaders, and the critical mass that is needed to support policy development, implementation, and evaluation is frequently lacking.

To build capacity for mental health policy, different and complementary approaches were taken in the past. Some countries developed capacity building activities at the national level, usually integrated into the training programs for mental health professionals. In most cases, however, capacity building in LMICs has been promoted in the context of international initiatives. WHO has had a leading role in this area during the last two decades, providing technical assistance to countries, developing training materials, organizing international conferences and seminars on mental health policy–related issues, and ensuring mental health policy–implementation supervision by consultants. However, other international organizations, such as the European Commission, governments, universities, and scientific and advocacy organizations have also had an important role in the development of these international initiatives.

Building capacity can be achieved through teaching programs of different sorts, ongoing support and supervision by consultants, and through the development of regional networks for mental health policy.

Teaching Programs

Most mental health policy teaching programs aim at developing the public health knowledge and skills of leaders, health professionals, and other people who may have a relevant role in mental health policy development. The format and duration of the programs can vary significantly in accordance with the specific objectives and targets to be attained and addressed. Some programs are carried out through short, intensive conferences, seminars, or courses; while others are diploma courses or post-graduate degree courses.

New information technologies have significantly facilitated the development of teaching programs involving students living in different countries. Using online-teaching methodologies, it is now possible to combine residential sessions with periods of web-based teaching, making it possible for students to continue living in their home countries.

Most programs address policy and service-development issues, as well as research capacity development. However, some programs especially focus on policy and service-development issues, specifically addressing the needs of leaders and workers involved in the implementation of mental health policy and services, while others are designed to develop research capacity (see Chapter 9, Capacity Building).

Ongoing Support and Supervision

In LMICs engaged in mental health policy development, ongoing support and supervision is indispensable for the success of the policy, and continued capacity building. Support and supervision must be provided to the unit responsible for the implementation of mental health policy, usually located at the Ministry of Health. It must address their main needs in areas such as how to conduct a situation analysis and needs assessment, the planning and organization of services, monitoring and evaluation, and human resources development.

Support can be provided through visits by local and international experts, and exchange of experiences with other countries. The Initiative for the Restructuring of Psychiatric Care in Latin America,[53] one of the more systematic, and better-documented, international initiatives providing support and supervision to LMICs on mental health policy development, included all these components. International consultants with broad experience of policy and services development visited the countries or regions engaged in mental health policy implementation at least twice a year. When necessary, experts on specific areas visited the countries to provide technical support or conduct training activities. The results of the initiative[54] show that this support, when organized and continued, can be extremely important for the success of policy implementation, and a valuable contribution to capacity building.

Developing Regional Networks for Mental Health Policy

The development of regional networks can also be a very effective strategy. In an initial phase, it allows the organization of capacity building activities benefiting several countries and the sharing of experiences. In later phases, as countries involved in the regional networks develop their capacities and experiences, more advanced countries can provide support to other countries in the conducting of capacity building activities.[55] These regional networks also create excellent opportunities to promote new projects involving two or more countries with similar problems and interests.

These benefits were particularly clear in Latin America and the Caribbean after 2001, when PAHO/WHO supported the development of regional networks, in continuation of the above-mentioned Initiative for the Restructuring of Psychiatric Care in Latin America, developed in the 1990s. The first step led to the creation of the Regional Mental Health Forum in Central America, which enabled the strengthening of the collaboration between Central American countries in the collection of data on mental health systems, implementation of mental health policy, and the development of mental health services and programs. Given the success of this first initiative, regional forums were subsequently organized in the Caribbean region, the Andean region, and South America, which had played, and continue to play, an important role in the development of collaborative projects on building capacity and other issues related to mental health policy and services development.[56]

In sub-Saharan Africa, a major initiative from 2005 to 2010 was the Mental Health and Poverty Project, a research program consortium including Ghana, South Africa, Uganda, and Zambia, with the objective of strengthening the development and implementation of mental health policy.[5] Partnerships were established between research institutions and ministries of health, and activities included the first major situational analyses of mental health policies and systems in each country, and the development of interventions to strengthen policy, legislation, and information systems in the study countries. Some major outcomes have included contributions to the reform of mental health legislation in Ghana, development of mental health policy and strategic plans in Uganda, development of a national mental health strategic plan in Zambia, and drafting of a new national mental health policy in South Africa. The development of the regional network, with a strong emphasis on building common approaches and strengthening capacity, were key ingredients to the success of this collaboration.

CONCLUSION

This chapter has described some of the key principles that should inform the development of mental health policies, the central components of such policies, and factors that are important to consider in their implementation. It has also emphasized the importance of continuing to build capacity for mental health policy at a national and regional level, and has described several recent initiatives in this regard.

Despite many challenges, there is increasing evidence from around the world that the development and implementation of evidence-based mental health policies is possible, even in low-resource settings. There is a growing international community of mental health leaders who have made substantial contributions to mental health policy and systems development in their own countries. Evidence for the growing international capacity for mental health policy is reflected in the growing number of training programs and support networks that build capacity in this field in an ongoing manner. It is also reflected in the growing number of countries with updated mental health policies. The WHO's *Atlas 2011* reports that, although only 60% of countries (covering 72% of the world's population) have a mental health policy, approximately 76% of countries that do have a policy have approved or updated that policy since 2005.[57] This appears to indicate that the problem is less one of updating mental health policies (although this of course remains an important issue), than one of persuading governments that have never put mental health on their policy agendas to do so.

A key challenge remains the capacity and motivation of ministries of health in LMICs, who are the principle change-agents in this field. This is particularly true in countries that do not yet have any mental health policy (neither as a stand-alone mental health policy document, nor one that is integrated into a general health policy document). Concerted efforts are required to improve, not only the mental health literacy of policymakers and public health practitioners, but also their capacity to use research evidence for policy and planning. It is crucial to bridge the gap between research and its utilization in ongoing policy and practice.[58] There is also an urgent need to lobby international development and health agencies, which frequently set the policy agendas for ministries of health in LMICs. While mental health remains excluded from international development initiatives such as the MDGs, and more recently the UN Declaration on Non-Communicable Diseases, it will be difficult to convince country-level political leaders of its importance.

REFERENCES

1. WHO. *Mental health policy, plans and programs: Mental health policy and service guidance package.* Geneva: WHO; 2005.
2. Roberts M, Hsiao W, Berman P, Reich M. *Getting health reform right: A guide to improved performance and equity* Oxford, UK: Oxford University Press; 2003.
3. Walt G. (1994). *Health policy. An introduction to process and power.* London: Zed Books; 1994.
4. Bird P, Omar M, Doku V, Lund C, Nsereko JR, Mwanza J, the MHaPP Research Programme Consortium Increasing the priority of mental health in Africa: findings from qualitative research in Ghana, South Africa, Uganda and Zambia. *Health Policy & Plan.* 2011;26(5):357–65. Available from: http://heapol.oxfordjournals.org/content/26/5/357.abstract.
5. Flisher AJ, Lund C, Funk M, Banda M, Bhana A, Doku V, et al. Mental health policy development and implementation in four African countries. *J Health Psychol.* 2007;12:505–16.
6. Sturm R. What type of information is needed to inform mental health policy. *J Ment Health Policy & Econ.* 1999;2:141–4.
7. Kleintjes S, Lund C, Swartz L, Flisher AJ, the MHaPP Research Programme Consortium. Mental health care user participation in mental health policy development and implementation in South Africa. *Int Rev Psychiatry.* 2010;22(6):568–77.
8. WHO. *Monitoring and evaluation of mental health policies and plans.* Geneva: WHO; 2007.

9. Thornicroft G, Tansella M. The mental health matrix: A manual to improve services. Cambridge, Cambridge University Press; 1999.

10. Pirkis J, Harris M, Buckingham B, Whiteford HA, Townsend-White C. International planning directions for provision of mental health services. *Admin & Policy Ment Health & Ment Health Serv Res.* 2007;34(4):377–87.

11. Thornicroft G, Tansella M. Components of a modern mental health service: a pragmatic balance of community and hospital care. *Br J Psychiatry.* 2004;185(4):283–90. Available from: http://bjp.rcpsych.org/content/185/4/283.abstract.

12. Patel V, Thornicroft G. (2009). Packages of care for mental, neurological, and substance use disorders in low- and middle-income countries: PLoS Medicine Series. *PLoS Med.* 6(10):e1000160. Available from: http://dx.doi.org/10.1371%2Fjournal.pmed.1000160

13. Atkins D, Best D, Briss PA, Eccles M, Falck-Ytter Y, et al. Grading quality of evidence and strength of recommendations. *BMJ.* 2004;328:1490.

14. Henderson AS, Andrews G, Hall W. Australia's mental health: an overview of the general population survey. *Aust N Z J Psychiatry.* 2000;34:197–205.

15. Hilton M.F. Scuffham PA, Vecchio N, Whiteford HA. Using the interaction of mental health symptoms and treatment status to estimate lost employee productivity. *Aust N Z J Psychiatry.* 2010;44:151–61.

16. Pirkis J, Ftanou M, Williamson M, et al. Australia's Better Access initiative: an evaluation. *Aust N Z J Psychiatry.* 2011;45:726–39.

17. Salize HJ, Dressing H. Epidemiology of involuntary placement of mentally ill people across the European Union. *Br J Psychiatry.* 2004;184:163–8.

18. Fistein EC, Holland AJ, Clare IC.H. & Gunn MJ. A comparison of mental health legislation from diverse Commonwealth jurisdictions. *Int J Law & Psychiatry.* 2009;32(3):147–55.

19. Ministry of Health. *Summary of consultation on Mental Health Policy for Sri Lanka.* Colombo, Sri Lanka: Ministry of Health; 2005.

20. Treatment Action Campaign. *Fighting for our lives: The history of the Treatment Action Campaign 1998–2010* Cape Town, SA: Treatment Action Campaign; 2010.

21. Murray CJL, Lopez AD. *The global burden of disease, Volume 1. A comprehensive assessment of mortality and disability from diseases, injuries and risk factors in 1990, and projected to 2020.* Cambridge, MA: Harvard University Press; 1996.

22. Lancet Global Mental Health Group. Scale up services for mental disorders: a call for action. *Lancet.* 2007;370:1241–52.

23. Whiteford HA. Shaping national mental health policies. In G Thornicroft et al., editors. *Oxford textbook of community mental health.* Oxford, UK: Oxford University Press; 2012: 273–80.

24. Thornicroft G, Brohan E, Kassam A, Lewis-Holmes E. Reducing stigma and discrimination: candidate interventions. *Int J Ment Health Syst.* 2008;2(3).

25. WHO. *WHO resource book on mental health, human rights, and legislation.* Geneva: WHO; 2005.

26. Prince M, Patel V, Saxena S, Maj M, Maselko J, Phillips MR, et al. No health without mental health. *Lancet.* 2007;370:859–77.

27. Collins PY, Holman AR, Freeman M, Patel V. What is the relevance of mental health to HIV/AIDS care and treatment programs in developing countries? A systematic review. *AIDS.* 2006;20(12):1571–82.

28. Freeman M. Using all opportunities for improving mental health—examples from South Africa. *Bull WHO.* 2000;78(4):508–10. Available from: PM:10885175.

29. Hogan MF. Transforming mental health care: realities, priorities and prospects. *Psychiatr Clin North Am.* 2009;31:1–9.

30. Skeen S, Kleintjes S, Lund C, Petersen I, Bhana A, Flisher AJ, the MHaPP Research Programme Consortium "Mental health is everybody's business": Roles for an intersectoral approach in South Africa. *Int Rev Psychiatry.* 2010;22(6):611–23.

31. Murthy RS, Lakshminarayana R. Mental health consequences of war: a brief review of research findings. *World Psychiatry.* 2006;5:25–30.

32. Arie S. (2011). Agencies prepare to deal with mental health problems in Libya after 42 years of repression. *BMJ.* 2011;343:d5653.

33. Lund C, De Silva M, Plagerson S, Cooper SD, Chisholm D, Das J, et al. Poverty and mental disorders: breaking the cycle in low-income and middle-income countries. *Lancet.* 2011;378:1502–14.

34. Friedli L. *Mental health, resilience and inequalities.* Copenhagen, Denmark: WHO Regional Office for Europe; 2009.

35. Shiffman J, Smith S. (2007). Generation of political priority for global health initiatives: a framework and case study of maternal mortality. *Lancet. 2007*;370:1370–9.
36. Shiffman J. Issue attention in global health: the case of newborn survival. *Lancet.* 2010;375:2045–9.
37. Jacob KS, Sharan P, Mirza I, Garrido-Cumbrera M, Seedat S, Mari JJ, et al. Mental health systems in countries: where are we now? *Lancet.* 2007;370:1061–77.
38. Patel V, Araya R, Chatterjee S, Chisholm D, Cohen A, De Silva M, et al. Treatment and prevention of mental disorders in low-income and middle-income countries. *Lancet.* 2007;370:991–1005.
39. Saraceno B, Van Ommeren M, Batniji R, Cohen A, Gureje O, Mahoney J, et al. Barriers to improvement of mental health services in low-income and middle-income countries. *Lancet.* 2007;370(9593):1164–74.
40. Department of Health *White paper for the transformation of the health system in South Africa.* Pretoria: Government Gazette; 1997.
41. Ministry of Health *The Mental Health Policy of Sri Lanka: 2005-2015.* Colombo, Sri Lanka: Ministry of Health; 2005.
42. Kakuma R, Minas H, Van Ginneken N, Dal Poz MR, Desiraju K, Morris J, et al. Human resources for mental health care: current situation and strategies for action. *Lancet. 2011*;378:1654–63.
43. WHO, World Organization of Family Doctors (WONCA). *Integrating mental health into primary care: A global perspective.* Geneva: WHO; 2008.
44. Cohen A. *The effectiveness of mental health services in primary care: The view from the developing world.* Geneva: World Health Organization; 2001.
45. Minas H, Kakuma R, Mahoney J. *Health for the South Community Mental Health Project: Evaluation report to World Vision Australia.* Melbourne: World Vision Australia; 2011.
46. WHO. *Mental Health Policy for Sri Lanka: Action Plan 2006.* Colombo, Sri Lanka: WHO Sri Lanka Country Office; 2005.
47. WHO. *WHO Sri Lanka country cooperation strategy 2006-2011.* Colombo, Sri Lanka: WHO Sri Lanka Country Office; 2006.
48. WHO. *Planning and budgeting to deliver services for mental health. Mental health policy and services guidance package.* Geneva: WHO; 2003.
49. Draper CLC, Lund C, Kleintjes S, Funk M, Omar M, Flisher A, the MHaPP Research Programme Consortium Mental health policy in South Africa: development process and content. *Health Policy & Plan.* 2009;24:342–56.
50. Lund C, Kleintjes S, Kakuma R, Flisher A, the MHaPP Research Programme Consortium. Public sector mental health systems in South Africa: inter-provincial comparisons and policy implications. *Social Psychiatry & Psychiatr Epidemiol.* 2010;45:393–404.
51. Ssebunnya J, Kigozi F, Ndyanabangi S. Developing a national mental health policy: a case study from Uganda. *PLoS Medicine.* 2012. doi: 10.1371/journal.pmed.1001319
52. WHO. *Mental health information systems.* Geneva: WHO; 2005.
53. Levav I, Restrepo H, Guerra de Macedo C. The restructuring of care in Latin America: a new policy for mental health services. *J Public Health Policy.* 1994;15:71–85.
54. Caldas de Almeida JM, Horvitz-Lennon M. Mental health care reforms in Latin America: an overview of mental health care reforms in Latin America and the Caribbean. *Psychiatr Serv.* 2010;61(3):218–21.
55. Caldas de Almeida JM. What can we learn from mental health reform in Latin America and the Caribbean? In JM Caldas de Almeida & A Cohen, editors. *Innovative mental health programs in Latin America and the Caribbean.* Washington DC: Pan American Health Organization; 2008: iv–xi.
56. Caldas de Almeida JM. Technical cooperation strategies of the Pan American Health Organization in the new phase of mental health services reform in Latin America and the Caribbean. *Panam J Public Health.* 2005;18:314–26.
57. WHO. *Mental Health Atlas 2011.* Geneva, WHO; 2011.
58. Yasamy MT, Maulik PK, Tomlinson M, Lund C, Van Ommeren M, Saxena S. Responsible governance for mental health research in low resource countries. *PLoS Med.* 2011;8(11):e1001126.

14 Scaling Up Services for Mental Health

Julian Eaton, Mary De Silva,
Graciela Rojas, and Vikram Patel

INTRODUCTION TO CONCEPTS

Mental disorders have generally been neglected as a global health priority, despite considerable evidence that they are at least as disabling as other non-communicable diseases.[1,2] As we have seen in chapters XX, there is now a growing evidence base for effective interventions and service models for delivery of health care in a variety of global contexts. A clear consensus as to the essential features of services that can meet the needs of people with mental health problems is emerging, and there is increasing accuracy in estimating costs of implementing such services. In this chapter, we examine the science of implementing health care interventions at large scales. This involves understanding how proven treatments perform when transferred to routine settings, and how the structures needed to deliver services play an essential role in maximizing benefits of such treatments when replicated for greater population coverage.

The Mental Health Treatment Gap

The *mental health treatment gap* is defined as the absolute difference between the true prevalence of a disorder and the proportion of affected individuals who are treated for the disorder.[3] In reality, obtaining an accurate estimate of the treatment gap is extremely difficult, as methods to measure both disorder prevalence and service utilization rely either on the analysis of data routinely collected at country-level, or on community-based epidemiological surveys, which may not be generalizable to national or regional levels.[4] Without accurate estimations of disorder prevalence or the number of people with a particular disorder who receive treatment, current estimates of the treatment gap should be viewed as no more than an approximation of the need for care.[3] There are also concerns, particularly in the context of mental health care—which often involves multiple treatments, intersectoral collaboration, and continuing care—whether "service utiliza-tion" is an adequate indicator of "treatment." At the very least, it should be considered a conservative estimate. There is also some uncertainty about whether having a "disorder" automatically signals a treatment "need," or how "treatment" is defined. There is a ten-dency to favor biomedical interventions in definitions of treatment, and the adequacy of treatment is often not considered. In the treatment of schizophrenia, for example, while a single visit to a medical clinic might qualify as a "treatment," in most cases this would not be an adequate response to the complex needs that people with the disorder often have. Clearly, in the context of mental disorders, these are critically important concerns, and it is important to strive for definitions that underlie research to be as accurate to the real world as possible.

In spite of these limitations, attempts at estimating the treatment gap for mental dis-orders have shown it to be extremely wide, particularly in lower-income countries (see Figure 14.1) This may reflect divergent perspectives on "need" or what constitutes "treat-ment," as suggested above.

Unfortunately, whilst the evidence for how to scale up services is improving, this evi-dence has not had a significant impact on the mental health treatment gap.[4,5] The gap is not the same for all disorders; people with the more overt and severe disorders, such as schizophrenia, are more likely to obtain services than those with depression and anxiety disorders. This may simply be because they are more easily identified, or because com-munities demand action from a family, particularly if a person's behavior has become disruptive to community life. Alcohol use disorders are particularly neglected,[6] which may be a reflection of the importance of attribution of cause to help-seeking behav-ior—people may consider alcohol misuse a moral failing rather than a medical condi-tion. Similarly, attribution of spiritual causes of many symptoms of mental disorders is a reason for the person's late presentation to health services. Levels of treatment access are also low for mental disorders in comparison to other non-communicable, chronic diseases such as diabetes.[7]

It is important to note that, even in countries that provide fairly comprehensive mental health services, the treatment gap remains large. For example, Table 14.1 shows that only around one-third of people with depression or bipolar disorder in high-income countries receive treatment. The figure is roughly one in 10 in LMICs. This suggests

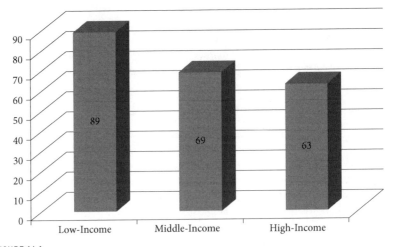

FIGURE 14.1
Percentage of people with a severe mental disorder (schizophrenia) not receiving care within previous 12 months.[20] Country Income Level (World Bank classification)

Table 14.1 12-Month Prevalence of Disorders and Treatment in High-, Low, and Middle-Income Countries

Disorders	Prevalence (%)		Treatment Prevalence (%)	
	High Income	Low Income	High Income	Low Income
Physical				
Arthritis	18.6	10.0	50.9	46.6
Asthma	10.0	3.5	51.0	61.4
Cancer	4.0	0.6	64.8	43.7
Chronic Pain	6.0	8.0	51.8	59.6
Diabetes	4.6	3.9	94.4	76.6
Heart Disease	4.7	5.9	77.7	50.9
Mental				
BPAD	1.4	0.7	29.1	13.4
Depression	5.7	5.2	29.3	8.1
GAD	2.4	1.4	31.6	7.2
Panic Disorder	1.6	0.7	33.1	9.4
PTSD	2.3	0.9	29.5	8.1

Adapted from Ormel et al., 2008.[7]

that the size of the treatment gap is affected by a range of factors in addition to service availability. Issues such as treatment acceptability (particularly biological treatments), stigma, and different attributions of causation, all affect the utilization of mental health services, even in contexts where they are affordable and available. Increasing the demand for mental health services will entail providing a more comprehensive range of interventions, which may include livelihoods and structured social support tailored to local needs, and, in addition, the availability of biomedical models of care in settings that are less associated with stigma.

SCALING UP SERVICES TO CLOSE THE TREATMENT GAP

In order to reduce the treatment gap, many more people need to have access to evidence-based mental health services, and also need to choose to use them. This can be done by not only providing good services, but ensuring that they are culturally appropriate ("acceptable"), and that social beliefs and attitudes that reduce service use are addressed.

The World Health Organization dedicated its annual *World Health Report* to mental health in 2001,[8] and whilst it set a positive tone with its title, "New Understanding, New Hope," over ten years later, most of its recommendations had only been implemented in wealthier nations, many of whom had already started this process in the 1980s. The report's recommendations included a wholesale shift from institutional to community-based care for most patients, and efforts to make services more holistic, including allowing more access to psychological treatments and creating better links to social services.

Since then, numerous reports[9,10,11] have recommended very similar reorganizations of services for low resource settings, including the first Global Mental Health Action Plan approved by the WHO's World Health Assembly in 2013. There has also been a significant strengthening of the evidence-base supporting this shift, which includes both proven interventions and the methods for delivering these interventions in practical

Box 14.1 The *World Health Report 2001* Recommendations[8]

1. PROVIDE TREATMENT IN PRIMARY CARE

   It was reinforced that the management and treatment of mental disorders should occur in primary care, ensuring greater access to care. Care should be delivered by general health personnel.

2. MAKE PSYCHOTROPIC DRUGS AVAILABLE

   Psychotropic drugs are an essential in delivery of comprehensive care but often not available. They should be provided as part of a country's essential drug list.

3. GIVE CARE IN THE COMMUNITY

   Due to better evidence of efficacy, cost-effectiveness, and reduction of stigma, there should be a shift from care in institutions to community-based settings.

4. EDUCATE THE PUBLIC

   The general public needs to be better educated about the nature and treatability of mental disorders, as well as to the human rights of people with mental health problems.

5. INVOLVE COMMUNITIES, FAMILIES, AND CONSUMERS

   Communities, service users and their caregivers should participate in implementation of services as well as creation of policies that affect them. Services will then better reflect the needs of those who rely on them.

6. ESTABLISH NATIONAL POLICIES, PROGRAMS, AND LEGISLATION

   Countries must develop relevant mental health policy and legislation as well as design programs that will improve provision of care. A greater proportion of health budgets needs to be devoted to mental health care.

7. DEVELOP HUMAN RESOURCES

   Expertise for delivery of services should be made more available, as well as improving the skills of general health care workers.

8. LINK WITH OTHER SECTORS

   Other sectors like education, social welfare, justice, and labor are important in the lives of people with mental health problems, and should be encouraged to recognize mental health needs in their programs of work.

9. MONITOR COMMUNITY MENTAL HEALTH

   Health information and reporting systems must include indicators for mental health care. This includes better mental health surveillance as well as measures of health care system effectiveness. This should improve the availability of information that can lead to greater resource allocation.

10. SUPPORT MORE RESEARCH

    More research would lead to a better understanding of prevalence, different characteristics of mental ill health in different regions, and an improved evidence base upon which to build services.

settings.[12,13] Why, then, has this evidence base not been translated into widely available services in many countries, and what can be done to promote a shift from evidence and recommendations to implementation?

What Is Meant by "Scaling Up Services"?

Scaling up services enables people with mental disorders to have the opportunity to access effective care that was previously not available to them. In a situation where the evidence of need is compelling, and there is a consensus of recommended best practice, the principles of justice and equity provide the imperative for action.

One accepted definition of scaling up is: "Deliberate efforts to increase the impact of health service innovations successfully tested in pilot or experimental projects so as to benefit more people and to foster policy and program development on a lasting basis."[14] The most widely accepted definitions of scaling up include five main components:[15]

1. Increase the number of people receiving services.
   - This might be through greater geographical coverage, a wider range of services (e.g., adding psychosocial care to biomedical services), or addressing more conditions.
2. Use the best available scientific evidence to design health care interventions and services.
   - Follow the principle that the most likely way of achieving the intended impact is to rely on the best evidence of effectiveness and cost-effectiveness of interventions, and how they can be delivered sustainably.
3. Use a service model shown to be effective in similar contexts.
   - The evidence of effectiveness in one context is not necessarily transferable to all. Practically, this means that interventions and service models should be tested in a pilot phase in the same or a similar setting prior to scaling up. This is particularly important because a high proportion of research is done in places that are most unlike the locales where the greatest treatment gaps exist.[16] While there are clearly significant similarities in different countries and cultures, it is easy (for convenience) to assume universality when in fact there is diversity; for example, in the way people explain mental symptoms, express their problems ("idioms of distress"), make decisions about accessing care, or value different types of treatments.
4. Integrate mental health services into existing health systems.
   - In order to ensure that mental health is considered an essential component of general health systems, it is important to emphasize the integration of such services into all levels of health care. This leads services in the evidence-based direction of deinstitutionalization, decentralization, and primary care-level based services. It also acts to reduce the stigma and exclusion suffered by people with mental disorders (processes that are mirrored at the individual and service level). "Health systems" are not only services, but the structures and processes that support them; for example, management, financing, and health information systems. This emphasis on integration into general health systems does not imply that other sectors are less important. In fact, the health system can only play a limited role in ensuring social inclusion of people with mental illnesses. Embedding mental health in the programs of organizations working in other sectors; e.g., education and justice, is a very effective way of not only reaching many people with needs who do not present to the health system, but also mobilizing resources towards the overall aim of promoting good mental health and increasing access to mental health care.

   In addition to the relevant formalized (government and professional private) structures is the informal sector. Most people with mental health problems turn first to sources of support that are accessible and fit in with their ideas of what will best resolve their problems. These include traditional or complementary medicine practitioners, as well as the care that people receive from friends, relatives, and non-health figures of authority such as religious or cultural leaders. Understanding this important set of care options is essential to developing effective, appropriate packages of service that complement the existing social resources that provide essential support, and build on them to provide a comprehensive response to the range of needs that people have.

5. Ensure sustainability of mental health services through policy formulation, implementation, and financing.
   - As discussed below, a major challenge to successfully scaling up services has been the difficulty of embedding services in a sustainable way in systems, particularly at

larger scales (for example, at the country level). The science and practice of implementation that encompasses engagement with political processes is therefore a priority if scaling up is to be successful.

This set of principles in health care has been adopted in mental health, but it was developed and has been taken further in other areas such as HIV/AIDS care and the maternal and child health field. There are many similar challenges and common solutions across different health fields. These similarities are particularly strong between services for mental health and chronic conditions such as HIV/AIDS or diabetes, which share many features in how to improve care and treatment outcomes. In fact, this has led

---

Case Study 14.1—"Epilepsy Management at a Primary Health Level" Program, China[18]

Epilepsy has a high burden of disability as the impact on the individual of repeated seizures and associated injuries is associated with the stigma attached to the disease. People with epilepsy have high rates of social exclusion and low employment levels. There is also a high economic impact from the condition, both on the family and on the health system.

Effective and affordable treatment is available for epilepsy, with 70% of people responding positively to simple and cheap medication regimens. Between 2000 and 2004, the World Health Organization (WHO), the International League Against Epilepsy (ILAE), and the International Bureau for Epilepsy (IBE), in association with Ministry of Health of China, carried out a demonstration project to improve epilepsy management in six provinces in rural China.

An initial survey found a lifetime prevalence of 7/1000, and a prevalence of active epilepsy of 4.6/1000. The treatment gap was 63% for people with active epilepsy.

The following interventions to address the identified needs of people with epilepsy were implemented in the six provinces: primary care physicians were trained to follow a simple treatment protocol using phenobarbital; and an educational program for families and the general public was carried out emphasizing the treatability of epilepsy.

A second epidemiological survey conducted after the intervention found that the treatment gap had reduced to 50% (a 13% reduction). Seventy percent of clients had an improvement in their condition, and 25% were seizure-free. It was also found that the economic burden on families had reduced, and the costs to the health system had fallen dramatically.

Based on these findings, a model of care was designed, which took account of issues such as public education and advocacy, improving medication supply, provision of human resources, development of training materials, and use of an evidence-based intervention package delivered in a feasible way.

Issues identified as crucial to success of the program were the inclusion of stakeholders in program design and implementation, formation of collaborative partnerships, engagement with government and ensuring political and financial support, and rigorous monitoring and evaluation. Effective communication of positive outcomes of the program led the government support for wider scaling up of the program, and as of 2008, the program had been scaled up in 79 counties in 15 provinces. By 2011, it was in 19 Chinese provinces, with plans to continue to expand coverage throughout China's rural health care system.

many to suggest that combining services for mental health with those for other chronic diseases may be a strategy for scaling up services for mental disorders.[17]

BARRIERS TO SCALING UP SERVICES

Having clarified the goal of evidence-based, quality, accessible care that is available to all, the most rational next step is to try to understand what might have prevented these goals from being achieved so far in most countries. The term "scaling up" has been used to refer to both an *objective* and a *process*. The practical considerations that can lead to success or failure in efforts to scale up services include a number of dynamic factors such as mobilizing political will, accessing sustainable financial resources, human resource development, availability of essential medicines, and monitoring and evaluation. The following sections cover major barriers to progressing in this process were identified through an extensive survey of experts from many countries.[19]

The Prevailing Public-Health Priority Agenda and Its Effect on Funding

In a world of limited resources, the allocation of competing needs should be rational and fair. The simplest way to look at whether the allocation of resources is fair is to compare the burden of mental disorders with the resources allocated to them as a proportion of total health needs. The proportion of the total burden of disability that can be attributed to mental health problems is over 12%. In contrast, governments typically spend far less than this percentage of their health budget explicitly on mental health—in Africa, it is typically less than 1% (see Figure 14.2).[20]

Chapter 9 describes in detail the iniquities in the availability and distribution of mental health resources, globally and at the level of countries. This stark imbalance is a clear indication of the low priority that mental health currently has on the agenda of politicians and other decision-makers. This low priority is a major challenge for advocates of service development, particularly as scaling up mental health services largely depends on securing adequate resources. It is important to point out that, in many countries, health services in general are underfunded, so reallocation of funds from elsewhere in the health budget is not the solution. Instead, there need to be new funds available, which should be used more efficiently (for example, used in primary rather than specialist care), and in an equitable manner.[21]

Health planning pays great attention to efficiency, so it is essential that evidence of cost-effectiveness be presented if resources are to be allocated. One argument against increasing resource allocation in a particular area may be that there are no interventions that are known to be cost-effective. In fact, the costs associated with providing effective mental health care in a variety of settings are becoming more accurately defined.[22,23] One way to compare cost-effectiveness is to use a common denominator for health benefit. One way of doing this is using the Disability Adjusted Life Year (DALY), a composite unit combining mortality and years lived with disability attributable to a disorder. The treatment for mental disorders has been found to compare favorably, in terms of cost per DALY averted, with interventions for other chronic diseases.[24] While this is significant, there are many other varieties of burden that are not covered by the DALY methodology used to compare disability attributed to different disorders, but are relevant to the lives of people with these disorders. These include burden to caregivers (time, financial resources, opportunity cost of caring for a sick relative), harm caused (a common consequence of alcohol and illicit drug use), and lost productivity at the individual, family, or society level. Economic cost is high, as

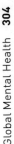
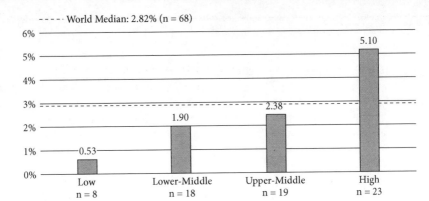

FIGURE 14.2
Proportion of health budget devoted explicitly to mental health, by country income level.[20]

many mental disorders disable people from a young age, and do so for many years. The evidence for cost-effectiveness for interventions in this area (usually using DALYs as a common denominator) is strong, but it is likely that the case would be even more persuasive if other sorts of burden were to be taken in account. (See Case Study 14.2 for an example of economic benefits of improved mental health being used to advocate for investment in scaling up services.)

In low-income countries, the typical per capita expenditure on mental health care is as low as $0.10–$0.20; that is, $100,000–$200,000 per year for a population of 1 million. The required expenditure to meet target coverage levels is estimated to be around $1.50–$2.00 per capita in low-income countries, and $3.00–$4.00 in middle-income countries.[11] The funding gap is therefore substantial, particularly in low-income countries. This gap is confounded by poor organization of the resources that do exist, and a lack of equitable mechanisms to distribute costs fairly (such as social insurance schemes). In the poorest countries in the world, "out-of-pocket" payment for services, the least equitable system, is the most common.[21] Scaling up mental health services to full coverage requires a tenfold increase from current levels of expenditure in many countries. Only large-scale redistribution of domestic resources and/or new investment from external sources is capable of overcoming the shortfall. Consequently, addressing the low priority afforded to mental health is essential both at the country level and on a global level (for example, raising the profile of mental health in funding allocation by governments or international donors), and must always be addressed as a practical issue as part of efforts to scale up services.

Complexity of and Resistance to Decentralization of Mental Health Services

Structures that are well established always resist change. The prevailing mental health system of the late twentieth century was one in which the main resources were focused in specialist centers (initially asylums, then psychiatric hospitals). This pattern was mirrored in countries colonized by European powers around the world. Many wealthier countries have made significant shifts in the makeup of mental health services towards a mixed range of services, including general hospital beds and more community-based care, since the 1980s (see Chapter 1). This shift has not occurred in lower-income countries, where there are still twice as many beds in psychiatric hospitals as in general hospitals.[20]

There are many justified criticisms of large psychiatric institutions. For example: they are inaccessible to most of the population, they are expensive to run, and the

Case Study 14.2—"Improving Access to Psychological Therapies" (IAPT) in the United Kingdom

For many years, advocates, including patients, for a more balanced approach to mental health treatment in the United Kingdom had argued for an increase in the availability of psychological therapies in the National Health Service. Despite strong clinical evidence for efficacy of specific psychological interventions for particular disorders, treatment options were limited, and biological treatments remained the dominant treatment modality. This changed with a radical scaling-up of psychological treatments in the United Kingdom following a landmark report by economist Professor Richard Layard, published in 2006.[27] Its most significant conclusion was that the costs to the national economy of depression and anxiety (mainly through absence from work) far outweighed the costs of providing evidence-based care for these conditions.

The IAPT was designed to increase the ease of access to psychological treatments at the PHC level, using a stepped-care approach, with defined care pathways, flexible referral routes (including self-referral), minimum quality standards, and routine monitoring of patient outcomes. The intervention package was approved by the U.K. National Institute for Health and Clinical Excellence (NICE), and largely focused on cognitive behavioral therapy (CBT). The single greatest challenge was to train an estimated 6000 new therapists required to provide services.

By 2011, the target of 900,000 people receiving treatment and of 25,000 coming off sickness benefit had been achieved. A recovery rate of around 50% was reported. Roughly 3600 therapists had been trained.[28]

A second phase of the program was launched in 2011, extending its scope to include children and young people, and people with chronic medical conditions, medically unexplained symptoms, or severe mental disorders. The government is committed to this ongoing funding, and to training the remaining therapists needed.

care they provide is often dehumanizing. So why have they proven so difficult to reform? The resistance to change is usually attributed to professionals whose interests are best served by working in large hospitals in cities. This is where they have a more comfortable quality of life and higher-status positions as hospital consultants and university professors. Until new decentralized structures are in place, there is no security in pursuing a career in anything other than the existing system. There is evidence, however, that the consistent messages from organizations such as the WHO, and the fact that more developed countries have decentralized services, has led to professionals recognizing the need to change, even if in practice the change will be gradual.[25] The fact nevertheless remains that in most countries there are far too few specialist beds.[20] There is need to *add* alternative, decentralized services *to* the specialist hospitals that exist, and not to reduce these services (unless the human rights situation is unacceptable and cannot be reformed). As we will see, decentralized and community-based services require oversight, supervision, and referral opportunities, and must be seen as complementary to, and not a substitute for, specialist hospital-based care.

Challenges to Implementation of Mental Health Care in Primary-Care Settings

In theory, primary health care (PHC) services offer the most accessible care available to most of the population. Since the 1978 Alma Ata declaration, "Health for All by 2000," this has been the accepted consensus of where mental health care should also be accessed. Other reasons why PHC is consistently recommended as the site where first-line services should be offered include:[10]

1. Mental and physical health needs are interwoven, so delivering care at the same point ensures holistic care is offered. The physical needs of people with mental health problems can be addressed, as well as the mental health needs of people who present with physical problems.
2. The high prevalence of mental health problems means that it is impossible for specialist (or even general) hospitals to meet these needs.
3. The great majority of the care that is needed is most appropriately delivered in a general health care setting, particularly the long-term routine follow-up that is a feature of chronic conditions. There is strong evidence of positive outcomes through care delivered at this level.
4. Availability of mental health care in PHC reduces the stigma that people experience when forced to use separate services outside of the usual system accessed by other people. In addition, hospitals have historically been sites where some of the worst human rights abuses have occurred.
5. Health care services at the PHC level are cost-effective both for service providers and for recipients and their families, due to reduced travel and expenses associated with inpatient services.

Despite the strong rationale for the integration of mental health care into PHC, there are relatively few examples of how this has been successfully implemented in practice and outside of wealthier nations. If a PHC system is struggling to meet basic general medical priorities, and many parts of it do not function well, it will be difficult to successfully integrate mental health. For example, in many countries where staff at this level are overburdened, referral systems do not function, and medications are not available, integrating mental health will not be successful without first considering how the overall system can be strengthened.

Low Numbers and Few Types of Workers Are Trained and Supervised in Mental Health Care

In many countries, workers with the skills to deliver mental health care are scarce at the various levels of health care, and the skilled workers who do exist often do not in work environments in which they are supported to provide mental health care (see Chapter 10, Human Resources).

Specialization in psychiatry is not a popular choice because of stigmatization of workers in the field, and because of perceived limited rewards in choosing this career pathway. There is both a shortfall of specialists being trained, and a low level of mental health skills among general clinical practitioners and managers. In low-income settings, specialists who do train are often tempted to work in wealthier countries, and even in wealthier countries, there is often a shortage of professionals in more rural or deprived areas. In many African countries, it is common to find ratios of less than one psychiatrist to 1 million people, and other professionals like occupational therapists, nurses, psychologists, special educationalists, or social workers who have specialized in mental health are even more limited in number.[26]

Scarcity of Public Mental Health Perspectives

In a context of limited numbers of professionals in mental health, their focus tends to be on fulfilling what are perceived as essential medical and administrative roles at the district, regional, or national level. As we have seen, the prevailing model is often biased towards specialist institutions, and professionals tend to migrate towards larger institutions like universities and tertiary hospitals. Their time and intellectual resources are therefore likely to be predominantly utilized in these roles; for example, running wards and outpatient clinics in hospitals, or carrying out teaching and research activities in universities. This often means that, despite being the experts in the field, often called upon by governments for technical advice, they do not have the public health perspective that is necessary to address policy and service development issues that focus on access and equity. The result is a perpetuation of biomedical top-down models of care that fall within the bounds of the experience of these experts. Of course, trainees in teaching institutions are also only exposed to existing models of care, and so will tend to emerge from training with similarly limited perspectives.

Coupled with this lack of public health perspective among mental health leaders is a lack of mental health knowledge among public health experts. Training in public health is often relatively weak on mental health, and public health departments advising governments or ministries may not be able to confidently provide up-to-date evidence about the epidemiology, mental health economics, or possible models for reform of services.

STRATEGIES TO OVERCOME BARRIERS

Specific ways of overcoming barriers will always depend on the situation in which a service is being scaled up. However, there are some common recommendations based on experience that have emerged to address barriers to successfully scaling up mental health care in an effective and affordable way.

Building Political Will

Understand the Political Environment Well, and Use a Tailored, Strategic Approach to Scaling Up

New interventions need to be implemented only after a proper situation analysis, so that evidence-based services are also appropriate to the needs of that country and the local context. There will be diverse solutions identified to address local problems, and any plan for scaling up services has to be tailor-made. In addition to understanding the epidemiological and resource context of the region where the scaling up is to take place, it is very important to understand what factors are likely to bring about change in relevant bodies, and what might motivate key persons in positions of power to support the scaling up process. For example, in many countries, it would be wrong to rely only on presenting convincing (even evidence-based) arguments about population needs that need to be met by the government health sector. In fact, individuals who hold senior positions in government ministries and, therefore, make important decisions about what is prioritized for budgetary allocation and implementation are much more likely to be inspired to act by personal contact with an individual who represents in a more visceral way the arguments being made.

It is also prudent to exploit timely opportunities as they arise. For example, significant progress might be made in gaining government approval for a mental health plan if it is joined to a plan for other non-communicable diseases and there is already political will for the latter. Similarly, there is growing recognition of the mental health consequences of humanitarian emergencies, and such extreme circumstances could offer a "foot in the door" to initiate mental health programs that are sustained beyond the acute emergency. This has been done in the Aceh province of Indonesia and in Sri Lanka after the 2004 tsunami.[29]

Enabling Policy Framework for Reorganization of Services

Address Issues Systemically, Not in Isolation

Specific interventions to increase coverage of mental health services need to be part of a broader process of change. That includes strong advocacy for financial commitment, and ensuring that relevant elements of health infrastructure are being strengthened to allow the services to flourish in the long term (for example, medication supply; relevant personnel to be trained, appropriately posted, and receive ongoing supervision). Sustained change will only occur if all the relevant issues, including identified barriers, in the local environment have been taken into account.

Policy and Legislation

A *policy framework* that gives a mandate for implementing change is an important part of a process of reform. It ensures that political support is documented and, if done well, is an opportunity to involve all relevant parties in a collaborative process of formulating ideas into a practical agenda for change. Unfortunately, many policies do not get translated into meaningful implementation. There are a number of reasons for this, including: insufficient political buy-in resulting in a lack of practical support in scaling up a service; failure to identify required resources at the planning stage and, as a result, programs are underfunded; and poorly thought-out policy recommendations that are not appropriate given the context or available resources. Chapter 13 provides more detailed information the development and implementation of mental health policies.

Alongside a policy that lays out what services should look like, it is essential that there be clear *mental health legislation* that sets out the rights and entitlements of people with mental health problems and how they engage with the state and health system. Without this, there is no way that rights and entitlements can be defended, not only from abuses that happen in the general social environment, but also in systematic ways in the health, education, and judicial systems. This "institutionalized discrimination" is the tendency of policymakers and administrators in these systems to assume that people with mental health problems (or "psychosocial disabilities") lack the capacity to make decisions on their own behalf, which in turn leads to their being at elevated risk of losing their property or inheritance rights, or being incarcerated with no legal protection.[30] People with mental health problems are particularly vulnerable when they are acutely unwell, so the relevant legislation needs to take into account the specific issues surrounding engagement with the healthcare system, such as confidentiality, consent to treatment, and the use of minimally restrictive practices in treatment. Medical, social work, and criminal justice personnel also need to have guidance on how to make decisions entrusted to them by society; for example, when judging a person's legal capacity, or with respect to consent to treatment in acute crises. Legislation should also lay out an independent system through which such decisions can be challenged in a transparent way. Similarly, situations in which people have committed crimes while mentally unwell, or are seen as a danger to society, need to be managed in a humane way that has been carefully considered and legally adopted by legislators. Chapter 8 provides more details on human rights in the context of global mental health. (See also Internet resources at the end of this chapter.)

Expertise and Sustained Advocacy at Different Levels Is Necessary to Ensure Continued Support for Changes

Even when a policy formulation process is carried out in a participatory and collaborative way, and is followed up with a costed, time-bound strategic plan, it is essential that there be a body clearly mandated with the long-term implementation of the policy on an ongoing basis. Unless this is the case, the tendency is for new initiatives to take over the attention of departments well before significant progress can be made on existing policy. This is particularly the case where policy or legislation has implications that cut across more than one government department (as is typically the case with mental health). Without proper coordination, implementation will always be patchy and inconsistent. For example, legislation related to offenders with mental health problems will require commitment from both legal and medical practitioners to implement.

One way to ensure sustained advocacy for mental health services is to have an *identified body with responsibility for mental health* (or a person in some settings) in government departments at national, district, and local levels. For example, the presence of a mental health committee at a district-level health authority will make it more likely that routine problems arising in the administration of mental health services will be resolved (e.g., ensuring supply of psychotropic drugs). Equally, a mental health representation in health (and other sector) governance structures means that opportunities to strengthen and integrate services are not missed (as discussed above). For example, if a new health information system is being designed, mental health can be included; or if a child and maternal health screening exercise is being planned, postnatal depression could be included.

Of course, advocacy and ideas for change do not only come from within the system. Others affected by how services run (such as service users and caregivers) can be extremely powerful catalysts for change if they are heard. One strategy for advocating for change therefore is to mobilize the voices of such groups, who, while clearly having a strong interest and a moral mandate to participate in processes of change, are all too often silent or are not listened to.

Integration into Primary Health Care

Find an Appropriate Mix of Services to Meet Local Needs

As we have seen, service delivery at the PHC level is essential. In many wealthy countries, this shift has largely taken place, with most basic care now being managed in primary care and community-based services.[31] One concept that has been influential in guiding new service models that aim to integrate mental health care into primary health care services is "collaborative care." The main components of this are close collaboration between mental health and PHC practitioners, including placement of mental health professionals in PHC settings, and a focus on addressing both the patient's needs as well as those of their family.[32]

Building on this, and emphasizing a rational provision of interventions and an efficient use of available human resources at different levels, is "collaborative stepped care." In this model, patients are treated at the lowest appropriate tier of services using clear guidelines for intervention, and are only referred for more specialist care if necessary; for example, if they have complications or do not respond to treatment. See Case Study 14.3 for one example of integrating mental health into PHC using the collaborative stepped care approach that has been successfully implemented in lower-income settings.

Unfortunately, in many low- and middle-income countries, provision of mental health care at this level is extremely limited. This is often a reflection of an overall weakness of the health system, and when attempting to improve mental health care provision at this level, it is necessary to use an approach that strategically identifies and addresses weaknesses in health systems.

Training of district-level and PHC staff is clearly necessary in order to improve the quality of care at this level. However, there is evidence to show that simply training personnel is not enough to bring about sustained change in practice and improved outcomes for clients. Without addressing the structural impediments to functioning services at this level, there is very little chance that even trained personnel will be able to implement any effective services. There is a need to create an environment in which they are enabled to remain motivated and work productively, not only through ongoing supervision and support, but also by ensuring that they have the resources necessary to carry out their duties. This includes having the time to see clients, physical space for private consultations, transportation if they are expected to see clients in the community, and a reliable and sufficient supply of medications.

In order to promote active collaborative relationships that fulfill functions that cannot be carried out by the PHC staff themselves, other levels in the system also need to function well. This may include engaging with traditional healers, or ensuring that community-based health workers carry out awareness-raising activities and identify clients. A referral system with district-level and hospital specialists who can accept referrals and refer back to the PHC for follow-up is also essential. The strength of the district level has been particularly emphasized in recent reviews, as this has often been neglected; and without input at this level, PHC services cannot receive the support they need to maintain services.[34]

As at other levels of the system, a clear plan has to be developed involving all those participating in the changes. The plan must be properly resourced, and be practical. Strong coordination must be in place to oversee systematic reform in PHC. Such coordination would ensure all components of such reform are completed, and that any advocacy that is needed when plans are not carried out, or resources reduced, is done. The coordinator (or team) would also be able to engage with other sectors to insure that mental health is involved, whenever it is relevant to other (government and civil society) activities. This might include programs that generally fall under the remit of health, education, justice, human rights, or social welfare, and engagement with local structures, such as youth or women's groups, or traditional healers.

The problem of giving more responsibilities to already overburdened PHC staff is often cited. A possible solution is to look more flexibly at how services might be better integrated into other services. One promising option is provision of combined services for people with chronic conditions, as they share many of the characteristics of services for mental and neurological disorders.[17] There are now examples of this being tried in the field, and models that promote integration rather than isolation of mental health care are to be encouraged.

Human Resources—See Chapter 10

Reallocation of Tasks Among the Personnel Available and Creating Additional Human Resources

There is clearly a need to respond to a lack of mental health workforce by increasing the number of people in the health care system who choose to specialize in mental health, and by making it easier for generalists to acquire and practice skills in the recognition and treatment of mental health problems. This, however, is not sufficient, and it will not be possible to meet need by continuing to pursue the idea of simply training more people.

Case Study 14.3—Stepped Care for Depression in Chile

Chile is a Latin American country with over 16 million inhabitants, and is regarded as a middle-income country according to the World Bank definition. During the 1990s, epidemiological studies demonstrated a high burden of mental disorders. This resulted in implementation of a process of reform of psychiatry services that emphasized the development of community care to treat mental disorders. Although the national public health system technically provided services to over 70% of the population, the efficiency of delivery of mental health care had historically been very low in this system.

From 2000 to 2002, a randomized controlled trial was carried out to compare the effectiveness of a stepped-care program with usual care to treat depressed women in primary care clinics.[33] The stepped-care program included a structured psychoeducational group headed by social workers and nurses, systematic monitoring of clinical progress, and structured pharmacotherapy for patients with moderate to severe depression, which was executed by trained general practitioners. A total of 240 adult women participated in this trial, and the results showed a large and significant difference in favor of the stepped-care program compared with the usual care across all assessed outcomes. This program was more effective and marginally more expensive than usual care. Women receiving the stepped-care program had a mean of 50 additional depression-free days over six months compared to patients allocated to usual care.

The results of this trial contributed to Chile's National Program for the Detection, Diagnosis and Treatment of Depression that started in 2001 in primary care clinics. The program began in 2001, and by 2004 it was implemented in primary care clinics throughout the country. The program follows clinical guidelines and algorithms for screening, diagnostic evaluation, delivery of psychosocial interventions and medications, follow-up, criteria to refer to secondary care, and consultation with specialists. The incorporation of psychologists into primary care, the evolution of general health centers into family health centers, and periodic consultations from specialists have facilitated the implementation of this program.

Among persons treated for depression in primary care, 90% were women, and most of them had a history of previous depressive episodes and low social support. Contrary to expectations, three quarters of female patients had a moderate or severe depression, a rate that is very similar to that observed in secondary care. An evaluation carried out in the first years of the program showed high compliance for pharmacological treatment (73.3%), but only moderate compliance for individual psychotherapy (47.4%) and group psychoeducation (37.8%). Furthermore, a significant decline was observed in the severity of symptoms at the three-month follow-up. The decline was greater among women with the most serious symptoms; a significant decrease in anxiety and somatic symptoms was also observed. From 2006, depression was incorporated into the program of "therapeutic health guarantees," which gave a legal right to persons with depression to receive treatment. This was delivered in primary care, with referral to specialist care for those with psychotic symptoms, a bipolar disorder, a high suicidal risk, or lack of response to two six-week courses of treatment with two different antidepressants at therapeutic doses plus psychosocial interventions.

Between July 2006 and June 2010, over 690,000 persons with depression had been treated through the national program.

When there are few specialists, "task sharing" is a means of efficiently using existing non-specialist personnel and reallocating their responsibilities at different levels. One example might be to provide staff at a primary health care level with the skills and resources to provide treatment for cases that they would previously have been expected to refer for specialty care. A high proportion of need can be met with simple packages of care delivered by non-specialists in settings outside of hospitals.[13] Primary health-level staff need to be better able (and more motivated) to manage mental disorders that their clients routinely present with, and be able, when necessary, to access specialist support as needed.[10]

This principle is now well established, and there are many specific examples of tasks that have been successfully allocated to particular groups of workers not traditionally given this role. Using this principle, Lady Health Workers in Pakistan have been able to provide psychosocial care for depressed mothers,[35] community health workers have been trained to provide care for people with schizophrenia in India,[36] and peer counselors have delivered psychological therapy for depression in Uganda,[37] among other examples. Indeed, a comprehensive review of the evidence from low- and middle-income countries identified 42 studies evaluating the effectiveness of task-shared interventions for mental health, with overwhelmingly positive results.[26] In the United Kingdom, nurses have developed a wide range of "extended roles," independently running diabetes and pain clinics, for example; while general practitioners have significantly increased the proportion of clients with mental disorders who are managed at the PHC level. Perhaps most innovative of all are services that have made increasing use of service users themselves (and their families) to provide peer support beyond the usual confines of medical services.

The science underpinning these ideas has largely arisen from other areas of global health and development. As more examples are implemented in mental health and evaluated, subsequent program design may be informed by the lessons learnt about, for example, what roles should be played, by whom, and what inputs are needed to make for better mental health services in low-resourced settings. However, at present, much of the evidence around service reform and scaling up is in the form of randomized controlled trials. Given that the principles of task-shifting must be applied in a wide range of settings, the challenge is to identify common factors for success that can guide planners in reforming services, whilst maintaining the capacity to integrate such reforms into existing services in a flexible way. This will enable the creation and use of an appropriate evidence-base without taking a one-size-fits-all approach that will not be sensitive to local peculiarities. One proposed method for doing this is to define essential "skill sets" that need to be fulfilled for a service to function. Different countries (or service environments) might assign these roles to different cadres in their system, and provide them with the skill sets, resources, and infrastructural environment they need to carry out these tasks (see Figure 14.3).

This system also outlines "implementation rules" for how the people so tasked might be supported to carry out their assigned roles. These rules include providing the enabling environment of policy support, mapping care pathways, providing clear tools to support decisions in clinical work, and using techniques that have been shown to improve quality of services and their capacity to adapt to improve their outcomes.[40]

The specific knowledge and skills that are needed for this and similar schema would usually be defined by an evidence-based "package of care." While several such sets of recommendations for services have been developed, probably the most widely recognized is the WHO's mhGAP program,[9] which includes recommendations not only for evidence-based clinical interventions, but also for training materials and program implementation guidelines, as well as being complemented by materials on policy and legislation development (see the online resources list at the end of this chapter). The evidence base for these packages of care has arisen largely from work in high-income countries, but recent examples (including mhGAP and the PLoS Medicine series on

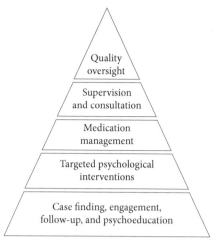

FIGURE 14.3
Skill sets necessary to deliver a mental health service.[40]

treatment packages for mental disorders) have explicitly sought to include the evidence arising from low-resource settings, despite its current relative scarcity.[41] Chapter 9 describes mhGAP and packages of care for specific mental disorders in more detail.

Public Mental Health Perspective

Evidence Base for Scaling Up Mental Health Services Needs to Be Applied in Practice

Advocates for scaling up activities to promote global mental health have recognized the need for collating good evidence and making it available for use at a local level. The experience of other global health advocacy initiatives is that if policymakers are to be persuaded of the importance of responding to a particular need, they require clear, focused, and practical messages. At present, mental health issues are perceived as complex and incomprehensible, reinforcing the myth that conditions are untreatable, and that services give poor value for money. Clearly presented evidence can change this perception, particularly if linked to guidance about how proven and practical interventions can be implemented.

This can only happen if the evidence is understood and made relevant for local use. This often requires the presence of persons suitably trained in public health aspects of mental health. This expertise is currently lacking in many settings, but as "global mental health" emerges as a discipline, this should change. In regions where there is a serious lack of mental health professionals and practitioners, it is unlikely that there will be the resources to have experts devoted solely to public mental health. Therefore, alongside improving the mental health expertise of public health officials, existing mental health professionals will need to broaden their roles from being traditional "clinicians," to including planning, training, supervision, and advocating with decision-makers in their areas of expertise.[42]

THE PROCESS OF SCALING UP SERVICES

We have seen that scaling up mental health services is necessary and that the evidence exists to defend the investment. The challenge is practical implementation. This section of the chapter presents practical guidance for those wishing to engage in scaling up services.

Case Study 14.4—Peer Support in High- and Low-Income Settings

There is a long-standing tradition recognizing the importance of shared experience in those recovering from alcohol and substance misuse, with Alcoholics Anonymous being the best-documented example of an organization autonomously run by people with, or recovering from, alcohol problems. Central to the Twelve-Step program of Alcoholics Anonymous are the principles of sharing failings and experiences with others in recognition of the strength that can be gained from this, and a commitment to help others in a similar situation (for no personal gain). The organization has grown in its 80-year history, and in 2010, there were 1.2 million people attending meetings in the United States, in 55,000 groups.

Despite this long tradition, and the early development of self-help and peer support for people with physical illness, it was only with the emergence of the Mental Health Service User, Survivor, or Consumer movement in the 1980s that formal groups for peer support for persons with mental illness were established. One of the achievements of this consumer movement has been to successfully argue for the greater participation of service users in their own care, and the inclusion of peer support as an accepted option in the range of treatment that can benefit people. Deinstitutionalization in many countries was another impetus for people to seek the support in community settings that they were previously able to find in hospitals and psychiatric institutions. Such groups are diverse in size, purpose, membership, and organizational structures. They have been shown to increase self-esteem and social functioning, although the evidence is not strong, and membership of such groups is still proportionately very low.[38]

As well as *peer-support groups,* two other ways that people who have experienced mental health problems have proven to have a valuable role in health services is through *consumer-run services* (often requiring funding by health authorities for financial viability), and through *employment in formal services.* Both these developments have the potential to lead to the availability of more positive role models for those in a process of recovery, as well as providing opportunities for people with mental health problems to influence services that affect them.

Self-Help Groups in Ghana

In 2008, clients of a community-based rehabilitation (CBR) program in the small town of Sandema in Northern Ghana decided to form a self-help group. Their shared priority initially was to try to improve their financial situation, as the stigma of mental illness meant that almost all of them found earning a living very difficult in this very poor region. They started meeting, initially facilitated by staff from the CBR program, on a monthly basis, and were able to form a committee and register as an organization, allowing them to open a bank account. Initially with small contributions from members, and later from external grants, they were able to give small loans to members, which were mainly used to invest in small farms or to buy animals (mainly goats and chickens) for rearing. These interventions have significantly improved the standard of living for members, who report:

- Better livelihood opportunities and family income
- Improved social status in the family and wider community
- Benefits of support in coping with distressing symptoms and improved treatment adherence among members
- Raised profile of issues that matter to them in political circles

There are now 23 such groups in the Upper East Region of Ghana, and they have developed to provide much more than just financial support. As well as discussing

(continued)

Case Study 14.4 Continued

common problems (and solutions) in the regular meetings, if a member is noted to have stopped attending, or to be becoming unwell, representatives from the group will visit their home to enquire what the problem is and advise or offer support. The group also keeps some money for those who have particular financial hardships, and they help pay for medication, for example, if a member is unable to do so. On several occasions, they have joined forces to complain to those in authority when members have been unfairly treated or abused.

The groups have focused more on advocacy in recent years. Their priorities have been challenging the regional authorities to improve access to services, particularly to employ psychiatric nurses in the local district health services, and to improve the availability of drugs in what is one of the poorest served parts of the country. In 2009, the nationwide Mental Health Society of Ghana (MEHSOG) was formed, and the groups from the Upper East Region were important founder members.[39]

Changes to services cannot happen in a vacuum. Extensive consultation and planning is necessary to ensure that the proposed change is supported by relevant stakeholders (including people in positions of power who may not consider mental health a priority), and that proposals fit into the reality of the local conditions. In addition, all the other factors that might affect the capacity of the personnel to implement their defined tasks must be considered. They need the necessary resources to carry out new tasks (transport, materials, medication); they must have sufficient remuneration and be motivated to follow this career; and there must be political commitment to effect change and maintain the service once it is established. Any innovations in services must have built-in systems for monitoring and evaluation so that successful and less successful aspects of the service design can be reflected upon and used as a basic for future improvement of services (see Figure 14.4).

Prioritizing Services

Packages of care such as mhGAP are disorder-based to enable locally implemented mental health care plans to choose, depending on local circumstances, needs and resources, the disorders on which to focus. The type of service that can be offered in different settings will largely depend on the human and financial resources available, as well as practical issues related to reforming the existing structures. It remains the case in many countries that whatever little care is available is limited to specialized care. While a gradual shift towards a more balanced range of services to meet different needs is often required, the exact range of services in a particular context will depend on historical, practical (resource), and political factors.[44]

Even in the lowest-resource settings where the priorities might be to address the most prevalent problems, it is important to ensure that the needs of the most vulnerable groups are not neglected. Groups requiring special consideration include, for example, homeless people with severe mental illness, prisoners, children with intellectual disabilities, or women in extreme poverty.

Ensuring the Quality and Sustainability of Scaled-Up Services

Two key issues that have historically been the most fundamental weaknesses in many programs are maintaining their key characteristics when taken to scale: ensuring that

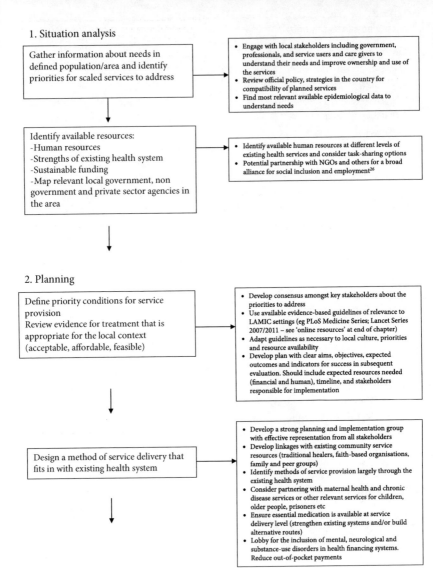

1. Situation analysis

Gather information about needs in defined population/area and identify priorities for scaled services to address

- Engage with local stakeholders including government, professionals, and service users and care givers to understand their needs and improve ownership and use of the services
- Review official policy, strategies in the country for compatibility of planned services
- Find most relevant available epidemiological data to understand needs

Identify available resources:
-Human resources
-Strengths of existing health system
-Sustainable funding
-Map relevant local government, non government and private sector agencies in the area

- Identify available human resources at different levels of existing health services and consider task-sharing options
- Potential partnership with NGOs and others for a broad alliance for social inclusion and employment[26]

2. Planning

Define priority conditions for service provision
Review evidence for treatment that is appropriate for the local context (acceptable, affordable, feasible)

- Develop consensus amongst key stakeholders about the priorities to address
- Use available evidence-based guidelines of relevance to LAMIC settings (eg PLoS Medicine Series; Lancet Series 2007/2011 – see 'online resources' at end of chapter)
- Adapt guidelines as necessary to local culture, priorities and resource availability
- Develop plan with clear aims, objectives, expected outcomes and indicators for success in subsequent evaluation. Should include expected resources needed (financial and human), timeline, and stakeholders responsible for implementation

Design a method of service delivery that fits in with existing health system

- Develop a strong planning and implementation group with effective representation from all stakeholders
- Develop linkages with existing community service resources (traditional healers, faith-based organisations, family and peer groups)
- Identify methods of service provision largely through the existing health system
- Consider partnering with maternal health and chronic disease services or other relevant services for children, older people, prisoners etc
- Ensure essential medication is available at service delivery level (strengthen existing systems and/or build alternative routes)
- Lobby for the inclusion of mental, neurological and substance-use disorders in health financing systems. Reduce out-of-pocket payments

FIGURE 14.4
(continued)

the service remains effective (quality), and sustaining these services at that level in the long-term (sustainability).

Maintaining Quality

By definition, the scaled-up version of a service involves provision of greater *quantities* of intervention; 100 health districts may be covered rather than five, or services expanded to address the needs of a wider population; for example, children or pregnant women. While it may be assumed that simply multiplying the number of units of the same intervention would have no effect on quality, in practice it is very difficult to maintain quality when services shift from their original format and scale, for a number of reasons.

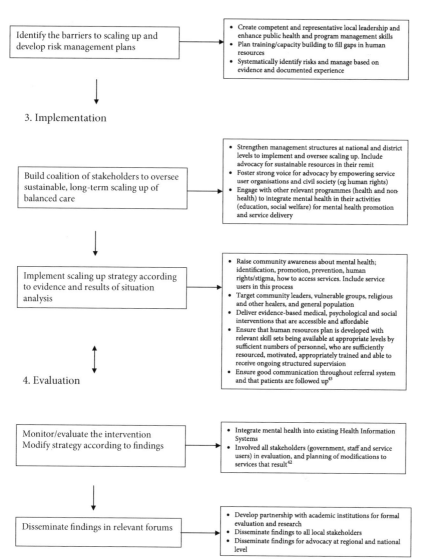

FIGURE 14.4
Important steps in strategically scaling up mental health services. (Based, with permission from Elsevier/*The Lancet,* on Eaton et al., 2011.[34])

(a) There may have been a charismatic figure who founded or sustained a service and who is impossible to replace. Even when there is no single identified person like this, a particularly dynamic and strong team is difficult to reproduce many times over, particularly in environments with fewer material and human resources.

(b) As a service is scaled up, it will inevitably cover a more diverse range of settings than in its original site. This means that there may be changes in the socio-demographic makeup of the target population, cultures represented, political environment, availability of resources, and a wide variety of other factors that may mean the service model does not function as effectively.

(c) There may have been aspects of the model that were considered to be incidental to the success at the small-scale, but are in fact essential to the success of the program at a larger scale. One frequent example is pilot programs that are well resourced, and have better outcomes, because they are part of carefully monitored research projects. When the program is scaled up, the competing demands of other services and the reduction in program oversight are likely to reduce the quality of the intervention.

Ensuring Sustainability

The initial project or program that is used as a model to scale up services is often financed in a way that cannot be replicated in a larger program. The different financial structure adopted for the scaled program may therefore not deliver the resources (or stability of resources) that are needed to implement all components of the model as required.

One particular example of this problem is when there has been a strong lead from a research perspective in the original project. In some ways, these projects are more likely to be seen as good candidates for scaling up; they have proven efficacy, may have had their cost-effectiveness determined, and often have strong advocates who are committed to their successful promotion. However, research-led projects have a particularly high level of support in the research phase, both financially and in terms of expertise and strong leadership. When considering scaling up such projects, and, even better, when designing them in the first place, it is important to recognize the risk that such strongly supported projects might not be replicable and that specific steps need to be put in place to address these risks; e.g., by ensuring that measures are put in place to provide strong leadership teams and close monitoring of progress.

It is worth noting that there are many countries with very limited internal resources, both financial and human. This means that it may not be possible to replicate across the country a very successful service delivery in one place, simply because there are not enough psychiatric nurses in the country to implement the program more widely. In fact, pilot projects are often sited in areas with more resources precisely *because* they are more likely to succeed in that environment. It is sometimes possible to mobilize external (donor) or extra governmental funds to run services, but these are often for time-limited programs that may only serve to postpone the time when the service can no longer be sustained.

Building sufficient human resources for scaling up is more challenging. Attracting workers from other countries is only an option in the very richest settings, and even this is not ideal, as such workers may be taken from environments in which they are equally (or more) needed. It also takes time to build human-resource capacity as there is a minimum period for training qualified personnel, and in the most under-resourced countries, the process may need to start at the level of creating such training opportunities in the first place.

Development of such personnel must be based on the principle of local capacity-building in order to ensure that people have relevant local knowledge and are available where they are needed, but are aware of evidence-based progress in practice. One way to do this is to develop partnerships between academic institutions (where much of the expertise and research capacity currently resides) and organizations delivering care. At the global level, many poorer countries suffer from loss of their experts to richer countries, and such partnerships carry with them the possibility of encouraging retention of experts in some of the more resource-poor settings where reform is most needed.

Ensuring sustainability is therefore a challenge that should be considered from the very beginning of services development. Inclusion of relevant stakeholders in evaluating needs and resources, and engagement with them in planning the scaling up process ensures greater "buy-in" and a sense of ownership from those involved. The importance of participation by all stakeholders, including service users, in service development also applies to setting priorities in evaluation and research. The different perspectives offered by including all stakeholders in development of the science that underpins the drive to improve the quality of and access to services can only make it stronger and more relevant to local settings.

Although wide consultation can initially be more challenging than running a service in isolation (often a temptation for externally funded services), in the long term, there are great benefits to having the support of a wide range of people when aiming to sustain a service. Engagement with key figures in government is essential, even if the service is mainly in the private or civil sector.

Using Theory of Change as a Tool to Scale Up Services

One strategic planning tool that can facilitate the process of scaling up services is Theory of Change (ToC). ToC is a visual way of deciding on and organizing the complex inter-related components of a service in the context of the setting in which the service is to be implemented. ToC is "a theory of how and why an initiative works,"[45] developed as a means to design, implement, and evaluate comprehensive community initiatives.

Based on this theory, stakeholders participate in a structured, goal-oriented, participatory planning process leading to the creation of a ToC map (see Figure 14.5 for an example of a ToC map). This is a diagram showing the causal pathways through which each component of a program leads to the intended outcomes. The participants come to a consensus about the logical steps needed to achieve a real-world impact, based on the constraints of the setting, available resources, and knowledge about what is possible and effective in this setting. Once the causal pathway is agreed on, specific strategies (components of the service) can be added, based on a rationale as to why each stage in the causal pathway logically leads to the next. Key assumptions that must be in place in order for the causal chain to remain intact are then added to the ToC map (e.g., PHC staff must have the time during patient consultations to identify patients with mental disorders). If these assumptions do not hold in a given setting, then additional strategies may need to be put in place to overcome them.

Additional assumptions that cannot be changed by the program (e.g., central government decisions to reduce funding for mental health services) should also be specified to highlight that the service maybe vulnerable to external pressures. Identifying the context-specific barriers to service implementation and reaching stakeholder consensus of the best strategies to address them may dramatically increase the chances that a service is both successful and sustainable.

Once developed, this road map can be used to plan the implementation of the service, guide its monitoring and evaluation, and be a useful visual tool for dissemination of results.[46]

EVALUATING THE SCALE-UP OF MENTAL HEALTH SERVICES

In order to improve services, it is necessary to have a good understanding of the population they are reaching (evaluation of coverage), whether services have been implemented appropriately (process evaluation), and whether they are of sufficient quality to have an impact upon peoples' lives and, perhaps, on society more broadly (evaluation of the quality of services). Apart from providing information that enables refinement in how services are designed and delivered, this evidence can be a powerful advocacy tool, especially when there is a component of economic evaluation associated with it.

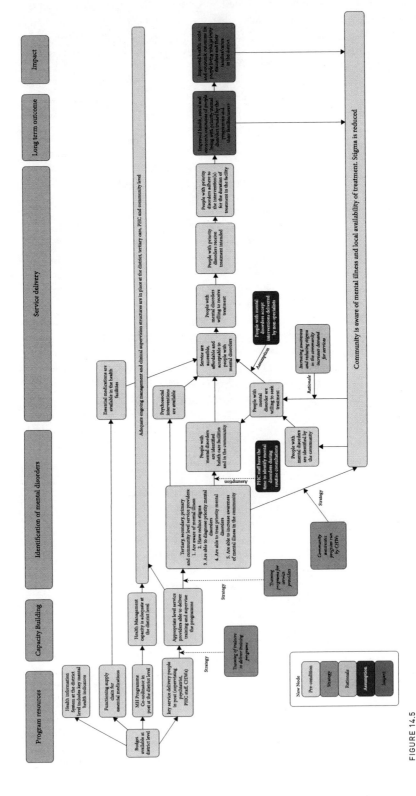

FIGURE 14.5

Simplified Theory of Change map for a PHC–based mental health services program. (With permission from PRIME—www.prime.uct.ac.za)

What to Evaluate

Coverage of Services

The main aim of scaling up services is to increase the number of people who access care. In order to determine whether this has been achieved, it is not sufficient just to know how many people are accessing the new service (compared to a previous time, or to a comparison site). We also need to know whether there has been a significant increase in the proportion of the target population who are receiving care. This requires knowledge of the denominator; i.e., the total number of people in need of services, which is often measured as the prevalence of the disorder in the target community. Ideally, this number should be obtained from epidemiological studies carried out in the same community; where these are not available, estimates from communities as geographically or culturally similar as possible may be used. In essence, one needs a numerator that accurately and reliably documents "cases" and an epidemiologically derived denominator to calculate coverage (Box 14.2). At present, in many countries, the existing systems for collecting numerator data are weak. Remember that whilst "scaling up" usually refers to expanding the geographical area served, in some cases it refers to widening the range of services in the same geographical area, and evaluation would seek to examine the coverage of the expanded range of services.

Box 14.2 A Hypothetical Example of Assessing Treatment Coverage

A previously small-scale service for priority mental disorders is scaled up to cover a district of 200,000 people. It aims to reach people at community level and enable them to access strengthened PHC services.

Prior to the program, a survey was carried out, which identified a prevalence of 3% of the population who had the priority disorders targeted by the service; i.e., 6000 people in the district. The survey determined that only about 200 people in the previous year had accessed care in the existing services. The proportion of the target population receiving care prior to the scaling up process was therefore:

200/6000 = 3%

After five years of the service, the total number of people receiving care in a year was 900, so as a proportion:

900/6000 = 15%

The treatment coverage therefore increased from 3% to 15% (or, conversely, the treatment gap fell from 97% to 85%). Without the denominator, the total number of patients accessing care in a year (200 increasing to 900) is much less meaningful. Imagine, for example, the prevalence of the priority disorders was only 0.5%. This would mean that the change in proportion of target population served changed from:

200/1000 = 20% to 900/1000 = 90%

These two results would obviously have very different meanings in real life.

It would be important to examine whether the reduction in the treatment gap could be reasonably attributed to the intervention (for example, whether the study was designed in a way that potential biases such as recall of treatment access in the baseline survey) and whether "receiving care" translated into improvements in health or social outcomes.

Implementation of Services

Process evaluation is used to determine whether the service has been implemented as intended, and how it worked in practice. The extent to which it succeeds in delivering the defined model of care in practice is referred to as its *fidelity*. As noted earlier, service models used for scaling up should be evidence-based and proved as having been successful in a similar context to the scale-up site. One way to judge how closely they replicate a given model is to measure their fidelity once being implemented. Specific tools are often designed to measure fidelity to specific components of a service model that are considered particularly important; for example, that the community nurses in a service have a caseload of less than a specific number.

Process evaluations measure service-level outputs such as what specific mental health interventions were offered, or what proportion of patients are followed up in community services. Broader issues that we have discussed above that have a bearing on success of scaling up services might also be a subject for evaluation. For example, what advocacy activities have been carried out; what training did primary care center staff receive; how frequently are mental health supervisors visiting clinics; in what way are service users engaged in the service, etc.?

Quality and Impact of Services

Simply accessing a service does not necessarily mean that the people benefit from the care they receive or that they are happy with it. The term "effective coverage" combines these two concepts of coverage and the quality of the intervention. More precisely, it is defined as the part of potential health gain that has been delivered to a population.[47] One method of assessing service quality, developed for the British National Health Service, defines a range of dimensions that give a broad framework for assessing quality of services more generally.[48]

Around these dimensions, it is suggested that a variety of indicators be used, depending on the service. For example, a clinical service might want to look at whether use of the service makes people better, as measured by symptom change, functional status, or quality of life. Social or community-level measures of quality include, for example, relevance to community needs and social acceptability of the interventions. The strongest arguments for investment in services tend to include the complete range of dimensions listed in Table 14.2. This involves demonstrating that services are (cost) effective, acceptable, and equitable.

How to Evaluate

Monitoring and Evaluation

Monitoring is the ongoing process of assessing the progress of a service against its expected results. *Evaluation* is a retrospective review of the outcomes of a service at a particular point in time; for example, annual, mid-term, or final evaluations. Internal monitoring and evaluation should be undertaken as standard by every program in order to continually assess whether the service being provided is meeting the needs of service users. It can also provide a regular review of implementation processes and allow appropriate changes to be made to address shortfalls.

Ongoing monitoring and evaluation provides a powerful, dynamic tool for allowing needs to be identified, stakeholders' voices heard, knowledge to be gained about the environment, and more to be learned about how aspects of the service interact with the local context and meet client and community needs. In this way, the principle aim of

Table 14.2 Maxwell's Dimensions for Assessing Quality of Health Care[48]

Dimensions of Health Care Quality	Brief Description
1 Access to services	Availability and ease of practical utilization of services
2 Relevance to need	The extent to which services address measured and expressed needs of individuals and the community
3 Effectiveness	The benefits of a service, measured by improvements in health
4 Equity	The fairness of distribution of benefits and burdens of a service between and within communities
5 Social acceptability	The degree to which interventions provide culturally sensitive responses to need and are welcomed by communities
6 Efficiency and economy	Whether the services are affordable (usually with reference to effectiveness). Includes affordability for providers as well as users of care

Reprinted with permission from BMJ Publishing Group Ltd.

evaluation can be achieved: to mold services to be more responsive to the real needs they set out to address. In the specific case of evaluating the process of scaling up services, evaluation would ideally clarify what aspects of the implemented model are working well towards this end, and what need to be changed.

The intended *outcomes* of the program should be set at the development stage, and usually follow logically from an assessment of need, through a participative process assessing, for example, stakeholder priorities and resources, to formulation of the overall *goal* of the program. Usually, in order to achieve this goal, a set of *specific objectives* that would lead to the overall goal are set. The intended outcomes are therefore a real-world description of what needs to be achieved in order to actualize (or move towards) the specific objectives. Such a process is often documented in a "logical framework matrix," which may also record other factors such as sources of verification of indicators, and assumptions and risks (see Table 14.3). If a ToC planning process has been used, this would be documented in a ToC map. In both cases, this record of the aims of the program or service, and the expected outcomes, provide a transparent benchmark against which it can be measured.

Indicators are used to assess whether outcomes have been achieved (in the expected timeframe and with the allocated resources). They should be set in advance, though they may require refinement, depending on what information is actually available when the evaluation is being carried out. Indicators are usually used to measure change, so it is vital to measure baseline indicators prior to the commencement of an intervention in order to show changes over time associated with the intervention. Some indicators may be very simple; for example, the proportion of children attending school in a village; but when the outcomes are more complex (for example, psychological symptoms in patients), it is usually necessary to use *tools* (sometimes called *instruments*) that will ideally provide an accurate, independent, and replicable measure of the extent to which a desired outcome has been achieved. Some indicators track change at individual level (e.g., change in symptoms or quality of life of treated patients), and some track changes at a larger scale, such as success in advocacy to improve medication supply in a district. Evaluations of services being scaled up would typically combine the two.

Table 14.3 Comprehensive Community Mental Health Program for Benue State, Nigeria. Sample of Logical Framework Matrix

	Project Description/ Narrative	Indicators	Source of Verification	Assumptions and Risks
Goal	Persons with psychosocial disability in Benue State are able to have access to good quality mental health care in their Local Government Area, and be empowered to fully participate socially and financially in their communities through peer support.			
Output 1: Establish government-funded CMH services in primary health care structure of state and district services	1.1. Establish a state-wide CMH service based in government PHC structures 1.2. Build staff capacity 1.3. Provide essential resources (e.g., motorcycles for community work, essential medication) 1.4. Establish referral and ongoing clinical supervision	1.1a. 20/23 Districts have a clinic by the end of year 3. 1.1b. Services reach 20%–40% of people with SMD and 5%–10% of people with CMD regularly by 5 years. 1.1c. Outcome measures for symptom change and function in sample of patients. 1.2. Two nurses in each PHC clinic receive standard 2-week training course. 1.3. Clinics, once established, always have a supply of essential psychotropic medication. 1.4. Nurses running services at district level receive quarterly training and supervisory visits.	1.1a. The number of clinics opened monitored with signed MOUs. 1.1b. Number of clients attending monitored, using the standard HIS. Baseline prevalence from existing published sources. 1.1c. Quality of care provided by CPN monitored in documentation of supervision process. Validated instruments to measure change in clinical state in sample of clients. 1.2. Attendance registers at training. Pre- and post-training knowledge measurements. 1.3. Pharmacy stock lists. 1.4. Attendance registers, supervision documentation.	**Assumption:** Government (state and local) cooperates as it has said it would in initial discussions. This is likely with good liaison. Also, there is little financial outlay on their part. **Risk:** That nurses will not want to work in rural areas (reduced by recruiting from these areas for training).

Output 2: Develop Self-Help Groups (SHG) in each district for persons with psychosocial disability	2.1. In order to foster self-advocacy and empowerment, service users in each district will be encouraged and equipped to establish Self-Help Groups. 2.2. These SHGs will provide peer support, a forum for advocacy, and livelihood activities. 2.3. They will receive ongoing support from a SHG/Economic Integration Project Officer.	2.1a. Self-Help Groups to be facilitated in 75% of districts within a year of clinic establishment. 2.1b. Member numbers from 10 to 50 in each group. 2.1c. All have democratic leadership structure, bank account, and constitution. 2.2. 50% have viable revolving loan schemes a year after establishment. 2.3. Project Officer will provide workshops in priority areas directed by group members on 4 occasions in first year.	2.1. Register of groups, their membership, and governance structures, maintained by Project Officer for SHGs. 2.2. Qualitative assessment of their benefit to members (focus group discussions with group members). Financial records for small loans. 2.3. Evidence of participatory process in planning workshops. Registers of attendance at workshops. Workshop evaluation reports from participants.	**Assumption:** Motivation among service users to form groups; stigma means that users may be unwilling to publicly admit their disability, particularly once overt symptoms are stabilized. **Risk:** Groups may not be financially independently sustainable as members are poor, so dependent on outside support. This can reduce independence and sense of ownership of groups.
Output 3	Etc.			

Based on Logframe for CBM/AusAID Community Mental Health Program for Benue State, Nigeria: www.cbm.org

Examples of indicators are:

- *Input indicators*: Measure the resources that went into the implementation of a program or service. The information for this should be available through a health information system, or it can be found though the financial or human-resource records of the program.
- *Process indicators* measure what was done by a program and how well it was done. In the case of evaluating scaling up services, the question is often whether the new service closely reflects the model it aimed to replicate (i.e., its fidelity; see above). An example of a process indicator would be to assess the regularity with which patients access services and whether they follow the recommended treatments.
- *Output indicators* are the easily measured results of what has been achieved by a program or service. Examples might be the number of patients seen or the number of districts covered in an awareness program.
- *Outcomes* should be distinguished from output, as they refer to the impact in the real world—what difference has been made—as opposed to just what the program has done. Indicators to measure the outcomes or impact of a program are effectiveness measures; for example, whether patients seen in a service have improved clinical and social outcomes. One common example that can illustrate these differences is training. An output from a training program might be how many people completed the course. A short-term outcome might be changed knowledge or attitudes in the trainees at the end of the course; a medium-term outcome might be change in their practice when they return to work in the field; and a long-term outcome might be better health in the patients they see.

Obviously it is preferable, when possible, to know the outcomes (ideally in the long-term and in a sustained way) of a program, but it tends to be more complex to do this than to gauge outputs, which can be measured easily and quickly. Outputs, and for that matter, any of the tools used to measure outcomes, are proxies, and it is always necessary to make a judgement as to how well they reflect the outcome they are intended to measure (their validity).

Methods to Reduce Bias in Evaluating Services

The main problem with the evaluation described above is its inability to assert that a particular service model is directly responsible for any changes in outcomes measured (as opposed to just occurring by chance or due to other factors). Ways to make an evaluation more robust include:

- To have an evaluation carried out by an independent, external body with no vested interest in the results.
- To use standardized tools, and ensure that they are valid and reliable in the local context.
- To include a comparison arm in the evaluation—i.e., to carry out the same outcome measures on a similar group who did not receive the novel intervention to see whether there is a difference in outcomes that can be attributed to the intervention.
- To allocate recipients of the service randomly to the intervention or comparison arm. This is a method that is designed to reduce bias in allocation (to the intervention group or the comparison group) and to ensure that known and unknown attributes that may be relevant to outcomes (i.e., confounding factors) do not confer bias to either group.

One way to evaluate a complex intervention is to try to mirror the methodology employed in a randomized controlled trial, where (as far as possible) the people exposed to the service and a comparison group have their progress measured in the same way to ascertain whether there is a significant difference in outcomes that cannot be explained by any other factor. Randomization to reduce the effect of bias is often done for services research using *cluster techniques*. This means that the unit randomly allocated to receive the intervention of interest or comparison intervention (the control) is larger than the individual. This may be PHC units, health districts, or hospitals. In practical terms, this can often be done through a staggered roll-out of the program whereby individual PHCs are randomized to receive the program first (the intervention group), and the second group of PHCs is randomly allocated to receive the program at a later date. The outcomes for patients in both sets of PHCs can then be tracked over time and compared to evaluate whether the service is effective at improving outcomes. Ideally, all programs in the first stages of scale-up would be randomized in this way in order to provide the most robust evidence on the effectiveness of the program. However, in practice, these types of naturalistic trials are very difficult to carry out, and the logistics of the data collection and analysis means they are costly and complex to implement, requiring external research funds and expertise to execute.

Mixed methods for evaluation of services Other research methods such as observational studies or case studies also yield valuable information about how well services are functioning, particularly if done in a standardized way that allows meaningful comparisons to be made.[49] Qualitative techniques are able to give the richest insights into why some things are working well, or not, in a service. Asking key informants connected to the service to share their knowledge and perspectives enables theories to be developed and tested about a particular aspect of the scaling up process under investigation. A combination of quantitative and qualitative work (mixed methods) can give stronger results and allow more defensible conclusions to be drawn than either method can achieve alone, and, indeed, should be standard practice in any evaluation of services.

Tools for Collecting Indicators

Techniques for collecting relevant data include interviews with relevant personnel, review of documents from the service and other relevant associated sources, collating service data from health facilities, and cohort studies following progress of cases at fixed time periods. Such techniques often represent an appropriate methodology in resource-poor contexts, particularly in regular monitoring, and internal periodic evaluations. In addition, the following tools allow data to be collected in a systematic way, but may be more resource-intensive than the simple techniques listed above.

Health Information Systems "Health information system" (HIS) is the collective term for the processes that allow routine collection, processing, and communicating of information related to the health system. A comprehensive HIS includes population-based surveillance data collected so as to understand needs and priorities (such as prevalence of disease and risk factors), as well as such information collected from health facilities. Information about how services are used, and resource availability and utilization (medication, human resources, finances) is also included. If the HIS is functioning well, it is an invaluable source for many of the indicators listed above (inputs, process, and output). Such data also have the advantage of being independent and long-term; allowing comparisons across time and establishing a sustainable model for evaluation in a service.

Evaluating services using routinely collected data is challenging, though. Health information systems in low- and middle-income settings routinely neglect mental health indicators, and the little information that is collected is patchy and inconsistent in methodology.[34] When establishing services in settings where the HIS is weak, it is important to devote advocacy efforts to ensure that the routine collection of relevant information on mental health is considered a standard part of a complete health system. This improves the visibility of a novel service, improves the integration of mental health into the standard health system, and increases its leverage in resource-allocation discussions. Without collecting and reporting relevant data, it is likely that mental health services will continue to be marginalized. For example, if numbers of clients seen by a service are not counted, health planners may conclude that there is no need for the service; or if psychotropic drugs are not included on records of service drug utilization, they will never be considered when orders are made.

Advances in communication technology have allowed more direct collection of information, its rapid and accurate collation and analysis, and widespread dissemination in useful formats. This technology, sometimes called *e-health* or *m-health,* has surprising utility in lower-income countries, which often have functioning mobile telephone (cell phone) networks, allowing such a system, if established in a program, to bypass many of the other infrastructural problems hampering HISs otherwise. One example of such a practical use of technology is the Millennium Villages Project, which, despite being based in very undeveloped countries, has made practical use of mobile telephones not only to collect information, but to exploit the wider possibilities of such technologies to aid decision-making based on the information entered.[50]

Use of existing tools There is a wide range of existing instruments that aim to measure aspects of these domains of service quality; for example, service-user outcome measures, which may be clinical (symptom change), social (for example, caregiver burden), or related to disability, functioning, or quality of life. There are advantages in using existing instruments that have been carefully developed for a particular purpose.[51] Of course, it is important to judge whether the instrument is relevant in a new context, and if necessary, adapt it for this purpose.[52] Using existing instruments also allows comparisons to be made across services and between different settings. On the other hand, there are also strong arguments for developing evaluation tools entirely based on the specific criteria considered important by those affected by the service.[37] This method has the advantage of being sensitive to priorities they may have that are different from those who have developed an instrument in a different cultural context.

The ability of instruments to measure what they are attempting to measure (their validity) may be severely compromised in a setting other than where they were developed and thus yield meaningless results. Their psychometric properties (e.g., how well they perform in terms of validity and reliability) should ideally be ascertained in new settings, and it may occasionally be necessary to develop new context-specific measures. Where it is felt appropriate to translate a measure, it is important that a systematic process of translation and back-translation be followed, as meanings typically change enormously in translation, and many of the issues relevant to mental health are understood in a very different way in different languages. (See Chapter 4 for a further discussion on the process of adaptation of tools.) It is always better to try to measure these prospectively by sampling at baseline and at appropriate times in the evaluation, rather than retrospectively, in order to reduce recall bias. Two methods of assessing outcomes in individuals are through surveys of a sample of beneficiaries, or by following a cohort.

Service-mapping tools While good, contextually appropriate services will always differ, it is useful to use common instruments and standards when evaluating programs for comparisons to be made: for example, standardized frameworks for assessing important features of programs,[49] and accepted outcomes by which to judge the success of different services' impact. This may highlight different strengths and weakness of programs, or expose inequitable resource allocation (for example, when comparing high- and low-income countries, or rural and urban areas within countries).[53] One standard set of criteria that have been proposed for evaluation of services at a larger (country) level uses data collected routinely by the World Health Organization through its Assessment Instrument for Mental Health Services (AIMS). It uses "core" and "secondary" indicators as a way of comparing differences in services among countries, as well as potential changes across time if repeated.[34,54] It should be noted that such country-level indicators are likely to be a consequence of broader social, political, and economic factors, and it must not be assumed that changes are a consequence of specific interventions, without substantial justification. Suicide rates, for example, are known to be much more strongly associated with broader social and economic factors than quality or accessibility of mental health services. The WHO-AIMS tool is also being used at the provincial level in some larger countries, such as India (see Table 14.4).

Evaluating Models of Care

Evaluation as described above tends to cover the question of *if* the scale up has been successful, but doesn't explore the question of *why* it has been successful (or failed), or look in more detail at what it is that determines the degree of success in this particular case. Service models are often described as "complex interventions," since they contain many different components that contribute to the outcome of the service. There are now clear frameworks for carrying out evaluations of such complex interventions in a rigorous, methodologically sound way,[55] which allow comparisons of outcomes of different models. Different relevant components can be thought of as "active ingredients," and in the design of a new service, these active ingredients are deliberately fitted to the local context in a way that attempts to maintain their proven efficacy in a different context. Specific aspects of a service that have been identified as active ingredients can be explored in more detail using qualitative techniques that systematically explore the experience of users of services and those working with the service.

It may also be valuable to compare service models that are theoretically similar when they have been implemented in different contexts to assess whether local factors affected their effectiveness in practice. One lesson that has emerged in recent years is that, because of great social inequalities even within richer countries, there may be many similarities between, for example, parts of Nairobi and New York, so that lessons learnt in poorer countries can have international applications.

CONCLUSION

The ethical mandate to scale up services for people with mental disorders globally is compelling. This is based not only on the evident need, but on the growing evidence that services can be cost-effective. The benefit of evidence-based treatment at an individual level and local service has been established for many years, but it has taken longer to translate this into meaningful reorganization of services in many countries, despite an emerging consensus of how scaling up should be structured and organized.

Drawing upon evidence about what works in mental health care, systematically addressing some of the recognized barriers to scaling up, and monitoring and evaluating the benefits of scaling up, it is possible to increase the coverage of the range of services for people with mental disorders in countries. This is only likely to succeed if done in a strategic way, and with the participation of relevant stakeholders, including government, health care workers, and service users.

Table 14.4 Indicators for Evaluation of Country-Level Services

	Proposed Indicators	*Existing Indicators**	*Sources of Data*
Core indicators			
Ensure that national and regional health plans pay sufficient attention to mental health.	1: Presence of official policy, programs, or plans for mental health, either including or accompanied by a policy on child and adolescent mental health.	Atlas, AIMS (1.1.1, 1.2.1)	National government
Invest more in mental health care.	2: Specified budget for mental health as a proportion of total health budget.	Atlas, AIMS (1.5.1)	National government
Increase trained staff to provide mental health care.	3: Mental health and related professionals per 100,000 population.	AIMS (4.1.1)	National government and professional bodies
Make basic pharmacological treatments available in primary care.	4: Proportion of primary health-care clinics in which a physician or an equivalent health worker is available, and at least one psychotropic medicine of each therapeutic category (antipsychotic, antidepressant, mood stabiliser, anxiolytic, and antiepileptic) is available in the facility or in a nearby pharmacy all year long.	AIMS (3.1.7)	National government
Increase the treatment coverage for people with schizophrenia	5: People treated each year for schizophrenia as a proportion of the total estimated annual prevalence of schizophrenia.	AIMS (2.2.4 2, 2.4.4.2, 2.6.5.2)	National government and statistical or academic organizations
Secondary indicators			
Balance expenditure in hospital and community services.	6: Proportion of total mental health expenditure spent on community-based services, including primary and general health-care services.	AIMS (1.5.2)	National government
Provide adequate basic training in mental health.	7: Proportion of the aggregate total training time in basic medical and nursing training degree courses devoted to mental health.	AIMS (3.1.1, 3.2.1)	National government and professional bodies

(continued)

Table 14.4 Continued

331 Chapter Fourteen: Scaling Up Services

	Proposed Indicators	Existing Indicators*	Sources of Data
Distribute staff equitably between urban and rural areas.	8: Proportion of psychiatrists nationally who work in mental health facilities that are based in or near the largest cities.	AIMS (4.1.7)	National government
Ensure least restrictive practice.	9: Involuntary admissions as a proportion of all annual admissions.	AIMS (2.4 5, 2.6.6)	National government
Protect the human rights of people with mental disorder.	10: Presence of a national body that monitors and protects the human rights of people with mental disorders, and issues reports at least every year.	AIMS (1.4.1)	National government, professional bodies, and civil-society groups
Reduce the suicide rate	11: Deaths by suicide and self-inflicted injury rate	WHO Mortality database[32]	National government and statistical organizations

*Atlas = WHO *Mental Health Atlas*.[17] AIMS = WHC Assessment Instrument for Mental Health Systems.[19] Figures in parentheses are AIMS indicator numbers.
(With permission from Elsevier/*The Lancet*; Lancet Global Mental Health Group, 2007.)

ONLINE RESOURCES

Available resources to support scaling up of mental health services:

WHO mental health Gap Action Programme (mhGAP):
http://www.who.int/mental_health/mhgap/en/
WHO Guidance on Mental Health Legislation
http://www.who.int/mental_health/resources/en/Legislation.pdf,   http://www.who.int/entity/mental_health/policy/fact_sheet_mnh_hr_leg_2105.pdf
PLoS Medicine Series on Packages of Care:
http://gmhmovement.org/articles_plos-medicine-series_174.html
Lancet Global Mental Health Series 2007:
http://www.thelancet.com/series/global-mental-health
Lancet Global Mental Health Series 2011:
http://www.thelancet.com/series/global-mental-health-2011
Movement for Global Mental Health:
http://www.globalmentalhealth.org

REFERENCES

1. Prince M, Patel V, Saxena S. No health without mental health. *Lancet*. 2007;370:859–77.
2. Murray CJL, Lopez AD. *The global burden of disease, Vol. 1. A comprehensive assessment of the mortality and disability from diseases, injuries and risk factors in 1990, and projected to 2020.* Harvard School of Public Health, WHO, and the World Bank. Cambridge MA: Harvard University Press; 1996.

3. Lora A, Kohn R, Levav I, McBain R, Morris J, Saxena S. Service availability and utilization and treatment gap for schizophrenic disorders: a survey in 50 low- and middle-income countries. *Bull WHO.* 2012;90:47–54B.

4. Kohn R, Saxena S, Levav I, Saraceno B. The treatment gap in mental health care. *Bull WHO.* 2004;82(11):858–66.

5. Wang PS, Guilar-Gaxiola S, Alonso J, Angermeyer MC, Borges G, Bromet EJ, et al. Use of mental health services for anxiety, mood, and substance disorders in 17 countries in the WHO World Mental Health surveys. *Lancet.* 2007;370(9590):841–50.

6. Alonso, J, Codony M, Kovess V, Angermeyer MC, Katz SJ, Haro JM, et al. Population level of unmet need for mental healthcare in Europe. *Br J Psychiatry.* 2007;190:299–306.

7. Ormel J, Petukhova M, Chatterji S, Aguilar-Gaxiola S, Alonso J, Angermeyer MC, et al. Disability and treatment of specific mental and physical disorders across the world. *Br J Psychiatry.* 2008;192:368–75.

8. World Health Organization. *The World Health Report 2001—New understanding, new hope.* Geneva: WHO; 2000.

9. World Health Organization. *Mental health Gap Action Program (mhGAP): Scaling up care for mental, neurological and substance abuse disorders.* Geneva: World Health Organization; 2008.

10. WHO, WONCA. *Integrating mental health into primary care. A global perspective.* Geneva: World Health Organization and World Organization of Family Doctors; 2008.

11. Lancet Global Mental Health Group. Scale up services for mental disorders: a call for action. *Lancet.* 2007;370(9594):1241–52.

12. Patel V, Araya R, Chatterjee S, Chisholm D, Cohen A, De Silva M, Hosman C, McGuire H, Rojas G, van Ommeren M. Treatment and prevention of mental disorders in low-income and middle-income countries. *Lancet.* 2007;370:991–1005.

13. Patel V, Thornicroft G. Packages of care for mental, neurological, and substance use disorders in low- and middle-income countries. *PLoS Med.* 2009;6:e1000160.

14. Simmons R, Fajans P, Ghiron L (eds.). *Scaling up health service delivery: From pilot innovations to policies and programs.* Geneva, World Health Organization; 2007:vii–xvii.

15. Mangham LJ, Hanson K. Scaling up in international health: what are the key issues? *Health Policy Plan.* 2010;25:85–96.

16. Patel V, Kim Y. Contribution of low- and middle-income countries to research published in leading general psychiatry journals, 2002–2004. *Br J Psychiatry.* 2007;190:77–8.

17. Patel V. Integrating mental health care with chronic diseases in low-resource settings. *Int J Public Health.* 2009;54(1):1–3.

18. WHO/ILAE/IBE. *Epilepsy management at primary health level in rural China: Global Campaign Against Epilepsy demonstration project.* Geneva: World Health Organization; 2009.

19. Saraceno B, van Ommeren M, Batniji R, Cohen A, Gureje O, Mahoney J, et al. Barriers to improvement of mental health services in low-income and middle-income countries. *Lancet.* 2007;370(9593):1164–74.

20. WHO. *Mental Health Atlas 2011.* Geneva: World Health Organization; 2011.

21. Saxena S, Thornicroft G, Knapp M, Whiteford H. Resources for mental health: scarcity, inequity, and inefficiency. *Lancet.* 2007;370:878–89.

22. Chisholm D. *Dollars, DALYs and decisions: Economic aspects of the mental health system.* Geneva: World Health Organization; 2006.

23. Gureje O, Chisholm D, Kola L, Lasebikan V, Saxena S. Cost-effectiveness of an essential mental health intervention package in Nigeria. *World Psychiatry.* 2007;6:42–8.

24. Chisolm D, Lund C, Saxena S: Cost of scaling up mental healthcare in low- and middle-income countries. *Br J Psychiatry.* 2007;191:528–35.

25. Patel V, Maj M, Flisher AJ, De Silva MJ, Koschorke M, Prince M, et al., and Member Society Representatives. Reducing the treatment gap for mental disorders: a WPA survey. *World Psychiatry.* 2010;9(3):169–76.

26. Kakuma R, Minas H, van Ginneken N, Dal Poz M, Desiraju K, Morris J, et al. Human resources for mental health care: current situation and strategies for action. *Lancet.* 2011;378:1654–63.

27. Layard R. The depression report: a new deal for depression and anxiety disorders. London: London School of Economics; 2006. Available at: http://cep.lse.ac.uk/textonly/research/mentalhealth/DEPRESSION_REPORT_LAYARD2.pdf. Retrieved Feb. 2012.

28. IAPT Programme Review December 2011. Improving Access To Psychological Therapies, NHS, UK http://www.iapt.nhs.uk/silo/files/iapt-programme-review-december.pdf

29. WHO. *Building back better: Sustainable mental health care after disaster.* Geneva: World Health Organization; 2012.

30. Thornicroft G. *Shunned.* Oxford: Oxford University Press; 2007.

31. Leff J, Trieman N, Gooch C. Team for the Assessment of Psychiatric Services (TAPS) Project 33: prospective follow-up study of long-stay patients discharged from two psychiatric hospitals. *Am J Psychiatry.* 1996;153:1318–24.

32. Von Korff M, Goldberg D. Improving outcomes in depression. *BMJ.* 2001;32:948–9.

33. Araya R, Rojas G, Fritsch R, Gaete J, Rojas M, Simon G, et al. Treating depression in primary care in low-income women in Santiago, Chile: a randomised controlled trial. *Lancet.* 2003;361:995–1000.

34. Eaton J, McCay L, Semrau M, Chatterjee S, Baingana F, Araya R, Ntulo C, Thornicroft G, Saxena S. Scale up of services for mental health in low-income and middle-income countries. *Lancet.* 2011;378(9802):1592–603.

35. Rahman A, Malik A, Sikander S, Roberts C, Creed F. Cognitive behaviour therapy-based intervention by community health workers for mothers with depression and their infants in rural Pakistan: a cluster-randomised controlled trial. *Lancet.* 2008;372:902–9.

36. Chatterjee S, Pillai A, Jain S, Cohen A, Patel V. Outcomes of people with psychotic disorders in a community-based rehabilitation programme in rural India. *Br J Psychiatry.* 2009;195(5):433–39.

37. Bolton P, Bass J, Neugebauer R, Verdeli H, Clougherty KF, Wickramaratne P, et al. Group interpersonal psychotherapy for depression in rural Uganda: a randomized controlled trial. *JAMA.* 2003 289(23):3117–24.

38. Davidson L, Chinman M, Kloos B, Weingarten R, Stayner, D, Tebes JK. Peer support among individuals with severe mental illness: a review of the evidence. *Clin Psychol.* 1999;6:165–87.

39. Cohen A, Raja S, Underhill C, Yaro B, Dokurugu A, De Silva M, Patel V. Sitting with others: mental health self-help groups in northern Ghana. *Int J Ment Health Syst.* 2012;6:1.

40. Belkin G, Unutzer J, Kessler R, Verdeli H, Raviola G, Sachs K, Oswald C, Eustache E. Scaling up for the "bottom billion": "5x5" implementation of community mental health care in low income regions. *Psychiatr Serv.* 2011;62(12):1494–502.

41. Barbui C, Dua T, van Ommeren M, Yasamy MT, Fleischmann A, Clark N, et al. Challenges in developing evidence-based recommendations using the GRADE approach: the case of mental, neurological, and substance use disorders. *PLoS Med.* 2010;7(8): e1000322. doi:10.1371/journal.pmed.1000322.

42. Thornicroft G, Alem A, Dos Santos RA, Barley E, Drake RE, Gregorio G, et al. WPA guidance on steps, obstacles and mistakes to avoid in the implementation of community mental health care. *World Psychiatry.* 2010;9(2):67–77.

43. Basic Needs 2009. Community mental health practice: seven essential features for scaling up in low- and middle-income countries. Available at: http://www.basicneeds.org. Accessed March 2012.

44. Thornicroft G, Tansella M. Balancing community-based, and hospital-based mental health care. *World Psychiatry.* 2002;1(2):84–90.

45. Weiss, C. Nothing as practical as good theory: exploring theory-based evaluation for comprehensive community initiatives for children and families. In Connell J, Kubisch AC, Schorr LB, Weiss C, editors. *New approaches to evaluating community initiatives: Concepts, methods, and contexts.* Washington, DC: Aspen Institute; 1995.

46. Anderson, AA. *The community builder's approach to Theory of Change. A practical guide to theory development.* Washington, DC: Aspen Institute; 2005.

47. Ravishankar N, Gubbins P, Cooley R, Leach-Kemon K, Michaud C, Jamison D, et al. Financing of global health: tracking development assistance for health from 1990 to 2007. *Lancet.* 2009;373:2113–24.

48. Maxwell RJ. Quality assessment in health. *BMJ.* 1984;288:1470–2.

49. Cohen A, Eaton J, Radtke B, George C, Manuel V, DeSilva M, Patel V. Three models of community mental health services in low-income countries. *Int J Ment Health Syst.* 2011;5:3.

50. Sachs JD. The millennium villages and ICT for development. *ITU News.* 2011; No. 8. Available at: https://itunews.itu.int/En/1683-The-Millennium-Villages-and-ICT-for-Development.note.aspx. Accessed March 2012.

51. Prince M, Stewart R, Ford T, Hotopf M, eds. *Practical psychiatric epidemiology.* Oxford, UK: Oxford University Press; 2005.

52. Thornicroft G. *Mental health outcome measures.* London: RCPsych Publications; 2010.

53. Lund C, Flisher A. Community/hospital indicators in South African public sector mental health services. *J Ment Health Policy & Econ.* 2003;6:181–7.

54. Saxena S, Lora A, van Ommeren M, Barrett T, Morris J, Saraceno B. WHO's assessment instrument for mental health systems: collecting essential information for policy and service delivery. *Psychiatr Serv.* 2007;58(6):816–21.

55. Craig P, Dieppe P, Macintyre S, Michie S, Nazareth I, Petticrew M. Developing and evaluating complex interventions: new guidance. *Med Res Coun.* 2008. Available at: http://www.mrc.ac.uk/Utilities/Documentrecord/index.htm?d=MRC004871D. Accessed March 2012.

15 Child and Adolescent Mental Health

Christian Kieling, Ana Soledade
Graeff-Martins, Hesham Hamoda, and
Luis Augusto Rohde

BURDEN

Global child and adolescent mental health is central to global mental health—and to global health in general. To achieve mental health equity across the globe, recognition and intervention have to start early, emphasizing transnational health issues, determinants, and multidisciplinary solutions (beyond the health sciences)[1]—all of which have been in the essence of the work of those who promote the health of children and adolescents.

The large burden imposed by mental disorders across the globe is largely attributable to their incidence early in life and to their persistence into adulthood and old age. Recent data from longitudinal studies and several retrospective investigations in adulthood have demonstrated that a substantial proportion of psychiatric diagnoses identified in adults have their roots in childhood and adolescence.[2] Even though a proportion of mental health problems remit after childhood and adolescence, a large number of individuals will continue to present similar (homotypic continuity) or new (heterotypic continuity) disorders after entering adulthood.[3]

Among the five leading causes of burden among individuals aged 10 to 24 years, three are formal psychiatric diagnoses, and the other two are closely related to mental health problems: unipolar depressive disorders account for 8.2% of all DALYs in this age group; road traffic accidents, 5.4%; schizophrenia, 4.1%; bipolar disorder, 3.8%; and violence, 3.5%.[4]

At the same time, new insights from developmental science indicate that the period of childhood and adolescence is a window of opportunity to prevent the onset and chronicity of mental health problems. For example, epigenetic modeling (in which environmental factors can regulate gene expression without changing the nucleotide sequence) might be a mechanism for neural and phenotypic plasticity that can lead to alterations that can be long-lasting, including transmission to subsequent generations.[5] This growing body of research supports the idea that attainment of early abilities enhances a person's competence in later challenges and that continuation along a maladaptive pathway increases the individual's risk for psychopathology and diminishes the chance of reclaiming a typical trajectory.[6]

Prevalence

Community-based studies conducted in both high-income countries (HIC) and in low and middle income countries (LMIC) document the high prevalence of mental health problems among children and adolescents. Although there is a large variability in terms of prevalence rates (in HIC and LMIC), most of the surveys estimate that 10% to 20% of young people have at least one diagnosable mental disorder according to the *Diagnostic and Statistical Manual of Mental Disorders* (DSM) or the *International Classification of Diseases* (ICD)[6]—see Table 15.1.

In general, studies that estimate the prevalence of mental health problems do not consider developmental disorders such as intellectual disability, autism spectrum disorders, and specific learning disabilities, which are all related to significant burden. An epidemiological study conducted in the United States evaluated the presence of developmental disabilities in a sample of 95,132 children 3 to 17 years of age, participants in the National Health Interview Surveys from 1997 to 2005.[7] The prevalence of mental retardation (0.7%), autism spectrum disorders (0.4%), and learning disabilities (7.0%) was estimated, and the three conditions were highly associated to mental health care in the last 12 months (40.5%, 54.8%, and 28.8%, respectively, versus 3.4% in children with no developmental disabilities). Unfortunately, there are very limited data available about developmental disorders in LMIC.

When comparing studies on the presentation of symptoms in children and adolescents from different cultures, investigators have always faced the difficulty of disentangling the methodological and cultural effects that may explain variability across studies.[8] Cultural aspects can influence the phenotypical presentation of mental health problems in several ways, such as, for example, defining and creating specific sources of distress and impairment, or determining the way people interpret and evaluate the symptoms. These aspects seem to be even more important for the majority of child mental health disorders in which the quality of the environment is crucial in shaping the expression of the biological vulnerability to the disorder.[9]

Culture has an important role to play in how child and adolescent mental health is perceived and how interventions are implemented in different countries and regions. What may be acceptable in one country may not be acceptable in another. Children's status in society may differ, and this leads to a lessening or heightening of concern to provide care or to expose children to interventions.[10] In the realm of research, it has been argued that the rigor of cross-cultural research is often less than would be expected,[11] and that the use of assessment instruments in populations that are significantly different than those for which they were developed creates methodological difficulties.[12] Betancourt and colleagues suggest that international studies more commonly investigate reliability rather than validity across cultural groups and are weak on cultural relevance.[13]

Despite these difficulties, dimensional scales have proven valuable as screening tools for emotional and behavioral problems in children and adolescents both in HIC and in LMIC (see Box 15.1). Importantly, recent research suggests that cross-national differences in scores do not necessarily reflect comparable differences in disorder rates.[14] It is expected that future research, combining dimensional and screening instruments and structured diagnostic interviews based on the DSM and/or the ICD will bring additional information in terms of case definitions across countries and cultures.

Table 15.1 Studies on the Global Prevalence of Child and Adolescent Mental Disorders in LMIC (extracted from Kieling et al. and used with permission from Elsevier.[6]

Study	Country	Income (WB)	Sample frame	Diagnostic systems and instruments	Information sources and strategy for combining information	Number of stages	N	Attrition	Age range/ mean (SD)	Prevalence rates in % (CI/SE)
Mullick & Goodman, 2005	Bangladesh	Low	Regional community, urban and rural	ICD-10; SDQ & DAWBA	Parents, children (<11y) and teachers; best estimate	2 stages	922	75	5–10y	15 (11–21)
Anselmi et al. 2010	Brazil	Upper-middle	Regional community, urban and rural	DSM-IV/ICD-10; SDQ & DAWBA	Parents and adolescents; best estimate	2 stages	4445	84.7	11 & 12y	10·8 (7·1–14·5)
Bilyk & Goodman, 2004	Brazil	Upper-middle	Regional school, urban and rural	DSM-IV; DAWBA	Parents, children (<11y) and teachers; best estimate	1 stage	519	83	7–14y	12·7 (9·8–15·5)
Goodman et al. 2005	Brazil	Upper-middle	Regional community, rural	DSM-IV; SDQ & DAWBA	Parents, children (<11y) and teachers; best estimate	2 stages	1251	94	5–14y	7 (2·3–11·8)
Guan et al. 2010	China	Lower-middle	Regional, school, urban and rural	DSM-IV; ISICMD & structured interview designed by authors	Parents	2 stages	9495	NA	5–17y	16·22 (15·49–16·97)

(continued)

Table 15.1 Continued

Study	Country	Income (WB)	Sample frame	Diagnostic systems and instruments	Information sources and strategy for combining information	Number of stages	N	Attrition	Age range/ mean (SD)	Prevalence rates in % (CI/SE)
Fekadu et al. 2006	Ethiopia	Low	Regional, school, urban	DSM-III-R; DICA	Children	1 stage	528	NA	5–15y	12·5 for school children; 20·1 for laborer children;[†] 16·5 combined
Hackett et al. 1999	India	Lower-middle	Regional community, rural	ICD-10; Rutter scales A/B & clinical assessment	Parents	2 stages	1403	95	8–12y	9·4 (7·9–10·8)
Malhotra et al. 2002	India	Lower-middle	Regional school, urban and rural	ICD-10; CPMS/ Rutter B scale & clinical interview	Parents and teachers; best estimate	3 stages	963	91·7	4–11y	6·33
Pillai et al. 2008	India	Lower-middle	Regional community, urban and rural	DSM-IV; DAWBA	Adolescent (half sample) and adolescent and parents (half sample)	1 stage	2048	76	12–16y	1·81 (1·27–2·48)

Study	Country	Income (WB)	Sample frame	Diagnostic systems and instruments	Information sources and strategy for combining information	Number of stages	N	Attrition	Age range/ mean (SD)	Prevalence rates in % (CI/SE)
Srinath et al. 2005	India	Lower-middle	Regional community, urban and rural	ICD-10; SCL and VSMS/ CBCL & DISC (4–16y) and clinical assessment (0–3y)	Parents and children; best estimate	2 stages	2064	90·5	0–16y	13·8 (10·6–17) for 0–3y; 12 (10·3–13·6) for 4–16y; combined = 12·5
Kasmini et al. 1993**	Malaysia	Upper-middle	Regional community, rural	ICD-9; RQC & FIC	Parents; best estimate	2 stages	507	99·6	1–15y	6·1
Benjet et al. 2009	Mexico	Upper-middle	Regional community, urban	DSM-IV; WMH-CIDI	Adolescents	1 stage	3005	71	12–17y	39·4 (38–40·9)
Abiodun et al. 1993*	Nigeria	Lower-middle	Regional community, rural	ICD-9; RQC & FIC	Parents	2 stages	200	NA	5–15y	15
Goodman et al. 2005	Russia	Upper-middle	Regional school, urban and rural	ICD-10; SDQ & DAWBA	Parents, children (< 11y) and teachers; best estimate	2 stages	448	74	7–14y	15·3 (10·4–20·1)

(continued)

Table 15.1 Continued

Study	Country	Income (WB)	Sample frame	Diagnostic systems and instruments	Information sources and strategy for combining information	Number of stages	N	Attrition	Age range/ mean (SD)	Prevalence rates in % (CI/SE)
Wacharasindhu et al. 2002	Thailand	Lower-middle	Regional, school, urban	DSM-IV	Parent, teacher, child#	2 stages	1480	83	8–11 y	37·58
Alyahri & Goodman, 2008	Yemen	Lower-middle	Regional, school, urban and rural	DSM-IV; SDQ & DAWBA	Parents and teachers; best estimate	2 stages	1210	91	7–10y	15·7 (11·7–20·2)

RQC = Reporting questionnaire for children; FIC = Follow-up interview for children; NA = not assessed or not available; CPMS = Childhood Psychopathology Measurement Scale (Indian adaptation of the CBCL); SCL = Structured Interview Schedule; VSMS = Vineland social maturity scale; ISICMD = Investigation Screening Inventory for Child Mental Disorders; GHQ-12 = General Health Questionnaire—12 questions version); CDI = child depression inventory.

* Although reported as a two-stage study, the second stage was not adjusted for the performance of the screening test in the first stage. So, technically it is a one-stage study (second stage = random subsample of the first stage).

** Only screening positives assessed in the second stage.

*** In the first stage, a short version of the KSADS-E with just the screening questions for each disorder was applied.

† This was a convenience sample.

Not clear how the information from different sources was combined.

When the study reported on prevalence rates from different waves of assessment, we opted for including the prevalence rate of the first wave. When, in addition to point prevalence/period prevalence (e.g. 12-month prevalence), lifetime prevalence was also presented, we included point prevalence/period prevalence to make findings comparable since the majority of studies report on this type of prevalence.

Box 15.1 Measurement of Child and Adolescent Mental Health Across the Globe

Instruments to assess the mental health of children and adolescents in a variety of countries and cultures have been developed and tested over the last decade. In general, those tools can be divided into two groups. There are questionnaires that assess psychopathology from a dimensional perspective, such as the Strengths and Difficulties Questionnaire (SDQ; translated into more than 75 languages and freely available at www.sdqinfo.com), and the Achenbach System of Empirically Based Assessment (the Aseba set of instruments, including the Child Behavior Checklist—CBCL, and the Teacher Report Form—TRF; translated into more than 80 languages and commercially available at www.aseba.org). These scales can be used either to measure the continuum from mental health to mental disorder or as screening instruments for subsequent confirmatory assessment. Diagnostic structured and semi-structured interviews such as the DAWBA (Development and Well-Being Assessment) are also available and validated in multiple languages, providing information on categorical diagnoses according to ICD and DSM criteria. There remains the need for multinational child and adolescent studies applying standardized criteria based on the ICD in different cultures, as is done for adults[15]—it is important that intellectual and developmental disorders not be excluded from these surveys. Another area of uncertainty is the variety of approaches that can be used to interpret and combine data from multiple informants. An increasing amount of data support the notion that combining information gathered with children and adolescents, parents, and teachers can increase the validity of the diagnostic process—since, for example, children tend to be better informants for internalizing syndromes, while parents report better on externalizing symptoms; also, the correlation between parents' and teachers' views on the child's behavior has been demonstrated to be very low.

Social and Economic Impact

The negative impact of mental disorders in childhood and adolescence results in a variety of negative outcomes, ranging from poor educational attainment to increased mortality rates. The WHO World Mental Health Survey Initiative evaluated the association between diagnoses and subsequent non-achievement of school milestones and found that substance-use disorders and impulse control disorders were associated with early termination of education both in HIC and in LMIC.[16] The condition most studied regarding this aspect is probably attention-deficit hyperactivity disorder (ADHD). In a longitudinal study that followed children with ADHD, children with sub-threshold ADHD, and controls for eight years, the two first groups presented a higher likelihood of repeating grades and graduation failure.[17] ADHD was also associated with higher rates of school flunking, suspensions, and expulsions in a community sample in Brazil.[18] Also in Brazil, school dropout in the first years of elementary school was associated with conduct disorders[19] and mental retardation.[20] Furthermore, children with developmental disabilities in United States had much greater need of special education services (80.8% of children with mental retardation, 87.1% of children with autism, and 52.9% of children with learning disabilities) than children with no developmental disabilities (1.5%).[7] Problematic substance use or dependence in adolescence—in concurrence or not with other psychiatric diagnoses—accounts for as many as one in every ten deaths between the ages of 15 to 29 worldwide.[21] Suicide, one of the leading causes of mortality among youth, is associated with depression in at least half of the cases in adolescence.[22]

However, the disproportionate burden that mental, neurological, and substance use disorders represent (accounting for 15%–30% of the disability-adjusted life-years— DALYs—lost in the first three decades of life) is not accompanied by investments in research and implementation targeting mental disorders among young people. Despite the fact that nine out of ten individuals under the age of 18 live in a low- or middle-income country (LMIC), the research focusing on the mental health of these individuals coming from these countries represented less than 10% of the scientific output on the subject in the last decade.[23]

RISK AND PROTECTIVE FACTORS

Modifiable factors that increase the risk towards the development of mental illness have been identified in LMIC as they have been in HIC. Ertem provided the basis for a conceptual approach that maps risk factors across the life-cycle, starting with prospective parents at the preconceptional period (Figure 15.1).[6] The identification of risk and protective factors at different developmental stages provides not only a framework for a conceptual model of the etiology of mental disorders, but also a practical guide to the implementation of preventative strategies at different developmental stages and in harmony with other programs beyond the mental health sector (e.g. early childhood programs, school-based interventions).

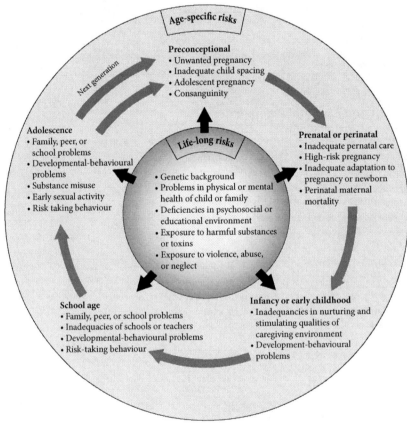

FIGURE 15.1

The life-cycle approach to risk factors for mental disorders (extracted from Ertem, adapted in Kieling et al.[6]).

There are several social factors that can have a negative impact on child and adolescent mental health. A strong body of evidence implicates child neglect, and emotional, physical, and sexual abuse as risk factors for mental illness. Abuse can lead to long-term psychological impairments—for example, children subjected to abuse and neglect are one and a half times more likely to use illicit drugs as adults.[24] Other social factors such as poverty also have an important role in child and adolescent mental health. For example, the landmark Great Smoky Mountains study showed that poverty greatly increased the likelihood of serious emotional disturbances[25] and that interventions to alleviate poverty had a major effect on some types of children's psychiatric disorders, such as conduct and oppositional defiant disorders, but not others, such as anxiety and depression.[26]

One of the current prevailing strategies in the search for the etiology of mental disorders is the assessment of the interplay between measured genetic and environmental factors. According to this view, gene–environment interactions (GxE) occur when environmental effects are conditioned by the individual's genetic background. Initial evidence for GxE was found between neurotransmitter-related genes and adverse experiences such as maltreatment, stressful events, and cannabis use for the development of antisocial behavior, depressive symptoms, and psychosis, respectively.[27]

Up to now, however, almost the totality of GxE studies focusing on mental health problems have been conducted in HIC. Considering the different levels of exposure to environmental risk and protective factors in LMIC, gene–environment interplay research in these contexts might be valuable to uncovering the determinants of mental health. Even if not feasible in many LMIC at the moment, the insights provided by these studies can be uniquely informative in terms of identifying confounding mechanisms such as gene–environment correlations (rGE); i.e. the case when genetic factors influence the likelihood that an individual will be exposed to a specific environment.

The scarcity of research on protective and resilience factors—especially in LMIC—should not reduce their relevance in the understanding of the origins of mental health problems. The concept of resilience goes beyond the notion of risk and protective factors, as it aims to incorporate innate qualities and differences in an individual that enable them to overcome adversity.[28] The identification of such factors can be extremely valuable in the design of interventions, as demonstrated, for example, in the development of a multi-strategic school-based intervention based on existing student resilience that reduced the prevalence of substance use.[29]

INTERVENTIONS

Prevention

The cost of long-term treatments and the lack of curative interventions for mental health problems have increased the relevance of preventive strategies to reduce the burden of mental disorders. Going beyond the traditional disease model, preventative interventions in the field of mental health are usually categorized as universal (directed at all children in a particular locality or setting), selective, or indicated (focused on children who are at high risk for development of a mental health problem because of the presence of either proximal risk factors or subclinical symptoms, respectively).[30] Although universal interventions have demonstrated limited effectiveness (even in HIC), interventions targeted at high-risk groups still need to be further developed, considering not only the limited availability of resources, but also the hazards of false-positive identification of at-risk individuals. Box 15.2 summarizes the experience in early intervention for psychotic disorders.

Evidence already exists from LMIC contexts that preventive interventions have the efficacy to prevent the development of emotional, behavioral, and intellectual disorders

Box 15.2 Early Intervention in Psychosis

Research on early identification and intervention for schizophrenia and other psychotic disorders has flourished over the last two decades. Following the Australian model of youth mental health, this strategy emphasizes the relevance of the transition period between late adolescence and the first years of adult life as a critical period for the occurrence of the first psychotic episode. Results from studies adopting criteria for identifying ultra-high-risk individuals (those at imminent risk for psychosis) suggest that, in general, around one-third convert to psychosis; about one-third do not convert but remain symptomatic and functionally impaired; and the remaining third achieve symptomatic and functional recovery.[32] Clinical trials, usually testing interventions that have already shown some benefit in full-blown cases (such as antipsychotics or cognitive-behavioral therapy), have assessed three major outcomes: the reduction of prodromal symptoms; the reduction of the risk to conversion to psychosis; and the reduction of the delay until initiation of antipsychotic treatment. While a number of positive findings have emerged, further studies addressing a better characterization of the pre-onset phase and novel treatment strategies are currently being conducted. Although the majority of studies on early intervention in psychosis have been conducted in Australia and other HIC, recent initiatives have also been implemented in LMIC—a review identified seven programs operating in urban areas of Latin America in 2011.[33]

through childhood and adolescence—and also into adulthood.[6] Both universal and selective/indicated interventions in early childhood (early stimulation, enhancement of caregiver responsiveness, high-quality preschool, conditional cash transfers) have been demonstrated to have beneficial non-specific effects on the mental health of children and adolescents in LMIC—including those exposed to risk factors such as poverty, institutionalization, low birth weight, stunting, and anemia. Universal interventions involving school-based teacher and parent training have been shown to reduce behavioral problems. Effective universal interventions to prevent intellectual deficits include maternal and child nutritional supplementation, immunization programs, reduction of exposure to toxins, malaria prevention, and early stimulation programs.[31]

Nonselective interventions, such as physical activity, have produced positive outcomes like decrease of anxiety and benefits for self-esteem, while psychosocial interventions have also demonstrated benefits for depression, hopelessness, and coping skills. Selectively offered child training and group interventions have been shown to be efficacious to reduce externalizing and internalizing problems for children with low symptomatology or risk factors for emotional problems, respectively. Home-visit strategies for mothers of disabled children in early-stimulation activities have shown some benefits to child development. The chapter "Mental Health Promotion and the Prevention of Mental Disorders" (Chapter 11) further discusses these strategies, and a detailed list of preventive interventions in LMIC can be found in a recent review.[6]

Treatment

Clinical trials assessing treatment options for childhood and adolescence mental health problems are extremely scarce in LMIC. In fact, despite the fact that 90% of all children and adolescents live in LMIC, 90% of randomized clinical trials for mental disorders in childhood and adolescence come from HIC.[6] Despite this imbalance, sufficient evidence exists to provide evidence-based data to inform the treatment of young people with a diagnosable mental disorder.

As detailed in the chapter "Treatment and Care of Mental Disorders," evidence-based guidelines have been established by the World Health Organization's mental health Gap Action Programme (mhGAP) for a variety of mental, neurological, and substance-use disorders, including child and adolescent mental health conditions.[34] The recommendations are organized in thirteen domains, encompassing parenting interventions (e.g. treatment of maternal depression, parental skills training for behavioral and developmental disorders); non-specialized detection of child abuse and intellectual disabilities; integration with the educational sector via school-based interventions; and cognitive behavioral and pharmacological interventions for a variety of disorders such as depression, anxiety, and ADHD. Such strategies are summarized in a very user-friendly intervention guide freely available online (www.who.int/mental_health/evidence/mhGAP_intervention_guide).

IMPLEMENTATION

Availability and Coverage of Services

Notwithstanding the impact and burden associated with mental health problems in children and adolescents, and the available strategies to prevent and treat these problems, most countries in the world are not able to provide adequate care to those in need.[35] In an attempt to obtain information about the available resources in the field in the 192 countries that are members of the World Health Organization, the Child and Adolescent Mental Health Atlas project was implemented in 2004. Very few countries reported having a system of services with adequate and permanent funding. There were scarce resources for professional training and, when it occurred, minimal standards were not designated. The problems seemed to be even worse in LMIC and in those where the child and adolescent population is proportionally larger.[35,36] More recently, a similar study was conducted in 42 LMIC, using a structured instrument developed by the World Health Organization to assess key components of mental health systems.[37] Despite the assessment of more clearly defined indicators, findings were similar to those from the previous study: mental health systems for children and adolescents in most countries are insufficient to provide needed care, and professional training is inadequate.

With greater availability of effective treatments to mental health problems of children and adolescents, the difficulties in accessing services become more significant.[38–40] The lack of specialized services in child and adolescent mental health is obviously the main cause of the problem, but other factors must be considered: stigma, lack of transportation, communication problems (when families and professionals are from different cultural backgrounds, for example), and deficient public awareness about children's and adolescents' mental health problems are important barriers to care.[41] Moreover, particularly associated with this age group, there are obstacles to accessing services. In first place, children and adolescents, in most cases, depend on their parents or other adults to identify the problem and look for help.[38,42–45] Secondly, the needs of children and adolescents with mental health problems frequently become apparent and are initially managed in other sectors, such as education, general health, social services, or justice.[35,36,46] Therefore, low recognition of problems by parents, teachers, or primary care professionals can also interfere in the adequate referral of children in need.[38,39,47]

Service Utilization

Understanding the factors associated with mental health service use by children and adolescents, as well as barriers to access, is essential to inform the planning of mental health services. Unfortunately, research about mental health service use is commonly a secondary product of epidemiological studies primarily interested in answering other questions. Thus, important conceptual variables to understanding mental health services access are frequently not collected.[48-50] A recent systematic review of literature[51] located 57 published studies with data from original investigations of use of mental health services based on non-referred samples (community or schools) of subjects 18 years of age or younger. Unfortunately, most of them were conducted in HIC, and limited information is available from LMIC.

The studies present four main different measures of prevalence of service use for mental health problems: use of any service by the general population, use of specialty mental health services by the general population, use of any service by individuals in need, and use of specialty mental health services by individuals in need. In many studies, these definitions are not clear. As a result, the variability of prevalence rates is enormous, and it is very difficult to summarize the findings, since they refer to different countries in different times, and to service use in different time frames, as reported by different informants.

The rates of service use varied between 2.2% (mental health service use by the general population, in a national representative sample of United States in 1977)[52] and 63.0% (specialty mental health service use in schools over the last two years, by adolescents in need, in a community sample in the United States).[53] These differences may be explained by sample characteristics. For example, lower rates of mental health service use were found in preschool children, an age group less predisposed to have emotional or behavioral problems identified and referred to treatment or evaluation. Lower rates were also identified among children with diagnoses of some disorder, but without impairment, an important factor associated with mental health service use.[25] The different types of services assessed are also determinants of lower (outpatient specialty services, for example) or higher rates of service use. The country of origin of a study is an important source of variability, since demand for and availability of services may depend on local cultural and political aspects. Finally, the timeframe of service use can determine lower or higher rates of prevalence.

Factors associated with the use of mental health services by children and adolescents can be classified in five different categories: child factors, socio-demographic characteristics, family factors, school factors, and factors associated with gatekeepers (Table 15.2). Interestingly, four studies have reported the prevalence rates of unmet need, or the proportion of people in need but who could not get treatment[54-57]—these rates vary between 17.1% and 87.1%. It is important to note that none of the studies included in this review reported data about mental health treatment or quality of services received; they reported only about any contact with services.

Innovative Models of Care

Higher mental health service-use rates by children and adolescents are associated with gatekeepers, which indicates that identification of the problem by parents, teachers, general practitioners, or pediatricians can lead to a more adequate approach to the problem. Some studies have shown that even if children do not have contact with specialized care, frequently they are seen in primary care,[53,58] justifying an investment in the training of these professionals in identification and management of mental health problems. In the same way, teachers should be trained to identify children and adolescents with mental health problems, and services located in schools should be considered.[50,53]

To address all the problems described above, mental health services for children and adolescents must be offered in innovative ways. One possibility is the use of telemedicine or telepsychiatry, which allows the communication between non-specialists in the community and specialists, facilitating discussion about and supervision of clinical cases. In

Brazil, one such project has made it possible for professionals from the National Institute of Developmental Psychiatry, located at University of São Paulo, to be in contact with family doctors from the north and the northeast, poorer, and traditionally under-served regions of the country (R. Lowenthal, personal communication).

THE WAY FORWARD

At best, child and adolescent mental health services across the globe remain weak and fragmented. Serious efforts and a constellation of changes are needed in order to have a positive impact on the mental health of our young population. The changes need to be tailored to meet the specific needs of LMIC populations, while considering local resources available to meet these needs. In the following section, we discuss changes that must take place in the areas of research, politics, public policy, systems of care, and professional development.

Research

There need to be more research efforts to demonstrate the cost-effectiveness of childhood and adolescence mental health interventions in LMIC. Without such studies, it will be hard to influence politicians and direct public policy towards supporting services[59] (see Chapter 17 on research priorities, capacity, and networks in global mental health in this book). A recent review also showed that, although there are large gaps in research into effective prevention and treatment, there is sufficient evidence from LMIC and from resource-poor settings in HIC to justify the establishment of services that can make these interventions available to a large number of children.[6]

Research also needs to focus on the imprecision of prevalence estimates to allow for improvement in services planning. In addition to epidemiology, other areas of focus identified in a study examining mental health research priorities in LMIC included health systems and social science as the highest priorities.[60]

Research on resilience and protective factors in LMIC is limited. In view of the increased exposure to many risk factors in these countries, the study of such positive elements can inform the design of interventions that aim to prevent or reduce risk factors at specific times in life. Because most risk factors were identified in cross-sectional or case-control studies, prospectively assessed cohorts are also needed to confirm and further understand the developmental trajectories of child and adolescent mental health problems from at-risk states to full-blown presentations.[6]

In addition, there are methodological challenges associated with applying existing instruments in populations that differ significantly from those for which they were developed. In light of these difficulties, studies conducted in LMIC should focus on developing instruments relevant to the local cultures or adapting international tools to become relevant to the culture where they are used.

Another relevant point is that researchers from LMIC should focus more on collaboration with other LMIC researchers and not only on HIC researchers. This is important since many LMIC have similar problems and similar resources, and there is a pressing need to develop local research capacity. Researchers and academicians from LMIC should also focus on building capacity for local and regional scientific journals as well as becoming more involved as reviewers and editorial board members of international journals. At the same time, together with investments in research, it is important for academicians not to lose sight of the real-world demands of the systems of care. As such, research efforts have to utilize the available scarce resources and prioritize on what research questions should be addressed first.

Table 15.2 Factors Associated with Mental Health Service Use by Children and Adolescents

Child factors

- Psychopathology / symptomatology
- Multiple disorders
- Impairment
- Internalizing disorders / externalizing disorders
- Chronic medical illness / health problem
- Developmental / language problems
- Stressful life events
- Mental health disability days
- Self-reported need of services

Sociodemographic characteristics

- Gender (male / earlier boys, later girls)
- Age
- White / African American
- Poverty
- Higher income / socioeconomic status
- Higher maternal education level
- Health insurance
- Other religions (vs. Catholic)

Family factors

- One-parent family / single mother household
- Living with others (vs. living with biological parents)
- Family conflict
- Change in family composition
- Parental psychopathology / parental history of MH treatment or visit
- Parental burden / impact of child problems on family
- Less traditional and restrictive parents
- Colder parents / parental criticism and hostility

School factors

- Poor school performance / academic problems

Factors associated with gatekeepers

- Parental report that child needs help
- Teacher report that child needs help
- Contact with primary health care / medical checkup
- Use of informal support

Extracted from Graeff-Martins.[51]

Health System Responses

Politics and Public Policy

Governmental child mental health policies are scarce worldwide.[35] LMIC, in particular, lack the policies to guide system implementation, thus hampering service development and undermining efforts to ensure accountability for the way resources for program development are allocated.[6] On many occasions in LMIC, child and adolescent mental health is low on the scale of priorities and is wrongfully considered to be a luxury rather than a necessity. To overcome such misperceptions, advocates for child and adolescent mental health need to be more agile in their advocacy efforts to navigate and influence the political process in their countries and, hence, ensure that child and adolescent mental health is on the agenda of policymakers.

Practice

Child and adolescent mental health, arguably more than any other field of medicine, needs a strong culture of collaboration between different systems of care. Some of these sectors are the educational system, child-protection agencies, the judicial system, and the health care system. In addition, within each of these systems there are usually multiple sectors that need to collaborate among them, which adds to the complexity of the situation. Jordans and colleagues described several challenges in the implementation of interventions for children in low-income settings: integration needs a high degree of intersectorial collaboration; interventions that work in one country may not work in another because of cultural differences; where schools are the entry-point for intervention, children who do not attend might be missed; and the cost-effectiveness of such a model has not been yet determined.[61]

In addition, there has not been enough collaboration among academic, private, non-governmental, and consumer groups. More integration and collaboration among systems of care is needed to ensure that the most efficient, effective, and compassionate CAMH care is delivered to those in need.

Human Resources

In addition to concerted efforts to garner investments for the development of youth mental health services, innovative approaches will be needed to maximize limited resources according to LMIC characteristics. An example is using physician "extenders" to deliver mental health services in developing countries that may have a shortage in highly qualified staff. Although key initiatives from global agents can offer research-based guidance on intervention strategies, the appropriate implementation of mental health services involves recognizing local demands and, possibly, international collaboration among LMIC.[10] Going beyond the health sector, school-based interventions constitute a promising approach given the increased investments in education in many LMIC. Intersectorial partnership can also be achieved throughout integration with other programs such as nutritional and prenatal care. Success is more likely to be achieved if this cooperation starts when training specialized, general, and non-health professionals.

While the role of specialists in child and adolescent mental health, including psychiatrists and psychologists, is important, in many countries specialists may only be available in major cities. The role of non-specialists in filling this void is essential. In all cases, parents, teachers, and peers also have an important role in the identification of mental health problems, making appropriate referrals, and providing the support system that patients need.

One of the most critical aspects in the delivery of child and adolescent mental health services is the presence of trained human resources. There need to be coordinated efforts for training multidisciplinary providers for child and adolescent mental health in LMIC. Training programs need to be well designed and adequately funded to foster the development of the next generation of clinicians and researchers. Presence of local training capacity may help limit the "brain drain" phenomenon in many LMIC. These countries should also seek to attract child and adolescent mental health professionals from their countries who have immigrated abroad. If such professionals cannot return, their expertise may still be valuable as consultants for program development in their home countries. Training resources and expertise should also be shared among countries in close proximity.

Programs in HIC that seek to train professionals from LMIC should focus on teaching skills that are applicable in LMIC.[10] For example, training someone in advanced psychopharmacology may be of little relevance if they return to their home country where the most basic medications may not be available. Other opportunities for knowledge-sharing between HIC and LMIC include establishing clinical collaborative networks through mentorship, teaching courses, giving presentations, and consulting on difficult cases. Considering longitudinal involvement with one country would allow for a better understanding of the unique challenges in that country and provide for a more meaningful collaboration.

There have also been challenges in collaboration among the numerous international professional organizations in CAMH.[10] More recently, there has been recognition among the leadership of these organizations of the need for collective action; therefore, many have joined in forming a global consortium to advance education and advocacy. The consortium includes the International Association for Child and Adolescent Psychiatry and Allied Professions (IACAPAP), the World Association for Infant Mental Health, the International Association for Adolescent Psychiatry and Psychology, the World Federation for Mental Health, and the International Association for Child Mental Health in Schools.[10]

CONCLUSION

Providing child and adolescent mental health is a global challenge, but a potentially rewarding one, as evidence accumulates to suggest that early interventions can provide large long-term health and socioeconomic benefits. As goals such as reducing child mortality are progressively being achieved in many LMIC,[62] new challenges surface. A focus on childhood and adolescent morbidity, for which mental health problems represent a disproportionate burden, will impact not only the third of the globe's population under the age of 18 years today—but also the other two-thirds in the next decades.

Addressing this becomes more relevant in LMIC, where, despite similar prevalence rates of mental disorders in comparison to HIC, the proportion of children and adolescents in the population is higher and the resources to reduce mental health burden are considerably fewer. To meet these needs, priorities will have to be set in order to provide culturally and contextually appropriate care, from early identification and diagnosis to intervention.

REFERENCES

1. Koplan JP, Bond TC, Merson MH, et al. Towards a common definition of global health. *Lancet.* 2009;373(9679):1993–5.
2. Kim-Cohen J, Caspi A, Moffitt TE, Harrington H, Milne BJ, Poulton R. Prior juvenile diagnoses in adults with mental disorder: developmental follow-back of a prospective-longitudinal cohort. *Arch Gen Psychiatry.* 2003;60(7):709–17.
3. Kasen S, Cohen P. What we can and cannot say about long-term longitudinal studies of childhood disorder. *Acta Psychiatr Scand.* 2009;120(3):165–6.
4. Gore FM, Bloem PJ, Patton GC, Ferguson J, Joseph V, Coffey C, et al. Global burden of disease in young people aged 10–24 years: a systematic analysis. *Lancet.* 2011;377(9783):2093–102.
5. Bagot RC, Meaney MJ. Epigenetics and the biological basis of gene x environment interactions. *J Am Acad Child Adolesc Psychiatry.* 2010;49(8):752–71.
6. Kieling C, Baker-Henningham H, Belfer M, et al. Child and adolescent mental health worldwide: evidence for action. *Lancet.* 2011;378(9801):1515–25.

7. Boulet SL, Boyle CA, Schieve LA. Health care use and health and functional impact of developmental disabilities among US children, 1997–2005. *Arch Pediatr Adolesc Med.* 2009;163(1):19–26.

8. Canino G, Alegría M. Psychiatric diagnosis—is it universal or relative to culture? *J Child Psychol Psychiatry.* 2008;49(3):237–50.

9. Rohde LA. Commentary: Do potential modifications in classificatory systems impact on child mental health in developing countries? Reflections on Rutter. *J Child Psychol Psychiatry.* 2011;52(6):669–70.

10. Hamoda H, Belfer M. Challenges in international collaboration in child and adolescent psychiatry. *J Child & Adolesc Ment Health.* 2010;22(2):83–9.

11. Saxena S, Paraje G, Sharan P, Karam G, Sadana R. The 10/90 divide in mental health research: trends over a 10-year period. *Br J Psychiatry.* 2006;188: 81–2.

12. Hollifield M, Warner TD, Lian N, Krakow B, Jenkins JH, Kesler J, et al. Measuring trauma and health status in refugees: a critical review. *JAMA.* 2002;288:611–21.

13. Betancourt TS, Bass J, Borisova I, Neugebauer R, Speelman L, Onyango G, et al. Assessing local instrument reliability and validity: a field-based example from Northern Uganda. *Soc Psychiatry Psychiatr Epidemiol.* 2009;44:685–92.

14. Goodman A, Heiervang E, Fleitlich-Bilyk B, et al. Cross-national differences in questionnaires do not necessarily reflect comparable differences in disorder prevalence. *Soc Psychiatry Psychiatr Epidemiol.* 2012;47:1321–31.

15. Demyttenaere K, Bruffaerts R, Posada-Villa J, et al. Prevalence, severity, and unmet need for treatment of mental disorders in the World Health Organization World Mental Health surveys. *JAMA.* 2004;291(21):2581–90.

16. Lee S, Tsang A, Breslau J, et al. Mental disorders and termination of education in high-income and low- and middle-income countries: epidemiological study. *Br J Psychiatry.* 2009;194(5):411–7.

17. Bussing R, Mason DM, Bell L, Porter P, Garvan C. Adolescent outcomes of childhood attention-deficit/hyperactivity disorder in a diverse community sample. *J Am Acad Child Adolesc Psychiatry.* 2010;49(6):595–605.

18. Rohde LA, Biederman J, Busnello EA, Zimmermann H, Schmitz M, Martins S, et al. ADHD in a school sample of Brazilian adolescents: a study of prevalence, comorbid conditions, and impairments. *J Am Acad Child Adolesc Psychiatry.* 1999;38(6):716–22.

19. Tramontina S, Martins S, Michalowski MB, Ketzer CR, Eizirik M, Biederman J, et al. School dropout and conduct disorder in Brazilian elementary school students. *Can J Psychiatry.* 2001;46(10):941–7.

20. Tramontina S, Martins S, Michalowski MB, Ketzer CR, Eizirik M, Biederman J, et al. Estimated mental retardation and school dropout in a sample of students from state public schools in Porto Alegre, Brazil. *Rev Bras Psiquiatr.* 2002;24(4):177–81.

21. Toumbourou JW, Stockwell T, Neighbors C, Marlatt GA, Sturge J, Rehm J. Interventions to reduce harm associated with adolescent substance use. *Lancet.* 2007;369(9570): 1391–401.

22. Thapar A, Collishaw S, Pine DS, Thapar AK. Depression in adolescence. *Lancet.* 2012;

23. Kieling C, Rohde LA. Child and adolescent mental health research across the globe. *J Am Acad Child Adolesc Psychiatry,* 2012;51:945–7.

24. Widom C, Marmorstein N, White H. Childhood victimization and illicit drug use in middle adulthood. *Psychol Addict Behav.* 2006;20(4):394–403.

25. Costello EJ, Angold A, Burns BJ, Erkanli A, Stangl DK, Tweed DL. The Great Smoky Mountains Study of Youth. Functional impairment and serious emotional disturbance. *Arch Gen Psychiatry.* 1996;53(12):1137–43.

26. Costello EJ, Compton SN, Keeler G, Angold A. Relationships between poverty and psychopathology: a natural experiment. *JAMA.* 2003;290(15):2023–9.

27. Rutter M, Moffitt TE, Caspi A. Gene–environment interplay and psychopathology: multiple varieties but real effects. *J Child Psychol Psychiatry.* 2006;47(3–4):226–61.

28. Rutter M. Implications of resilience concepts for scientific understanding. *Ann NY Acad Sci.* 2006;1094:1–12.

29. Hodder RK, Daly J, Freund M, Bowman J, Hazell T, Wiggers J. A school-based resilience intervention to decrease tobacco, alcohol and marijuana use in high school students. *BMC Public Health.* 2011;11:722.

30. Institute of Medicine U.S. Committee on Prevention of Mental Disorders and Substance Abuse Among Children Youth and Young Adults. *Preventing mental, emotional, and behavioral disorders among young people: Progress and possibilities.* Washington, DC: National Academies Press; 2009.

31. Flament MD, Nguyen H, Furino C, et al. Evidence-based primary prevention programmes for the promotion of mental health in children and adolescents: a systematic worldwide review. In: Remschmidt H, Nurcombe B, Belfer ML, Sartoirius N, Okasha A. *The mental health of children and adolescents: An area of global neglect.* West Sussex, UK: Wiley; 2007.

32. Yung AR, Nelson B. Young people at ultra high risk for psychosis: research from the PACE clinic. *Rev Bras Psiquiatr.* 2011;33(Suppl 2):s143–60.

33. Brietzke E, Araripe Neto AG, Dias A, Mansur RB, Bressan RA. Early intervention in psychosis: a map of clinical and research initiatives in Latin America. *Rev Bras Psiquiatr.* 2011;33(Suppl 2):s213–24.

34. Dua T, Barbui C, Clark N, et al. Evidence-based guidelines for mental, neurological, and substance use disorders in low- and middle-income countries: summary of WHO recommendations. *PLoS Med.* 2011;8(11):e1001122.

35. Belfer ML, Saxena S. WHO Child Atlas project. *Lancet.* 2006;367(9510):551–2.

36. Belfer ML. Child and adolescent mental disorders: the magnitude of the problem across the globe. *J Child Psychol Psychiatry.* 2008;49(3):226–36.

37. Morris J, Belfer M, Daniels A, et al. Treated prevalence of and mental health services received by children and adolescents in 42 low-and-middle-income countries. *J Child Psychol Psychiatry.* 2011;52(12):1239–46.

38. Costello EJ, Egger H, Angold A. 10-year research update review: the epidemiology of child and adolescent psychiatric disorders: I. Methods and public health burden. *J Am Acad Child Adolesc Psychiatry.* 2005;44(10):972–86.

39. Satcher DS. Executive summary: a report of the Surgeon General on mental health. *Public Health Rep.* 2000;115(1):89–101.

40. Williams R, Hazell P. Implementing guidance and guidelines for developing and delivering equitable child and adolescent mental health services. *Curr Opin Psychiatry.* 2009;22(4):339–44.

41. Patel V, Flisher AJ, Nikapota A, Malhotra S. Promoting child and adolescent mental health in low and middle income countries. *J Child Psychol Psychiatry.* 2008;49(3):313–34.

42. Angold A, Messer SC, Stangl D, Farmer EM, Costello EJ, Burns BJ. Perceived parental burden and service use for child and adolescent psychiatric disorders. *Am J Public Health.* 1998;88(1):75–80.

43. Pavuluri MN, Luk SL, McGee R. Help-seeking for behavior problems by parents of preschool children: a community study. *J Am Acad Child Adolesc Psychiatry.* 1996;35(2):215–22.

44. Pescosolido BA, Jensen PS, Martin JK, Perry BL, Olafsdottir S, Fettes D. Public knowledge and assessment of child mental health problems: findings from the National Stigma Study–Children. *J Am Acad Child Adolesc Psychiatry.* 2008;47(3):339–49.

45. Shepherd M, Oppenheim A, Mitchell S. Childhood behaviour disorders and child-guidance clinic—epidemiological study. *J Child Psychol & Psychiatry.* 1966;7(1):39–52.

46. Glied S, Cuellar A. E. Trends and issues in child and adolescent mental health. *Health Aff (Millwood).* 2003;22(5):39–50.

47. Graeff-Martins AS, Flament MF, Fayyad J, Tyano S, Jensen P, Rohde LA. Diffusion of efficacious interventions for children and adolescents with mental health problems. *J Child Psychol Psychiatry.* 2008;49(3):335–52.

48. Langner TS, Gersten JC, Greene EL, Eisenberg JG, Herson JH, McCarthy ED. Treatment of psychological disorders among urban children. *J Consult Clin Psychol.* 1974;42(2):170–9.

49. McKinlay JB. Some approaches and problems in the study of the use of services—an overview. *J Health Soc Behav.* 1972;13(2):115–52.

50. Ford T. Practitioner review: how can epidemiology help us plan and deliver effective child and adolescent mental health services? *J Child Psychol Psychiatry.* 2008;49(9):900–14.

51. Graeff-Martins A. *Serviços de saúde mental para crianças e adolescentes: recomendações para o planejamento de políticas de saúde mental.* PhD thesis. São Paulo, Brazil: Universidade Federal de São Paulo; 2010.

52. Horgan CM. Specialty and general ambulatory mental health services. Comparison of utilization and expenditures. *Arch Gen Psychiatry.* 1985;42(6):565–72.

53. Burns BJ, Costello EJ, Angold A, et al. Children's mental health service use across service sectors. *Health Aff (Millwood)*. 1995;14(3):147–59.

54. Flisher AJ, Kramer RA, Grosser RC, et al. Correlates of unmet need for mental health services by children and adolescents. *Psychol Med.* 1997;27(5):1145–54.

55. Goodman SH, Lahey BB, Fielding B, Dulcan M, Narrow W, Regier D. Representativeness of clinical samples of youths with mental disorders: a preliminary population-based study. *J Abnorm Psychol.* 1997;106(1):3–14.

56. Kataoka SH, Zhang L, Wells KB. Unmet need for mental health care among U.S. children: variation by ethnicity and insurance status. *Am J Psychiatry.* 2002;159(9):1548–55.

57. Sturm R, Ringel JS, Andreyeva T. Geographic disparities in children's mental health care. *Pediatrics.* 2003;112(4):e308.

58. Sawyer MG, Sarris A, Baghurst PA, Cornish CA, Kalucy RS. The prevalence of emotional and behaviour disorders and patterns of service utilisation in children and adolescents. *Aust N Z J Psychiatry.* 1990;24(3):323–30.

59. Collins PY, Patel V, Joestl SS, et al. Grand challenges in global mental health. *Nature.* 2011;475(7354):27–30.

60. Sharan P, Gallo C, Gureje O, et al. Mental health research priorities in low- and middle-income countries of Africa, Asia, Latin America and the Caribbean. *Br J Psychiatry.* 2009;195(4):354–63.

61. Jordans MJ, Tol WA, Komproe IH, et al. Development of a multi-layered psychosocial care system for children in areas of political violence. *Int J Ment Health Syst.* 2010;4: 15.

62. Lozano R, Wang H, Foreman KJ, et al. Progress towards Millennium Development Goals 4 and 5 on maternal and child mortality: an updated systematic analysis. *Lancet.* 2011;378(9797):1139–65.

16 Women's Mental Health

Jane Fisher, Helen Herrman,
Meena Cabral de Mello, and
Prabha S. Chandra

INTRODUCTION

From conception, the life experiences of girls and women differ from those of boys and men. Some of these pertain to the intrinsic biological differences in female and male reproductive potential, but the more prominent differences are gender-based and reflect disparities in opportunities, responsibilities and roles throughout the life course. These have consequences for all aspects of health, including mental health.

BURDEN OF MENTAL DISORDERS EXPERIENCED BY WOMEN

The burden and determinants of the morbidity of mental disorders carried by women differ consistently from those experienced by men.

Prevalence

Mental health surveys to estimate population prevalence of disorders vary by catchment area: districts, states or nations, and some are extrapolated from in-patient populations or sub-groups defined by sociodemographic characteristics such as age or migration status. Conceptualizations of the nature of conditions have become more comprehensive and specific and recognition has increased over time (see Box 16.1 for illustrative example). Point, period, lifetime and life stage prevalence data are reported, but not always specified, they are not always disaggregated by sex and most are from high income settings.[1] Together these lead to diverse prevalence estimates.

Box 16.1 Recognition of Mental Health Problems Related to Pregnancy and Childbirth

The World Health Organization's Making Pregnancy Safer initiative aims to reduce pregnancy-related deaths in women and improve newborn survival through addressing hemorrhage, infection, unsafe abortion, pregnancy illnesses, and complications of childbirth by ensuring skilled perinatal healthcare. However as yet there is no consideration of mental health as a determinant of maternal mortality or morbidity in the initiative.

In high-income settings, as pregnancy and childbirth became safer and maternal mortality rates declined, particularly in the decades following World War II, awareness of the psychological aspects of pregnancy, childbirth, and the postpartum period grew. While there are historical references to disturbed behavior among women who had recently given birth, it was not until the 1960s that systematic reports were published of elevated rates of admission to psychiatric hospital in the first postpartum month.[2] In 1964, Paffenberger reported the nature and course of postpartum psychoses,[3] and in 1968, Pitt[4] described an atypical depression observable in some women following childbirth. These reports stimulated the very substantial research of the past five decades into psychological functioning and the nosology of psychiatric disorder associated with pregnancy, birth, and early motherhood in women. It is not agreed whether rates of mental health problems are higher at this than at other life stages.

Severe Mental Disorders

Between 0.2% and 2.0% of adults develop schizophrenia, and 0.4% to 1.6%, a bipolar mood disorder across the life span. There are some sex differences in the presentation of these serious mental disorders.[5] Women tend to have a later age of onset of schizophrenia and, in addition to disturbed cognition, to present with mood or affective symptoms.[6] Among women, the first episode of a bipolar disorder is likely to be marked by depressed or severely lowered mood, whereas mania or elevated mood and an overactive state is more typical among men. Women with bipolar disorders have more depressive episodes, more mixed affective and dysphoric manic states, and higher chances of rapid cycling.[6] Nevertheless, in a systematic review of 188 studies, Saha et al.[1] found no difference in the lifetime prevalence of schizophrenia between females and males and concluded that the overall prevalence of severe psychotic mental illnesses in adult populations appears similar in women and men. Women experience an increased risk of psychosis after having a baby, but men do not (see Box 16.2).

Common Mental Disorders

Non-psychotic "common mental disorders," for example depressive, anxiety, adjustment and somatoform disorders, which compromise day-to-day functioning, are more prevalent among women than men.[14]

Lifetime prevalence of major depression is 1.6 to 2.6 times higher among women, and the prevalence ratio of chronic mild depression or dysthymia in women and men is 2:1.[15–17] Piccinelli and Homen found higher rates of depression in women than men in all then-available population–based epidemiological studies, from 12 middle- and high-income countries.[18] Kessler asserts that the "higher prevalence of depression among women than men is one of the most widely documented findings in psychiatric epidemiology."[8] Lifetime prevalence rates of generalized anxiety disorder, panic disorder, and

Box 16.2 Prevalence of Severe Perinatal Mental Disorders

New onset of psychotic disorders during pregnancy is very rare, estimated to be about 7.1 per 10,000 pregnancies.[7] In women with bipolar affective disorder, acute episodes occur at the same rates during pregnancy as they do at other life phases, and risk of recurrence is increased if antipsychotic medication is ceased.[8]

About 1 or 2 per 1000 women experience psychosis within the first month after giving birth. The risk for women of experiencing a psychotic illness is elevated for the first thirty days postpartum (Kendell, Chalmers, Platz, 1987). Clinical characteristics include acute onset and extreme affective variation, with mania and elation as well as sadness, thought disorder, delusions, hallucinations, disturbed behavior, and confusion.[9,10] Postpartum psychoses are commonly regarded as episodes of bipolar affective disorder; rates of schizophrenic psychotic episodes are not elevated postnatally.[9] Risk of recurrence after subsequent pregnancies is between 51% and 69%.[9]

Systematic international comparisons are not available, but in all countries from which there is evidence, psychotic disorders following childbirth have been identified.[11] Schizophrenia is reported more commonly than affective disorder in low-income settings, but these patterns may reflect inter-country differences in diagnostic criteria.[12] In low-income countries, confusional states related to fever from infections or poor nutrition are associated with organic disorder, but can be mislabeled as psychoses.[12] Ndosi and Mtawali[13] described a case series of 86 women who developed psychosis within six weeks of giving birth in the United Republic of Tanzania; the incidence rate was 3.2 per 1000. Most were in young primiparous women with coexisting anemia and infectious disorders, and 80% were categorized as organic psychoses.

simple phobias are two to three times higher among women than men.[19] In both low- and high-income countries, unipolar depression is the leading cause of years lived with disability in adults, but women carry a 50% higher burden than men.[20] Comorbidity or the co-occurrence of more than one diagnosable condition in particular the common mental disorders is associated with higher disability and observed more frequently among women than men.[19,21]

The substantial focus on the prevalence of common mental disorders, in particular depression and to a lesser extent anxiety, associated with pregnancy and childbirth demonstrates the burden of these conditions experienced by women. Systematic reviews conclude that in high-income settings, about 10% of women who are pregnant and 13% who have recently given birth[22] experience depression.[23] Equivalent research about women living in low- and lower-middle income countries has only been conducted more recently, most published since 2000.[24] This is in part because of competing health priorities, including high rates of maternal deaths from obstetric emergencies. Research attention has also been slowed by beliefs that traditional confinement and post-partum practices, including social seclusion, prescribed rest, increased practical support from female family members, provision of specific foods and herbal preparations, gift giving, and an honored status are protective. This is now known to be an oversimplification: the presumption that culturally prescribed postnatal care is available to all, and welcome, does not reflect reality for many women. A systematic review of the evidence from these settings revealed that the weighted mean average prevalence of antenatal mental disorders (15.6%, 95% CI 15.4%–15.9%) and postnatal disorders (19.8%, 95% CI 19.5%–20.0%) was substantially higher than in HIC.[24] However, there is a significant difference in prevalence estimates by study sites: lowest from urban tertiary teaching hospitals, accessible to relatively advantaged women and highest from women in rural communities (see Figure 16.1). This indicates a social gradient in which prevalence is highest amongst the most socially and economically disadvantaged women, especially those living in crowded households in rural areas.

Somatisation is the experience of clinically significant symptoms, which cannot be explained by a known medical condition; disproportionate anxiety about physical symptoms, or "psychogenic" or idiopathic symptoms. *Dissociation* is a state in which psychological stress leads to loss of "normal psychological integration." These are presumed to be a means of communicating psychosocial distress and are diagnosed ten times more frequently in women (point prevalence of 2%) than in men (0.2%).[25]

Substance Abuse

In general women begin to use alcohol at a later age, consume less alcohol per occasion, and have lower rates of alcohol dependence and heavy episodic or binge drinking than men.[26] However, compared to men, women have a more rapid progression to alcohol dependence and to alcohol-related brain volume reduction.[26] WHO estimates that 1.4%

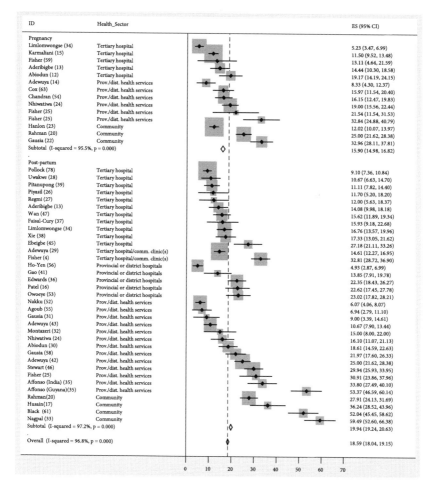

FIGURE 16.1

Meta-analysis of individual study and overall prevalence of common mental disorders (CMD) in women in low- and lower-middle-income countries during pregnancy and after childbirth. Used with permission from the World Health Organization.[24]

of the global burden of disease in women is attributable to alcohol use.[27] In many countries, women have not traditionally used tobacco, but their rates of use are increasing, in particular among young women.[28] Overall women are estimated to smoke or use smokeless forms of tobacco at about a quarter the rate of use by men.[28]

The prevalence of illegal drug use has not been established in most regions of the world. However, it is estimated that the prevalence worldwide of drug use disorders among women is about 0.4% (compared to ≥ 1.6% of men) with substantial interregional variation.[27]

Eating Disorders

Prevalence estimates of the clinical eating disorders of anorexia nervosa (0.5%–1.0%), bulimia nervosa (0.9%–4.1%), and sub-syndromal abnormal eating behaviors (5%–13%) have been derived from studies undertaken in high-income settings. It remains unclear to what extent these are observable in low-income settings, where food insufficiency and malnutrition are widespread. Eating disorders are rare, but concerns about being overweight are emerging among young women in societies undergoing rapid development, including China and India.[29] Eating disorders occur most commonly in adolescent and young adult women and at rates ten times higher than among men.[30] In addition to morbidity, the risk of premature death is substantially increased among women with disordered eating. In a recent meta-analysis of 36 studies reporting mortality associated with eating disorders, Arcelus et al. found that the weighted annual mortality rate for females with anorexia nervosa (data from 14 studies) was 5.39 (95% CI, 3.57–7.59) and of bulimia nervosa (data from five studies) was 2.22 (95% CI, 0.73–4.72) per 1000 person-years.[31]

Suicide

Ascertaining prevalence of suicide is difficult in countries where vital registration systems are weak, and suicide, as a socially stigmatized cause of death, which in some settings is illegal, may be recorded in a non-specific category. It is one of the three leading causes of death among people aged 15–44 years, and the second for the 10–24 years age group.[32] Overall, rates of suicide appear to be increasing.[33] In almost all countries, more males than females die by suicide. In China in the decade from 1990–1999, suicide rates were 25% higher in females than males, mostly accounted for by young women in rural areas.[34] This disparity diminished in the subsequent decade, attributed in a case-control study by Zhang et al. (2010) to improvements in standard of living in rural areas, including greater opportunities for women to participate in education and to migrate to urban areas for income-generating work.[35] However, it remains higher than in men (AOR 1.14, 95% CI 0.79–1.64). In general, women are more likely to use self-poisoning than other forms of self–harm and the difference in male-to-female ratios in Asia has been attributed in part to access to agricultural chemicals, which when ingested are fatal.[36] Suicide during pregnancy and following childbirth has been investigated comprehensively in high-income settings, but there is much less evidence available from low- and lower-middle income countries (see Box 16.3 and Box 16.4).

Although completed suicide may be rare, suicidal behaviors, including thoughts about suicide, plans to commit suicide and attempts to self-harm are 10 to 40 times more common.[39,43,44] Estimates of suicidal behaviors vary by the specificity of definitions, but prevalence is higher in females than males in all settings that have evidence.[39,43] In a review of surveys of more than 8000 school-attending adolescents in China, Thailand, El Salvador, and Egypt, thoughts of death, a "death wish," contemplation of suicide, planning for suicide, or acts of self-harm were reported by between one in three and one in eight participants. In all investigations suicidal thoughts and acts of self-harm were

Box 16.3 Suicide in the Perinatal Period

Maternal deaths are defined as those occurring in women during pregnancy or up to 42 days after pregnancy ends. In most high-income settings, sophisticated and comprehensive systems to investigate such deaths have identified suicide as a contributor to maternal mortality. The British Centre for Maternal and Child Enquiries reviewed maternal deaths from 2006–2008 and found that there were 0.57 deaths by suicide per 100,000 maternities and that this increased to 1.27 when the period of ascertainment was extended to the first six postpartum months.[37] The most significant risks were a past personal history of psychotic disorder (apparent in 59%) and substance abuse (31%). About half were well-educated, partnered women who were members of the dominant ethnic group, but had a past history of severe psychiatric disorder. The others were young, unemployed, and marginalized women whose lives were complicated by substance abuse.

Socially stigmatized causes of death are less reliably recorded and probably under-reported.[38] Postmortem examinations after suicide do not always include the uterine examination necessary to confirm pregnancy and studies that have examined obstetric records in addition to death certificates have identified significant under-recognition.[39] Investigations of suicide in women often fail to consider or report pregnancy status, and specific data regarding suicide in pregnancy are generally poorly documented.[39] Antenatal suicide is disproportionately associated with adolescent pregnancy, and appears to be the last resort for women with an unwanted pregnancy in settings where single women do not have access to contraception and legal pregnancy termination services are unavailable.[40]

In low-income countries, young women who fear parental or social sanction, who lack the financial means to pay for an abortion, or who cannot obtain a legal abortion may attempt to induce abortion themselves. Women who do this by self-poisoning, use of instruments, self-inflicted trauma, or herbal and folk remedies are at increased risk of death by misadventure.[41] In a population survey of mortality associated with abortion in Maharashtra, India, death rates from abortion-related complications were found to be disproportionately higher among adolescents, because they were more likely than older women to use untrained service providers. In addition, a number of adolescents had committed suicide to preserve the family honor without seeking abortion.[42]

significantly more common in girls than boys.[45] Although suicidal behaviors in women are stereotyped as help-seeking behaviors rather than a desire to die, there are no sex differences in intent.[46]

There is a small body of literature that suggests that postpartum suicidal behaviors are more common among women in low- than in high-income countries. Rahman and Hafeez[51] report that more than one-third (36%) of mothers caring for young children and living in refugee camps in the North West Frontier Province of Pakistan had a mental disorder, and that, of these, 91% had suicidal thoughts. Fisher et al.[52] found that, among a consecutive cohort of 506 women attending infant health clinics six weeks postpartum in Ho Chi Minh City, Viet Nam, 20% acknowledged thoughts of wanting to die.

DETERMINANTS OF MENTAL DISORDERS IN WOMEN

It is generally agreed that mental health problems are multifactorially determined by interactions among biological, psychological, and social risk and protective factors.

Box 16.4 Maternal Deaths by Suicide in Low and Lower-Middle Income Countries

In high-income countries, pregnancy suicide rates have declined because of the increased availability of contraception, affordable and accessible pregnancy termination services, and reduction in the stigma associated with births outside marriage.[40] However, where data are available, they indicate that suicide makes a substantial contribution to maternal deaths:

- In Haryana, India, 20% of 219 deaths among 9894 women who had given birth in rural areas in 1992 were due to suicide or accidental burns.[47]
- At Maputo Central Hospital, Mozambique, 9 of 27 (33%) postpartum deaths (1991–1995) not attributable to pregnancy or coincidental illness were by suicide, 7 of these in women aged less than 25 years.[48]
- In Viet Nam, verbal autopsies of all maternal deaths in seven provinces (2000–2001) found that overall 8%, but in some provinces 16.5% were by suicide, with problematic "community behaviors towards women" a contributing factor.[49]
- In Nepal, the Department of Health Services examined maternal deaths 1998–2008 in eight districts and found that, while there was an overall reduction from 539 to 229 per 100,000 live births, suicide was the leading cause, accounting for 16%.[50]

A number of hypotheses related to these risks are proposed to explain the similarities and differences in sex differences in the prevalence of mental disorders between women and men.

Biological

Causal models of psychotic disorders that are described as "hypercomplex" include that risk is associated with place and season of birth; and genetic, epigenetic, intrauterine, and environmental factors; but as yet, the interactions among them are unclear. Heritability is estimated to be 64% for schizophrenia and 59% for bipolar disorder. It is not suggested that there are different causal pathways in women and men,[53] but gender is a relevant determinant of the course of disorders, via interactions with family members, health services, and healthcare professionals. While acknowledging potential intercultural differences, Nasser et al.[54] propose that, as expectations of educational achievements and occupational roles are often lower for females, women with schizophrenia are less likely to experience family disapproval for being unable to meet aspirations in these domains than men are. Women experience greater symptomatic improvement if families are involved in treatment than if they are not, attributed to a reduction in rejecting behaviors.

The timing of onset of postpartum psychoses, family history, and molecular genetic studies support an underlying biological etiology, with circumstances of childbirth the precipitating factor.[9] Circumstances that have been associated with postpartum psychosis include primiparity, personal or family history of affective psychosis, unmarried status, perinatal death of an infant, caesarean birth, and most strongly, a past history of psychosis and marital difficulties.[55]

Many investigators have presumed that sex differences in rates of common mental disorders are biologically determined. Hormonal differences, especially those associated with puberty, the menstrual cycle, pregnancy and childbirth, and menopause, are assumed to be responsible and to render women intrinsically vulnerable to poor mental health. Patel[56] argues that sex differences in the prevalence of depression and anxiety cannot be attributed to "over-simplistic biological or hormonal explanations for the female excess because few biological parameters show this degree of variability." While biological differences may contribute, particularly through different individual sensitivities to hormonal fluctuations, systematic reviews conclude consistently that depression and anxiety in women are not related to sex hormones.[21,57]

Psychological

A second group of theories ascribes women's greater vulnerability to mental disorders as attributable to individual psychological functioning. In particular, there is a presumption that women tend to have maladaptive ways of thinking, to catastrophize, personalize and worry excessively, and to be "neurotic," with more "emotion-focused" and less "solution-focused" coping styles in the face of adverse life events.[19,21] However, critics of these theories argue that women's propensity to worry reflects entrenched patterns of socialization in which girls and women are confined to passive roles and are given fewer developmental opportunities to develop mastery and experience agency than their male counterparts, rather than to intrinsic psychopathology.[21]

It is also proposed that clinicians and researchers, who are socialized and shaped within cultures, form stereotypes about what constitutes normality in females and males and therefore what divergence from these should be classified as abnormal (see Box 16.5).

Social

The last general explanation covers social causation hypotheses, which argue that aspects of women's and men's lives make them more or less vulnerable to different patterns of ill health, including mental health. Thus, the contribution of the different social position occupied by women is integral to both the higher level of risk factors for poor mental health that they face and the lower levels of protective factors to which they have access. The World Health Organization's Commission on the Social Determinants of Health (CSDH) concludes that both structural factors and everyday circumstances are associated with disproportionate burdens of illness.[32, p5]

The CSDH conceptualizes the structural determinants of health as those reflecting the unequal distribution of power, income, goods, and services within and between

---

Box 16.5 Gender-Based Stereotypes Held by Clinicians

Broverman et al.'s[58] classic study demonstrated that 79 currently active mental health professionals' clinical judgements about what constituted healthy adult functioning were governed significantly by gender stereotypes. Similar characteristics were assigned by both male and female clinicians to a notionally healthy man and a healthy adult whose sex was not specified. However, a healthy female was characterized by being more submissive, suggestible, non-aggressive, non-competitive, concerned about appearance, emotional, excitable, and uninterested in mathematics and science than a healthy man or adult of unspecified sex.

Nearly thirty years later, Heesacker et al.[59] found, in a series of experiments with trainee and counseling psychologists, that unacknowledged stereotypes persisted. These included that women are "hyper-emotional," easily emotionally aroused, and have difficulties with emotional regulation, and that men are "hypo-emotional," have problems with emotional expression, and are "unable to feel emotionally alive." Diagnostic decisions are significantly influenced by the gender of the patient, with women being more likely than men to be diagnosed as depressed and prescribed antidepressants than men presenting with the same symptoms.[60]

countries. Mental health cannot be realized without justice; equality of human rights; inclusion of all; fairness of opportunity and access to adequate resources on which to live.[20] These are intrinsically gendered. The roles and rights of women have undergone major changes in some parts of the world, but women's rights to equality of participation, personal safety, reproductive choice, and freedom from discrimination are not recognized universally. Girl children and women face discrimination across the lifespan in many settings. These include female feticide, preference for male children leading to lower survival and worse nutritional status and health in young girls, female genital mutilation, no or limited education for females, restrictions on income-generating activities, forced marriage, adolescent marriage, polygamy, and "honor killing." Girls and women are also subject to more controlling social influences about achieving an ideal appearance, including shape, weight, and eating, than boys. Discrimination, inequality, and subordination have inevitable adverse effects on individual development and health, including mental health.[61]

Illustrative evidence was provided by Chen et al.,[62] who investigated the links between structural determinants and self-reported depressive symptoms in American women. Data were drawn from surveys of more than 7700 women and publicly available information from the 50 states in which they lived. These data included: political participation (number of female elected officers, availability of a legislative body for the status of women, and number of females registered to vote); reproductive rights (state-supported access to legal abortion, modern contraception and fertility treatment); economic autonomy (legislated right to equal employment, number of female-owned businesses, and proportion of women with incomes below the poverty line) and employment and earning (median female income and rates of female labor-force participation). Women who lived in states in which female political participation was high, reproductive rights recognized, and employment and economic autonomy assured had significantly lower average levels of depressive symptoms. It was concluded that, as it is safe to assume that women in general are biologically and psychologically the same across the states, structural social determinants outweighed both intrinsic biological and individual psychological factors in explaining gender differences in rates of depression.

The CSDH conceptualizes the other social determinant of health as being people's living circumstances, including their access to education, health care, and leisure, and the conditions of their work, housing, family relationships, and community resources.

In World Bank–defined high-income countries,[63] women have universal access to schooling and almost all complete at least secondary education. There is commitment in most school curricula in these settings to education about sexual health, reproductive rights, and interpersonal skills. Most women participate in income-generating work and have access to social protection, including maternity leave and state benefits for those who are un-partnered parents or are not wage-earners. They have ready access to comprehensive family planning services, technically sophisticated prenatal care, well-resourced hospitals in which to give birth, and skilled multidisciplinary teams of birth attendants. The political environments promote individual autonomy and endorse and protect women's rights to safety, equality, and full social and economic participation. However, most women live in the world's resource-constrained low- and lower-middle income countries.[63] In these settings, girls often lack access to primary, secondary, and post-secondary education and have little opportunity to learn about their sexual and reproductive health. Women may live in crowded housing, undertake hard physical work, and are malnourished and vulnerable to communicable diseases. Their lives can be constrained by rigid gender stereotypes about roles and responsibilities, including opportunities to earn money and make financial decisions. Women in these settings often lack access to family planning services, skilled birth attendants, health care facilities in which to give birth, and basic and emergency obstetrical care. These are all relevant to considerations of women's mental health (see Box 16.6 for illustration of a multifactorial model of suicide).

Poverty

Although definitions of "poverty" vary, including whether it is absolute (below the international poverty line) or relative (individual or household income in relation to median or mean income in the population), people occupying lower positions on the socioeconomic spectrum have fewer resources to be able to obtain basic commodities. Women invariably occupy lower socioeconomic positions than men and are therefore more likely to experience both absolute and relative poverty.[21] In the context of poverty, women are more vulnerable than men to CMD.[67] Even when there are sufficient financial resources in a household, women are less likely than men to be able to govern financial decisions or to have access to money to spend on discretionary rather than essential items.

Gender-Based Violence

Interpersonal violence is a global public health problem. The World Health Organization[68,69,70] defines any act of violence against women in their families, the general community, or perpetrated by the state as *gender-based violence*. The Declaration and Platform for Action of the Fourth World Conference on Women in Beijing in 1995, building on an earlier declaration,[69,70] elaborated this in defining gender-based violence as acts that *result in physical, sexual or psychological harm or suffering to women, including threats of such acts, coercion or arbitrary deprivation of liberty, whether occurring in public or private life.*

Violence Against Girls

Violent transgressions of the human rights of females begin prior to birth. Since the early 1980s, when ultrasound technologies that could be used to determine fetal sex were first available, selective abortion of female fetuses has increased. It occurs predominantly in countries with a strong cultural preference for sons rather than daughters, including China, India, Korea, and Pakistan.[71] It is regarded as one of the leading cause of "missing girls" or disproportions of males to females in the population. In India it has been

---

Box 16.6 Multifactorial Model of Suicide and Suicidal Behaviors

Suicide and suicidal behaviors are determined by multiple factors including social adversity, personality factors, depression, substance abuse and possible inherited risk for mental disorder or suicidality.[64,65] Herrera et al.[65] propose a theoretical model of the pathway to suicidal behaviors in resource-constrained settings. It includes material conditions: poverty, social inequality, and dangerous neighborhoods; and family factors: conflicted or abusive relationships and neglect or absence of care. Risk is amplified if there is no access to an alternative trusted adviser in the community or the primary health care system. Triggering events can include physical or sexual abuse, rejections, or experiences of failure, major loss, shame, humiliation or powerlessness. In pregnancy, suicidal ideas and behaviors are more common in women with than without a history of childhood sexual abuse, and in those who have experienced gender-based violence.[66]

established that female fetuses conceived in families that already have one or two female children are most at risk.[72]

One of the most common violations of girls is sexual abuse. The impact of childhood sexual abuse on adult mental health has been investigated comprehensively, but is difficult to elucidate, as it often co-occurs with other risks to adult mental health, including neglect, exposure to conflict, and emotional and physical abuse. Estimates of exposure to sexual abuse perpetrated by an adult against a child vary by definition, age cut-off, and method of assessment. Disclosures are governed by shame, health literacy, and availability of an adult in whom to confide.[73] It is experienced by boys, but much more commonly by girls. Anderson et al.[74] found that almost a third of a randomly selected cohort of 3000 women in New Zealand reported having had at least one unwanted sexual experience by the age of 16. Finkelhor and Dziuba-Leatherman,[75] in a review of the then-available epidemiological studies, including nationally representative surveys, found that 7%–36% of girls had experienced sexual abuse, most commonly perpetrated by a male they knew. Childhood sexual abuse often co-occurs with threats to a girl's life or personal safety if she discloses it to another adult. All unwanted sexual experiences in childhood are potentially problematic, but girls who have experienced genital contact or sexual penetration, perpetrated by a family member or known caregiver (especially when the abuse is conducted repeatedly and over sustained periods) are at highly elevated risk of mental health problems, including depression, anxiety, substance abuse, and comorbid occurrence of these conditions in adolescence and adulthood.[21,76] Somatization and dissociation are closely linked to experiences of traumatic events, which involve actual or witnessed threats to life coupled with helplessness and horror.[77] Seriousness and chronicity of exposure to childhood sexual abuse and severity of mental health problems have a dose–response relationship.[21]

Intimate-Partner Violence

There is still inconsistency in language as evidenced by the multiple descriptors used for violence in the intimate-partner relationship: spousal abuse, wife abuse, intimate-partner violence, sexualized violence, domestic violence, and family violence. Gender-based violence occurs in all societies, but especially in cultures in which there are rigid gender-role restrictions and women have low status, and their rights are not respected. Psychological and sexual violence in intimate partnerships are experienced much more commonly by women than by men. Intimate partner violence (IPV) is a clear and consistent predictor of depression, anxiety, trauma symptoms, suicidal ideas, and substance abuse in women, regardless of circumstances.[21] Mental health problems are even more common than physical injuries following IPV.[78] In the WHO Multi-Country study (2005), women who had experienced IPV were at two to three times higher risk of suicidal thoughts and suicide attempts compared to those who had not (see Box 16.7).[79] Depression diminishes in women who have left violent relationships and are living in refuges; this improvement is attributed to the benefits associated with cessation of violence, provision of professional and peer support, and an environment in which personal agency is promoted.[78]

Neighborhood Violence and Women

Neighborhood violence, which involves witnessing, hearing about, or being directly exposed to community violence involving serious injury or death, or hearing gunshots, observing fights, knife attacks, and shootings, is also problematic. It increases the likelihood of experiencing common mental disorders in women, even when the effects of intimate-partner violence and neighborhood poverty are controlled for.[80] Garcia and

> **Box 16.7** The World Health Organization's Multi-Country Study on Domestic Violence and Women's Health Household Survey
>
> This study collected data from more than 24,000 women from randomly selected households in ten countries using face-to-face interviews. There were wide inter-country variations in lifetime prevalence of experiences of violence from current or ex-husbands or boyfriends: from 13% in Japan to 61% in Peru, with most countries in the range of 23% to 49%.[79] Co-occurrence of violence was widespread: 94% of women experiencing physical violence also experienced verbal insults and humiliations, and 36%, forced sex. This study has established the gold standard for ascertainment of exposure to physical, emotional, and sexual violence in women. It demonstrates that it is essential to address specific behaviors and not just general self-reports of whether or not abuse has been experienced.

Herrero[81] investigated attitudes towards reporting gender-based violence among a nationally representative sample of 14,994 Spaniards. They found that people in neighborhoods with high social disorder had less favorable attitudes to reporting violence against women. They conclude that where disadvantage and social disorder are concentrated in neighborhoods, there is less trust or willingness to assist others, including women in perilous personal predicaments.

Trafficking and Violence

There are very few systematic data about the mental health consequences for women of being trafficked and forced into sex work, including in resource-constrained countries, but personal testimonies illustrate the serious psychological harm this incurs (see Box 16.8). Tsutsumi et al.[82] investigated prevalence and determinants of symptoms of depression, anxiety, and post-traumatic stress disorder (PTSD) in female victim survivors of trafficking aged 15 to 44 who were receiving services from non-governmental agencies in Kathmandu, Nepal. Comparisons were made between women who had been forced into sex work and those who had been forced into domestic service or to perform as circus entertainers. While not stratified by age group, there were extremely high rates of common mental disorders in all participants. However, rates of depressive and PTSD symptoms were significantly higher in women forced into sex work: all had clinically significant depressive symptoms, 97.7% anxiety symptoms, and 29.5% symptoms indicating PTSD.

Sexual Violence Against Girls and Women During Armed Conflict

During and in the aftermath of armed conflict, when law and social order are often absent, it has been common for armed groups to *loot, pillage and rape with impunity, treating women as the "spoil of war."*[83] Although not a recent phenomenon, mass rape of girls and women was witnessed and documented following recent wars in Bosnia, Rwanda, the Democratic Republic of Congo, and Sierra Leone. In response, the UN Security Council unanimously adopted, in 2008, Resolution 1820, which recognizes sexual violence as a weapon of war and calls for its cessation. Sexual violence is profoundly damaging to women, not only because of the direct physical and psychological consequences of rape, but also because of the follow-on consequences of stigmatization in which victim-survivors are regarded as unmarriageable, or are accused of adultery and

---

Box 16.8 A Personal Account of Trafficking and Sexual Violence

I am 23 years old. I was working in a factory in Moldavia and it closed down. My brother moved to England and I wanted to be there with him. A friend told me about an agency: they were offering jobs in Italy. I thought it would be a good way to meet my brother. We traveled across the border into Serbia. As we entered the apartment they locked the door. I went to run out of the door, but one of the buyers caught me, he hit me hard across the face, the blood moved into my mouth fast. Then he pushed me onto the bed, he ripped my clothes as if they were paper and as I fought it became worse, he bit me hard on my breast. He told me to shut up, that he would kill me if I screamed again.

He forced me night after night. They had guns...they told me "you are going to Kosovo." We were forced to have sex with up to five men every night, the owner also used any of the girls whenever he wanted to. We were not allowed to go out and we were locked into one small room all day long. There were eight of us in the room, there was...hardly anything to eat.

From: International Office of Migration, Counter Trafficking Unit, Pristina, Kosovo (1999). Information leaflet: You pay for a night—she pays with her life. (Cited in Watts and Zimmerman, 2002)[73]

---

rejected by their husbands. Women who conceive may be accused of damaging family honor and are frequently ostracized (see Box 16.9).

Unpaid Work and Caregiving

Women carry primary responsibility for the unpaid work of household tasks and caregiving throughout the world. This work is not dignified with the descriptors or language of *work* and is therefore essentially unrecognized. Gendered roles underpin the division of routine household labor. The essential daily tasks of cleaning, food preparation, laundering clothes, and the care of dependent children are stereotypically regarded as female responsibilities. The invisibility and low social value of this work is that women who are primary caregivers are described invariably in public, clinical, and domestic discourses as "not working" or as having "given up work." The actual unpaid workload of infant care and coincidental household tasks has proved difficult to define and measure (see Box 16.10).

This evidence suggests that women are at high risk of work-related fatigue, which is the subject of substantial scholarly research, most focused on the military, manufacturing,

---

Box 16.9 Mental Health Consequences of War-Related Sexual Violence

The mental health consequences of war-related sexual violence were examined in 573 women living in displaced person's camps as a result of war in Northern Uganda. Overall, 28.6% had experienced at least one form of sexual violence. Being younger than 44 and Catholic (thought to be taken as an indicator by perpetrators that the victim was less likely to be HIV-positive) increased their risk of violence. Gynecological morbidities were common among victim-survivors, and 69.4% had significant psychological distress.[84]

Box 16.10 Quantifying the Unpaid Work of Mothering an Infant

Smith et al.[85] attempted to quantify the unpaid "caring workload" in a community-based sample of 188 mothers of infants. Data were collected by a portable electronic recording device in which each of 25 defined activities was programmed to individual buttons that could be pressed at activity initiation and completion. Each woman collected data for seven consecutive 24-hour periods. The device records the date and duration of each activity, but can only capture one task at a time, so it underestimates actual work.

Infant-care activities alone were very frequent. When the infants were aged three months there were on average 49 feeds a week, lasting a mean of 20 minutes each. On average there were 70 other 13–18 minute occasions a week when infants were carried, held, or soothed. Smith et al.[85] conclude that it is inaccurate to define infant sleep times as leisure, not only because there are always other household tasks, but also because essential primary responsibility for the infant precludes rest or the pursuit of leisure activities. Active and passive infant care occupied about 165.4 of the 168 hours of the week.

transport, media and communications, and health sectors. Occupational fatigue is known to affect both health and performance. It has adverse effects on emotional, cognitive, and physical domains. However, there are no occupational health and safety provisions that recognize the occupational fatigue associated with the home as a workplace or that it might contribute to mental health problems in women (see Box 16.11).[15]

The burden of caregiving for people who are ill, frail, or disabled falls disproportionately on women. Eighty percent of caregivers are women who are diverse in age and relationship to care recipients. Most are middle-aged or elderly; two-thirds are caring for someone in a different generation, many giving 24-hour care, seven days a week.[87–89] In sub-Saharan Africa, most people with AIDS are cared for by elderly women and girls.[90] In high-income countries, about one in five households is providing some care to a person with a chronic condition or disability, and one in twenty, primary care.[87,91,92] In low-income countries and, with the closure of custodial institutions, increasingly in high-income countries, families are the predominant primary-care providers for people with serious mental disorders.[93] Caregiving can be long-term, with little respite, and it carries significant adverse consequences.

There are both indirect and direct economic costs. In addition to supporting the care-recipient, who might not have an income, it is more difficult for caregivers to maintain their own income-generating activities. Medicines and special equipment are costly and usually not state-subsidized. This is especially problematic in low- and lower-middle income countries where, even if caregiving is shared in a multigeneration household, it

Box 16.11 Women's Causal Explanations of Mental Distress in Goa, India

As I keep doing my work I keep thinking. So I feel mentally tired. I have no time other than my house work. All that takes time and I don't get time for myself. I told my husband to take me somewhere but he has no time. When you don't have time for yourself you get irritated and angry. I could have been so relaxed if I had help. I need help. I tell my husband to go late for work and help me with the cleaning. But he says no.

—Participant, in Pereira et al. [86]

Box 16.12 Mental Health Burden of Caregiving in an AIDS-Endemic Community in South Africa[94]

Kuo and Operario recruited 1599 adult caregivers in a household survey in Umlazi Township, Kwazulu Natal, where prenatal prevalence of HIV is 41.9%, and 19.8% of children are orphaned. Overall, 33% were caring for orphaned children. Comparisons were made between adults (86.4% of whom were female) caring for AIDS-orphans and those caring for non-orphans. These revealed that caregivers of orphans had:
- significantly worse general health;
- were more likely to be clinically depressed (OR 1.39, 95% CI 1.12–1.75)
- and had higher rates of post-traumatic stress than those caring for non-orphans;

Overall:
- female caregivers had worse health and were poorer than male caregivers; and
- 74.1% scored above the threshold for moderate anxiety.

is associated with significant economic disadvantage because families are often already surviving at near-subsistence levels (see Box 16.12).[89]

There is consistent evidence that caregivers have worse mental health than non-caregivers. In the Nurses' Health Study with 37,000 participants across 11 American states, women who provided at least 36 hours of care per week for spouses who were ill or had a disability were six times more likely than non-caregivers to experience symptoms of depression or anxiety.[95] Elsewhere, caregivers report consistently greater medication use and worse self-rated health, life satisfaction, affect, energy, and access to social support than non-caregivers.[96] High care-recipient needs, problematic family functioning, lack of support, and financial hardship are all associated with diminished confidence, lowered vitality, and increased risk of social isolation and mental health problems in caregivers.[97,98] These are, in turn, associated with caregiver self-reports of potentially harmful behavior towards the care-recipient, a precursor to mistreatment.[99] Caregivers in Italy who received more support from their social network and mental health professionals had lower levels of "family burden."[100] Despite these needs, in most countries, family caregivers receive little recognition or support from governments, clinical services, or others in the community.[89,93,95]

Reproductive Health

There are multiple intersections between women's reproductive lives and their mental health. Reproductive health conditions, which occur within the political, economic, cultural, and social contexts in which women live, can carry adverse consequences for mental health. In turn, women with mental health problems are vulnerable to poor reproductive health. In 1994, the International Conference on Population and Development (ICPD) declared that rights to sexual and reproductive health, which include bodily integrity, security, privacy, and the benefits of scientific progress, were human rights.[21] Women can experience reproductive health morbidities from early life, including those associated with menarche and the menstrual cycle, fertility and fertility management, pregnancy and childbirth, and menopause. These can either be prevented or easily assisted in settings where there is ready access to affordable, "friendly," confidential psychologically and gender-informed health services.

The demands of pregnancy, childbirth, and adjustment to the responsibilities of caring for a dependent infant for a woman's psychological resources and her intimate relationships have been investigated in detail and are discussed through this chapter. The following examples illustrate in particular the adverse consequences for mental health that can occur when reproductive rights are transgressed, women's needs are unrecognized and there is limited or no access to services.

Female Genital Mutilation

Female genital mutilation (FGM), sometimes termed "female circumcision," is defined as all procedures that involve non-therapeutic and irremediable partial or total removal of, or injury to, external female genital organs.[101] The practice is most common in countries of sub-Saharan Africa, parts of the Eastern Mediterranean, Indonesia, and Malaysia. Approximately 130 million women alive today have experienced some form of this procedure, and at least three million girls are at risk or are subjected to it each year. Estimates of prevalence in different population groups in which it is practiced vary; but in Egypt, Eritrea, Ethiopia, Somalia, and Sudan, 70%–98% of women have undergone the procedure, with higher rates among those with lower literacy and socioeconomic position. A WHO systematic review[102] found that only 15% of the available studies of the health effects of FGM considered mental health; most of these were case reports. Young women, who want to conform to parental and societal expectations by complying with FGM, but who are thereby exposed to fear, pain, complicated recovery, and possible long-term health problems experience conflict. Chronic depression and anxiety in response to genital disfigurement and gynecological dysfunction, and specific fears that cysts or scars were cancer or that the genitals were regrowing have been observed.[103] In Senegal, 47 women from Dakar (half of whom had experienced FGM), completed semi-structured interviews about the events of circumcision and their reactions to it in structured psychiatric diagnostic interviews.[104] FGM had been performed on girls between the ages of five and 14 years, and when interviewed, participants were aged 15 to 40 years. The events of circumcision were recalled as "appalling and traumatic" by most, and intrusive re-experiencing in thoughts and images was almost universal. Overall, 80% met current criteria for depression and anxiety, and 30.4% post-traumatic stress disorders. In the non-circumcised group, only one person had symptoms of mood disorder, and none had PTSD.[104] Elnasha and Abdelhady[105] surveyed 264 newly married women, 75.8% of whom had been circumcised, in Benha, Egypt. Overall, 40 (20%) of the circumcised group had been married by the age of 20, while none of the non-circumcised group had married in adolescence. The circumcised group had higher rates of somatization, general anxiety, and phobias than the non-circumcised group.

Obstetric Fistulae

One of the consequences of adolescent pregnancy, including in the context of female genital mutilation, is obstructed childbirth, leading to stillbirth of the baby and genitourinary and/or anorectal fistulae, which often result in an uncontrolled flow of urine and or feces. These can lead to social ostracizing. Ojanuga,[106] in an early series of case descriptions, reported that the psychological consequences were profound and involved depression, grief, and reduced self-confidence. These were worse in women who were rejected and abandoned. Women attending the Dhaka Medical College Hospital Fistula Unit in Bangladesh and the Addis Ababa Fistula Hospital in Ethiopia were surveyed prior to reparative surgery, and almost all (97%) met criteria for psychiatric caseness. A substantial proportion (38%) had actively contemplated killing themselves, and another 40% experienced suicidal ideation.[107] It was estimated from the distribution of scores that up to 38.8% had major depression, with the rest experiencing less severe psychiatric morbidities. Kabir et al.[108] assessed 120 women aged from 10 to 36 attending the Laure fistula center at a specialist hospital in northern Nigeria. More than half had experienced social exclusion, and a third were "mentally depressed."

Vaginal Discharge

Vaginal discharge can be a symptom of reproductive tract infections, but the association is not strong, and many women reporting problematic discharge do not, when investigated and tested, have an infection. In Goa, India, Patel et al.[109] investigated 2494 women recruited from the community using structured interviews about psychosocial risks, common mental disorders, and gynecological and laboratory testing, and reassessed 91% six and 86.9% twelve months later.[109,110] At baseline, the 14.5% who reported an abnormal vaginal discharge were more likely than the rest of the sample to report CMD (OR 2.16, 95% CI 1.4–3.2) and somatoform disorders (OR 6.23 95% CI 4.0–9.7). Incidence of this complaint in the follow-up period was associated with these two risks and being younger, illiterate, of the religious minority, and concerned about their husband's extramarital relationships. These findings were interpreted as indicating that reported vaginal discharge could in this setting indicate somatization of psychological distress, a cultural idiom to explain fatigue and low mood, or a mechanism to avoid sexual intercourse or to legitimize professional help seeking.

Spontaneous Pregnancy Loss

The rate of miscarriage or spontaneous pregnancy loss in the population cannot be ascertained exactly, because these outcomes are not usually recorded in national data, and women do not always seek clinical care in this circumstance. However, it is thought to occur in the first trimester of about 20% of pregnancies. Mental health consequences of miscarriage reflect both individual characteristics and sociocultural context. Pregnancy loss can lead to anxiety, guilt, powerlessness, self-blame, and sadness in women, which are amplified if miscarriages are recurrent. The most widespread conceptual framework to understanding responses to miscarriage is grief or bereavement reactions, which reflect the loss of an emotional attachment formed between a women and her fetus from conception.[111] Grief is a normal if intense response to loss, which is expected to reduce with time and is generally assisted by empathic support. It is more problematic if the pregnancy has not yet been announced and, therefore, the loss can be unrecognized, leading to disenfranchised or unacknowledged grief in which the loss is experienced, but there is no public recognition or increased support. This can be amplified when health professionals respond to miscarriage as a routine event of relatively minor psychological significance. In some women, more sustained mental health problems can develop following miscarriage. Neugebauer et al.[112] compared prevalence of major depressive disorder in 229 women in the first six months after miscarriage with 230 women in the community. They found that relative risk was 2.5% (95% CI 1.2–5.1), with rates being highest in both groups among those with a prior history of depression or experiencing coincidental adverse life events. In settings where women have access to few adult roles apart from motherhood, miscarriage can be experienced as a profound loss, which arouses fear of abandonment by the partner and rejection from the extended family.[111]

Reproductive Health of Women with Serious Mental Disorders

The complex reproductive mental and physical health needs of women with preexisting chronic severe mental disorder are not well investigated. Among those with severe chronic mental disorder, frequency of sexual activity may be normal, but contraceptive use and autonomous reproductive decision-making are compromised.[113] Women with schizophrenia who are pregnant tend to present late for prenatal care and are at risk for poor obstetric outcomes. The multiple psychosocial difficulties experienced by those with severe chronic mental disorders can have adverse effects on the formation of mother–infant attachments.

The interactions among risk and protective factors for mental health problems are illustrated by the evidence about the determinants of perinatal common mental disorders (see Box 16.13).

Mechanisms Linking Risk Factors and Women's Mental Health

The mechanisms by which poverty, violence, unpaid caregiving, and poor reproductive health contribute to mental health problems in women reflect theories about the social origins of depression. Brown and Harris (1978) concluded from systematic investigations of women living in situations of chronic adversity in public housing in London that depression is a consequence of co-occurring experiences of entrapment and humiliation.[116] Broadhead and Abas (1998) confirmed that severe adverse events were "particularly depressogenic" among women in Zimbabwe if they involved humiliation and entrapment in a situation from which there is no apparent escape.[117]

Unpaid caregiving reduces income-generating opportunities and thereby financial and personal autonomy. It is generally undervalued and unrecognized. Home is optimally a haven, in which there is physical and psychological safety and in which people can trust that they will be responded to with sensitivity and care. Intimate-partner violence is a complete contravention of this and involves inability to escape (entrapment) and breach of trust (subordination and humiliation).[117,118] It violates women's rights to liberty, security of person, and freedom from fear, and thereby constitutes a major rights transgression.[119] Neighborhood violence similarly invokes feelings of helplessness and powerlessness, usually because of shame about poverty, which reduces a person's ability to escape. Reproductive health problems often invoke shame as a result of limited understanding of the normal and healthy functioning of the reproductive system and attribution of causation of health problems like infertility or sexually transmitted infections to women. In contexts in which there is limited access to health services, these conditions can be untreated and lead to social exclusion.

IMPACT

As the nature, course, determinants, and behavioral changes associated with mental health problems are generally poorly understood, people with these conditions can experience mistrust, insensitivity, and being ostracized. Among women, this amplifies the gender-based discrimination that women experience in many settings where their rights to equality of participation are not recognized.

Stigma and Discrimination

Stigmatization is the attribution of undesirable or objectionable characteristics to a person on the basis of their circumstances or qualities. These are used to justify hostile and discriminatory responses and behaviors towards the affected person, which carry clear adverse consequences for their emotional well-being and social functioning.[120] There has been less attention to gender-based than other forms of stigmas related to

Box 16.13 Determinants of Perinatal Common Mental Disorders in Women

Perinatal mental health problems are thought to be the outcome of the interaction of multiple risk and protective factors rather than being attributable to a single factor. These are comparable between high- and low-income settings, but risks are more prevalent and access to protective factors more limited in the latter.

Biological

- general health
  - nutritional status
  - coincidental burden of infectious or chronic disease
  - substance use
  - adverse obstetric events, including life-threatening complications and perinatal loss

Psychological

- cognitive capability and learning style
  - personality, including capacities for emotional regulation and adaptation to new experiences
  - interpersonal skills, including capacity to trust and form sustained relationships
  - past experience of neglect or sexual, physical or emotional abuse
  - past mental health problems

Social

- low socioeconomic position
  - exposure to interpersonal violence
  - income insecurity, lack of maternity benefits, and pregnancy-related discrimination
  - criticism, coercion, and lack of empathic support from the intimate partner
  - role restrictions regarding housework and infant care, and excessive unpaid workloads
  - insufficient access to social resources, including practical and emotional support
  - crowded housing
  - lack of access to family planning services to enable reproductive choice about when and how many children to have
  - in some settings, having a female baby

Women's perinatal mental health is protected by having better education, paid work, maternity leave, sexual and reproductive health services, including family planning, and supportive, non-judgemental family relationships.

Sources:[10,45,114,115]

serious mental disorders. Loganthan and Murthy[121] investigated perceptions of stigma in narrative interviews with 118 men and 82 women with schizophrenia in India. Stigma related to marriage and childbearing was more common and problematic among women than men. Women reported experiences like being forced to terminate a pregnancy because of family beliefs that a child would be similarly affected, or coerced not to conceive, forcibly divorced, or separated from their children. Many had experienced verbal abuse, rejection, and social ostracizing. In several low-income countries, it is common for married women with schizophrenia to be abandoned by their spouses or families. They are then doubly stigmatized and highly vulnerable to becoming homeless and destitute because of social exclusion and limited access to social protection.[122]

Violence Against Women With Serious Mental Disorders

Women with severe mental disorders are an especially vulnerable group who report experiencing high rates of physical and sexual violence, but low rates of accessing violence-specific services.[123,124] Women with schizophrenia who are victims of violence are often disbelieved by police and health care professionals, who can attribute their accounts to delusions, thereby increasing a sense of powerlessness in the victims.[123]

The psychological consequences of sexual violence among women with severe mental disorder are rarely investigated. A study among consecutive female inpatient admissions ($N = 146$) to a large psychiatric hospital in southern India found that sexual coercion was reported by 30% of the 146 women. The most commonly reported experience was sexual intercourse involving threatened or actual physical force (reported by 14% of women), and the most commonly identified perpetrator was the woman's husband or intimate partner (15%), or a person in a position of authority in their community (10%). Women with a history of abuse were more likely to report risky sexual behavior (p < 0.001). In contrast to the 30% of women who reported sexual coercion during interviews, only 3.5% of the medical records contained this information.[124] A marked gender difference has been found with very few men with severe mental disorder reporting sexual violence.[125]

Consequences for Fetal and Infant Development

In addition to the consequences for women, there is increasing evidence that both fetal and infant development can be compromised if their mothers are experiencing mental health problems. Maternal cortisol, a stress-response hormone, can pass through the placenta. Even though the placenta has a mechanism to protect the fetus, if the mother is experiencing chronic anxious arousal, this is thought to influence the level of fetal cortisol, which in turn has adverse consequences for fetal development.[126] In high-income countries, prenatal anxiety is associated with increased risk of child behavioral/emotional problems at four years of age[127]; and has a negative association with cognitive ability.[128,129] In Pakistan, when socioeconomic status and maternal body mass index were controlled, infants of depressed mothers weighed on average 2910 grams and of non-depressed mothers, 3022 grams (p < 0.01); the relative risk of birth weight less than 2500 grams was 1.9 (95% CI 1.3–2.9).[130] The interpersonal functioning of mothers who are depressed is compromised, and the quality and sensitivity of mother–infant interaction are disrupted.[131] Poor maternal psychological state can reduce sensitivity and responsiveness through neglect or inaccurate interpretation of infant cues, developmentally inappropriate expectations, and hostile or inconsistent responses. In resource-constrained settings, maternal depression has been linked directly to higher rates of stunting in infants, higher rates of diarrheal diseases, infectious illness and hospital admission, reduced completion of recommended schedules of immunization, and worse social, behavioral, and emotional development in children.[132–134]

PROMOTION, PREVENTION AND TREATMENT

Complex ecological explanatory models are therefore required to understand mental health problems in women and to inform mental health promotion, primary prevention, early intervention, and treatment strategies to address them.

Promotion

Promotion of the mental health of girls and women clearly requires cross-sectoral approaches in which the protective factors of equality of participation in primary, secondary, and post-secondary education; access to income-generating occupations; safety from family and community violence, and recognition of the unpaid workload are secured in legislative and policy frameworks with clear mechanisms to ensure implementation.

Prevention

Recognition and Modification of Gender-Based Risks

Structural interventions seek to modify contextual risk factors and thereby reduce the likelihood that mental health problems will occur. The Intervention with Microfinance for AIDS and Gender Equity (IMAGE) was tested in a cluster-randomized trial in villages in the rural South African Limpopo province. The aim was to reduce HIV infection, but it addressed risk factors that are also salient to women's mental health: poverty and intimate-partner violence. The multi-component intervention included microfinance support (provision of loans and business planning, guidance, and review) for the poorest households, fortnightly center-based meetings for women in the village, and community mobilization. The meetings covered the 10-session "Sisters for Life" Gender and HIV program, which were facilitated by trained local community members and covered topics including gender roles, women's work, rights to bodily integrity, and empowerment. Local leaders were identified and support to initiate solutions to local problems through community action. Women used loans to establish small retail businesses selling produce, clothing, or services like tailoring, and 99.7% were repaid. Women in the intervention group had improved household wealth, social capital, and indicators of empowerment (e.g., more equitable attitudes to gender roles and capacity to communicate about sexual matters) compared to women in the control group. Over the two-year follow-up period, levels of intimate-partner violence were reduced by 55% in women in the intervention group compared to those in the control condition. While mental health per se was not measured as an outcome, it is likely that these benefits would be reflected in improved mental health. This approach provides powerful evidence of the potential benefits for women of initiatives to reduce poverty and intimate-partner violence and improve economic autonomy and promote gender equity at a local level.

Access to health services and care are also determined by gender. Women who either lack financial resources or are unable to influence financial decision-making in a household are less able to make autonomous decisions to seek health care or to purchase prescribed medications.

Probably as a result of this, women with mental health problems are, when other factors are controlled for, less likely to use essential preventive health care like micronutrient supplements in pregnancy.[135] In countries like Pakistan and Afghanistan, where many women are unable to leave the household unless accompanied by a man, they are less likely to attend a health service for assistance with either gynecological or mental health problems. Many women prefer to consult female practitioners, but because opportunities for women to be trained as health professionals are severely limited in many settings, there are fewer women in the health workforce, especially as medical specialists.[136]

Support for Women Caregivers

Many countries have yet to plan financial, legal, and policy responses to chronic disorder and disability. The needs of women and girls who provide care for family members with these conditions, in particular those who are additionally marginalized through poverty or being from an ethnic minority, are a priority. Prince and colleagues (2007)[89] regard it as likely that the greatest obstacle to providing effective support and care for older persons with mental disorder and their families in low-income countries is the lack of awareness of the problem among policymakers, health care providers, and the community.

Low-income countries lack the economic and human capital to provide widespread specialist services. The most cost-effective way to manage people with these conditions will be through supporting, educating, and advising family caregivers, adding respite care, in day centers or in residential or nursing homes where feasible.[89] Ideally, primary care services with the supports available can respond to the mental and physical health needs of ill and disabled people and their family caregivers, and collaborate in providing care with the patients and families.

In a number of countries, caring for people who have a disability or are frail and aged is recognized in social policy, and systems are established for caregivers to receive help. For example, in Australia, government-supported home and community care program and carers' support packages are well established. These allow for short and longer-term respite care, information, financial support for caregivers, and education and employment assistance. The rationale includes reducing the risk of residential care through early intervention and support for the well-being of caregivers. Government, private, and voluntary agencies each have a part to play. The government aims to work in partnership with families and other caregivers to help older and disabled people stay in their own homes.

In countries of all income levels, this partnership is important. The World Health Organization recommends psycho-education to help caregivers and families to understand the disorder, encourage treatment adherence, and recognize early signs of relapse as an important community-based strategy to promote mental health.[93]

Treatment

Mental health services in many settings are experienced by women as unsafe, perpetuating the power disparities they experience in their domestic lives, and lacking in warmth or compassion for the contribution of circumstances to their predicaments (see Box 16.14).[136] Women benefit from services in which staff members have been educated about the ways in which gender stereotypes influence their language and behavior, and this knowledge is then translated into practice.[136] Gender-sensitive mental health services for women are those in which stigma is addressed, empowerment and autonomy are promoted, staff are respectful and non-judgemental, safety is assured, and comprehensive care, including care for general and sexual and reproductive health, is provided.[136] In most parts of the world, rehabilitation services are also not gender-sensitive. Women with severe mental disorders have specific needs, which are more often relational and social and not limited just to income-generation. Nasser et al.[54] conclude that as the *disease* becomes the focal point, the *experience* of the individual with the disease is ignored, but it is nevertheless highly relevant to effective service provision.

Effective treatment of mental disorders requires multiple strategies, including in countries where recognition is low and there are few services. Patel et al.[137] reviewed the evidence about "packages" of care to treat depression effectively. They concluded that, in addition to accurate recognition and the provision of evidence-informed treatments: increasing consumer awareness and demand for services, improving health care provider skills, adapting programs to maximize acceptability, having both clinic and community based approaches, and addressing psychosocial disability were essential. In low-income settings, it was recommended that packages include screening to detect symptoms, psycho-education, generic antidepressants, and problem-solving therapy.

Box 16.14 Barriers to Mental Health Care for Women with Serious Mental Disorders

Lack of coordination between health and social services constitutes a significant barrier to care for women with serious mental disorders, particularly in low-income countries, which leads to:

• Delayed help-seeking
• Inadequate community and outpatient treatment and more admissions into a psychiatric hospital, adding to stigma
• Lack of family inputs and family education regarding mental disorder
• Delay in discharge from hospital and lack of after-care services
• Loss of skills and identity
• Abandonment
• Inadequate access to legal services
• Destitution

Source: [136]

In general, women prefer to have mental health care integrated with general or specialized health care (see Box 16.15 for an illustrative example).

Women throughout the world have at least some contact with health services during pregnancy, which provides opportunities to assess their mental health and intervene if

Box 16.15 Comprehensive Sexual and Reproductive Health Care for Women with Serious Mental Disorders: A Working Model in Bangalore, India

Planned pregnancies are advocated in women with severe mental disorders. However, rates of unintended pregnancies can be quite high owing to lack of contraceptive advice and knowledge about family planning services. Across the world, there are few examples of specialized services for women with severe mental disorder who want to conceive and have children.

In Bangalore, India, a specialized perinatal and parenting assistance service has been developed in National Institute of Mental Health and Neuro Sciences, a public hospital, for women with severe mental disorder. The service provides advice and counseling for women with severe mental disorder and their partners. Women from across the region are referred to the service for advice regarding—planned conception, readiness for parenting and becoming a mother, advice to spouses and families on support to the woman when pregnant, liaison with gynecologists and obstetricians when planning pregnancy; and, once pregnant, enhancing maternal–fetal bonding, and monitoring side effects of psychotropic drugs and effects of drugs on the fetus. Written information in local languages in the form of booklets on pre-pregnancy counseling, pregnancy-related and postpartum mental health is provided. Following birth, assessments and interventions related to mother–infant bonding, sleep hygiene, managing safe lactation, and future family planning advice are also provided. In addition, the service also conducts assessments among women with schizophrenia and other severe mental disorders who have young children, and offers parenting training.

The service, which does not receive any extra funds and is run by the regular adult psychiatry team, also offers an opportunity for training in gender-sensitive care for women with severe mental disorders.[138]

necessary. There is a small group of randomized controlled trials of interventions to treat perinatal depression in women in primary health care in resource-constrained settings, which have promising findings.

Rojas et al.[139] developed a multi-component intervention which included eight weekly structured psycho-educational groups covering symptoms and treatments, problem-solving and behavioral activation strategies, cognitive techniques, and a cost-free pharmacotherapy protocol of fluoxetine (20–40mg per day) or sertraline (50–100mg per day) for women who did not respond to fluoxetine or were lactating. They tested it in primary care clinics providing prenatal and postnatal health care to women in Santiago, Chile, against standard care. Participants were women who had been diagnosed with major depression within a year of giving birth. Mean Edinburgh Postnatal Depression Scale (EPDS)scores were lower in the multi-component intervention at three months' follow-up (–4.5 difference in mean scores between groups, 95% CI –6.3 to –2.7, $p <$ 0.0001) and were at least 3 points lower at six months than at baseline in 73% of the intervention group and 57% of the usual care group (95% CI 3–29).

Rahman et al.[140] undertook a trial of the Thinking Healthy Program (THP), a manualized intervention incorporating cognitive and behavioral techniques of active listening, problem solving, collaboration with the family, non-threatening enquiry into the family's health beliefs and substitution of alternative information when required, and inter-session practice activities. It was implemented by trained, supervised Lady Health Workers (LHWs) who are community-based primary health workers in a rural area in Pakistan. The intervention group received 16 sessions in scheduled household visits from late pregnancy on, and the control group received the same number and schedule of home visits, but from an untrained LHW. Study participants were pregnant married women aged 16–45 years, diagnosed as experiencing a major depressive episode. After adjusting for covariates, women in the intervention group were less likely to be depressed and experiencing disability and had better global functioning and perceived social support at six and twelve months after the initiation of the intervention ($p < 0.0001$). Infants of intervention group mothers had fewer episodes of diarrhea at 12 months ($p = 0.04$); and were more likely to be fully immunized ($p = 0.001$).

CONCLUSION

Women's [mental] health is inextricably linked to their status in society. It benefits from equality and suffers from discrimination. Today the status and well-being of countless millions of women worldwide remains tragically low. As a result, human well-being suffers, and the prospects for future generations are dimmer....[141]

Mental health problems in women are prevalent and multifactorially determined, including by structural factors and circumstances of day-to-day life that are beyond individual control, and by gender-based risks. They are associated with significant disability, reduced quality of life, lower life satisfaction, and compromised capacity to participate. However, because of competing health priorities, stigma, gender-based role restrictions, low emotional literacy, and limited services, recognition and effective responses remain inadequate in many settings, but especially in low- and lower-middle-income countries. A comprehensive cross-sectoral approach is crucial. Addressing social causes through the realization of girls' and women's human rights to education, nutrition, health care, equal social and economic participation, safety, individual autonomy, and freedom from discrimination is an essential first step. In the health sector, an approach is required that focuses on gender-sensitive mental health promotion and evidence-informed strategies for prevention in addition to early intervention and treatment. In order to achieve these, gender-informed clinical and public health research is necessary to provide local evidence and monitor and evaluate interventions. Mental health workers and researchers who advocate for these strategies and implement these approaches can be powerful agents of empowerment for women.

REFERENCES

1. Saha S, Chant D, Welham J, McGrath J. A systematic review of the prevalence of schizophrenia. *PLoS Med.* 2005;2(5):0413–33.
2. Robinson GE, Stewart DE. Postpartum disorders. In: Stotland N, Stewart D, editors. *Psychological aspects of women's health care: The interface between psychiatry and obstetrics and gynecology.* 1st ed. Washington, DC: American Psychiatric Press; 1993;115–138.
3. Paffenbarger RS. Epidemiological aspects of parapartum mental illness. *Br J Prev & Soc Med.* 1964;18:189–95.
4. Pitt B. "Atypical" depression following childbirth. *Br J Psychiatry.* 1968;114:1325–35.
5. American Psychiatric Association. *Diagnostic and statistical manual of mental disorders, 4th edition.* Washington, DC: American Psychiatric Association; 1994.
6. Castle DJ, McGrath J, Kulkarni J. *Women and schizophrenia.* New York: Cambridge University Press; 2000.
7. Watkins ME, Newport DJ. Psychosis in pregnancy. *Obstet Gynecol.* 2009;113(6):1349–53.
8. Viguera A, Cohen L, Baldessarini R, Nonacs M. Managing bipolar disorder during pregnancy: weighing up the risks and benefits. *Can J Psychiatry.* 2002;47:426–36.
9. Pfuhlmann B, Stoeber G, Beckmann H. Postpartum psychoses: prognosis, risk factors, and treatment. *Curr Psychiatry Rep.* 2002;4:185–90.
10. Scottish Intercollegiate Guidelines Network. *Postnatal depression and puerperal psychosis. A national clinical guideline.* Royal College of Physicians; 2002 [cited 2010]; available from: http://www.sign.ac.uk/guidelines/fulltext/60/index.html.
11. Kumar R. Postnatal mental illness: a transcultural perspective. *Soc Psychiatry & Psychiatr Epidemiol.* 1994;29:250–64.
12. Husain N, Bevc I, Husain M, Chaudhry IB, Atif N, Rahman A. Prevalence and social correlates of postnatal depression in a low income country. *Arch Women Ment Health.* 2006;9(4):197–202.
13. Ndosi NK, Mtwali ML, Ndosi NK, Mtwali MLW. The nature of puerperal psychosis at Muhimbili National Hospital: its physical co-morbidity, associated main obstetric and social factors. *Afr J Reprod Health.* 2002;6(1):41–9.
14. Goldberg D, Huxley P. *Common mental disorders: A biosocial model.* London: Tavistock / Routledge; 1992.
15. Fisher J, Herrman H. Gender, social policy and implications for promoting women's mental health. In: Chandra PS, Herrman H, Fisher J, Kastrup M, Niaz U, Rondon MB, et al, editors. *Contemporary topics in women's mental health: Global perspectives in a changing society.* Chichester, West Sussex: John Wiley & Sons; 2009:499–506.
16. Kessler RC. Epidemiology of women and depression. *J Affect Disord.* 2003;74(1):5–13.
17. Kessler RC, McGonagle KA, Zhao S, Nelson CB, Hughes M, Eshleman S, et al. Lifetime and 12-month prevalence of DSM-III-R psychiatric disorders in the United States. Results from the National Comorbidity Survey. *Arch Gen Psychiatry.* 1994;51(1):8–19.
18. Piccinelli M, Homen FG. *Gender differences in the epidemiology of affective disorders and schizophrenia.* Geneva: World Health Organization; 1997.
19. Kadri N, Alami KM. Depression and anxiety among women. In: Chandra PS, Herrman H, Fisher J, Kastrup M, Niaz U, Rondón MB, et al, editors. *Contemporary topics in women's mental health: Global perspectives in a changing society.* Chichester, West Sussex: John Wiley & Sons; 2009:37–64.
20. Mathers CD, Lopez AD, Murray CJL. The burden of disease and mortality by condition: data, methods and results for 2001. In: Lopez AD, Mathers CD, Ezzati M, Murray CJL, Jamison DT, editors. *Global burden of disease and risk factors.* New York: Oxford University Press; 2006:45–240.
21. Astbury J, Cabral de Mello M. *Women's mental health: An evidence based review.* Geneva: World Health Organization; 2000.
22. Hendrick V. Evaluation of mental health and depression during pregnancy. *Psychopharmacol Bull.* 1998;34(3):297–9.

23. O'Hara M, Swain A. Rates and risks of postpartum depression—a meta-analysis. *Int Rev Psychiatry.* 1996;8:37–54.

24. Fisher J, Cabral de Mello M, Patel V, Rahman A, Tran T, Holton S, et al. Prevalence and determinants of common perinatal mental disorders in women in low- and lower-middle-income countries: a systematic review. *Bull WHO.* 2012;90(2):139G–49G.

25. American Psychiatric Association. *Diagnostic criteria from DSM-IV-TR.* Washington, DC: American Psychiatric Association; 2000.

26. Mann K, Ackermann K, Croissant B, Mundle G, Nakovics H, Diehl A. Neuroimaging of gender differences in alcohol dependence: Are women more vulnerable? *Alcoholism.* 2005;29(5):896–901.

27. World Health Organization. *Atlas on substance use (2010)—Resources for the prevention and treatment of substance use disorders.* Geneva: World Health Organization; 2010.

28. World Health Organization. *World report on the global tobacco epidemic, 2008: The MPOWER package.* Geneva: World Health Organization; 2008.

29. Fisher J, Cabral de Mello M, Izutsu T, Vijayakumar L, Belfer M, Omigbodun O. Adolescent mental health in resource-constrained settings: a review of the evidence of the nature, prevalence and determinants of common mental health problems and their management in primary health care. *Int J Soc Psychiatry.* 2011;57(1 Suppl):v–vii, 9–116.

30. Abbas S, Palmer RL. Eating disorders. In: Chandra PS, Herrman H, Fisher J, Kastrup M, Niaz U, Rondón MB, et al, editors. *Contemporary topics in women's mental health: Global perspectives in a changing society.* Chichester, West Sussex: John Wiley & Sons; 2009:97–116.

31. Arcelus J, Mitchell AJ, Wales J, Nielsen S. Mortality rates in patients with anorexia nervosa and other eating disorders. A meta-analysis of 36 studies. *Arch Gen Psychiatry.* 2011;68(7):724–31.

32. World Health Organization. *Closing the gap in a generation: Health equity through action on the social determinants of health.* Geneva: World Health Organization; 2008.

33. Bertolote J, M., Fleischmann A, De Leo D, Bolhari J, Botega N, De Silva D, et al. Suicide attempts, plans, and ideation in culturally diverse sites: the WHO SUPRE-MISS community survey. *Psychol Med.* 2005;35:9.

34. Phillips MR, Li X, Zhang Y. Suicide rates in China, 1995–1999. *Lancet.* 2002;359(9309):835–40.

35. Zhang J, Xiao S, Zhou L. Mental disorders and suicide among young rural Chinese: a case-control psychological autopsy study. *Am J Psychiatry.* 2010;167(7):773–81.

36. Fleischmann A, Bertolote JM, De Leo D, Botega N, Phillips M, Sisask M, et al. Characteristics of attempted suicides seen in emergency-care settings of general hospitals in eight low- and middle-income countries. *Psychol Med.* 2005;35(10):1467–74.

37. Cantwell R, Clutton-Brock T, Cooper G, Dawson A, Drife J, Garrod D, et al. Saving mothers' lives: Reviewing maternal deaths to make motherhood safer: 2006–2008. The Eighth Report of the Confidential Enquiries into Maternal Deaths in the United Kingdom. *BJOG.* 2011;118 Suppl 1:1–203.

38. Graham W, Filippi V, Ronsmans C. Demonstrating programme impact on maternal mortality. *Health Policy & Plan.* 1996;11(1):16–20.

39. Brockington I. Suicide in women. *Int Clin Psychopharmacol.* 2001;16:S7–19.

40. Frautschi S, Cerulli A, Maine D. Suicide during pregnancy and its neglect as a component of maternal mortality. *Int J Gynaecol & Obstet.* 1994;47:275–84.

41. Smith J. Risky choices: the dangers of teens using self-induced abortion attempts. *J Pediatr Health Care.* 1998;12(3):147–51.

42. Ganatra B, Hirve S. Induced abortions among adolescent women in rural Maharashtra, India. *Reprod Health Matters.* 2002;10(19):76–85.

43. Lopez AD, Mathers CD, Ezzati M, Jamison, DT, Murray CJL. Global and regional burden of disease and risk factors, 2001: systematic analysis of population health data. *Lancet* 2006;367:1747–57.

44. Scmidtke A, Bille-Brahe U, De Leo D, Kerkhof A. *Suicidal behaviour in Europe: Results from the WHO/EURO Multicentre Study on Suicidal Behaviour.* Gottingen: Hogrefe & Huber; 2004.

45. Fisher J, Cabral de Mello M, Patel V, Rahman A, Tran T, Holton S, et al. Prevalence and determinants of common perinatal mental disorders in women in low- and lower-middle-income countries: a systematic review. *Bull WHO.* 2011.90;139–49.

46. Hjelmeland H, Hawton K, Nordvik H, Bille-Brahe U, De Leo D, Fekete S, et al. Why people engage in parasuicide: a cross-cultural study of intentions. *Suicide Life Threat Behav.* 2002;32(4):380–93.

47. Lal S, Satpathy S, Khanna P, Vashisht B, Punia M, Kumar S. Problem of mortality in women of reproductive age in rural area of Haryana. *Indian J Matern & Child Health*. 1995;6(1):17–21.

48. Granja A, Zacarias E, Bergstrom S. Violent deaths: the hidden face of maternal mortality. *BJOG*. 2002;109:5–8.

49. World Health Organization. *Maternal mortality in Viet Nam, 2000–2001: An in-depth analysis of causes and determinants*. Manila: World Health Organization, Regional Office for the Western Pacific; 2005.

50. Karki C. Suicide: Leading cause of death among women in Nepal. *Kathmandu Univ Med J (KUMJ)*. 2011;9(35):157–8.

51. Rahman A, Hafeez A. Suicidal feelings run high among mothers in refugee camps: a cross-sectional survey. *Acta Psychiatr Scand*. 2003;108(5):392–3.

52. Fisher J, Morrow M, Ngoc N, Anh L. Prevalence, nature, and correlates of postpartum depression in Vietnam. *BJOG*. 2004;111:1353–60.

53. Sullivan PF. The genetics of schizophrenia. *PLoS Med*. 2005;2(7):e212.

54. Nasser EH, Walders N, Jenkins JH. The experience of schizophrenia: what's gender got to do with it? A critical review of the current status of research on schizophrenia. *Schizophr Bull*. 2002;28(2):351–62.

55. Marks MN, Wieck A, Checkley SA, Kumar R. Contribution of psychological and social factors to psychotic and non-psychotic relapse after childbirth in women with previous histories of affective disorder. *J Affect Disord*. 1992;29:253–64.

56. Patel V. *Gender in mental health research*. Geneva: World Health Organization; 2005.

57. Piccinelli M, Wilkinson G. Gender differences in depression: critical review. *Br J Psychiatry*. 2000;177:486–92.

58. Broverman I, Broverman D, Clarkson F, Rosencrantz P, Vogel S. Sex-role stereotypes and clinical judgments of mental health. *J Consult & Clin Psychol*. 1970;34(1):1–7.

59. Heesacker M, Wester SR, Vogel DL, Wentzel JT, Mejia-Millan CM, Goodholm Jr CR. Gender-based emotional stereotyping. *J Counseling Psychol*. 1999;46(4):483–95.

60. Dowrick C. *Beyond depression: A new approach to understanding and management*. Oxford, UK: Oxford University Press 2004.

61. Kastrup M, Niaz U. *The impact of culture on women's mental health*. In: Chandra PS, Herrman H, Fisher J, Kastrup M, Niaz U, Rondón MB, et al, editors. *Contemporary topics in women's mental health: Global perspectives in a changing society*. Chichester, West Sussex: John Wiley & Sons; 2009:463–84.

62. Chen Y-Y, Subramanian SV, Acevedo-Garcia D, Kawachi I. Women's status and depressive symptoms: A multilevel analysis. *Soc Sci Med*. 2005;60:49–60.

63. The World Bank. *The World Development Report 2011: Conflict, security, and development*. Washington, DC: The World Bank; 2011.

64. Hadlaczky G, Wasserman D. Suicidality in women. In: Chandra PS, Herrman H, Fisher J, Kastrup M, Niaz U, Rondón MB, et al, editors. *Contemporary topics in women's mental health*. Chichester, UK: John Wiley & Sons; 2009:117–37.

65. Herrera A, Dahlblom K, Dahlgren L, Kullgren G. Pathways to suicidal behaviour among adolescent girls in Nicaragua. *Soc Sci Med*. 2006;62(4):805–14.

66. Stark E, Flitcraft. Killing the beast within: Woman battering and female suicidality. *Int J Health Serv*. 1995;25(1):43–64.

67. Lund C, Breen A, Flisher AJ, Kakuma R, Corrigall J, Joska JA, et al. Poverty and common mental disorders in low and middle income countries: A systematic review. *Soc Sci Med*. 2010;71(3):517–28.

68. World Health Organization. *World report on violence and health*. Geneva: WHO; 2002.

69. United Nations General Assembly. *The United Nations Declaration on the Elimination of Violence against Women* 1993 [cited December 20, 1993]; available at: http://www.un.org/documents/ga/res/48/a48r104.htm.

70. United Nations General Assembly. *Declaration on the Elimination of Violence against Women*; 1993 [cited December 9, 2011]; available at: http://www.unhcr.org/refworld/docid/3b00f25d2c.html.

71. Miller BD. Female-selective abortion in Asia: patterns, policies, and debates. *Am Anthropol*. 2001;103(4):1083–95.

72. Jha P, Kumar R, Vasa P, Dhingra N, Thiruchelvam D, Moineddin R. Low female[corrected]-to-male [corrected] sex ratio of children born in India: national survey of 1.1 million households. *Lancet*. 2006;367(9506):211–8.

73. Watts C, Zimmerman C. Violence against women: global scope and magnitude. *Lancet.* 2002;359(9313):1232–7.

74. Anderson J, Martin J, Mullen P, Romans S, Herbison P. Prevalence of childhood sexual abuse experiences in a community sample of women. *J Am Acad Child Adolesc Psychiatry.* 1993;32(5):911–9.

75. Finkelhor D, Dziuba-Leatherman J. Children as victims of violence: a national survey. *J Pediatr.* 1994;94(4 Pt 1):413–20.

76. Finkelhor D, Hotaling G, Lewis IA, Smith C. Sexual abuse in a national survey of adult men and women: prevalence, characteristics, and risk factors. *Child Abuse & Neglect.* 1990;14(1):19–28.

77. Chaturvedi SK, Rajkumar RP. Somatisation and dissociation. In: Chandra PS, Herrman H, Fisher J, Kastrup M, Niaz U, Rondón MB, et al, editors. *Contemporary topics in women's mental health: Global perspectives in a changing society.* Chichester, West Sussex: John Wiley & Sons; 2009:65–98.

78. Kamo T. The adverse impact of psychological aggression, coercion and violence in the intimate partner relationship on women's mental health. In: *Contemporary topics in women's mental health.* Chichester, UK: John Wiley & Sons; 2009:549–58.

79. Garcia-Moreno C, Jansen H, Ellsberg M, Heise L, Watts C. *WHO multi-country study on women's health and domestic violence against women: Initial results on prevalence, health outcomes and women's responses.* Geneva: World Health Organization; 2005.

80. Clark C, Ryan L, Kawachi I, Canner M, Berkman L, Wright R. Witnessing community violence in residential neighborhoods: a mental health hazard for urban women. *J Urban Health.* 2008;85(1):22–38.

81. Gracia E, Herrero J. Perceived neighborhood social disorder and attitudes toward reporting domestic violence against women. *J Interpers Violence.* 2007;22(6):737–52.

82. Tsutsumi A, Izutsu T, Poudyal AK, Kato S, Marui E. Mental health of female survivors of human trafficking in Nepal. *J Interpers Violence.* 2008;66(8):1841–7.

83. United Nations. *Annual parliamentary hearing at the United Nations.* 2008. Available at: http://www.ipu.org/splz-e/unga08.htm

84. Kinyanda E, Musisi S, Biryabarema C, Ezati I, Oboke H, Ojiambo-Ochieng R, et al. War related sexual violence and its medical and psychological consequences as seen in Kitgum, Northern Uganda: A cross-sectional study. *BMC Int Health Hum Rights.* 2010;10:28.

85. Smith JR, Ellwood MCL. The Australian Time-Use Survey of New Mothers—implications for policy. *Australian National University.* 2009.

86. Pereira B, Andrew G, Pednekar S, Pai R, Pelto P, Patel V. The explanatory models of depression in low income countries: listening to women in India. *J Affect Disord.* 2007;102(1–3):209–18.

87. Schofield H, Bloch S, Herrman H, Murphy B, Nankervis J, Singh B, editors. *Family caregivers: Disability, illness and ageing.* St. Leonard's, NSW: Allen & Unwin; 1998.

88. Grant JS, Elliott TR, Weaver M, Bartolucci AA, Giger JN. Telephone intervention with family caregivers of stroke survivors after rehabilitation. *Stroke.* 2002;33(8):2060–5.

89. Prince M, Livingston G, Katona C. Mental health care for the elderly in low-income countries: a health systems approach. *World Psychiatry.* 2007;6(1):5–13.

90. Kipp W, Tindyebwa D, Rubaale T, Karamagi E, Bajenja E. Family caregivers in rural Uganda: The hidden reality. *Health Care Women Int.* 2007;28(10):856–71.

91. Howe AL, Schofield H, Herrman H. Caregiving: a common or uncommon experience? *Soc Sci Med.* 1997;45(7):1017–29.

92. Butterworth P, Pymont C, Rodgers B, Windsor TD, Anstey KJ. Factors that explain the poorer mental health of caregivers: results from a community survey of older Australians. *Aust N Z J Psychiatry.* 2010;44(7):616–24.

93. World Health Organization. *The world health report 2001: Mental health: New understanding, new hope.* Geneva: WHO; 2002.

94. Kuo C, Operario D. Health of adults caring for orphaned children in an HIV-endemic community in South Africa. *AIDS Care.* 2011;23(9):1128–35.

95. Cannuscio CC, Jones C, Kawachi I, Colditz GA, Berkman L, Rimm E. Reverberations of family illness: A longitudinal assessment of informal caregiving and mental health status in the nurses' health study. *Am J Public Health.* 2002;92(8):1305–11.

96. Schofield HL, Bloch S, Nankervis J, Murphy B, Singh BS, Herrman HE. Health and well-being of women family carers: a comparative study with a generic focus. *Aust N Z J Public Health.* 1999;23(6):585–9.

97. Biadgilign S, Deribew A, Amberbir A, Deribe K. Adherence to highly active antiretroviral therapy and its correlates among HIV infected pediatric patients in Ethiopia. *BMC Pediatrs.* 2008;53.

98. Edwards B, Higgins DJ. Is caring a health hazard? The mental health and vitality of carers of a person with a disability in Australia. *Med J Aust.* 2009;190(7 SUPPL.):S61–S65.

99. MacNeil G, Kosberg JI, Durkin DW, Dooley WK, Decoster J, Williamson GM. Caregiver mental health and potentially harmful caregiving behavior: the central role of caregiver anger. *Gerontologist.* 2010;50(1):76–86.

100. Fiorillo A, Del Vecchio HG, De Rosa C, Malangone C, Del Vecchio V, Giacco D, et al. P02–30—Family burden in major depression: a multicentric survey in 30 Italian mental health centres. *European Psychiatry.* 2011;26, Suppl 1:625.

101. UNICEF. *Female genital mutilation/cutting: A statistical exploration.* New York: UNICEF; 2005.

102. Fisher J Female genital mutilation. In World Health Organization. *Mental health aspects of women's reproductive health. A global review of the literature.* Geneva: World Health Organization and United Nations Population Fund; 2009:147–154.

103. Toubia N. Female circumcision as a public health issue. *N Engl J Med.* 1994;33(11):712–6.

104. Behrendt A, Moritz S. Post-traumatic stress disorder and memory problems after female genital mutilation. *Am J Psychiatry.* 2005;162(5):1000–2.

105. Elnashar A, Abdelhady R. The impact of female genital cutting on health of newly married women. *Int J Gynaecol Obstet.* 2007;97(3):238–44.

106. Ojanuga D. Preventing birth injury among women in Africa: case studies in northern Nigeria. *Am J Orthopsychiatry.* 1991;61(4):533–9.

107. Goh JT, Sloane KM, Krause HG, Browning A, Akhter S. Mental health screening for women with genital tract fistulae. *Br J Obstet & Gynaecol.* 2005;112:1328–30.

108. Kabir M, Iliyasu Z, Abubakar IS, Umar UI. Medico-social problems of patients with vesicovaginal fistula in Murtala Mohammed Specialist Hospital, Kano. *Ann Afr Med.* 2003;2:54–7.

109. Patel V, Pednekar S, Weiss H, Rodrigues M, Barros P, Nayak B, et al. Why do women complain of vaginal discharge? A population survey of infectious and pyschosocial risk factors in a South Asian community. *Int J Epidemiol.* 2005;34(4):853–62.

110. Patel V, Weiss HA, Kirkwood BR, Pednekar S, Nevrekar P, Gupte S, et al. Common genital complaints in women: the contribution of psychosocial and infectious factors in a population-based cohort study in Goa, India. *Int J Epidemiol.* 2006;35(6):1478–85.

111. Rowe H. Spontaneous pregnancy loss. In: World Health Organization. *Mental health aspects of women's reproductive health. A global review of the literature.* Geneva: World Health Organization and United Nations Population Fund; 2009:67–74.

112. Neugebauer R, Kline J, Shrout P, Skodol A, O'Connor P, Geller PA, et al. Major depressive disorder in the 6 months after miscarriage. *JAMA.* 1997;277(5):383–8.

113. Cole M. Out of sight, out of mind: female sexuality and the care plan approach in psychiatric inpatients. *Int J Psychiatry Clin Pract.* 2000;4(4):307–10.

114. Flach C, Leese M, Heron J, Evans J, Feder G, Sharp D, et al. Antenatal domestic violence, maternal mental health and subsequent child behaviour: a cohort study. *BJOG.* 2011;118(11):1383–91.

115. Fottrell E, Kanhonou L, Goufodji S, Behague DP, Marshall T, Patel V, et al. Risk of psychological distress following severe obstetric complications in Benin: the role of economics, physical health and spousal abuse. *Br J Psychiatry.* 2010;196(1):18–25.

116. Brown GW, Harris T. *The social origins of depression. A study of psychiatric disorder in women.* London: Tavistock Publications; 1978.

117. Broadhead JC, Abas MA. Life events, difficulties and depression among women in an urban setting in Zimbabwe. *Psychol Med.* 1998;28(1):29–38.

118. Abas MA, Broadhead JC. Depression and anxiety among women in an urban setting in Zimbabwe. *Psychol Med.* 1997;27(1):59–71.

119. Da Costa IER, Ludemir AB, Avelar I. Violence against adolescents: differentials by gender and living conditions strata. [*Violência contra adolescentes: Diferenciais segundo estratos de condição de vida e sexo*]. 2007;12(5):1193–200.

120. Thornicroft G, Brohan E, Rose D, Sartorius N, Leese M. Global pattern of experienced and anticipated discrimination against people with schizophrenia: a cross-sectional survey. *Lancet.* 2009;373(9661):408–15.

121. Loganathan S, Murthy RS. Living with schizophrenia in India: gender perspectives. *Transcult Psychiatry*. 2011;48(5):569–84.

122. Thara R, Kamath S, Kumar S. Women with schizophrenia and broken marriages—doubly disadvantaged? Part II: family perspective. *Int J Soc Psychiatry*. 2003;49(3):233–40.

123. Rice E. Schizophrenia and violence: the perspective of women. *Issues Ment Health Nurs*. 2006;27(9):961–83.

124. Chandra PS, Carey MP, Carey KB, Shalinianant A, Thomas T. Sexual coercion and abuse among women with a severe mental illness in India: an exploratory investigation. *Compr Psychiatry*. 2003;44(3):205–12.

125. Shack AV, Averill PM, Kopecky C, Krajewski K, Gummattira P. Prior history of physical and sexual abuse among the psychiatric inpatient population: a comparison of males and females. *Psychiatr Q*. 2004;75(4):343–59.

126. Weinstock M. The potential influence of maternal stress hormones on development and mental health of the offspring. *Brain Behav Immun*. 2005;19(4):296–308.

127. O'Connor TG, Heron J, Glover V. Antenatal anxiety predicts child behavioral/emotional problems independently of postnatal depression. *J Am Acad Child Adolesc Psychiatry*. 2002;41(12):1470–7.

128. Bergman K, Sarkar P, O'Connor TG, Modi N, Glover V. Maternal stress during pregnancy predicts cognitive ability and fearfulness in infancy. *J Am Acad Child Adolesc Psychiatry*. 2007;46(11):1454–63.

129. Bergman K, Sarkar P, Glover V, O'Connor TG. Maternal prenatal cortisol and infant cognitive development: moderation by infant-mother attachment. *Biol Psychiatry*. 2010;67(11):1026–32.

130. Rahman A, Bunn J, Lovel H, Creed F. Association between antenatal depression and low birthweight in a developing country. *Acta Psychiatr Scand*. 2007;115(6):481–6.

131. Murray L, Cooper P. The impact of postpartum depression on child development. *Int Rev Psychiatry*. 1996;8(1, March):55–63.

132. Patel V, Desouza N, Rodrigues M. Postnatal depression and infant growth and development in low income countries: a cohort study from Goa, India. *Arch Dis Childhood*. 2003;88(1):34–7.

133. Rahman A, Iqbal Z, Harrington R. Life events, social support and depression in childbirth: perspectives from a rural community in the developing world. *Psychol Med*. 2003;33:1161–7.

134. Rahman A, Bunn J, Lovel H, Harrington R. Impact of maternal depression on infant nutritional status and illness: a cohort study. *Arch Gen Psychiatry*. 2004;61:946–52.

135. Fisher J, Tran T, Biggs B, Dwyer T, Casey G, Tho DH, et al. Iodine status in late pregnancy and psychosocial determinants of iodized salt use in rural northern Viet Nam. *Bull WHO*. 2011;89(11):813–20.

136. Rondón MB. Gender sensitive care for adult women. In: *Contemporary topics in women's mental health*. Chichester, UK: John Wiley & Sons; 2009:323–36.

137. Patel V, Simon G, Chowdhary N, Kaaya S, Araya R. Packages of care for depression in low- and middle-income countries. *PLoS Med*. 2009;6(10):e1000159.

138. Chandra PS. *Comprehensive sexual and reproductive health care for women with serious mental disorders: a working model in Bangalore, India*. National Institute of Mental Health and Neurosciences 2011 (personal communication).

139. Rojas G, Fritsch R, Solis J, Jadresic E, Castillo C, Gonzalez M, et al. Treatment of postnatal depression in low-income mothers in primary-care clinics in Santiago, Chile: a randomised controlled trial. Lancet. 2007;370(9599):1629–37.

140. Rahman A, Malik A, Sikander S, Roberts C, Creed F. Cognitive behaviour therapy-based intervention by community health workers for mothers with depression and their infants in rural Pakistan: a cluster-randomised controlled trial. *Lancet*. 2008;372(9642):902–9.

141. World Health Organization. *The world health report 1998—Life in the 21st century: a vision for all*. Geneva: World Health Organization; 1998.

17 Mental Health and Psychosocial Support in Humanitarian Settings

Wietse A. Tol, Pierre Bastin,
Mark J. D. Jordans, Harry Minas,
Renato Souza, Inka Weissbecker, and
Mark Van Ommeren

INTRODUCTION

Humanitarian settings—areas affected by armed conflicts, natural and industrial disasters—are widespread. In 2010 alone, 30 active armed conflicts were recorded in 25 locations.[1] In the same year, 385 natural disasters killed more than 297,000 people, affected over 217 million others, and were associated with US$124 billion in economic damage.[2] Humanitarian crises have wide-ranging impacts on the mental health and psychosocial well-being of affected populations, ranging from resilience (good mental health despite exposure to significant adversity) to normal psychological distress reactions and increased prevalence of mental disorders.[3,4]

Most epidemiological studies on mental health in humanitarian settings have focused on the more limited agenda of establishing prevalence rates of symptoms of major depression, post-traumatic stress disorder (PTSD), and anxiety disorders. For example, a recent meta-analysis of studies of populations affected by armed conflict found pooled prevalence rates of 30.6% for PTSD and 30.8% for depression. Study methodology, however, accounted for significant variations in prevalence rates. In a subset of rigorous studies, prevalence rates were 15.4% for PTSD (30 studies using representative sampling and diagnostic interviews) and 17.3% for depression (26 studies using representative sampling and diagnostic interviews) respectively.[5] A meta-analysis of studies of children affected by armed conflict reported rates of 47%, 43%, and 27% for PTSD, depression, and anxiety, respectively. Similar to studies with adults, heterogeneity in rates could partly be attributed to the choice of measurement instruments for PTSD. In both studies, a longer time since conflict was predictive of lower rates of PTSD. In adults, having been

The views expressed in this article are those of the authors and not necessarily those of the institutions that they serve.

tortured, cumulative exposure to potentially traumatic events, and higher levels of political terror were associated with higher levels of PTSD, whereas in children, the location of the conflict was a significant predictor (studies in the Middle East showed higher rates).

In addition to methodological concerns, researchers and practitioners have been critical of the general approach underlying the current body of psychiatric epidemiology in humanitarian settings. First, criticism has focused on the strong emphasis this body of research places on exposure to circumscribed crisis-related events in the past (e.g., past exposure to bomb blasts, cross-fire, rape, witnessing sudden death of loved ones) as the key predictors of mental health problems. Comparatively limited attention is paid to risk and protective factors, besides gender and age. For example, we know little of how individual risk and protective factors (e.g., coping, religious beliefs, help-seeking behavior) and variables in the socio-ecological contexts of humanitarian crises (e.g., parenting styles, community social support systems, power dynamics) affect mental health and well-being over time, despite a significant body of social science literature emphasizing the importance of such factors.[6] Highlighting the importance of this gap are emerging findings with armed conflict–affected children showing that, in addition to conflict-related events, current family adversity and social marginalization are strong predictors of psychological symptoms over time.[7,8] Researchers have pointed to the important role of ongoing stressors, such as a lack of access to resources to meet basic needs, domestic and community violence, and continued threats for human rights abuse, for mental health in humanitarian settings.[9,10] Second, our current knowledge of the mental health impacts of humanitarian crises is limited by an overreliance on symptom checklists that have not been validated for use in local contexts. Research with such checklists generally shows higher prevalence rates than research conducted with diagnostic interviews[5] and obscures the possibility of distinguishing between normal psychological distress and psychiatric disorders.[11] Third, research has consistently shown variety across sociocultural contexts in the way that psychological distress is expressed and addressed, but this has received little attention in epidemiological studies.[12,13] Finally, little attention has been given in psychiatric epidemiological research in humanitarian settings to mental disorders other than PTSD and depression. Primary health care clinics in humanitarian settings often see people presenting with neuropsychiatric disorders such as epilepsy, psychotic disorders, bipolar disorder, and substance use,[4] and a study in Timor-Leste showed that psychosis was associated with the largest impairment in functioning.[14]

Despite these important methodological and substantive concerns, the available literature strongly suggests that mental health and psychosocial well-being are crucial public health concerns in humanitarian settings. In response, mental health and psychosocial support (MHPSS) programs, defined as "any type of local or outside support that aims to protect or promote psychosocial well-being and/or prevent or treat mental disorder," are increasingly integrated in humanitarian programs.[15, p.1] Although there appears to be an emerging consensus on best practices in this field, controversy has remained with regard to a number of key policy and research questions.[16]

In post-disaster settings, the importance of mental health as part of a comprehensive recovery and public health response comes into focus for governments, populations, and disaster response and development agencies, often for the first time. Such recognition of the central place of mental health in recovery efforts can represent an opportunity to take a longer-term approach to mental health system development in addition to providing the short- and mid-term mental health and psychosocial support programs that are often desperately needed.

Based on a number of recent policy and research efforts, this chapter aims to provide the following: an overview of current consensus on best practices; the evidence base for mental health and psychosocial support interventions in humanitarian settings; and consensus on research priorities. We also comment on the possibility of moving from disaster response to mental health system development, an area in which experience is accumulating but where there is very little research. Based on this overview, we highlight gaps in knowledge and provide recommendations for practice and research. The chapter is focused on populations in low- and middle-income countries, as this is where the largest populations affected by humanitarian crises reside.

CONSENSUS ON BEST PRACTICES

The field of MHPSS is relatively new, with large ideological cleavages between agencies' perspectives on best practices up to a few years ago. To improve coordination among actors, prevent harmful interventions, and overcome polarized positions in the field, the World Health Organization (WHO) took the initiative to establish inter-agency consensus by proposing the development of Inter-Agency Standing Committee (IASC) Guidelines. The IASC is a committee of heads of United Nations (UN) and non-UN international humanitarian agencies responsible for humanitarian policy in accordance with UN General Assembly Resolution 46/182.[17] An IASC task force of staff of 27 agencies co-chaired by the WHO and InterAction subsequently developed "Guidelines on Mental Health and Psychosocial Support in Emergencies."[15] These guidelines focus on high-priority responses that should be implemented as soon as possible in emergencies. Core principles advocated by the guidelines include: promotion of human rights; equity in availability and accessibility of services; attention to avoiding unintended consequences of humanitarian activities (i.e., the "Do No Harm" principle); and active participation of affected populations in the design and implementation of MHPSS programs. Furthermore, to promote sustainability, the guidelines recommend that humanitarian actors from the beginning focus on strengthening of local resources and building on government and civil society capacities. The guidelines also recommend that MHPSS interventions be integrated as much as possible into existing systems of support (e.g., health, education, protection systems) for increased accessibility and sustainability. Descriptions of best practice are provided in "action sheets" that cover: (a) activities important across different programs (coordination, needs assessment, monitoring and evaluation, protection and human rights standards, and human resource considerations); (b) core MHPSS domains (community mobilization and support, health services, education, and dissemination of information); and (c) social considerations in other humanitarian sectors such as nutrition, water, sanitation, shelter, and site planning. In terms of interventions, the guidelines advocate against stand-alone services for specific disorders or target groups, but rather recommend a multilayered system of care, including diverse levels of care (i.e., social considerations in basic services and security, strengthening community and family supports, focused non-specialized supports, and specialized supports—see Figure 17.1).[15] Boxes 17.1 through 17.4 provide illustrations of MHPSS programs implemented across these levels of care in diverse recent crises. An overriding conclusion of these boxes is that, despite significant challenges, it is feasible to implement programs that are in line with current consensus. Program evaluations show overall acceptability of interventions and benefits to mental health.

Following the publication of the 2007 Guidelines, a new IASC Reference Group on Mental Health and Psychosocial Support was established to promote dissemination and implementation of the IASC Guidelines, and has issued specific guidance for actors in the health sector[18] and protection sector.[19]

In addition, a revised version of the "Humanitarian Charter and Minimum Standards for Disaster Response" was published in 2011.[20] This is the influential handbook of the Sphere Project, a group governed by non-governmental organizations. The 2011 revision

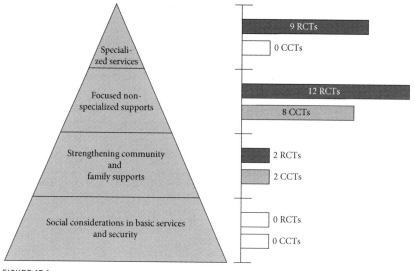

FIGURE 17.1

Evidence for MHPSS interventions.

Box 17.1 Social Considerations in Basic Services and Security

Intervention: Protection and assistance programs for victims of sexual violence

Location: North and South Kivu, Democratic Republic of Congo (DRC)

Implementing organization: International Committee of the Red Cross (ICRC)

Author: Renato Souza

Background: Since 1996, Congo has been experiencing a prolonged armed conflict characterized by extreme violence, mass population displacements, widespread sexual violence, and a collapse of public health services. In the Kivu region, many women after surviving sexual violence are rejected by their partners and family, obliged to leave their house, and sometimes expelled from their village.

Objectives: During the last three years, the ICRC has implemented a program based on the development and reinforcement of community efforts to protect and assist victims of sexual violence. The main objectives are to: (1) reduce levels of stigma and discrimination and (2) reduce the immediate risks after sexual violence.

Methods: Activities are aimed at (a) changing communities' negative perceptions related to victims and developing a community-based information and support system in order to prevent social exclusion, as well as (b) providing access to immediate assistance via a network of community-based ICRC supported "Houses of Listening." Activities under (a) are developed at two levels by community members called *sensitizers* and include mass communication campaigns such as lectures and radio programs, door-to-door communication activities and leaflet distribution, and meetings with community leaders in which they are asked to become advocates against stigmatization and exclusion of victims. Community leaders are encouraged not to tolerate social rejection of victims in their villages. In the Houses of Listening the following activities are offered: psychological first aid; food, shelter, and clothing for women in need; direct referral to medical structures where medical care after sexual violence can be offered.

Houses of Listening do not only offer services to victims of sexual violence to avoid the risk that victims will be identified or stigmatized while looking for help.

(continued)

Box 17.1 Continued

To complement the above-mentioned approach, the ICRC is continuously seeking to develop its dialogue with weapon-bearers on respect of international humanitarian law and human rights with the aim to prevent violations such as sexual violence.

Evaluation: The complete network of Houses of Listening is visited on a monthly basis by ICRC delegates for data collection (sexual violence typology, demographics, psychosocial consequences) and supervision. A preliminary evaluation showed that this strategy has been well accepted by victims and communities alike. Regular data collection shows that women are able to access the Houses of Listening and are successfully linked to immediate support services. In the absence of other services, the Houses of Listening and their network of support seem to have provided immediate protection and assistance to victims of sexual violence in the midst of armed conflict.

Box 17.2 Strengthening Community and Family Supports

Intervention: Family-based psychosocial intervention for children affected by armed conflict

    Location: Burundi

    Implementing organization: HealthNet TPO

    Authors: Mark J. D. Jordans, Wietse A. Tol

    Background: In recent years, HealthNet TPO has been involved in an effort to develop a multilayered psychosocial and mental health care package for children affected by political violence. In Burundi, the absence of a family-based intervention was considered a major gap in the care package, as well as in the published literature on interventions for children in complex emergencies.[40]

    We developed a research strategy to make informed decisions for intervention selection, particularly relevant in low- and middle-income countries, including qualitative research and stakeholder meetings, expert consultation, and systematic selection of intervention components from evidence-based treatments.[41] Application of this strategy resulted in a stepped family-intervention protocol. We highlight the first step (as step 2 is considered a focused intervention, exceeding the focus of this section), which comprises community-level interventions for families at risk.

    Objectives: The following objectives were developed as a result of the followed procedures: (a) to improve a sense of connectedness of families within the larger communities; (b) to increase parental support, understanding, and coping towards dealing with children's psychosocial problems; and (c) to strengthen the health care system in identifying and responding to family health, child development, and child protection issues.

    Methods: The interventionists for the first steps were local lay community counselors, who had received a training course of a few weeks on generic psychosocial support skills and concepts. Specifically, they were trained to provide a range of services, including community-sensitization, psycho-education groups, case-management, and individual counseling. This type of task-shifting—a process of delegation whereby tasks are moved to less specialized health workers—needed to make care provision feasible in resource-poor settings.

(continued)

Box 17.2 Continued

Evaluation: Consistent with the overall aim of developing an evidence-based care package, HealthNet TPO is in the process of evaluating the developed family intervention. As a first step, the effect of a two-session parenting psycho-education intervention (covering the second objective as outlined above) on children who had been screened for elevated psychosocial distress was assessed. The intervention had a beneficial effect on controlling behavioral problems, especially among boys, while not showing impact on emotional complaints or family social support. Parents evaluated the intervention positively, with increased awareness of positive parenting strategies and appropriate disciplinary techniques reported as the most common learning points. Further and more rigorous research is needed to demonstrate efficacy of the entire stepped family intervention for children with psychosocial complaints.

Box 17.3 Focused Non-Specialized Supports

Intervention: Mental health services provided by primary care health workers in disaster-affected areas

Location: Sierra Leone, Haiti, Indonesia, Sri Lanka, Afghanistan, Jordan, Syria, occupied Palestinian territories (oPt), Iraq, Turkey, and Lebanon

Implementing organization: International Medical Corps (IMC)

Author: Inka Weissbecker

Background: Integrating mental health into primary health care (PHC) is especially relevant in the context of humanitarian crises where the number of people with mental health problems increases while those with preexisting mental health problems often lack access to continued care and are especially vulnerable.[4]

Objectives: The objectives of IMC PHC integration programs include making mental health care more accessible and less stigmatizing, and building capacity of general health staff to identify, manage, and refer cases of mental disorders.

Methods: Steps in the integration of mental health (MH) into PHC include: (a) working with local governments and authorities; (b) assessing the existing system of providing general health and specialized mental health services, including types and distribution of clinics, human resource allocations, roles, responsibilities, and existing MH training and capacities of staff; and (c) designing a program that builds on the existing system and has potential for scale-up and sustainability within the county context. IMC usually adapts existing training materials and guidelines such as the WHO mhGAP Intervention Guide to the local social and cultural context and to existing training needs. Local health professionals then receive intensive theoretical training sessions (about 12 full days) over the course of 2–4 months to recognize, treat and refer cases of mental disorders. Theoretical training is followed up with mentorship, on-the-job supervision and case discussions to ensure that the content of training is effectively put into practice. In some countries (e.g., oPt, Chad, Jordan) we also have facilitated activities to change attitudes towards those affected by mental illness through community awareness-raising and psycho-education and strengthening support networks among those affected by mental illness and the community. In addition, integration of mental health care has been stimulated through

(continued)

Box 17.3 Continued

implementing quality standards; supporting data collection; holding referral workshops[42]; and working with traditional healers.[33,43,44]

Evaluation: IMC evaluates the results of PHC MH programming through: (a) assessment of trainees (pre-and post-tests, on-the-job-supervision checklists, institutional quality checklists[45]; (b) assessment of training (e.g., feedback from trainees, managers, and other stakeholders through daily and general training evaluation; (c) institutional-level changes (e.g., staff roles, availability of psychotropic medication, knowledge and use of referral pathways, and health system data collection); and (d) beneficiary outcomes (client and family satisfaction surveys, client improvement). In Iraq, for example, we found that trained PHC providers had better observed clinical skills and more satisfied patients than untrained providers.[45] IMC shares lessons learned among country teams and makes modifications for new trainings. In Lebanon, for example, we conducted refresher trainings to address knowledge gaps that emerged from the training evaluation. Our MH PHC integration program in Lebanon is now informing national policy.[42]

Box 17.4 Specialized Services

Intervention: Psychiatric care for new arrivals into a protracted refugee situation
 Implementing organization: Médecins sans Frontières Suisse (MSF-CH)
 Location: Dagahaley camp, Dadaab, Kenya
 Author: Pierre Bastin
 Background: Dagahaley, located 80 kilometers from the Kenya-Somalia border, has had a continuously increasing population from the originally intended 30,000 to a peak of about 125,000, given escalating conflict and drought within Somalia. An estimated one in three Somali refugees suffers from mental disorders, including severe mental disorders and epilepsy (WHO, 2010). MSF-CH observed stigmatization and human rights abuse (e.g., severe restraint) against people with mental disorders, with limited capacity to respond in outpatient departments (OPD).[46,47]

Objectives: The main objective of the program was to integrate a mental health component in decentralized primary care sites (health posts) and improve awareness and case management at community outpatient and camp hospital levels. Furthermore, we aimed to prevent high levels of stress and burnout amongst MSF staff.

Methods: Two Kenyan psychiatric nurses were trained on consultation and psychotropic medication prescription and started a scheduled rotation to five health posts. In addition, one refugee staff of MSF-CH per health post was trained to function as an auxiliary psychosocial nurse. All the refugee camp health staff received training on screening and referral of common and severe mental disorders. The 70 community health workers already working in the camp were additionally trained to perform "IEC" activities on mental disorders through group sessions and home visits. Finally, hospital staff received training on admissions (i.e., management of severe mental disorders in a general hospital setting) under supervision of an expatriate psychiatrist

Evaluation: MSF-CH has evaluated this program through (a) obtaining a Global Assessment of Functioning (GAF) score of patients at each visit to health posts and

(continued)

Box 17.4 Continued

hospitals; (b) monthly data analysis of GAF, number of consultations, and diagnosis; and (c) tracing of patients not returning for consultation by community health workers. Results showed 1450 patients were admitted to date, with the following diagnoses: epilepsy 40%; schizophrenia 16%; depression 16%; bipolar disorder 7%; PTSD 4%; anxiety 2%; drug-induced psychosis (*khat*) 1.5%. Furthermore, 86 patients with severe mental disorders received home visits and intermittent inpatient hospital-based care. Particularly the treatment of severe mental disorders and the release of people with mental disorders who were chained were received positively, with reduction of stigma and increased acceptance of MSF-CH medical interventions in the camp. It was observed that the integrated setup (i.e., a combination of community health workers, health posts, and hospital-based care) allows new arrivals to be assisted promptly.

places central emphasis on understanding and supporting local responses to disasters. The standards contain four areas of particular relevance to MHPSS:

(a) a new chapter outlining four protection principles, two of which highlight psychosocial issues (Protection Principle 3: Protect people from physical and psychological harm arising from violence and coercion; Protection Principle 4: Assist people to claim their rights, access available remedies, and recover from the effects of abuse);

(b) a core standard that emphasizes building on community capacities and strengthening self-help (Core Standard 1: People-centered humanitarian response);

(c) integration of psychosocial and social considerations as a cross-cutting issue in the writing of all standards throughout the handbook; and

(d) a specific standard focused on mental health as a health sector activity (Essential Health Services—Mental Health Standard 1).

The mental health standard emphasizes community self-help and social support, the provision of psychological "first aid" (i.e., non-intrusive and practically oriented form of support, including assessment of needs, attending to basic needs, supportive listening, and protecting people from further harm), capacity building of the primary health care system, care for people with mental disorders in institutions, minimizing harm related to substance use, and initiating plans for developing a community mental health system.[20]

EMPIRICAL EVIDENCE FOR MHPSS INTERVENTIONS

Despite this consensus on best practices, the 2007 "Lancet Series on Global Mental Health" reported a specific gap in evidence for mental health interventions in emergencies.[21] The second "Lancet Series on Global Mental Health" included a paper on MHPSS in humanitarian settings that focused on low- and middle-income countries.[22] This paper provides an overview of popular practices and funding for this field, as well as a systematic review and meta-analysis of evaluation studies. In total, the systematic review identified 32 controlled studies (studies using a pre- and post-test and comparing with active other treatments, no treatment, standard care, or waitlist control groups) and randomized controlled trials (same as controlled studies but with participants randomized across study conditions) of a variety of MHPSS interventions. As can be seen in Figure 17.1, most studies evaluated focused on non-specialized support interventions and specialized treatment, with very few studies evaluating interventions at the bottom two layers of the intervention pyramid. This lack of studies at the bottom of the pyramid signifies a considerable gap between science and practice, because such interventions are among the most commonly implemented in practice. For example, community-based support for vulnerable individuals, child-friendly spaces, supporting community-initiated programs, and structured social activities all featured in the top 10 of most-often-reported MHPSS activities between 2007 and 2009. This picture of popular practices was confirmed by data collected through the "Who Does What, Where, and until When" coordination tool in three recent humanitarian settings (Haiti, Jordan, Nepal). In these settings, organizations most frequently reported implementing structured social activities, basic counseling, and MHPSS in general humanitarian sectors (e.g., shelter, protection, education), whereas specialized care was infrequently reported.[22]

In addition, the authors report on meta-analyses with a subset of studies identified through the systematic review; that is, those that applied a no-treatment or waitlist control condition. The most commonly reported outcomes across studies were PTSD for adults, and for children, both PTSD and internalizing symptoms. Meta-analysis of the outcome "psychosocial well-being" was not possible because it was not measured consistently across studies, if it was included at all. Three meta-analyses were conducted. First, meta-analysis focused on adults with PTSD symptoms. This meta-analysis included diverse psychological treatments, including:

(a) brief control-focused behavioral therapy with earthquake survivors in Turkey;
(b) psychosocial support groups with war-affected mothers in Bosnia-Herzegovina (mother outcomes);
(c) one to two sessions of testimony therapy in rural areas affected by prolonged civil war in Mozambique;
(d) Narrative exposure therapy with widow and orphan survivors of the genocide in Rwanda, as well as with Rwandan and Somali refugees in Uganda; and
(e) three-day trauma healing and reconciliation workshops with one follow-up session in Burundi.

An overall effect of treatment on PTSD symptoms was observed, with no statistically significant heterogeneity between studies. Second, meta-analysis of studies focused on school-based interventions for children with PTSD symptoms in armed conflict–affected areas in Indonesia, Nepal, and the occupied Palestinian territories (oPt), and with children affected by the 2004 tsunami in Sri Lanka. This meta-analysis failed to show an overall effect of treatment, with very high statistical heterogeneity of treatment effects across studies. Third, meta-analysis was conducted on a broader group of psychological interventions for children with internalizing symptoms (depression and anxiety), including aforementioned school-based interventions, as well as: (a) interpersonal group therapy and creative play for armed conflict–affected adolescents in Uganda, and (b) a supportive group intervention for mothers of young children in war-affected areas in Bosnia-Herzegovina (child outcomes). An overall effect of treatment was observed, with high statistical heterogeneity of treatment effects among studies.

In summary, although the evidence base for MHPSS interventions is increasing, there is a wide gap between knowledge and practice. It appears that the most rigorous evidence has focused on interventions and outcomes that have received less attention from practitioners, whereas the most popular interventions (e.g., counseling, structured social activities, psycho-education and awareness raising) have received little scientific scrutiny.[22]

In addition to identifying if (and how) interventions may be effective, research may support MHPSS interventions through answering other essential questions; such as, "How is distress expressed across socio-cultural settings?" "What are the availability and quality of health systems in humanitarian settings?" "How can methods for assessment, monitoring and evaluation be improved?" However, as among practitioners, polarized views have existed on major research priorities in this field. Moreover, the research agenda has had little input from practitioners and researchers outside of humanitarian settings.[23] The Mental Health and Psychosocial Support in Humanitarian Settings—Research Priority Setting (MH-SET) study aimed to remedy this situation.[24,25] The MH-SET initiative aimed to develop a consensus-based research agenda for the next 10 years, through two phases. First, focus group discussions were held in capitals and remote humanitarian settings in Nepal, Peru, and Uganda with local stakeholders ($N = 114$) representing a range of academic expertise (psychiatry, psychology, social work, child protection, anthropology) and organizations (governments, universities, non-governmental organizations, United Nations). Participants in both capitals and remote humanitarian settings were asked to agree on the 10 leading research priorities, and discuss hampering and facilitating factors for research in humanitarian settings in their respective countries. A promising finding of this study was that prioritization of research themes was remarkably similar across countries and between capitals and remote settings. Five major research themes received high priority (in order of frequency):

(1) the prevalence and burden associated with mental health and psychosocial difficulties;
(2) how MHPSS implementation can be improved;
(3) evaluation of specific MHPSS interventions;
(4) the determinants of mental health and psychological distress; and
(5) improved research methods and processes.

Although researchers and practitioners agreed on major research themes, they had differing views on how research should be implemented. This disconnection was interpreted in terms of "excellence" and "relevance"; i.e., academic researchers gave more weight to scientific validity of methods and results (excellence), whereas policymakers and practitioners emphasized the utilitarian value of research (relevance).[26] This difference in emphasis resulted in different appreciation of aspects of the research process, such as time taken for research activities (e.g., academic researchers were more comfortable spending a longer time on analyzing all aspects of a phenomenon over time, *vs.* pressure for timely information to influence policy and programs), language and communication (policymakers and practitioners valuing comprehensible language in an accessible format, *vs.* technical language in specialized communications), and the ideal research product (a frequently cited journal article *vs.* a policy or program influenced by data). In addition, participants across countries raised concerns about research often being conducted by outsiders, particularly by universities in high-income countries, and therefore not being optimally geared towards the concerns on the ground. Moreover, participants raised concerns about findings not being disseminated after data collection, research findings not being translated into programs, and the validity of findings resulting from the use of tools originating in Western settings in non-Western contexts.[25]

In the second phase, 136 people—representative of the regions in which humanitarian crises occur—were invited to list their top five research priorities. This group consisted of 43.3% women, two-thirds of whom originated from low- and middle-income countries, were working in 47 different languages in both academic and implementation settings, and were focusing on both mental disorders and psychosocial well-being. This advisory group generated a list of 733 research questions, which was consolidated into a list of 74 unique research questions. More than half of the original participants ($N = 72$) together with the steering committee ($N = 10$) subsequently rated this list of 74 research questions, using five criteria (significance, answerability, applicability, equity, ethics). The 10 leading prioritized research questions scored above 80% endorsement as "essential" on all of these criteria. In accordance with results from the first phase, the resulting agenda favors research initiatives that:

(a) take a *fresh look at problem analysis*—analyzing the key stressors facing populations in humanitarian settings (#1); identifying local perceptions on mental health and psychosocial problems (#3); identifying the major protective factors for mental health and psychosocial well-being (#7); identifying the most common mental health and psychosocial problems in the general population (#10);

(b) a strong potential for *translation of knowledge into MHPSS programming*—identifying appropriate methods of needs assessment (#2); identifying appropriate indicators to monitor and evaluate programs (#4); evaluation of family- and school-based MHPSS (#6, #8), and

(c) *participation of and sensitivity to the socio-cultural contexts of populations affected by humanitarian settings*—e.g., identifying ways to adapt MHPSS to differing socio-cultural contexts (#5); evaluating the extent to which current MHPSS meets locally perceived needs (#9).

It should also be noted that MHPSS research in humanitarian settings requires careful consideration of various ethical issues. Allden et al. (2009) have outlined an ethical framework for conducting research in humanitarian settings. Their recommendations suggest that research should:

(a) benefit the affected population;

(b) use culturally valid assessment instruments and measures;

(c) consider power dynamics and the relative social statuses of researchers and beneficiaries;

(d) "do no harm" by protecting participants from potential negative effects of participation, such as stigmatization, discrimination, and security threats;

(e) minimize psychological risks, such as raised expectations and labeling, while ensuring review of research by affected communities;

(f) protect confidentiality;

(g) involve affected communities in selection of research topics;

(h) obtain genuine informed consent (e.g., understandable explanations, avoiding inappropriate incentives, repeating consent as appropriate); and

(i) share findings with affected communities and make reports accessible to relevant stakeholders and others in the field.

The authors argue that it would be unethical not to conduct research and evaluations on MHPSS interventions in emergencies, given the need for more evidence in this field; while it would also be unethical to conduct such research without benefit to beneficiaries. These sentiments are summarized in the statement "No survey without service, and no service without survey." It should be said, however, that this aspiration is rarely achieved.

The experience of recent decades has been that major disasters in low- and middle-income countries have occurred in contexts where there are very poorly developed mental health and social support systems. Just two examples are the prolonged conflicts in Sri Lanka and Aceh and the additional catastrophe of the 2004 tsunami in both places. A brief account of the development of mental health policy and community mental health services in Sri Lanka[27,28] is given in Chapter 13 (Mental Health Policy Development). Here we will briefly outline some mental health system development issues confronted in Aceh, Indonesia, in the context of the massive humanitarian response that followed the earthquake and tsunami on December 26, 2004.

Eleven of Indonesia's 22 districts were directly affected by the tsunami, with 160,000 dead and more than 500,000 of the 4 million population of Aceh displaced. There was very early recognition by the government of Indonesia that mental health would be a major issue following the disaster. In January of 2005, the Mental Health Department of WHO in Geneva, and the Centre for International Mental Health, University of Melbourne, at the invitation of the Indonesian government, worked with the Ministry of Health to prepare the ministry's mental health response to the disaster.[29] The only mental health service in Aceh at the time was the mental hospital in the capital city, Banda Aceh. Among the WHO recommendations accepted by the Ministry of Health and by the Provincial Health Office of Aceh was the suggestion to develop a comprehensive community-focused mental health system.

In the immediate post-tsunami period, more than 400 NGOs, large and small, and military disaster-response teams from many countries were operating in Aceh, most of which left soon after the end of the early emergency response phase. The psychosocial support response was an uncoordinated, unregulated, and unaccountable free-for-all.

A great deal of "psychosocial" work, of widely varying kinds and quality, is already being conducted in Aceh. There is currently no reliable information concerning the theoretical underpinnings for these interventions, the skills of practitioners, or the extent of beneficial or harmful impact of the work being carried out. There is a pressing need to understand what is being done and the impact of what is being done in the psychosocial/mental health arena.[30, p. 2]

The chaotic post-disaster response and disparate "psychosocial" programs experienced in Aceh was one among many similar post-disaster experiences that provided an impetus for the development of the IASC Guidelines on Mental Health and Psychosocial Support in Emergency Settings.[15]

Implementation of the WHO recommendation to move from the initial disaster response phase to a process of mental health system development was challenging.[30]

Agreement has now been reached to establish a community mental health system in the 11 tsunami-affected districts of Aceh. The process whereby this agreement was reached engaged the three levels of government (ministry, province and districts) and other key stakeholders, including key UN agencies, universities, national and international NGOs, and professional associations.

The establishment of community mental health services will occur in a complex and challenging environment. A number of challenges and obstacles to the success of this process must be considered. District health officials are under enormous pressure in all areas of health planning and implementation. They are required to deal with multiple national and international agencies, each pursuing somewhat different agendas. While considering the reconstruction of the health system they are also engaged in reconstructing the DHOs [District Health Offices], with shortages of personnel, inadequate office space and equipment, and shortages of the skills necessary for the massive task they face. At the same time, many officials are dealing with the aftermath of personal losses. A key issue for the development of the mental health system is that district health officials generally have no experience of planning or implementing mental health services and there is variable appreciation of what this undertaking means and what it will entail. The concept of community mental health services is almost entirely unfamiliar. In such a context, district health officials will require significant and sustained support to successfully undertake planning, implementation, monitoring and evaluation of the proposed community mental health services.

Key challenges in the establishment of district level community mental health services will be the lack of trained clinical staff (particularly nurses and doctors with adequate mental health training) and the limited capacity at Province and District levels to design and implement such services. A critical element in carrying out this process successfully will be to identify, train and support people at Province and District levels who will be able to assume leadership roles in the development of the new system of mental health service delivery.

It is vital that the process of establishing community mental health services is informed by evidence and that the services that are established are rigorously evaluated. This is particularly important since the possibility has already been flagged at high levels of the Ministry of Health that the system that is developed in Aceh could serve as a model for other provinces in Indonesia.[30, p.2]

The mental health system development program initiated in 2005[31–33] continues, and has served as a model for community mental health system development in other Indonesian provinces. Among the positive outcomes are the availability of primary care–based mental health services in every district of the province, the implementation of an effective task-shifting human resources for mental health strategy,[34] and provincial and national government commitment to protection of the human rights of people with severe mental disorders.[35,36] As was demonstrated in Sri Lanka,[28] initiating and sustaining a process of mental health system development, as well as providing the more immediate mental health and psychosocial support that is required immediately after a disaster, is possible even in difficult and severely resource-constrained circumstances.

WAYS FORWARD

Despite the emerging nature of the field of mental health and psychosocial support in humanitarian settings, and the polarized views that have accompanied its nascence, recent initiatives are starting to show more unified perspectives on best practices in research and intervention. For example, the IASC and Sphere Guidelines provide a consensus-based policy framework that unites actors across diverse sectors (e.g., education, health, nutrition, protection) to respond to the wide range of mental health and psychosocial needs in humanitarian crises (see boxes 17.1–17.4).[15,20] Similarly, researchers and practitioners have been shown to agree on a research agenda that focuses on: (a) research questions that may inform practice (e.g., identifying major stressors; evaluation studies; strengthening measurement of indicators for monitoring and evaluation); (b) broad assessment of diverse mental health needs; and (c) sensitivity to local sociocultural contexts and participation of affected populations.[24,25] Despite this progress, major obstacles continue to impede the delivery of evidence-based

MHPSS interventions. In the following paragraphs, we identify a few important gaps in knowledge and practice that we feel need to be addressed.

First, it is clear that there is a critical need for a stronger evidence base that supports MHPSS interventions. Currently, there is a dearth of studies that have evaluated some of the most frequently implemented interventions, including specific forms of counseling, community-based social support, structured creative and recreational activities, child-friendly spaces, and psycho-education. The limited available evidence for these interventions has been inconsistent. For instance, psycho-education was not associated with improvement in two of three randomized controlled trials.[37,38] Furthermore, evaluation studies have focused on a limited range of mental health concerns in humanitarian settings (PTSD, depressive, and anxiety symptoms); seem lacking for the Latin American, western and central African regions; and have mostly neglected the early childhood period.[22]

Second, and related to the first point, a major obstacle remains in the gap between the main interests of researchers and practitioners. For example, much of the mental health literature on humanitarian crises has focused on establishing prevalence rates for mood and anxiety disorders, particularly PTSD. Of the 733 research questions that were sent in as part of the first step of the MH-SET initiative, however, only 42 (6%) focused specifically on trauma. A better alignment of the priorities of researchers and practitioners may be stimulated by "bringing research into practice" as well as "bringing practice into research." The former would involve implementation of interventions that have been proven effective where applicable. Also, bringing research into practice may be stimulated by upgrading the basic research skills of humanitarian practitioners in order to improve data collection as part of ongoing programming. Although the randomized controlled design remains in our opinion the gold-standard design for outcome evaluation, other less-stringent designs may provide crucial information on the effectiveness of interventions. Bringing practice into research would involve ensuring that researchers focus on answering research questions that matter to practitioners; for instance, the research agenda resulting from the MH-SET initiative, for which there was strong consensus between researchers and practitioners. Furthermore, strengthening partnerships between universities and humanitarian organizations would help narrow the gap between science and practice.

Third, a key obstacle relates to the sustainability of humanitarian interventions after the immediate crisis period. Humanitarian crises most often affect populations in low- and middle-income countries, or settings suffering from a lack of mental health system resources even before major crises emerged. Ideally, humanitarian interventions—from the early-recovery phase onwards—contribute to strengthening mental health and psychosocial systems beyond generally time-bound humanitarian assistance.[39] A recent financial analysis, however, found that only 5.2% of all identified MHPSS funding was spent through medical services, and 2.9% through the education system. Much more effort is necessary to strengthen local and national health, education, social service, and protection systems as part of humanitarian assistance in order to ensure sustainability of MHPSS services over time.

Fourth, while it is often necessary to strengthen existing primary care and other community-based social infrastructure, it may not be desirable to strengthen some existing institution-based mental health and social protection systems. The challenge is frequently one of initiating and sustaining a process of substantial reform of existing systems of mental health, rehabilitation, and social support, in order to develop integrated, effective, and equitable hospital and community-based mental health and social support services. A particular focus in such work, difficult everywhere, is to promote and enable effective collaboration among health, social, education, justice, and other relevant sectors.

Fifth, as well as the need for effective and evidence-based post-disaster psychosocial response, there is usually also the need to embark on more sustained mental health system development. Experience in Aceh and Sri Lanka demonstrates that even in very challenging humanitarian settings this is possible.

REFERENCES

1. Themnér L, Wallensteen P. Armed conflict, 1946–2010. *Journal of Peace Research.* 2011;48(4):525–36.
2. Guha-Sapir D, Vos F, Below R, Ponserre S. *Annual disaster statistical review 2010: The numbers and trends.* Brussels, Belgium: Centre for Research on the Epidemiology of Disasters (CRED), Université catholique de Louvain; 2010.
3. Masten AS, Narayan AJ. Child development in the context of disaster, war, and terrorism: pathways of risk and resilience. *Annu Rev Psychol.* 2012;63:227–57.
4. Jones L, Asare JB, El Masri M, Mohanraj A, Sherief H, Van Ommeren M. Severe mental disorders in complex emergencies. *Lancet.* 2009;374:654–61.
5. Steel Z, Chey T, Silove D, Marnane C, Bryant RA, van Ommeren M. Association of torture and other potentially traumatic events with mental health outcomes among populations exposed to mass conflict and displacement. *JAMA.* 2009;302(5):537–49.
6. Tol WA, Kohrt BA, Jordans MJ, Thapa SB, Pettigrew J, Upadhaya N, et al. Political violence and mental health: a multi-disciplinary review of the literature on Nepal. *Soc Sci Med.* 2010;70(1):35–44. Epub 2009/10/17.
7. Panter-Brick C, Goodman A, Tol WA, Eggerman M. Mental health and childhood adversities: a longitudinal study in Kabul, Afghanistan. *J Am Acad Child Adolesc Psychiatry.* 2011;50(4):349–63.
8. Betancourt TS, Borisova II, Williams TP, Brennan RT, Whitfield TH, de la Soudiere M, et al. Sierra Leone's former child soldiers: a follow-up study of psychosocial adjustment and community reintegration. *Child Dev.* 2010;81(4):1077–95.
9. Rasmussen A, Nguyen L, Wilkinson J, Vundla S, Raghavan S, Miller KE, et al. Rates and impact of trauma and current stressors among Darfuri refugees in eastern Chad. *Am J Orthopsychiatry.* 2010;80(2):227–36.
10. Fernando G, Miller KE, Berger DE. Growing pains: the impact of disaster-related and daily stressors on the psychological and psychosocial functioning of youth in Sri Lanka. *Child Dev.* 2010;81(4):1192–210.
11. Rodin D, van Ommeren M. Commentary: explaining enormous variations in rates of disorder in trauma-focused psychiatric epidemiology after major emergencies. *Int J Epidemiol.* 2009;38(4):1045–8.
12. Ambramowitz SA. Trauma and humanitarian translation in Liberia: the tale of Open Mole. *Cult Med Psychiatry.* 2010;34:353–79.
13. Tol WA, Reis R, Susanty D, de Jong JT. Communal violence and child psychosocial well-being: qualitative findings from Poso, Indonesia. *Transcult Psychiatry.* 2010;47(1):112–35. Epub 2010/06/01.
14. Silove D, Bateman CR, Brooks RT, Fonseca CA, Steel Z, Rodger J, et al. Estimating clinically relevant mental disorders in a rural and an urban setting in post-conflict Timor Leste. *Arch Gen Psychiatry.* 2008;65(10):1205–12.
15. Inter-Agency Standing Committee [IASC]. *IASC guidelines on mental health and psychosocial support in emergency settings.* Geneva: IASC; 2007.
16. van Ommeren M, Saxena S, Saraceno B. Mental and social health during and after acute emergencies: emerging consensus? *Bull WHO.* 2005;83(1):71–5; discussion 5–6.
17. Wessells M, van Ommeren M. Developing inter-agency guidelines on mental health and psychosocial support in emergency settings. *Intervention: International Journal of Mental Health, Psychosocial Work & Counselling in Areas of Armed Conflict.* 2008;6(3/4):199–218.
18. IASC Reference Group for Mental Health and Psychosocial Support in Emergency Settings. *Mental health and psychosocial support in humanitarian emergencies: What should humanitarian health actors know?* Geneva: IASC; 2010.
19. IASC Reference Group for Mental Health and Psychosocial Support in Emergencies. *Mental health and psychosocial support in humanitarian emergencies: What should protection programme managers know?* Geneva: IASC; 2010.

20. Sphere Project. *Humanitarian charter and minimum standards in disaster response—2011 edition.* Geneva: The Sphere Project; 2011.

21. Patel V, Araya R, Chatterjee S, Chisholm D, Cohen A, De Silva M, et al. Treatment and prevention of mental disorders in low-income and middle-income countries. *Lancet.* 2007;370(9591):991–1005.

22. Tol WA, Barbui C, Galappatti A, Silove D, Betancourt TS, Souza R, et al. Mental health and psychosocial support in humanitarian settings: linking practice and research. *Lancet.* 2011;378(9802):1581–91. Epub 2011/10/20.

23. Allden K, Jones L, Weissbecker I, Wessells M, Bolton P, Betancourt TS, et al. Mental health and psychosocial support in crisis and conflict: report of the Mental Health Working Group. *Prehosp Disaster Med.* 2009;24(4):s217–27.

24. Tol WA, Patel V, Tomlinson M, Baingana F, Galappatti A, Panter-Brick C, et al. Research priorities for mental health and psychosocial support in humanitarian settings. *PLoS Med.* 2011;8(9):e1001096. Epub 2011/09/29.

25. Tol WA, Patel V, Tomlinson M, Baingana F, Galappatti A, Silove D, et al. Relevance or excellence? Setting research priorities for mental health and psychosocial support in humanitarian settings. *Harv Rev Psychiatry.* 2012;20(1):25–36.

26. Frenk J. Balancing relevance and excellence: organizational responses to link research with decision making. *Soc Sci Med.* 1992;35(11):1397–404.

27. Mahoney J, Chandra V, Gambheera H, De Silva T, Suveendran T. Responding to the mental health and psychosocial needs of the people of Sri Lanka in disasters. *Int Rev Psychiatry.* 2006;18(6):593–7. Epub 2006/12/13.

28. Minas H, Mahoney J, Kakuma R. *Health for the south community mental health project, Sri Lanka: Evaluation report.* Melbourne: World Vision Australia, 2011.

29. Saraceno B, Minas H. *WHO recommendations for mental health in Aceh.* Geneva: World Health Organization, 2005.

30. Minas H. *Disaster to development: A community mental health system for Aceh.* Melbourne: Centre for International Mental Health, University of Melbourne, 2005.

31. Prasetiyawan Test, Viora E, Maramis A, Keliat BA. Mental health model of care programmes after the tsunami in Aceh, Indonesia. *Int Rev Psychiatry.* 2006;18(6):559–62. Epub 2006/12/13.

32. Irmansyah I. Mental health problems after tsunami disaster in Aceh and Nias; immediate responses and future programs. *Seishin Shinkeigaku Zasshi.* 2005;107(11):1178–83. Epub 2006/01/18.

33. Jones L, Ghni H, Mohanraj A, Morrison S, Smith P, Stube D, et al. Crisis into opportunity: setting up community mental health services in post-tsunami Aceh. *Asia Pac J Public Health.* 2007;19:60–8.

34. Miller G. Who needs psychiatrists? *Science.* 2012;335(6074):1294–8.

35. Puteh I, Marthoenis M, Minas H. Aceh Free Pasung: releasing the mentally ill from physical restraint. *Int J Ment Health Syst.* 2011;5:10. Epub 2011/05/17.

36. Irmansyah I, Prasetyo YA, Minas H. Human rights of persons with mental illness in Indonesia: more than legislation is needed. *Int J Ment Health Syst.* 2009;3(1):14. Epub 2009/06/24.

37. Yeomans PD, Forman EM, Herbert JD, Yuen E. A randomized controlled trial of a reconciliation workshop with and without PTSD psychoeducation in Burundian sample. *J Traum Stress.* 2010;23(3):305–12.

38. Neuner F, Schauer M, Klaschik C, Karunakara U, Elbert T. A comparison of narrative exposure therapy, supportive counseling, and psychoeducation for treating posttraumatic stress disorder in an African refugee settlement. *J Consult Clin Psychol.* 2004;72(4):579–87.

39. Patel PP, Russell J, Allden K, Betancourt TS, Bolton P, Galappatti A, Hijazi Z, Johnson K, Jones L, Kadis L et al: Transitioning mental health & psychosocial support: from short-term emergency to sustainable post-disaster development. Humanitarian Action Summit 2011. *Prehosp Disaster Med* 2011;26(6):470–81.

40. Jordans MJD, Tol WA, Komproe IH, de Jong JTVM. Systematic review of evidence and treatment approaches: psychosocial and mental health care for children in war. *Child & Adolesc Ment Health.* 2009;14(1):2–14.

41. Jordans MJD, Tol WA, Komproe IH. Mental health interventions for children in adversity: pilot-testing a research strategy for treatment selection in low-income settings. *Soc Sci Med.* 2011;73:456–66.

42. Hijazi Z, Weissbecker I, Chamnay R. The integration of mental health into Primary Health Care in Lebanon. *Intervention: International Journal of Mental Health, Psychosocial Work & Counselling in Areas of Armed Conflict*. 2011;9(3):265–78.

43. Asare J, Jones L. Tackling mental health in Sierra Leone. *BMJ*. 2005;331:720.

44. Rose N, Hughes P, Ali S, Jones L. Integrating mental health into primary health care settings after an emergency: lessons from Haiti. *Intervention: International Journal of Mental Health, Psychosocial Work & Counselling in Areas of Armed Conflict*. 2011;9(3):211–24.

45. Sadik S, Abdulrahman S, Bradley M, Jenkins R. Integrating mental health into primary health care in Iraq. *Ment Health Fam Med*. 2011;8:39–49.

46. MSF CH. *Field visit report Dabaab Project (internal report)*. Geneva: MSF CH, 2009.

47. Reggi M. *Mental health survey in Dadaab refugee camps—final report*. Milan, Italy: Laboratory of Anthropology of Migration and Transnationalism, University of Milan-Bicocca & Gruppo per le Relazioni Transculturali; 2010.

18 Stigma, Discrimination, and Promoting Human Rights

Nisha Mehta and Graham Thornicroft

INTRODUCTION

The effects of stigmatization upon people with mental illness are common and result in profound social exclusion. The *Oxford English Dictionary* states that the word *stigma* has, since the 1620s, meant "a mark of disgrace or infamy." Goffman described stigma as "an attribute that is deeply discrediting," leading the affected person to be "reduced...from a whole and usual person to a tainted or discounted one."[1] More recently stigma has come to mean "any attribute, trait or disorder that marks an individual as being unacceptably different from the 'normal' people with whom he or she routinely interacts, and that elicits some form of community sanction."[1–3] At the same time, the forms of exclusion that are the discriminatory consequences of stigmatization have serious negative implications for many aspects of social participation, in effect reducing the ability of many people with mental illness to obtain the full enjoyment of their fundamental human rights. In this chapter, we examine, in turn, these two closely interrelated aspects of the social reality of having a mental illness: the experience of stigma and discrimination, and the violation of human rights. We then go on to consider what needs to be done.

DEFINITIONS AND CONCEPTS

What Are Stigma and Discrimination?

A considerable literature now refers to stigma.[1,4–15] For the purposes of this chapter, we consider stigma as an overarching term including three elements:

- problems of knowledge (ignorance or misinformation)

Cape Town Declaration of the Pan African Network of People with Psychosocial Disabilities

We recognize that people with psychosocial disabilities have been viewed in bad ways, with derogatory words being used to describe us such as mentally disturbed, having unsound minds, idiots, lunatics, imbeciles and many other hurtful labels.

We are people first! We have potentials, abilities, talents and each of us can make a great contribution to the world. We in the past, presently and in the future have, do and will continue to make great contributions if barriers are removed.

We believe in an Africa in which all people are free to be themselves and to be treated with dignity. We are all different, unique and our differences should be appreciated as an issue of diversity. We need all people to embrace this diversity, Diversity is beautiful.

The can be no mental health without our expertise. We are the knowers and yet we remain the untapped resource in mental health care. We are the experts. We want to be listened to and to fully participate in our life decisions. We must be the masters of our life journeys.

We want, like everyone else, to vote. We want to marry, form relationships, have fulfilled family lives, raise children, and be treated as others in the workplace with equal remuneration for equal work.

For as long as others decide for us, we do not have rights. No one can speak for us. We want to speak for ourselves.

We want to be embraced with respect and love.

We are deeply concerned about the extent of suffering experienced by our brothers and sisters on our vast continent. Poverty, human rights violations and psychosocial disability go hand in hand. We know that there can be no dignity where poverty exists. No medicines or sophisticated western technology can eradicate poverty and restore dignity.

The history of psychiatry haunts our present. Our people remain chained and shackled in institutions and by ideas which our colonizers brought to our continent.

We want everyone to acknowledge their participation in calling us names and treating us a lesser beings. These are the barriers to our full enjoyment of life. These barriers are disabling us and these prevent us from fully participating in society.

We wish for a better world in which all people are treated equally, a world where human rights below to everyone. We invite you to walk beside us. We know where we want to go.

Cape Town
October 2011

- problems of attitudes (prejudice)
- problems of behavior (discrimination).[3,16–18]

Ignorance: The Problem of Knowledge

There is a great deal of information in the public domain, but the level of accurate knowledge about mental illness (sometimes called "mental health literacy") is relatively poor.[19] In a population survey in England, for example, most people (55%) believe that the statement "someone who cannot be held responsible for his or her actions" describes a person who is mentally ill.[20] Most (63%) thought that fewer than 10% of the population would experience a mental illness at some time in their lives.

Measures taken to improve public knowledge about mental illness can be successful, and can reduce the effects of stigmatization. At the national level, social marketing campaigns have produced positive changes in public attitudes towards people with mental illness, as shown in New Zealand and Scotland.[21,22] In a campaign in Australia to increase knowledge about depression and its treatment, some states and territories received an intensive, coordinated program, whilst others did not. In the former, people more often recognized the features of depression, were more likely to support help-seeking for depression, or to accept treatment with counseling and medication.[23] Similarly evidence comparing trends between Scotland and England in public attitudes towards mental illness are consistent with a positive effect of the Scottish "See Me" anti-stigma campaign.[24] A larger and more wide-ranging campaign now running in England entitled "Time to Change" aims to fundamentally reduce stigma and discrimination.[25–27] However, whilst anti-stigma programs raise public awareness, there is no evidence to suggest that programs lasting less than a year have any real effect on stigma.[28]

Prejudice: The Problem of Negative Attitudes

The term *prejudice* is used to refer to the negative beliefs or opinions of social groups about people with a particular characteristic; for example, minority ethnic groups, yet it is employed rarely in relation to people with mental illness. The reactions of a host majority to act with prejudice in rejecting a minority group usually involve not just negative thoughts but also emotion such as anxiety, anger, resentment, hostility, distaste, or disgust.

There is not much in the literature which describes emotional reactions to people with mental illness apart from that which describes a fear of violence.[18,29] That said, fear of violence is probably one of the leading causes of stigma and discrimination. In 1987, Link et al. reviewed several studies and concluded: "When a measure of perceived dangerousness of mental patients is introduced, strong labeling [stigma] effects emerge...the interaction between labeling and perceived dangerousness is highly significant...Such individuals find former patients threatening and prefer to maintain a safe distance from them."[30] Similarly, an increase in social distance towards people with mental illness was noted in Germany after the attempted murder of two prominent politicians by mentally ill individuals in 1990.[31] Broader examples of such negative labeling are the terms used by school students towards people with mental health problems, and in one English study, among 250 such terms, none were positive and 70% were negative.[32] The content of newspaper reporting about mental illness provides other examples of negative labeling.[33]

Discrimination: The Problem of Rejecting and Avoidant Behavior

Discrimination occurs at both an individual and interpersonal level as well as at a systemic level within societies and can be considered the natural outcome of the combined elements of problems of knowledge and negative attitudes, as discussed above.

"Systemic" or "institutional" discrimination is common in relation to mental illness and refers, for example, to how funding decisions appear to more often favor more investment (and less disinvestment) in physical than in mental health care services. Another example of "institutional" discrimination was described by Corrigan et al., who examined all of the relevant bills introduced in the United States in 2002 in the 50 states and found that about one-quarter of the bills reviewed were relevant to protection from discrimination in general. Within this group, they found that half of all the legal bills actually reduced protection for people with mental illness, including restriction of parental rights.[34]

Institutional discrimination is by no means limited to mental illness and is well established as an issue in U.K. race relations, from which important lessons can be learned for the stigma movement in mental illness. In 1999, the U.K. government published the Macpherson Report, which described the failings of the London Metropolitan Police in handling the investigation of the racially motivated murder of black teenager Stephen Lawrence. Now widely regarded as a seminal work in the fight against racial discrimination in the United Kingdom, the Macpherson report tied police failings to the issue of institutional racism in the police, defined as follows: "The collective failure of an organization to provide an appropriate and professional service to people because of their color, culture, or ethnic origin." It can be seen or detected in processes, attitudes, and behavior that amount to discrimination through unwitting prejudice, ignorance, thoughtlessness, and racist stereotyping, which disadvantage minority ethnic people.[35]

As a result of this, there emerged a notable determination by central government to take the Macpherson recommendations seriously. The U.K. government has imposed targets on police authorities requiring the modernization and diversification of the police to boost numbers of black, minority ethnic (BME) officers. In addition, the Home Office "Strength in Diversity" agenda[36] is actively pursued within all strands of policing policy development, and the Macpherson recommendations continue to be reproduced in official documents and their implementation monitored in all aspects of policing. The Macpherson ethos has permeated other public institutions, and has been enshrined in legislation (Race Relations Amendment Act, 2000), meaning that the identification and elimination of institutional racism as defined by this report is now firmly on the agenda of every U.K. government department and of every U.K. public body.

The lessons learned from the successes of this movement may be applied to the concept of "structural discrimination" identified by Corrigan et al. The authors argue that an understanding of macro-societal determinants of stigma are just as important as the individual experience of the person with mental illness. *Structural discrimination* is defined as:

the policies of private and governmental institutions that intentionally restrict the opportunities of people with mental illness and policies of institutions that yield unintended consequences that hinder the options of people with mental illness.[10]

This definition is similar in many ways to Macpherson's definition of institutional racism. Corrigan et al. argue for further methodological and conceptual work to understand structural discrimination, and this will be of undoubted benefit. Additionally, we argue that by publicizing structural discrimination in bold terms, and by relating macro-level analyses to the plight of individuals (in the way that was achieved in the wake of the Lawrence Inquiry into a murder that was motivated by racism), the stigma agenda may achieve similar prominence. People affected by stigma and mental illness are as numerous if not more so than those affected by institutional racism. We can learn important lessons from the successes of the U.K. race relations struggle and apply them for ourselves to each institution and each system. Coupled with the impact of powerful domestic and European anti-discrimination law and proven centrally driven goodwill and resources (e.g., the "See Me" anti-stigma Campaign in Scotland and "Time to Change" in England), it seems that at the very least the European anti-stigma movement has the ingredients to empower governments and institutions to tackle the problem of stigma and mental illness head-on.

At an interpersonal level, understanding the direct effects of discrimination using quantitative methods has historically been problematic. Attitude and social-distance surveys (of unwillingness to have social contact) usually ask either students or members of the general public what they would do in imaginary situations or what they think "most people" would do, for example, when faced with a neighbor or a work colleague with a mental illness. Although such research is useful, it does not assess behavior and discrimination directly. Evidence-based outcomes are required to demonstrate tangible reductions in discrimination, namely the behavior and social excluding implications of stigma.[37–39] A quantitative approach to this question was taken by one large global study that developed and used the Discrimination and Stigma Scale (DISC) in a cross-sectional survey in 27 countries using language-equivalent versions of the instrument in face-to-face interviews between research staff and 732 participants with a clinical diagnosis of schizophrenia.[38] The most frequently occurring areas of negative experienced discrimination were making or keeping friends (47%), discrimination by family members (43%), keeping a job (29%), finding a job (29%), and intimate or sexual relationships (29%). Positive experienced discrimination was rare. Anticipated discrimination was common for: applying for work or training or education (64%), looking for a close relationship (55%); and 72% felt the need to conceal the diagnosis. Anticipated discrimination was commoner than experienced discrimination. This study suggests that rates of discrimination are high across countries. Qualitative research is very powerful in helping understand the burden of discrimination at an individual level when aimed against people with mental illness. A growing body of qualitative evidence considers how people with mental illness, and their caregivers, subjectively experience, describe, and cope with stigma. This has allowed an enhanced understanding of the scope and dimensions of stigma; the personal consequences of stigma; mental health service users views on anti-stigma campaign priorities; and the impact of stigma on the family, along with the development of related scales to measure stigma.[40]

STIGMA AND HUMAN RIGHTS

Human rights are entitlements set out in international law (for example, the International Covenant on Civil and Political Rights) or national law (for example, a constitution or a specific law). The state is the primary "body" that has a responsibility to respect, protect, and fulfill full enjoyment of human rights. The word *state* includes central government, local government, other governmental and quasi-governmental agencies, as well as courts and tribunals.

Under international law, states must respect, protect and fulfill human rights. "The obligation to respect" means that states must not interfere with or curtail the enjoyment of human rights. To give one example, states must not interfere with the right to vote of persons in social-care institutions. The obligation to protect requires states to protect individuals and groups against human rights abuses. For example, institutions must ensure that there are procedures in place to prevent violence and abuse. The obligation to fulfill means that states must take positive action to facilitate the enjoyment of basic human rights. For example, a mental health professional needs to provide written and verbal information to a person in a language and format the person understands before asking that person to consent to, or refuse, any type of treatment.

People with mental health problems or intellectual disabilities may be exposed to a range of issues, many of which are interlinked with stigma, and which can be thought of in human rights terms. Violation of these rights is likely to exacerbate any preexisting mental health problems, rather than make them better. Some human rights abuses are obvious: a male nurse raping female psychiatric patients, for example, is an issue for which it is easy to point a finger at a perpetrator who carries out the abuse with intent.

Instead, systemic violations may be the result of a faulty law or policy, a law or policy that has not been implemented at all or properly, a national or regional or institutional culture, systemic under-funding of services, or funding the wrong type of service—for example, a large psychiatric hospital instead of community-based mental health services. It is in these instances that it is particularly useful to remember that "the state" has obligations to respect, protect and fulfill human rights for all people in its territory without discrimination. It is important to remember that human rights monitoring is not necessarily about demonizing service-providers—who often do the best they can under difficult conditions—but rather about objectively and accurately measuring the reality against human rights standards.

Worldwide, many people with mental illness–related disability have little or no access to supportive systems that provide talking therapies, pharmacological, or social assistance.[41] Many such people live in conditions outside of the purview of the local, national, or international communities. In many countries, laws facilitate exclusion and stigmatization against people with disabilities. In 2006, the United Nations General Assembly adopted the Convention on the Rights of Persons with Disabilities (CRPD).[42] This convention represents a paradigm shift in the perspective on human rights for people with disabilities, and it uses a social model of disability, one that sees disability not as something that defines a person, but rather as one variation on the spectrum of human experiences. People are not disabled—society fails to enable them. As such, individuals are seen not as recipients of charity but as persons who are entitled to assert their rights autonomously, and where needed, with reasonable accommodation or support by others. The Convention also makes it clear that its provisions extend to people with mental health problems as well as people with intellectual disabilities (Article 1, CRPD). While the CRPD does not include any new rights, it does explicitly define the protections and entitlements for the estimated 800 million people with disabilities worldwide.[42,43] The CRPD serves, for example, as the normative framework for the development of the Institutional Treatment, Human Rights and Care Assessment (ITHACA) Toolkit to assess the observation or violation of human rights in mental health institutions.[44]

The regulatory bodies within each European country vary widely and are beyond the scope of this paper. However, various mechanisms exist within Europe to monitor and document the human rights of people in psychiatric and social care institutions, including the right to health.[43,45] The Committee for the Prevention of Torture and Inhuman or Degrading Treatment or Punishment (CPT) is a body of the 47-member Council of Europe. The CPT visits states each year and carries out a mission during which it monitors several places of detention, including prisons, police stations, and psychiatric and social care institutions. Its mandate is to prevent torture and other forms of ill-treatment. After each visit, it writes a report to the relevant government on its findings. The government may authorize publication of the report, and if this happens, the report is uploaded to the CPT's website (see http://www.cpt.coe.int/en/). The importance of human rights monitoring is increasingly recognized. Paul Hunt, a former UN Special Rapporteur on the right of everyone to the enjoyment of the highest attainable standard of physical and mental health, has pointed out that "lack of monitoring of psychiatric institutions and weak or non-existent accountability structures allow these human rights abuses to flourish away from the public eye."[46–49] Guidelines for monitoring of human rights will be discussed further in the section titled "Interventions."

PREVALENCE AND PATTERNS OF STIGMA

There are few countries, societies, or cultures in which people with mental illness are considered to have the same value as people who do not have mental illness. Consistent findings describing the existence of stigma have emerged from evaluating stigma in Africa,[50–53] Asia,[54–58] South America,[59] North America,[10,60–62] in Islamic countries of North Africa and the Near East,[63] Australasia,[64,65] and Europe.[13]

Much of the early work in stigma over the last 50 years has been carried out in high-income country settings, with much published work on stigma coming from authors in the United States, Canada, and the United Kingdom.[2,7,8,16–18,30,66–81] Much of this work is about knowledge, attitudes, or intended behavior towards people with mental illness, a problematic approach which has been discussed earlier in the chapter. Much of the interest focuses on specific conditions such as depression or schizophrenia (with other conditions such as bipolar disorder relatively neglected), or takes mental illness to be a generic concept.[82] Anti-stigma research in high-income country settings is now beginning to focus on identifying and adapting the active ingredients of anti-stigma campaigns, and this will be discussed in further detail below.

More recently, the attention of research describing the patterns and prevalence of stigma has focused on the 153 low- and middle-income countries (LAMIC) which are home to 85% of the world's population.[83] There is now a rich literature on stigma in some low- and middle-income countries, and this rapidly expanding field merits specific attention in this paper.

One study in Ethiopia investigated the perceived stigma amongst family members of people with schizophrenia using a community-based sample and the Family Interview Schedule. Stigma was found to be common (reported by 75%), and few differences were found among sociodemographic groups. Popular attitudes about causes of mental illness included supernatural forces (27%), and preferred methods of dealing with psychosis included praying (65%).[84]

A large study in Nigeria randomly sampled 350 doctors from eight hospitals in three states. They were found to hold stigmatizing attitudes towards their patients, and beliefs in supernatural causes were very prevalent. Other outcomes showed a common belief in dangerousness, poor prognosis, and high social distance, and those more likely to stigmatize were found to have less than 10 years of clinical experience, were more likely to be female and aged under 45. A large study in Malawi of patients and carers attending hospital outpatient clinics found respondents most commonly attributing mental illness to drug and alcohol use, "brain disease," spirit possession, and psychological trauma.[85]

A recent descriptive study in Uganda found stigma to be one factor in a study trying to understand the relative barriers to help-seeking behavior and accessing of services.

In India there is a wealth of descriptive work about stigma.[54,56,86–88] For example, among relatives of people with schizophrenia in Chennai, South India, the main concerns were lack of marital prospects, fear of rejection by neighbors, and a need to conceal the condition from others. Higher levels of stigma were seen against women and younger people with the condition.[56] Women with mental illness have been found to be at a particular disadvantage in India, because of concerns that they will pas along the trait to their children, lack of financial support from husbands or ex-husbands, and the additional stigma attached to being divorced, which is a common outcome for women who become mentally ill.[87,89] Using standardized instruments, a study in Vellore, South India, aimed to understand, among patients and their relatives, the association between explanatory models of mental illness and stigma. The study found that multiple contradictory models of illness and treatment were held. Stigma scores were significantly associated with male gender, poor literacy, rural residence, and beliefs that the illness was due to "karma." A majority of patients had used at least two medicine systems. It is postulated (though not proven) that some explanatory models held by patients are an adaptive mechanism to reduce stigma.[57] A large study of 2040 people at the community level in Nigeria found widespread negative attitudes (96% believing that people with mental illness are violent) and poor knowledge levels about causation of mental illness.[90]

In China, a large-scale survey was undertaken of over 600 people with a diagnosis of schizophrenia and over 900 of their family members. Over half of family members said that stigma had an important effect on them and their family, and levels of stigma were higher in urban areas and for people who were more highly educated.[91,92]

Little is written in the English-language literature on stigma in Islamic communities, but despite earlier indications that the intensity of stigma may be relatively low, [93,94] detailed studies indicate that, on balance, it is no less than we have seen described elsewhere.[95–97] A study of 100 family members of people with schizophrenia in Morocco found that 76% had no knowledge about the condition, and many considered it chronic (80%), handicapping (48%), incurable (39%), or linked with sorcery (25%).[98]

It is clear from these findings that "rejection and avoidance of people with mental illness appear to be universal phenomena."[18]

SOURCES AND DETERMINANTS OF STIGMA

Experiences of stigma can be usefully considered to originate from both internal and external sources. Internal stigma can be further broken down into "experienced" (actual) discrimination (for example, being unreasonably rejected in a job application), or they can be consequences of "anticipated" discrimination (for example, when an individual does not apply for a job because he or she fully expects to fail in any such application).[99] This is a global phenomenon: in the global study using the DISC described earlier,[38] anticipated discrimination was more common than experienced discrimination, and positive experienced discrimination was rare. This has important implications: disability discrimination laws may not be effective without also developing interventions to reduce anticipated discrimination, such as by enhancing the self-esteem of people with mental illness so they will be more likely to apply for jobs. This distinction between experienced and anticipated discrimination is closely related to what has been described as the difference between "enacted" and "felt" stigma. "Enacted" stigma refers to events of negative discrimination, whilst "felt" stigma includes the experience of shame at having a condition and the fear of encountering "enacted" stigma,[100] and is associated with lower self-esteem. It is worth noting, however, that not all groups of mentally ill people suffer from internal stigma, including some ethnic minority groups and children with physical disabilities,[99] and that at the opposite end of the scale is the concept of empowerment, which will be covered in more detail below.

As discussed above, external stigma comes from a variety of sources and can occur at a variety of levels, including institutional and systemic. Stigma against people with mental illness comes from all directions, including family, friends, employers, the police, the criminal justice system, and the health care system, to name but a few.[18] A potent external source of stigma is the media. Most people gather what they know about mental illness either from personal contact with people with such conditions, or from the mass media.[101] Strong evidence exists to demonstrate that negative information predominates in newspaper coverage about mental illness. A careful evaluation of one month's newspaper stories about mental illness in New Zealand found 600 items. Ninety-four percent were editorials or news items, and the remainder were letters, cartoons, or advertisements. In results similar to an earlier Australian study,[102] more than half of the items depicted the mentally ill person as dangerous, and the key traits that emerged were that the mentally ill were dangerous to others (61%), criminal (47%), unpredictable (24%), and dangerous to themselves (20%). The authors concluded that "print media portrayals are negative, exaggerated and do not reflect the reality of most people with mental illness."[102–104] Similar studies have reproduced similar findings across several countries, including Canada,[105] the United Kingdom,[106] the United States,[107] and Germany.[108]

As previously discussed, work in Germany also described a significant increase in social distance towards those with schizophrenia after extensive media coverage of two violent attacks by people with mental illness on prominent politicians.[109] On a more positive note, a recent study concluded that between 1992 and 2008, there was a significant reduction in negative coverage about mental illnesses in several newspapers in the United Kingdom. Coverage improved for depression, but it remained largely negative for schizophrenia.[110]

In addition to external and internal stigma, it is useful to consider that determinants of stigma may be rooted in other sociological constructs, such as poverty and gender. This is an area about which we know relatively little, but there are some good studies from low-income settings in particular that highlight these issues. The link between poverty and stigma has been elaborated by useful work from Uganda. Qualitative interviews with key stakeholders and informants across a variety of sectors produced findings pointing to the link between poverty and mental illness, with stigma as a "mediator" between the two.[111] The complex interaction between female gender, mental illness, stigma, and divorce in India has already been discussed.[87] Within cultures, it seems that factors determining stigma are linked in complex ways that merit further attention in future research.

IMPACT OF STIGMA

I have lost all my friends since the onset of my mental illness. My ex-colleagues at work have also ceased all contact with me. I lost my career, my own flat, my car. Mental illness has destroyed my life. (Fiona)[18]

The problems resulting from stigma—those of knowledge, attitudes, and behavior—can have a profound and devastating impact on people with mental illness, their families, caregivers, health services, and the wider society at large. At a systemic level, stigma causes a "vicious cycle" of under-investment in services leading to under-treatment, leading to worsening stigma, leading to further under-investment. Furthermore, stigma is responsible, to a large degree, for significantly poorer physical and mental health outcomes in affected populations, and we shall consider this issue in the following two sections.

Stigma, Discrimination and "Diagnostic Overshadowing" in the Health Care System

There is strong evidence that people with mental health disabilities and intellectual disabilities receive worse treatment for physical disorders. One of the factors contributing to this is "diagnostic overshadowing," which is defined as the process by which people with mental health disabilities and intellectual disabilities receive poorer physical health care because general health care staff are poorly informed or misattribute physical symptoms to mental health disabilities and intellectual disabilities; "diagnostic overshadowing" has been best investigated in people with learning disabilities in medical settings.[112,113] This concept has been explored in the literature on people with intellectual disabilities for over two decades, but it is an area that has received very little attention in the mental health literature, although mental health service users have extensively reported the occurrence of this phenomenon.[114]

Among the implications of such discrimination and neglect are higher mortality rates among people with mental health disabilities and intellectual disabilities.[115,116] For example, in regard to cardiac infarctions, after adjusting for other risk factors such as socio-economic status, depression in men was found to be associated with an increase in cardiovascular-related mortality.[117] Those with a diagnosis of psychosis are particularly affected by high mortality rates. A study followed up 2723 patients who presented in three areas of the United Kingdom with first-episode psychosis. They were followed over a period of four decades in total, and the mean length of follow-up in the group was 11.5 years. Investigators found that the groups in question had an excess mortality risk of nearly double that of the general population, that their deaths were mostly from natural causes (mainly from respiratory causes and infectious diseases), and that the mortality gap had widened over recent decades.[118] The overall reduction in life expectancy for people with mental illness is now well established—what is yet to be clarified is how far such early death rates are attributable to stigma related factors.[119,120]

Indeed, the reasons for this health care disparity are not well understood. One major associated factor is the stigmatizing approaches of physicians and other health care staff, which reveal negative stereotypes.[121] However, more recent studies suggest that another important factor may be that clinicians make different diagnostic and treatment decisions in relation to people with mental illness. "Treatment overshadowing" is a term that has been proposed to describe possible biases in actual treatment decisions. For example, this may include a clinician's deciding against certain treatment because of an assumption that a person's mental illness precludes such an intervention. It has been shown, for example, that people with comorbid mental disorders were "substantially less likely to undergo coronary re-vascularization procedures" than those without mental disorders.[122] Similarly, people with comorbid mental illness and diabetes who presented to an emergency department were less likely to be admitted to hospital for diabetic complications than those with no mental illness.[123]

It is also clear that many health care professionals are not sufficiently trained to recognize and treat people with mental health and intellectual disabilities (including, for example, epilepsy), and to recognize the many interactions between physical and mental health problems. For example, a toothache can present as "challenging behavior" in a person with limited communication skills. Furthermore, social factors such as bereavement and other losses, or changes in social structure like moving from one home to another, incompatibility with other residents, disrespectful handling from carers, environmental causes like noise or disruption of routine, can also manifest as "challenging behavior." The use of medication in these cases is not only contraindicated, but may add to the distress already experienced. "Treatment" for such situations is often simply achieved by manipulating the environment: that is, by removing the stress-inducing situation for the individual.

Barriers to Access to Mental Health Care

One of the consequences of both negative attitudes and the resulting discrimination is that people with mental health problems commonly avoid seeking help for their problems, often for fear of receiving a mental health–related diagnosis.[15] It is only relatively recently that the full potency of such barriers to finding treatment and care has been recognized.[124,125] For example studies from several countries have consistently found that even after a family member has developed clear-cut signs of a psychotic illness, on average it is over a year before the unwell person first receives assessment and treatment.[126] A survey of almost 10,000 adults in 17 countries has added more detail to this picture. The results showed that the majority of people with mental disorders eventually contact treatment services, but they often wait a long time before doing so: with average delays before seeking help of eight years for mood disorders, and at least nine years for anxiety disorders. People who wait longer than average before receiving care are more likely to be young, old, male, poorly educated, or a member of a racial or ethnic minority.[127,128]

The following common beliefs reduce the likelihood that an individual will seek help: that psychiatric treatments are ineffective[129]; others would react with avoidance; a person should solve his own problems; lack of perceived need, not knowing where to go for help; thinking the problem will resolve itself; and fear of being hospitalized against one's will.[130] Nevertheless, strong family encouragement to go for mental health assessment and treatment does often work.[131]

One reason that stigma and discrimination has received increasing research attention is their potential to act as barriers to access to health care–seeking. Of four reviews that examined the impact of stigma on access to mental health care, each concluded that it had a significant detrimental effect.[132] Prospective studies provide evidence that stigma may have a negative impact on service use.[133] Non-stigma-related barriers to accessing mental health care can include poor funding for public mental health services, centralized mental health services, low numbers of adequately trained health care staff, and poor advocacy and mobilization of informal resources.[134] Other barriers might include financial, geographical, and language barriers, as well as lack of awareness of services and poor mental health literacy, to name but a few. Thus it is clear that both non-stigma-related barriers (such as inadequate service provision) and stigma-related barriers limit access to mental health care, but what is not currently known is the relative influence of these different types of barriers.

MEASUREMENT OF STIGMA—RESEARCH METHODS

We have devoted a considerable amount of attention to defining and understanding what we mean by "stigma." A consideration of different ways by which we can measure stigma is important to help provide an evidence base for what does and does not work in stigma-reduction research.

A 2010 review[135] of 57 studies of survey measures of stigma constructs revealed 14 survey measures. Of these, seven studies examined perceived stigma, 10 examined experienced stigma, and five examined self-stigma.[136,137] "Stigma" was used as an overarching term to cover stigma, prejudice, and discrimination. Perceived stigma was most frequently assessed (79% of studies), experienced stigma in 46% of studies, and self-stigma in 33% of studies. Furthermore, the relationship between the "knowledge and attitudes" elements of stigma and discrimination is not clear. For example, changes in legislation may decrease discrimination, but negative attitudes may remain the same, or even increase. In addition, the definition of "stigma" is not necessarily the same in all communities and cultures across the world. Thus, such measures may well have little relevance and possibly even risk doing more harm than good if applied in a Western-philosophical style to a non-Western culture. As one study puts it, "such intersections and translations may inadvertently exacerbate stigma and create obstacles to care for mental illness."[58] In the rapidly expanding field of global mental health, it is therefore of the utmost importance that anti-stigma work in culturally unique and distinct settings be informed by anthropological and ethnographic field work.

ANTI-STIGMA INTERVENTIONS

We have discussed some of the vast global literature describing stigma. Early in the chapter we stated that most research in stigma reduction has focused on intended behavior and hypothetical outcomes, and called for more evidence-based discrimination-reduction interventions with measurable successes. In this section, we will first consider what we know so far to be the active ingredients of anti-stigma interventions. We will then turn our attention to examples of anti-stigma interventions that have been carried out at national, district, facility, and community levels, from which we can learn lessons going forward. Finally, we will highlight areas where we have a significant knowledge gap in stigma reduction work, and suggest avenues for future research.

Active Ingredients of Anti-Stigma Interventions

There is an increasing body of evidence about the evaluation of anti-stigma interventions. A meta-analysis of the literature of anti-stigma campaigns focused on methods that included four strategies: protest, social activism, education, and contact.[138] Taking an approach to stigma based on lessons learned from ethnic minority and gender discrimination, Corrigan and colleagues state that the principles behind a review of effective interventions can usefully be divided into these four approaches to stigma reduction efforts. They conducted a meta-analysis of studies examining the effects of anti-stigma campaigns that included one of the above strategies. Seventy-two articles and reports met their inclusion criteria of assessing change in public stigma and were sufficiently statistically powerful to include in the meta-analysis. They found that interventions including both education and contact reduced stigma for adults and adolescents with mental illness. Contact was better at reducing stigma for adults, and education was more effective for adolescents. Face-to-face contact was more effective than video contact, but video contact has the advantage of being potentially cheap with wide coverage, and it was found that both types of contact significantly reduce stigma. A recent RCT in fact concluded that video contact with nursing students was as effective as face-to-face contact in reducing stigma. [139]

The promising avenues of contact and education have been considered by the Queensland Alliance,[140] and the suggestions for development of such anti-stigma interventions from this report are provided below:

DIRECT CONTACT

- Common, although disclosure is rare
- Most effective when there is (a) a relationship of equal status; (b) it occurs in the context of active cooperation and the pursuit of shared goals; (c) there is an opportunity for interaction and discussion; (d) coexisting relationships are better (e.g., friend, neighbor, work colleague); (e) message and messenger need to be culturally appropriate; (f) contact dispels common myths; (g) the presenter should be "credible"; (h) celebrity disclosure is useful.

EDUCATION

- Education must "build understanding of the human experience of living with mental health problems," therefore information alone is insufficient.
- Education interventions should be: (a) delivered by people with experience of mental health problems (contact plus education is best); (b) multifaceted and confront myths; (c) stories that "touch the heart and mind of the listener," describing challenges, overcoming discrimination, and conveying hope and optimism; (d) promoting respect, rights, and shared responsibility to tackle discrimination; (e) targeted, segmented, delivered locally to specific audiences (there is no such thing as the "general public"); (f) use creative art, theater, comedy, photo stories, poetry, first-person narratives.

In the Corrigan et al. meta-analysis discussed above, there were few studies measuring the impact of social protest; but of those that were included, significant effect sizes were not seen. Social protest focuses on shaming people for their prejudicial views and foregrounding the injustice and harm that is done to people who experience stigma— although it should be noted that some forms of protest have been shown to increase social distance from the affected group through an inadvertent "rebound" effect.[141,142] Examples of anti-stigma interventions to date help to illustrate the type of evidence we currently have in the promising fields of education and contact and in the less-well-evidenced field of social protest. However, there is little evidence overall demonstrating real and sustained change resulting from anti-stigma interventions, which highlights an area in need of further research.

A further active ingredient of anti-stigma campaigns is empowerment. This may be seen as the antithesis of self-stigma, and a way to enhance self-confidence which is the opposite end of the spectrum from self-stigma.[136,143] Empowerment is thus a powerful tool for addressing internalized stigma, which results in poorer outcomes, anticipated discrimination, and low self-esteem. The literature is increasingly pointing towards approaches for self-stigma-reduction as a successful method of stigma intervention. A paper discussed definitions of self-stigma and reviewed self-stigma-reduction strategies, finding 14 key articles with eight reporting an improvement in self-stigma outcomes.[144–152] Mittal et al. suggest that the most promising interventions are of two types: firstly, interventions that "enhance skills for coping with self-stigma through improvements in self-esteem, empowerment, and help seeking behavior"; and secondly, and less popular amongst current stigma-intervention designers, "interventions that attempt to alter the stigmatizing beliefs and attitudes of the individual." Empowerment was also highlighted as an important tool that can cross national boundaries, allowing for the active leadership of people with mental illness through organized groups such as Mad Pride, the National Empowerment Centre, the Hearing Voices Network, and New Zealand's "Out of Their Minds."[140]

Anti-Stigma Interventions at National, District, Facility, and Community Levels

Having considered the probable active ingredients of anti-stigma interventions, we now turn to a review of the work in the field that has been carried out at different levels of society. In considering global evidence, it should be noted that the vast majority of the work to date has been carried out in high-income settings, and the authors call for more work to be carried out in this field in low- and middle-income settings.

In national and international policy terms, there needs to be a sustained attack upon discrimination through an emphasis on social inclusion. Some conceptual, system-level approaches to reducing stigma were suggested by the Queensland Alliance in 2009.[140] Their suggestions include improving mental health literacy (with emphasis on social connectedness to produce best outcomes); teaching young people about mental illness (improved empathy, pro-social behavior, attitudes); and moving away from the biomedical model, which worsens pessimism and social distance in most settings. But this may not be the case in all settings. In Nigeria, for example, people with a biomedical understanding of mental illness had relatively low levels of stigmatizing attitudes.[90] Also discussed in the report by the Queensland Alliance is the "social inclusion model" at a policy level:

the development of policies and targeted approaches which deal with the economic causes of social exclusion... work, education, training, health inequalities, early intervention, poverty, housing, civil rights, trauma, abuse, neglect... promoting a client centred approach to the design and delivery of services... fostering connections with people through community resources.[140,p.16]

The Australian government established the Social Inclusion Ministry and made discrimination reduction a priority in 2007–2012. Table 18.1[153] summarizes actions needed at a national level to systematically tackle system-level stigma.

Action at the highest level as displayed above should be seen in the context of the international setting, in which organizations such as the WHO can contribute to better

Table 18.1 Strategies to Reduce System-Level Stigma

Action	By whom
Use a social model of disability that refers to human rights, social inclusion, and citizenship.	Governments and NGOs to change core concepts
Apply the anti-discrimination laws to give parity to people with physical and mental disabilities.	Parliaments and governments
Inform all employers of their legal obligations under these laws.	Ministry of Employment or equivalent
Interpret anti-discrimination laws in relation to mental illness.	Judiciary and legal profession
Establish service-user speakers' bureaus to offer content to news stories and features on mental illness.	NGOs and other national-level service-user groups
Provide and evaluate media-watch response units to press for balanced coverage.	Statutory funding for NGOs to provide media watch teams
Share between countries the experience of disability discrimination acts.	Legislators, lawyers, advocates, and consumer groups
Understand and implement international legal obligations under binding declarations and covenants.	NGOs to communicate legal obligations of all stakeholders, and health and social care inspection agencies to audit how far these obligations are respected in practice
Audit compliance with codes of good practice in providing insurance.	Associations of insurers with service-user organizations and mental health NGOs
Providing economic incentives rather than disincentives to disabled people ready to return to work.	Employment ministries to introduce new and flexible arrangements for disabled people to work with no risk to their income
Change laws to allow people with a history of mental illness to serve on juries with a presumption of competence.	Justice ministries to amend the laws relating to jury service

care and less discrimination by indicating the need for national mental health policies and by giving guidance on their content.

It is useful to describe national level anti-stigma initiatives to illustrate the principles above with some examples of national-level social protest. In the United States, the "StigmaBusters" group targets and challenges stigma in the media, and successfully had several episodes of a television drama cancelled because they contained stigmatizing content about people with mental illness.[80] Similar success has been seen in Germany where a group called "BASTA—The Alliance for Mentally Ill People" uses email to alert members about stigmatizing advertisements and media messages and encourages them to take collective action. Eighty percent of the cases that they took on were eventually dropped with apologies issued from the offending institutions.[99]

Another noteworthy national-level attempt to tackle stigma has been carried out in South Africa. South Africa's Department of Health coordinates provincial anti-stigma initiatives with the help of three NGOs (South African Federation for Mental Health, South African Depression and Anxiety Group, and Mental Health Information Centre) and other bodies.[154] The anti-stigma drive from the national level coexists with a plethora of local and regional initiatives, and all nine provinces in South Africa ran some form of campaign between 2000 and 2005. The authors call for peer-reviewed evaluation of the stigma work being carried out in order to help share best practices and inform policy elsewhere.

There are many examples of national-level mass-media campaigns aimed at improving mental health awareness and reducing stigma. The "See Me" Campaign in Scotland began in 2002, and during 2002–2004, the Scottish government supported a well-funded, high-profile campaign that delivered specific messages ("See me—I'm a person") to the Scottish population using all forms of media as well as cinema advertising, libraries, prisons, schools, youth groups, and health care settings. Comparing public attitudes towards people with mental illness in England and Scotland between 1994 and 2003, one study has found that although attitudes did not improve, they did not deteriorate as much as they did in England, with a greater difference seen during the first year of this campaign.[82] Another large national campaign is currently underway in England. The "Time to Change" Campaign in England was started in 2009, funded with £18 million by two large U.K. charities (the Big Lottery Fund and Comic Relief). "Time to Change" uses coordinated action at national and local levels to engage individuals, communities, and stakeholder organizations—such as statutory health services and professional membership groups—to take part. For example, mass physical exercise events held annually during Mental Health Awareness Week (called "Get Moving!") facilitate social contact between people with and without experience of mental health disorders. The national campaign uses bursts of mass-media advertising and public relations exercises. Its key messages are:

(1) Mental illnesses are common, and people with such disorders can lead meaningful lives.
(2) Mental illness is our last taboo, such that the accompanying discrimination and exclusion can affect people in a way that many describe as worse than the illness itself.
(3) We can all do something to help people with mental illness.

This call to action encourages people to support those they know with mental illness—e.g., by maintaining social contact.[155] The full evaluation and results of this campaign are yet to emerge, but both "See Me" and "Time to Change" are good examples of national anti-stigma interventions using mass media approaches.

At the district or provincial level, there is a peer-reviewed study reporting outcomes from a stigma intervention in a low-income setting. It describes a mental health training program for community health workers in Bangalore Rural District, in the Indian state of Karnataka, and reports a small reduction in stigmatizing attitudes.[156] The authors designed an intervention for 70 community health workers in the district, in which they attended a four-day training course designed to increase their recognition of mental disorders, improve responses and referral rates, and improve support provided to patients and families, as well as improve mental health promotion within communities. The training program was underpinned by production of a facilitator's manual. Analysis of effectiveness was carried out by asking participants to complete a pre-intervention and post-intervention (immediately and then three months later) mental health literacy survey that has been used in other studies and contains two vignettes describing depression and psychosis. Participants were asked to identify "the problems, their causes, and effective sources of help. They were also asked about attitudes towards people with mental disorders, and anticipated outcomes for them." Following the course, there was a small but statistically significant improvement in recognition of disorders, a sustained improvement in the perceived helpfulness of pharmacological interventions rather than non-evidence-based non-pharmacological interventions, and a very small improvement in some aspects of stigmatizing attitudes in depression more than psychosis, though no real convincing evidence for either condition of sustained and meaningful change.

The "facility" level describes interventions that occur within specific settings, such as hospitals, primary care centers, schools, or police forces. These interventions therefore often target a specific group of people, an approach of some merit, as certain groups may have specific anti-stigma training needs and anti-stigma instruments can be more finely tuned than broader campaigns targeting the "general" public. There are many such examples of "facility"-level interventions in the literature, and we will turn our attention to two of these.

The results of an initiative in the United Kingdom (West Kent) demonstrate a successful education-based intervention: Pinfold et al.[157–160] carried out an anti-stigma program targeting secondary school students, police officers, Citizen's Advice Bureau volunteers, school nurses, and local borough council staff. A systematic training program was developed and presented to 600 school students and 200 police officers. Before the training took place, a focus group was conducted to establish a core set of messages to be delivered by the program. These included: (a) people do recover from mental health problems; (b) we all have mental health needs; (c) one in four people will seek help for a mental health problem at some point; (d) schizophrenia is not "split personality"; (e) anyone can be violent—violence is not a symptom of mental illness; and (f) mental health problems differ from learning disabilities. Findings from the initiative in West Kent demonstrated that educational workshops can have a small but positive impact on attitudes; women are more receptive than men to educational workshops in police and students; improvements in knowledge are weakened over time, but the impact of hearing personal experiences is reported to be longer lasting; people with personal experiences of mental illness hold more positive views than those without—through family, friends, or work colleagues; and young people who have personal experiences learn more from the workshops.

A contact-based anti-stigma intervention targeting specific groups of people was carried out in Brazil as part of the World Psychiatric Association's Program to reduce stigma and discrimination. In 2002, a team of mental health professionals, patients, and family members met and developed content for a series of educational meetings, including a 12-week educational program for families and caregivers (15 in the group) and a larger, open educational meeting that consisted of patients with schizophrenia, families, caregivers, and clergy (250 per group). Two hundred twenty-two evaluations from the larger group meetings showed a 33% self-reported increase in knowledge and 63% self-reported significant increase in knowledge. Self-reported attitude change was demonstrated: 86% were more positive, 14% reported no change. There was no reported increase in negative attitudes. After this success, these meetings continued at a frequency of twice a month, and a communications team have developed informational resources, a website, and a booklet for journalists. There is a regular column in the Brazilian Psychiatric Association Quarterly Bulletin.[3]

Finally, anti-stigma interventions can be carried out at the community level amongst smaller groups of people who are not necessarily identified as being part of larger organized groups or at a population level. In low-income settings, there is a great deal of excellent work being carried out at the community level by a variety of NGOs and charities, much of which is written about only in the "gray" literature (materials not published commercially), and it is worth highlighting the efforts of such groups. A great deal of groundbreaking work is being carried out in India, and anti-stigma work is often done by the groups that have been working with consumers for years. These include the well-established Schizophrenia Research Foundation (SCARF) in Chennai, which carries out a variety of support, empowerment, awareness, and treatment work in and beyond the city. Sangath is an NGO based in Goa that works to improve priority areas of child development, youth health, and mental health, and also develops, runs, and evaluates local anti-stigma initiatives. One study in Nigeria[161] did not directly measure stigma, but delivered a mental health awareness program to village health workers (VHWs) in three states over four years (training a total of 2310 VHWs). Knowledge about treatability of mental illness is poor in these areas. The intervention resulted in a jump in referral rates to services, possibly because of increased awareness of the treatment facilities available, which tailed off in the following months although the benefits were still sustained to some extent. Although not measuring stigma directly, the intervention is likely to have had an effect on attitudes, which would normally center around traditional belief systems of "spiritual attack," and which in themselves may propagate stigma. A community-level anti-stigma intervention in the United States[162] targeted self-stigma among family members of people with severe mental illness: "In Our Own Voice" (IOOV) compared a peer-led family companion intervention to a didactic clinician-led education session. The peer-led group intervention was rated highly as acceptable (culturally, respect, relevance, technical quality) and a substantial reduction in self-stigma and secrecy was seen compared to the clinician-led intervention.

CONCLUSION

After several decades of relative neglect, there has been a resurgence of practical and research interest in recent years in the nature of stigma and discrimination in relation to people with mental illness, the implications for violations of human rights, and in the investigation of methods for the reduction or elimination of stigma and discrimination that are suitable for scaling up, within the context of a recent drive to scale up mental health services globally.[163] There is now a rapidly growing literature on effective candidate interventions to reduce stigma via social contact methods (at the community and facility levels) and via social marketing interventions (at the regional and national levels). The challenge for the next decade is to test whether these or different methods are effective in low-resource settings, how far these are affordable and sustainable, whether they truly reverse human rights inequities, and to what extent they accelerate progress towards meeting the aspirations of the "Cape Town Declaration of the Pan African Network of People with Psychosocial Disabilities." Global partners are now joining forces to develop unified anti-stigma interventions in earnest, using lessons learned from the anti-stigma movement as discussed to date.[164–166] The stage is now set for stigma reduction research to continue in earnest.

REFERENCES

1. Goffman E. *Stigma: Notes on the management of spoiled identity.* Harmondsworth, Middlesex: Penguin Books; 1963.
2. Hinshaw SP, Cicchetti D. Stigma and mental disorder: conceptions of illness, public attitudes, personal disclosure, and social policy. *Dev Psychopathol.* 2000;12(4):555–98.
3. Scambler G. Stigma and disease: changing paradigms. *Lancet.* 9/26/1998;352(9133):1054–5.
4. Mason T. *Stigma and Social Exclusion in Healthcare.* London: Routledge; 2001.
5. Falk G. *Stigma: How we treat outsiders.* New York: Prometheus Books; 2001.
6. Heatherton TF, Kleck RE, Hebl MR, Hull JG. *The social psychology of stigma.* New York: Guilford Press; 2003.
7. Corrigan PW, Thompson V, Lambert D, Sangster Y, Noel JG, Campbell J. Perceptions of discrimination among persons with serious mental illness. *Psychiatr Serv.* 2003;54(8):1105–10.
8. Corrigan PW. *On the stigma of mental illness.* Washington, DC: American Psychological Association; 2005.
9. Corrigan PW. Mental illness stigma as social injustice: yet another dream to be achieved. In: Corrigan PW, editor. *On the stigma of mental illness: Practical strategies for research and social change.* Washington, DC: American Psychological Press; 2005:315–20.

10. Corrigan PW, Markowitz FE, Watson AC. Structural levels of mental illness stigma and discrimination. *Schizophr Bull.* 2004;30(3):481–91.

11. Wahl OF. Mental health consumers' experience of stigma. *Schizophr Bull.* 1999;25(3):467–78.

12. Pickenhagen A, Sartorius N. *The WPA global programme to reduce stigma and discrimination because of schizophrenia.* Geneva: World Psychiatric Association; 2002.

13. Sartorius N, Schulze H. *Reducing the stigma of mental illness. A report from a global programme of the World Psychiatric Association.* Cambridge, UK: Cambridge University Press; 2005.

14. Callard F, Sartorius N, Arboleda-Florez J, Bartlett P, Helmchen H, Stuart H, et al. *Mental illness, discrimination and the law: Fighting for social justice.* London: Wiley Blackwell; 2012.

15. Thornicroft G, Brohan E, Rose D, Sartorius N, Group TIS. Global pattern of anticipated and experienced discrimination against people with schizophrenia. *Lancet.* 2009;373(9661):408–15.

16. Hinshaw S. *The mark of shame.* Oxford, UK: Oxford University Press; 2007.

17. Link BG, Phelan JC. Conceptualizing stigma. *Annual review of sociology.* 2001;27:363–85.

18. Thornicroft G. *Shunned: Discrimination against people with mental illness.* Oxford, UK: Oxford University Press; 2006.

19. Crisp A, Gelder MG, Goddard E, Meltzer H. Stigmatization of people with mental illnesses: a follow-up study within the Changing Minds campaign of the Royal College of Psychiatrists. *World Psychiatry.* 2005;4:106–13.

20. Department of Health. *Attitudes to mental illness 2003 report.* London: Department of Health; 2003.

21. Vaughn G. Like minds, like mine. In: Saxena S, Garrison P, editors. *Mental health promotion: Case studies from countries.* Geneva: World Health Organization; 2004:62–6.

22. Dunion L, Gordon L. Tackling the attitude problem. The achievements to date of Scotland's "see me" anti-stigma campaign. *Ment Health Today.* 2005:22–5.

23. Jorm AF, Christensen H, Griffiths KM. The impact of beyondblue: the national depression initiative on the Australian public's recognition of depression and beliefs about treatments. *Aust N Z J Psychiatry.* 2005;39(4):248–54.

24. Mehta N, Kassam AML, Butler GGT. Public attitudes towards people with mental illness in England and Scotland, 1994–2003. *Br J Psychiatry.* 2009;194(3):278–84.

25. Henderson C, Thornicroft G. Stigma and discrimination in mental illness: Time to Change. *Lancet.* 2009 Jun 6;373(9679):1928–30.

26. Evans-Lacko S, Henderson C, Thornicroft G. Strengthening the evidence base to support PSAs. *Psychiatr Serv.* 2012;63(1):3.

27. Henderson C, Corker E, Lewis-Holmes E, Hamilton S, Flach C, Rose D, et al. England's Time to Change antistigma campaign: one-year outcomes of service user-rated experiences of discrimination. *Psychiatr Serv.* 2012;63(5):451–7.

28. Sartorius N. Short-lived campaigns are not enough. *Nature.* 2010;468(7321):163–5.

29. Graves RE, Cassisi JE, Penn DL. Psychophysiological evaluation of stigma towards schizophrenia. *Schizophr Res.* 2005;76(2–3):317–27.

30. Link BG, Cullen FT, Frank J, Wozniak J. The social rejection of ex-mental patients: understanding why labels matter. *Am J Sociol.* 1987;92:1461–500.

31. Angermeyer MC, Matschinger H. Violent attacks on public figures by persons suffering from psychiatric disorders. Their effect on the social distance towards the mentally ill. *Eur Arch Psychiatry Clin Neurosci.* 1995;245(3):159–64.

32. Rose D, Thornicroft G, Pinfold V, Kassam A. 250 labels used to stigmatize people with mental illness. *BMC Health Serv Res.* 2007;7:97.

33. Goulden R, Corker E, Evans-Lacko S, Rose D, Thornicroft G, Henderson C. Newspaper coverage of mental illness in the UK, 1992–2008. *BMC Public Health.* 2011;11(1):796.

34. Corrigan PW, Watson AC, Heyrman ML, Warpinski A, Gracia G, Slopen N, et al. Structural stigma in state legislation. *Psychiatr Serv.* 2005;56(5):557–63.

35. UK Government. The Stephen Lawrence Inquiry: The Report of an Inquiry by Sir William Macpherson of Cluny. Advised by Tom Cook, The Right Reverend Dr John Sentamu, Dr Richard Stone. Presented to Parliament by the Secretary of State for the Home Department by Command of Her Majesty: The Stationery Office; 1999.

36. UK Home Office. Home Office "Strength in Diversity" Agenda. http://wwwhomeofficeg-ovuk/documents/cons-strength-in-diverse-170904/ [serial on the Internet]. 2009: Available from: http://www.homeoffice.gov.uk/documents/cons-strength-in-diverse-170904/.

37. Thornicroft G, Rose D, Kassam A, Sartorius N. Stigma: ignorance, prejudice or discrimination? *Br J Psychiatry.* 2007;190:192–3.

38. Thornicroft G, Brohan E, Rose D, Sartorius N, Leese M. Global pattern of experienced and anticipated discrimination against people with schizophrenia: a cross-sectional survey. *Lancet.* 2009;373:408–15.

39. Lasalvia A, Zoppei S, Van BT, Bonetto C, Cristofalo D, Wahlbeck K, et al. Global pattern of experienced and anticipated discrimination reported by people with major depressive disorder: a cross-sectional survey. *Lancet.* 2013;381(9860):55–62.

40. King M, Dinos S, Shaw J, Watson R, Stevens S, Passetti F, et al. The Stigma Scale: development of a standardised measure of the stigma of mental illness. *Br J Psychiatry.* 2007;190(3):248–54.

41. World Health Organization. *WHO resource book on mental health, human rights and legislation.* Geneva: World Health Organization; 2005.

42. United Nations. *Convention on the Rights of Persons with Disabilities.* New York: United Nations; 2006.

43. Bartlett P, Lewis O, Thorold O. *Mental disability and the European Convention on Human Rights.* Leiden: Martinus Nijhoff; 2006.

44. ITHACA Study Group. *The ITHACA toolkit for monitoring human rights and general health care in mental health and social care institutions.* London: King's College London: http://www.ithacastudy.eu; 2011.

45. Council of Europe. *Recommendation CM/Rec (2009)3 of the Committee of Ministers to member states on monitoring the protection of human rights and dignity of persons with mental disorder.* Brussels: Council of Europe; 2009.

46. Drew N, Funk M, Tang S, Lamichhane J, Chavez E, Katontoka S, et al. Human rights violations of people with mental and psychosocial disabilities: an unresolved global crisis. *Lancet.* 2011;378(9803):1664–75.

47. Hunt P. *Economic, cultural and social rights. Report of the Special Rapporteur on the right of everyone to enjoyment of the highest attainable standard of physical and mental health.* Commission on Human Rights, 61st Session, Item 10 on the provisional agenda. New York: United Nations Economic and Social Council; 2005.

48. Hunt P, Mesquita J. Mental disabilities and the human right to the highest attainable standard of health. *Human Rights Q.* 2006;45:332–56.

49. Mental Disability Advocacy Center. *Building the architecture for change: Guidelines on Article 33 of the UN Convention on the Rights of Persons with Disabilities.* Budapest: Mental Disability Advocacy Centre (available at http://www.mdac.info/webfm_send/77); 2011.

50. Alem A, Jacobsson L, Araya M, Kebede D, Kullgren G. How are mental disorders seen and where is help sought in a rural Ethiopian community? A key informant study in Butajira, Ethiopia. *Acta Psychiatr Scand Suppl.* 1999;397:40–7.

51. Nsereko JR, Kizza D, Kigozi F, Ssebunnya J, Ndyanabangi S, Flisher AJ, et al. Stakeholder's perceptions of help-seeking behaviour among people with mental health problems in Uganda. *Int J Ment Health Syst.* 2011;5(1):1–9.

52. Ssebunnya J, Kigozi F, Lund C, Kizza D, Okello E. Stakeholder perceptions of mental health stigma and poverty in Uganda. *BMC International Health and Human Rights.* 2009;9(1):5.

53. Adewuya AO, Oguntade AA. Doctors' attitude towards people with mental illness in Western Nigeria. *Soc Psychiatry & Psychiatr Epidemiol.* 2007;42(11):931–6.

54. Thara R, Kamath S, Kumar S. Women with schizophrenia and broken marriages—doubly disadvantaged? Part I: patient perspective. *Int J Soc Psychiatry.* 2003;49(3):225–32.

55. Thara R, Kamath S, Kumar S. Women with schizophrenia and broken marriages—doubly disadvantaged? Part II: family perspective. *Int J Soc Psychiatry.* 2003;49(3):233–40.

56. Thara R, Srinivasan TN. How stigmatising is schizophrenia in India? *Int J Soc Psychiatry.* 2000;46(2):135–41.

57. Charles H, Manoranjitham SD, Jacob KS. Stigma and explanatory models among people with schizophrenia and their relatives in Vellore, south India. *Int J Soc Psychiatry.* 2007;53(4):325–32.

58. Kohrt BA, Harper I. Navigating diagnoses: understanding mind-body relations, mental health, and stigma in Nepal. *Culture, Med & Psychiatry.* 2008;32(4):462–91.

59. de Toledo Piza PE, Blay SL. Community perception of mental disorders—a systematic review of Latin American and Caribbean studies. *Soc Psychiatry Psychiatr Epidemiol.* 2004;39(12):955–61.

60. Henderson S, Stacey CL, Dohan D. Social stigma and the dilemmas of providing care to substance users in a safety-net emergency department. *J Health Care Poor Underserved.* 2008;19(4):1336–49.

61. Corrigan PW. The impact of stigma on severe mental illness. *Cognitive and Behavioral Practice.* 1998;5(2):201–22.

62. Corrigan PW, Watson A, Gracia G, Slopen N, Rasinski K, Hall L. Newspaper stories as a measure of structural stigma. *Psychiatr Serv.* 2005;56 (5):551–6.

63. Al-Krenawi A, Graham JR, Dean YZ, Eltaiba N. Cross-national study of attitudes towards seeking professional help: Jordan, United Arab Emirates (UAE) and Arabs in Israel. *Int J Soc Psychiatry.* 2004;50(2):102–14.

64. Vaughan G, Hansen C. "Like Minds, Like Mine": a New Zealand project to counter the stigma and discrimination associated with mental illness. *Australas Psychiatry.* 2004;12(2):113–7.

65. Lyons M, Ziviani J. Stereotypes, stigma, and mental illness: learning from fieldwork experiences. *Am J Occup Ther.* 1995;49(10):1002–8.

66. Link B, Phelan J, Bresnahan M, Stueve A, Moore R, Susser E. Lifetime and five-year prevalence of homelessness in the United States: new evidence on an old debate. *Am J Orthopsychiatry.* 1995;65(3):347–54.

67. Link B, Castille DM, Stuber J. Stigma and coercion in the context of outpatient treatment for people with mental illnesses. *Soc Sci Med.* 2008;67(3):409–19.

68. Link BG, Susser E, Stueve A, Phelan J, Moore RE, Struening E. Lifetime and five-year prevalence of homelessness in the United States. *Am J Public Health.* 1994;84(12):1907–12.

69. Link BG, Struening EL, Neese-Todd S, Asmussen S, Phelan JC. Stigma as a barrier to recovery: the consequences of stigma for the self-esteem of people with mental illnesses. *Psychiatr Serv.* 2001;52(12):1621–6.

70. Link BG. Understanding labeling effects in the area of mental disorders: an assessment of the effects of expectations of rejection. *Am Sociol Rev.* 1987;52:96–112.

71. Link BG, Yang LH, Phelan JC, Collins PY. Measuring mental illness stigma. *Schizophr Bull.* 2004;30(3):511–41.

72. Link BG, Struening EL, Rahav M, Phelan JC, Nuttbrock L. On stigma and its consequences: evidence from a longitudinal study of men with dual diagnoses of mental illness and substance abuse. *J Health Soc Behav.* 1997;38(2):177–90.

73. Link BG, Struening EL, Neese-Todd S, Asmussen S, Phelan JC. On describing and seeking to change the experience of stigma. *Psychiatr Rehabil Skills.* 2002;6(2):201–31.

74. Link BG, Cullen FT, Struening EL, Shrout PE, Dohrenwend BP. A modified labeling theory approach in the area of mental disorders: An empirical assessment. *Am Sociol Rev.* 1989;54:100–23.

75. Corrigan PW. Beat the stigma: come out of the closet. *Psychiatr Serv.* 2003;54(10):1313.

76. Corrigan P, Thompson V, Lambert D, Sangster Y, Noel JG, Campbell J. Perceptions of discrimination among persons with serious mental illness. *Psychiatr Serv.* 2003;54(8):1105–10.

77. Corrigan PW, Lundin R. *Don't call me nuts.* Tinley Par, IL: Recovery Press; 2001.

78. Corrigan PW, Markowitz FE, Watson A, Rowan D, Kubiak MA. An attribution model of public discrimination towards persons with mental illness. *J Health Soc Behav.* 2003;44(2):162–79.

79. Corrigan PW. How stigma interferes with mental health care. *Am Psychol.* 2004;59(7):614–25.

80. Corrigan PW, Gelb B. Three programs that use mass approaches to challenge the stigma of mental illness. *Psychiatr Serv.* 2006;57(3):393–8.

81. Estroff SE, Penn DL, Toporek JR. From stigma to discrimination: an analysis of community efforts to reduce the negative consequences of having a psychiatric disorder and label. *Schizophr Bull.* 2004;30(3):493–509.

82. Mehta N, Kassam A, Leese M, Butler G, Thornicroft G. Public attitudes towards people with mental illness in England and Scotland, 1994–2003. *Br J Psychiatry.* 2009;194(3):278–84.

83. Jacob KS, Sharan P, Mirza I, Garrido-Cumbrera M, Seedat S, Mari JJ, et al. Mental health systems in countries: where are we now? *Lancet.* 2007;370(9592):1061–77.

84. Shibre T, Negash A, Kullgren G, Kebede D, Alem A, Fekadu A, et al. Perception of stigma among family members of individuals with schizophrenia and major affective disorders in rural Ethiopia. *Soc Psychiatry Psychiatr Epidemiol.* 2001;36(6):299–303.

85. Crabb J, Stewart R, Kokota D, Masson N, Chabunya S, Krishnadas R. Attitudes towards mental illness in Malawi: a cross-sectional survey. *BMC Public Health.* 2012;12(1):541.

86. Thara R, Srinivasan TN. Outcome of marriage in schizophrenia. *Soc Psychiatry Psychiatr Epidemiol.* 1997;32(7):416–20.

87. Thara R, Kamath S, Kumar S. Women with schizophrenia and broken marriages—doubly disadvantaged? Part II: family perspective. *Int J Soc Psychiatry.* 2003;49(3):233–40.

88. Thara R, Srinivasan TN. Outcome of marriage in schizophrenia. *Soc Psychiatry Psychiatr Epidemiol.* 1997;32(7):416–20.

89. Raguram R, Raghu TM, Vounatsou P, Weiss MG. Schizophrenia and the cultural epidemiology of stigma in Bangalore, India. *J Nerv Ment Dis.* 2004;192(11):734–44.

90. Gureje O, Lasebikan V, Ephraim-Oluwanuga O, Olley BO, Kola, L. Community study of knowledge of and attitude to mental illness in Nigeria. *Br J Psychiatry.* 2005;186:436–41.

91. Kleinman A, Mechanic D. Some observations of mental illness and its treatment in the People's Republic of China. *J Nerv Ment Dis.* 1979;167(5):267–74.

92. Phillips MR, Pearson V, Li F, Xu M, Yang L. Stigma and expressed emotion: a study of people with schizophrenia and their family members in China. *Br J Psychiatry.* 2002;181:488–93.

93. Fabrega H, Jr. The culture and history of psychiatric stigma in early modern and modern Western societies: a review of recent literature. *Compr Psychiatry.* 1991;32(2):97–119.

94. Fabrega H, Jr. Psychiatric stigma in non-Western societies. *Compr Psychiatry.* 1991;32(6): 534–51.

95. Karim S, Saeed K, Rana MH, Mubbashar MH, Jenkins R. Pakistan mental health country profile. *Int Rev Psychiatry.* 2004;16(1–2):83–92.

96. Al-Krenawi A, Graham JR, Kandah J. Gendered utilization differences of mental health services in Jordan. *Community Ment Health J.* 2000;36(5):501–11.

97. Cinnirella M, Loewenthal KM. Religious and ethnic group influences on beliefs about mental illness: a qualitative interview study. *Br J Med Psychol.* 1999;72 (Pt 4):505–24.

98. Kadri N, Manoudi F, Berrada S, Moussaoui D. Stigma impact on Moroccan families of patients with schizophrenia. *Can J Psychiatry.* 2004;49(9):625–9.

99. Rusch N, Angermeyer MC, Corrigan PW. Mental illness stigma: concepts, consequences, and initiatives to reduce stigma. [Review] [106 refs]. *Eur Psychiatry.* 2005;20(8):529–39.

100. Jacoby A. Felt versus enacted stigma: a concept revisited. Evidence from a study of people with epilepsy in remission. *Soc Sci Med.* 1994;38(2):269–74.

101. Wahl OF, Kaye A. Mental illness topics in popular periodicals. *Community Ment Health J.* 1992;28(1):21–8.

102. Coverdale J, Nairn R, Claasen D. Depictions of mental illness in print media: a prospective national sample. *The Australian and New Zealand J psychiatry.* 2002;36(5):697–700.

103. Nairn R, Coverdale J, Claasen D. From source material to news story in New Zealand print media: a prospective study of the stigmatizing processes in depicting mental illness. *Aust N Z J Psychiatry.* 2001;35(5):654–9.

104. Williams M, Taylor J. Mental illness: media perpetuation of stigma. *Contemp Nurse.* 1995;4:41–6.

105. Day DM, Page S. Portrayal of mental illness in Canadian newspapers. *Can J Psychiatry.* 1986; 31(9):813–7.

106. Lawrie S. Newspaper coverage of psychiatric and physical illness. *Psychiatr Bull.* 2000;24: 104–6.

107. Corrigan PW, Watson AC, Gracia G, Slopen N, Rasinski K, Hall LL. Newspaper stories as measures of structural stigma. *Psychiatr Serv.* 2005;56(5):551–6.

108. Angermeyer MC, Schulze B. Reinforcing stereotypes: how the focus on forensic cases in news reporting may influence public attitudes towards the mentally ill. *Int J Law Psychiatry.* 2001; 24(4–5):469–86.

109. Angermeyer MC, Matschinger H. The effect of violent attacks by schizophrenic persons on the attitude of the public towards the mentally ill. *Soc Sci Med.* 1996;43(12):1721–8.

110. Goulden R, Corker E, Evans-Lacko S, Rose D, Thornicroft G, Henderson C. Newspaper coverage of mental illness in the U.K., 1992–2008. *BMC Public Health.* 2011;11:796.

111. Ssebunnya J, Kigozi F, Lund C, Kizza D, Okello E. Stakeholder perceptions of mental health stigma and poverty in Uganda. *BMC Int Health Hum Rights.* 2009;9:5.

112. Disability Rights Commission. *Equal treatment: Closing the gap. A formal investigation into physical health inequalities experienced by people with learning disabilities and/or mental health problems.* London: Disability Rights Commission; 2006.

113. Disability Rights Commission. *Equal rights: Closing the gap: The evidence base.* London: Disability Rights Commission; 2006.

114. Jones S, Howard L, Thornicroft G. "Diagnostic overshadowing": worse physical health care for people with mental illness. *Acta Psychiatr Scand.* 2008;118(3):169–71.

115. Desai MM, Rosenheck RA, Druss BG, Perlin JB. Mental disorders and quality of diabetes care in the Veterans Health Administration. *Am J Psychiatry.* 2002;159(9):1584–90.

116. Desai MM, Rosenheck RA, Druss BG, Perlin JB. Mental disorders and quality of care among post-acute myocardial infarction outpatients. *J Nerv Ment Dis.* 2002;190(1):51–3.

117. Gump BB, Matthews KA, Eberly LE, Chang YF. Depressive symptoms and mortality in men: results from the Multiple Risk Factor Intervention Trial. *Stroke.* 2005;36(1):98–102.

118. Dutta R, Murray RM, Allardyce J, Jones PB, Boydell JE. Mortality in first-contact psychosis patients in the U.K.: a cohort study. *Psychol Med.* 2012;42(8):1649–61.

119. Wahlbeck K, Westman J, Nordentoft M, Gissler M, Laursen TM. Outcomes of Nordic mental health systems: life expectancy of patients with mental disorders. *Br J Psychiatry.* 2011;199(6):453–8.

120. Thornicroft G. Physical health disparities and mental illness: the scandal of premature mortality. *Br J Psychiatry.* 2011;199:441–2.

121. Filipcic I, Pavicic D, Filipcic A, Hotujac L, Begic D, Grubisin J, et al. Attitudes of medical staff towards the psychiatric label "schizophrenic patient" tested by an anti-stigma questionnaire. *Coll Antropol.* 2003;27(1):301–7.

122. Druss BG. Cardiovascular procedures in patients with mental disorders. *JAMA.* 2000;283(24):3198–9.

123. Sullivan G, Han X, Moore S, Kotrla K. Disparities in hospitalization for diabetes among persons with and without co-occurring mental disorders. *Psychiatr Serv.* 2006;57:1126–31.

124. Amaddeo F, Jones J. What is the impact of socio-economic inequalities on the use of mental health services? *Epidemiol Psichiatr Soc.* 2007;16(1):16–9.

125. Cooper AE, Corrigan PW, Watson AC. Mental illness stigma and care seeking. *J Nerv Ment Dis.* 2003;191(5):339–41.

126. Compton MT, Kaslow NJ, Walker EF. Observations on parent/family factors that may influence the duration of untreated psychosis among African American first-episode schizophrenia-spectrum patients. *Schizophr Res.* 2004;68(2–3):373–85.

127. Wang PS, Aguilar-Gaxiola S, Alonso J, Angermeyer MC, Borges G, Bromet EJ, et al. Use of mental health services for anxiety, mood, and substance disorders in 17 countries in the WHO world mental health surveys. *Lancet.* 2007;370(9590):841–50.

128. Thornicroft G. Most people with mental illness are not treated. *Lancet.* 2007;370(9590):807–8.

129. Corrigan PW. *On the stigma of mental illness: Practical strategies for research and social change.* Washington, DC: American Psychological Association; 2004.

130. Kessler RC, Berglund PA, Bruce ML, Koch JR, Laska EM, Leaf PJ, et al. The prevalence and correlates of untreated serious mental illness. *Health Serv Res.* 2001;36(6 Pt 1):987–1007.

131. Link BG, Cullen FT, Struening EL, Shrout PE, Dohrenwend BP. A modified labeling theory approach in the area of mental disorders: an empirical assessment. *Am Sociol Rev.* 1989;54:100–23.

132. Schomerus G, Angermeyer MC. Stigma and its impact on help-seeking for mental disorders: what do we know? *Epidemiol Psichiatr Soc.* 2008;17(1):31–7.

133. Sirey JA, Bruce ML, Alexopoulos GS, Perlick DA, Friedman SJ, Meyers BS. Stigma as a barrier to recovery: perceived stigma and patient-rated severity of illness as predictors of antidepressant drug adherence. *Psychiatr Serv.* 2001;52(12):1615–20.

134. Saraceno B, Van OM, Batniji R, Cohen A, Gureje O, Mahoney J, et al. Barriers to improvement of mental health services in low-income and middle-income countries. *Lancet.* 2007;370(9593):1164–74.

135. Brohan E, Slade M, Clement S, Thornicroft G. Experiences of mental illness stigma, prejudice and discrimination: a review of measures. [Review]. *BMC Health Serv Res.* 2010;10:80.

136. Brohan E, Gauci D, Sartorius N, Thornicroft G. Self-stigma, empowerment and perceived discrimination among people with bipolar disorder or depression in 13 European countries: The GAMIAN-Europe study. *J Affect Disord.* 2011;129(1–3):56–63.

137. Brohan E, Elgie R, Sartorius N, Thornicroft G. Self-stigma, empowerment and perceived discrimination among people with schizophrenia in 14 European countries: the GAMIAN-Europe study. *Schizophr Res.* 2010;122(1–3):232–8.

138. Corrigan PW, Morris S, Michaels P, Rafacz J, Rusch N. Challenging the public stigma of mental illness: a meta-analysis of outcome studies. *Psychiatr Serv.* 2012;63(10):963–73.

139. Clement S, van NA, Kassam A, Flach C, Lazarus A, de CM, et al. Filmed vs. live social contact interventions to reduce stigma: randomised controlled trial. *Br J Psychiatry.* 2012;201: 57–64.

140. Queensland Alliance. *From discrimination to social inclusion. A review of the literature on anti stigma initiatives in mental health.* Australia: Queensland Alliance; 2009.

141. Wegner D, Erber R, Zanakos S. Ironic processes in the mental control of mood and mood-related thought. *J Pers Soc Psychol.* 1993;65:1093–104.

142. Macrae C, Bodenhausen G, Milne A. Out of mind but back in sight: stereotypes on the rebound. *J Pers Soc Psychol.* 1994;67:808–17.

143. Sibitz I, Unger A, Woppmann A, Zidek T, Amering M. Stigma resistance in patients with schizophrenia. *Schizophr Bull.* 2011;37(2):316–23.

144. Mittal D, Sullivan G, Chekuri L, Allee E, Corrigan PW. Empirical studies of self-stigma reduction strategies: a critical review of the literature. *Psychiatr Serv.* 2012;63(10):974–81.

145. Adler AB, Bliese PD, McGurk D, Hoge CW, Castro CA. Battlemind debriefing and battlemind training as early interventions with soldiers returning from Iraq: randomization by platoon. *J Consult Clin Psychol.* 2009;77(5):928–40.

146. Griffiths KM, Christensen H, Jorm AF, Evans K, Groves C. Effect of web-based depression literacy and cognitive-behavioural therapy interventions on stigmatising attitudes to depression: randomised controlled trial. *Br J Psychiatry.* 2004;185:342–9.

147. Shin SK, Lukens EP. Effects of psychoeducation for Korean Americans with chronic mental illness. *Psychiatr Serv (Washington, DC).* 2002;53(9):1125–31.

148. Lucksted A, Drapalski A, Calmes C, Forbes C, DeForge B, Boyd J. Ending self-stigma: pilot evaluation of a new intervention to reduce internalized stigma among people with mental illnesses. *Psychiatr Rehabil J.* 2011;35(1):51–4.

149. Wade NG, Post BC, Cornish MA, Vogel DL, Tucker JR. Predictors of the change in self-stigma following a single session of group counseling. *J Couns Psychol.* 2011;58(2):170–82.

150. MacInnes DL, Lewis M. The evaluation of a short group programme to reduce self-stigma in people with serious and enduring mental health problems. *J Psychiatr & Ment Health Nurs.* 2008;15(1):59–65.

151. Luoma J, Kohlenberg B, Hayes S, Bunting K, Rye A. Reducing self-stigma in substance abuse through acceptance and commitment therapy: model, manual development and pilot outcomes. *Addict Res Theory.* 2008;16:149–65.

152. Hammer J, Vogel D. Men's help seeking for depression: the efficacy of a male-sensitive brochure about counseling. *Couns Psychol.* 2010;38(296):313.

153. Thornicroft G, Brohan E, Kassam A, Lewis-Holmes E. Reducing stigma and discrimination: candidate interventions. *Int J Ment Health Syst.* 2008;2:doi:10.1186/752–4458-2-3.

154. Kakuma R, Kleintjes S, Lund C, Drew N, Green A, Flisher AJ, et al. Mental health stigma: What is being done to raise awareness and reduce stigma in South Africa? *Afr J Psychiatry.* 2010;13: 116–24.

155. Henderson C, Thornicroft G. Stigma and discrimination in mental illness: Time to Change. *Lancet.* 2009;373(9679):1928–30.

156. Armstrong G, Kermode M, Raja S, Suja S, Chandra P, Jorm AF. A mental health training program for community health workers in India: impact on knowledge and attitudes. *Int J Ment Health Syst.* 2011;5(1):17.

157. Pinfold V, Thornicroft G, Huxley P, Farmer P. Active ingredients in anti-stigma programmes in mental health. *Int Rev Psychiatry.* 2005;17(2):123–31.

158. Pinfold V, Huxley P, Thornicroft G, Farmer P, Toulmin H, Graham T. Reducing psychiatric stigma and discrimination—evaluating an educational intervention with the police force in England. *Soc Psychiatry & Psychiatr Epidemiol.* 2003;38(6):337–44.

159. Pinfold V, Toulmin H, Thornicroft G, Huxley P, Farmer P, Graham T. Reducing psychiatric stigma and discrimination: evaluation of educational interventions in U.K. secondary schools. *Br J Psychiatry.* 2003;182:342–6.

160. Pinfold V, Huxley P, Thornicroft G, Farmer P, Toulmin H, Graham T. Reducing psychiatric stigma and discrimination—evaluating an educational intervention with the police force in England. *Soc Psychiatry Psychiatr Epidemiol.* 2003;38(6):337–44.

161. Eaton J, Agomoh AO. Developing mental health services in Nigeria: the impact of a community-based mental health awareness programme. *Soc Psychiatry Psychiatr Epidemiol.* 2008;43(7):552–8.

162. Perlick DA, Nelson AH, Mattias K, Selzer J, Kalvin C, Wilber CH, et al. In our own voice-family companion: reducing self-stigma of family members of persons with serious mental illness. *Psychiatr Serv.* 2011;62(12):1456–62.

163. Eaton J, McCay L, Semrau M, Chatterjee S, Baingana F, Araya R, et al. Scale up of services for mental health in low-income and middle-income countries. *Lancet*. 2011;378(9802):1592–603.

164. World Health Organization. *World Mental Health Day*. 2012 [updated 2012; cited 10/23/2012]; available from: http://www.who.int/mediacentre/events/annual/world_mental_health_day/en/index.html.

165. Department for International Development. *Programme for Improving Mental Health Care (PRIME)*. 2012 [updated 2012; cited 10/23/2012]; available from: http://www.dfid.gov.uk/R4D/Project/60851/Default.aspx?utm_source=email&utm_medium=newsletter&utm_campaign=April2012newsletter.

166. Grand Challenges Canada. *Global Mental Health*. 2012 [updated 2012; cited 10/23/2012]; available from: http://www.grandchallenges.ca/grand-challenges/gc4-non-communicable-diseases/mentalhealth/.

19 Research Priorities, Capacity, and Networks in Global Mental Health

Pamela Y. Collins, Mark Tomlinson,
Ritsuko Kakuma, Jude Awuba, and
Harry Minas

INTRODUCTION

An article in the *Jakarta Post* informed Indonesian readers about one of the most severe forms of human rights abuses for people with mental illness.[1,2] The reporter wrote:

Eradicating the practice of *pasung*, or shackling the mentally ill, in Central Java is ambitious, but can be done, according to a top official. "The target of zero shackling cases by 2012 can be achieved if data on victims can be gathered properly," Central Java Deputy Governor Rustriningsih said.... According to the Central Java Health Agency, the reported number of people shackled in the province was 458 as of September 2011. "After data on patients has been collected through *puskesmas* [community health centres] and social offices in the respective districts, only then can we fetch them," she said. Families sometimes regarded [mental illness] as a disgrace to be hidden, leading them to confine their relatives. A person who is shackled is typically bound to a long wooden plank, although others are confined to a single room or place.[1]

Thousands of miles around the globe, Bridget O'Shea wrote of the Midwestern state of Illinois in the United States:

The sounds of chaos bounce off the dim yellow walls. Everywhere there are prisoners wearing orange, red, and khaki jumpsuits. An officer barks out orders as a thin woman tries to sleep on a hard bench in a holding cell. This is a harsh scene of daily life inside what has become the state's largest de facto mental institution: the Cook County Jail. Of the 11,000 prisoners awaiting trial and serving sentences for crimes committed, Cook County Sheriff, Tom Dart, estimated that about 2000 of them suffer from some form of serious mental illness, far more than at the big state-owned Elgin Mental Health Center, which has 582 beds.

O'Shea explains, "The city [Chicago] plans to shut down 6 of its 12 mental health centers by the end of April, to save an estimated $2 million.... Not treating people with mental illness is bad enough, but treating them like criminals? Please, what have we become?"[3]

These two stories highlight practices that interfere with provision of safe, effective, quality mental health services in two very different contexts: a lower-middle-income country where lack of resources and community mental health services contributes to abuses, and a wealthy country where limited resources allocated to mental health similarly lead to inhumane treatment. Stories such as these raise the question of whether and how research can be relevant when the need for greater resources for better services seems so apparent. Research plays a central role. In the Indonesian example, the article describes a practice on which, until recently, there had been very little research or policy guidance about how to eradicate the practice throughout Indonesia.[2] Policy success depends upon research on the prevalence and determinants of shackling, as well as evaluation of the effectiveness of interventions and the implementation of the policy. The Central Java Health Agency official gives precise numbers of people who have been subjected to the practice of *pasung* and reports how mental health service officials have responded. She makes a clear link between data collection and capacity to respond effectively. Similarly, in the North American example, health services researchers can play a role in aiding state health systems to solve the problems of effective linkage to efficient care interventions.

   This chapter will examine the role of research in global mental health, with a focus on low-resource settings around the world. Many of our examples come from low- and middle-income countries (LMICs) in an attempt to highlight recent data and research developments emerging from these settings. We will demonstrate the need to integrate research and research capacity building across the spectrum of research activities. Our discussion rests on several assumptions. First, mental health research covers a vast array of activities, including, but not limited to, basic neuroscience, genomics, type 1 translational studies that link basic science discoveries to clinically relevant interventions, implementation and dissemination research, as well as studies of mental health policy and health economics. The research examples in this chapter primarily feature one segment of the research enterprise: implementation and dissemination research. The translation of research findings to public health practice and policy occurs through these activities, and targeted research capacity-building efforts in these areas may multiply the public health impact of science. Second, the desired endpoint of mental health research around the world is the improvement of mental health outcomes in individuals and communities. The conduct of research and the development of research capacity are integral to this process. Third, achieving this desired endpoint requires an understanding of the processes and consequences of global health research priority setting within and outside of the mental health arena.

   This chapter explores the role of research: why research should be central to global mental health activities; research capacity building, a prerequisite for a research program (i.e., how we define it and the resources required to support robust, sustainable scientific activities); research priority-setting: how stakeholders determine research priorities and the implications of these activities; and uptake and demand for research: how research is implemented and translated to practice (i.e., what efforts ensure that research priorities can best meet local needs).

WHY IS RESEARCH IMPORTANT TO GLOBAL MENTAL HEALTH?

Conducting basic research, translating it into the development of new health tools, and delivering products to patients in need of them are core functions of an effective global health system.[4]

Research is an integral part of global health.[4] A functioning global health system generates knowledge through discovery research; identification of intervention targets; and the development, testing, implementation, and scale-up of effective interventions. This issue has gained importance in tandem with growing investments in global health; in fact, the World Health Organization selected the topic as a focus for its 2012 World Health Report, "No Health Without Research." More than 20 years ago, the Commission on Health Research for Development put forth the argument for conducting research globally with equitable inclusion of LMICs. The report articulated four reasons for research. First, research guides action, thereby minimizing the likelihood of wasteful and ineffective activity for organizations and for individual health. Research findings can fruitfully shape health policies and health system strategies. Second, research leads to the development of new tools to fight disease. In the context of mental health, a pertinent example is that research has established a set of effective evidence-based psychotherapies for depression and has demonstrated their effectiveness in vastly different sociocultural settings. Third, research enables effective planning and judicious use of resources. Global research efforts are particularly valuable in this respect, as effective, low-cost interventions developed in one country can be disseminated and lead to savings for many countries. Fourth, research contributes to development. Societies that cultivate a culture of science and problem-solving enhance their capabilities for discovering and implementing solutions to existing problems and anticipating new ones.

Despite the clearly articulated benefits of global health research, the Commission highlighted the striking scarcity of research investments in LMICs. Greater research investments have occurred in high-income countries, and limited investment in lower-income countries may have contributed to the ongoing health problems specific to these settings, and, in some cases, to vulnerable communities in high-income countries. The Commission report confirmed that, where disease burden was greatest, the conduct of research was minimal, even though research is crucial for addressing equity in development.

Mental health research investments in LMICs largely reflect this disparity; i.e., research funding is low despite the significant disease burden attributable to mental disorders. To date, the most comprehensive study on mental health research workforce activities in LMICs was conducted in 2004 by the Global Forum for Health Research and the WHO. The investigators surveyed and categorized mental health researchers in 114 LMICs based on gender, age, profession, work place, and training.[5] A significant proportion of the research workforce in LMICs were academics or clinicians or professionals acting in both capacities, but the majority of the participating countries contributed few research products to the broader scientific community. Only six countries stood out among the others as significant producers of research.

Whereas financial data on mental health research expenditures may not be readily available in every country, research publications indicate, to some degree, the availability of support for research. In general, mental health research publications from LMICs make up a small proportion of the total research output on mental health from the world.[6] Databases from the Institute of Scientific Information (ISI) and Medline contained no psychiatric journals from low-income countries as recently as 2007, and only 4.1% of journals were from upper-middle-income countries.[7]

PREREQUISITES FOR RESEARCH: BUILDING CAPACITY AND IDENTIFYING RESOURCES IN LOW-RESOURCE SETTINGS

A cadre of researchers, capacity building, enabling environments for researchers, functioning research infrastructure, and sustained research funding provide the foundations for successful national research programs. A mental health research workforce is critical for conducting the research necessary to guide policy development, program planning, and the provision of mental health services.[8]

Human Resources and Capacity Building

Research capacity is the "ongoing process of empowering individuals, institutions, organizations and nations to: (1) define and prioritize problems systematically; (2) develop and scientifically evaluate appropriate solutions; and (3) share and apply the knowledge generated."[9] Importantly, research capacity does not end with the ability to secure funding, conduct research, and publish the findings; rather, the task extends to equipping investigators with the skills to apply their findings in policy and practice contexts.[10]

In a review of research capacity-building for global mental health, Thornicroft and colleagues note that the lack of mental health research output in the majority of LMICs can be related to the shortage of mental health professionals, lack of graduate programs, and the fact that research and education are "additional" activities to clinical work.[10] Other obstacles include limited funding for mental health research, a lack of individual- and institutional-level research capacities, limited trained mental health research personnel, and inadequate infrastructural support and research networks.[11]

The barriers to optimal research capacity require intervention at multiple levels. Strategies aimed at individuals, institutions, and nations typically depend upon one another to produce a sustainable research infrastructure. Common approaches include *targeted capacity development* initiatives, which refer to initiatives that solely focus on building research capabilities; and *integrated capacity development*, in which training activities occur within the context of development or research programs.

Targeted Capacity Development Initiatives

Over the past decade, greater investment in training researchers has boosted the development of mental health research in low-resource settings. Programs such as the Universidade Nova de Lisboa's International Master's on Mental Health Policy and Services draw students from the Americas, Asia, Africa, Europe, and the Middle East. The curriculum's focus on policy, planning, and program development and implementation, as well as organization of services, is accompanied by training in research methods. Funders in the United States, United Kingdom, Portugal, and Canada, to name a few, support programs that enable trainees from countries with less research infrastructure to train in research intensive settings in middle- or high-income countries. Programs supported by the U.S. National Institutes of Health enable U.S. universities to host and train mental health researchers from China, Indonesia, Vietnam, and other settings; however, increasingly, funds support training activities based in LMICs that benefit others in their region. Targeted capacity-building activities range from short, intensive courses to longer degree-granting programs for master's and doctoral students. In these contexts, balanced training efforts should include support and training in scientific writing skills, translating research results into policy, public speaking, presentations, and dissemination of research.[12] Training opportunities are not limited to LMIC investigators. A growing number of HIC mental health research trainees seek careers focused on global communities. Training opportunities are increasing in both LMICs and HICs. (Please see Box 19.1 for examples of selected programs.)

Box 19.1 Examples of Existing Initiatives/Programs in Research Capacity Strengthening in Mental Health

- International Mental Health Leadership Program—Melbourne, Australia (http://www.cimh.unimelb.edu.au/pdp/imhlp)
- International Mental Health Research—Methods and Applications, London School of Hygiene and Tropical Medicine / Institute of Psychiatry (http://www.lshtm.ac.uk/prospectus/short/simh.html)
- Leadership in Mental Health—Goa, India (http://www.sangath.com/sangath/files/otherpdfs/leadership_in_mental_health_course_announcement_for_registration.pdf)
- Leadership in Mental Health—Ibadan, Nigeria http://mhlap.org/
- International Master on Mental Health Policy and Services, Lisbon (http://www.fcm.unl.pt/gepg/index.php?option=com_content&task=view&id=400&Itemid=420)
- Interdisciplinary Postgraduate Training in Mental Health Policy and Economics Research—Venice, Italy (http://www.icmpe.org/test1/training/index.htm)
- International Diploma in Mental Health Law and Human Rights (http://www.mentalhealthlaw.in/)
- University of Cape Town–Stellenbosch University Joint Postgraduate Diploma and Master's (Mphil) degree in Public Mental Health (http://www.cpmh.org.za)
- Global Mental Health: Trauma and Recovery Training Programme—Orvieto, Italy (http://hprt-cambridge.org/?page_id=31)
- Global Mental Health: Methods and Applications, London School of Hygiene and Tropical Medicine, London, U.K. (Centre for Global Mental Health) (http://www.centreforglobalmentalhealth.org/msc)
- Masters of Science in Global Mental Health, Centre for Global Mental Health, London, U.K. (http://www.centreforglobalmentalhealth.org/)
- Master of Science in Global Mental Health, University of Glasgow, Scotland (http://www.gla.ac.uk/postgraduate/taught/globalmentalhealth/)
- Columbia University Global Mental Health Post-Doctoral Fellowship (http://columbiapsychiatry.org/research/global_mental_health)
- Massachusetts General Hospital Chester Pierce Department of Global Mental Health Fellowship Program (http://www.mghglobalpsychiatry.org/our-work/postdoctoral_training.html)
- Expanded from Thornicroft et al.[10]

Integrated Capacity Development

Capacity development activities are often integrated within research or development projects. Also known as "learn by doing" approaches,[9] they may support research staff in obtaining graduate degrees and include opportunities for co-learning by mentors and protégés. The mental health system development program of the Centre for International Mental Health at the University of Melbourne is an integrated program of capacity-building, combining training and research with mental health system development projects in the context of continuing collaboration and partnerships.[13–15]

Although integrated research capacity development frequently occurs in university settings, a minority of global mental health non-governmental organizations also conduct research and train potential investigators. The Institute for Development, Research, Advocacy and Applied Care provides one such example.[16] The organization, dedicated to mental health in Lebanon and the Arab world, trains physicians, psychologists, and public health professionals in research and survey methods through coursework in epidemiology and biostatistics and through participation in ongoing clinical studies, treatment trials, and population studies. Mentors tailor a program of research training to the needs and level of experience of individual trainees, with a goal of developing principal investigators.

The Mental Health and Poverty Project program of research funded by the U.K. Department for International Development (DFID), also provides an example of "learning by doing" approaches. The project aimed to evaluate mental health care systems in Ghana, Uganda, South Africa, and Zambia; assist in the development and implementation of mental health policies in those countries; and evaluate policy implementation. The MHaPP team investigated strategies for making mental health care accessible to poor communities through primary health care and non-health sectors.[17–21] Each of the academic institutions in the four countries partnered with their respective ministries of health to harmonize the research with country priorities and also collaborated with WHO and the University of Leeds for technical assistance.

MHaPP integrated capacity development into its overall program, and partners engaged in a range of training activities, beginning with identification of training and development needs. Capacity development activities—linked to specific research activities—included workshops on designing instruments, semi-structured interview skills, qualitative data analysis, academic writing for peer review publication, and other communication skills (policy briefs, press releases, etc.). MHaPP members made special efforts to enable all Consortium members (principal investigators [PIs], research officers, and ministry partners) to publish as first authors in peer-review journals and also actively sought opportunities to publish special journal issues (e.g., *African Journal of Psychiatry*, *International Review of Psychiatry*) that focused on MHaPP outputs.

Thornicroft and colleagues suggest a series of stages of research capacity development that can occur in targeted or integrated programs.[10] First, an introduction to research allows non-researchers (e.g., clinicians and health policy workers) to learn about the existence and uses of the evidence base. Second, these students learn about the work of research teams by attending research symposia or other activities where research results are shared. Third, learners with an interest in mental health research can benefit from short courses that provide training in research methods, leadership, fundraising, and delivering scientific presentations, and equip participants with other relevant transferable skills. Fourth, students may enroll in master's degree programs that deepen and broaden their set of transferable research relevant skills. Next, a subset of these students may opt to pursue pre-doctoral or doctoral fellowships in order to pursue a Ph.D. Finally, postdoctoral researchers learn to lead smaller projects and develop grant applications for such studies while also participating as co-investigators on larger studies.

Identification, Recruitment, and Retention of Researchers

In concert with building capacity, institutions must recruit and retain human resources in order to create a research workforce. Outreach efforts that target both potential researchers and existing investigators at various career levels can create a pipeline for the workforce in biomedical and behavioral research.[22] Such efforts must target and recruit promising researchers in a transparent and competitive selection process with appropriate gender balance and other considerations relevant to each context (e.g., ethnic diversity, social economic diversity), but resources for sustaining a career must be available.

The "brain drain" poses complicated training and retention questions for the research community in LMICs. In LMICs, where research budgets are not allocated to finance researchers' salaries, many researchers work as volunteers. Institutional and systemic capacities to support research careers are therefore essential in order to minimize brain drain. Initiatives such as the Medical Education Partnership Initiative (MEPI), funded by the NIH and the President's Emergency Fund for AIDS Relief (PEPFAR), afford some opportunities for clinical training in psychiatry as well as research training, thus attracting students to the mental health field and offering professional development options that may increase retention.

Additional factors play a role in retention and success: the ability of trainees to utilize and access resources, to develop a sense of efficacy and competence in academics, and to acquire skills (e.g., time management, productive work habits, and research writing and presentation abilities) that develop one as a scientist.[23] Mentors help trainees to navigate the terrain. They demonstrate that one attains writing skills and presentation skills with practice; they provide trainees with a "roadmap" of a research career and help to correct naïve assumptions and enable them to assess the costs and benefits of pursuing various career directions.[23] University of Zimbabwe's MEPI-supported mental health program, Improving Mental Health Education and Research Capacity in Zimbabwe (IMHERZ), pairs trainees with mentoring teams—a locally based mentor and an international mentor—for career development.

However, the limited number of available mentors for the large number of young scientists that need mentors, and the lack of protected time allocated to mentorship, impede career development in many areas.[24] In many LMICs, the dearth of researchers translates to a dearth of mentors. A corresponding need exists in HICs: fewer potential mentors exist for trainees dedicated to research in global contexts. In both of these situations, "geographic and intellectual isolation" that can result from being at an institution or in a region where no researchers who share one's interests reside underscores the importance of mentors.[25]

Without appropriate incentives, effective mentorship is difficult to implement and maintain. In HICs, researchers can receive concrete benefits for mentoring students through increased scientific publications and assistance with grant writing, thus contributing towards faculty members' career development and advancement. Similar incentives are not always present in many academic institutions in LMICs, and more often than not, research and mentorship create demands in addition to heavy clinical and administrative responsibilities.

An additional problem occurs globally in settings that lack research intensive institutions: senior faculty members may also require mentoring in order to be able to secure grants from national or international funders. Thus, the individuals who are expected to develop strong research programs in their institutions may not have been exposed to the kinds of training that their junior colleagues seek and need. In this context, collaborative relationships with experienced partners can provide some benefits. Box 19.2 identifies relevant lessons from the MHaPP program.

Partnerships and Networks

The connections of people through formal and informal channels, diaspora communities, virtual global networks and professional communities of shared interests are important drivers of international collaboration. Yet little is understood about the movements and networks of scientists and what they mean for global science.[26]

For both targeted and integrated capacity-building activities, various forms of partnerships (e.g., international, interdisciplinary, or intersectoral) play a key role. Institutional partnerships between LMICs and HICs provide platforms for developing individual research capacity; however, their benefits extend beyond individual trainees, as they increase exposure to new methodologies, ideas, technical expertise, and sustainable

---

Box 19.2 Lessons Learned From International Research Capacity-Building Initiatives in LMICs

- Train senior and junior investigators—senior investigators may need updated training as well as new skills for seeking funding from a variety of agencies.
- Build skills that are career phase-specific.
- Use diverse methods for international communication: email, teleconferences, Skype, face-to-face meetings.
- Stimulate site visits between research centers.
- Identify a lead person at each site who is responsible for local capacity development and is a liaison with other network members.
- Adopt train-the-trainer approaches so that local staff can provide ongoing training and support to team members.
- Implement an online journal club to discuss and critique key articles.
- Identify specific strengths of each partner that can be shared with the rest of the collaborative group.
- Provide opportunities for junior staff to practice key skills (e.g.. oral presentations, poster presentations, grant applications) and receive feedback from peers and senior staff.

Adapted from Thornicroft et al.[10]

---

funding.[9] National and international collaborations to produce research networks, and Centers of Excellence constitute an additional platform for capacity building and fundraising. Centers frequently provide opportunities for fellowships, exposure to research grant writing, and numerous collaborative possibilities. Recently, the U.S. National Institute of Mental Health (NIMH) funded a new initiative, Collaborative Hubs for International Research on Mental Health in Low- and Middle-Income Countries (CHIRMH), through which international partnerships both amongst LMICs and between LMICs and HICs will strengthen mental health research capacity in LMICs at individual and institutional levels. HICs also stand to benefit from such partnerships. HICs also face shortages of mental health specialists and inequitable access to services across communities. These countries, like their low-income partners, seek innovative strategies to provide cost-effective and equitable care. Given their increasingly culturally diverse communities and in-country inequities, international research collaborations could provide opportunities for HIC researchers to build and utilize an evidence base that may extend efficient, effective, culturally appropriate, and equitable services in their own countries. Furthermore, such collaborations support the training of global mental health researchers in HICs. The increasing number of HIC research centers focusing on global mental health will not be sustainable without ongoing successful collaborations with colleagues in LMIC settings.

As collaborative relationships increasingly span great distances, members of research partnerships, mentoring dyads, and others utilize networks to sustain connections. A "network" exists when two or more elements (people, groups, organizations, or databases) are connected for some purpose that is larger or more complex than either could manage on their own.[27] Ideally, research networks link groups of people by common goals, making use of personal relations and ties of mutual interest, sharing, reciprocity, and trust. Links may occur through coordination meetings, conferences, newsletters, and joint projects. Individuals, groups, teams, or organizations form the nodes of the network. They are global (e.g., Global Network for Research in Mental and Neurological Health,), regional (e.g., European Observatory on Health Systems and Policies), and national (e.g., Indian Council for Medical Research). Technology plays a critical role and enables network activities to occur virtually (through email and other means) as well as supporting face-to-face encounters.[27]

At the global level, networks contribute to transnational cooperative activities such as priority setting and advocacy to support global mental health research. Global research networks such as the Council on Health Research for Development harmonize national and donor priorities to ensure that global support addresses country/regional specific needs and strengthens local research capacity.[28] Regional research networks interface with national and global networks and serve as platforms for advocating regional and national research priorities to the funders, policymakers, and the research community. At the national level, networks may form from the need to better define and strengthen national priorities and coordinate research efforts.

Networks can advance and improve research by bringing together a wide range of stakeholders (e.g., research institutions, policymakers, civil society organizations, medical research councils, business organizations, and donors) whose broad representation and participation is critical for building public consensus on research priorities, support for its practice, and trust in its findings and implications.[26] In this way, networks also help narrow the gulf between research and practice and facilitate the uptake of research findings. Ultimately, networks can be useful for strengthening collaboration and galvanizing the efforts of multiple stakeholders towards the advancement of research for public benefit. One such network, the International Observatory on Mental Health Systems,[13] builds the capacity of member countries to track mental health system performance in order to provide evidence-based advice to policy makers, service planners, and implementers.

The ASEAN Mental Health Taskforce

Member states of the Association of Southeast Asian Nations (ASEAN) endorsed the region's Strategic Framework for Health Development (2010–2015) in 2010. Mental health is included under the Framework section, "Promote ASEAN Health Lifestyle." An ASEAN meeting on mental health held in June 2011 led to the establishment of the ASEAN Mental Health Taskforce and the development of a Taskforce work plan. The mission of the Taskforce is to strengthen mental health in ASEAN and promote cooperation among ASEAN member states. The objectives of the Taskforce work plan are to strengthen collaboration on mental health to promote healthy lifestyles; promote effective, affordable, accessible, and sustainable mental health services and sharing of lessons learned and best practices; to generate and share mental health information and research; and to enhance human resource development in mental health prevention, promotion, treatment, and rehabilitation within ASEAN member states.

Research figures among the strategies identified to achieve the objectives of the work plan: develop ASEAN policy advocacy on mental health; facilitate the integration of mental health into the health care system and strengthen capacity building; facilitate and strengthen the mental health data information system, knowledge management, and research among ASEAN member states; and establish an ASEAN Network on mental health.

The ASEAN Mental Health Taskforce provides a clear policy-relevant and policy-led opportunity to develop and evaluate current programs, develop strategies to integrate mental health into general health care, and to strengthen capacity of researchers and decision makers at individual and organizational levels. The Taskforce is an inter-governmental body, endorsed by the health ministers of the ten ASEAN member states, with Taskforce members appointed by ministries of health. The research that has been incorporated into the Taskforce work plan is already identified as being both important and relevant by the ministries of the member states. The Taskforce, therefore, has the possibility of very closely linking research, policy development and implementation, and mental health service development.

Monitoring and Evaluating Capacity Building Activities

After the elements for developing capacity have been established, how can outcomes for capacity building be evaluated? Can initiatives for strengthening research capacity be evidence-based? How have existing training programs affected the career trajectories of the trainees thereafter? Systematic monitoring and evaluation of capacity building allows program implementers to assess whether the objectives of the capacity building activities have been achieved and to maximize the sustainability of effective capacity building strategies.

Intended outcomes should be determined prior to initiating training activities. These could include authorship of peer-reviewed publications, number of conference presentations, number of successful research grants, multiplier funds generated for mental health research, researchers trained in mental health research methods, linkages with other regional health research capacity training programs, support for mental health research by public health institutions, establishment of mental health research courses in each country, establishment of new collaborations between network partners, and the use of research by decision makers and other stakeholders.[10]

In 2011 ESSENCE on Health Research, a network of funding agencies working together to harmonize their programs and monitoring and evaluation (M&E) strategies, published a M&E framework for health research capacity development that includes a set of indicators to assess activities, outputs, and outcomes at the individual, organizational, and national-regional research system levels.[29] The Canadian Academy of Health Sciences has also developed a framework that outlines specific indicators for evaluating the impact of investing in health research.[30] Although these frameworks (like many other such frameworks) were developed through methods such as review of the literature and consensus among panel members, they have yet to be validated, particularly in LMIC contexts. Indicators such as numbers of academic outputs, involvement with grant applications, training programs, available resources, and number of partnerships in LMICs may reflect only part of the available research capacity.[10] In addition to simply reporting numbers of products (such as published manuscripts), time-dependent measures such as shifts in roles to first author on manuscripts or principal investigator on grant applications; increase in teaching, supervisory, and mentorship roles; and change in confidence to conduct research and publish papers must also be captured. Furthermore, if we want to examine the impact of research on policy and practice, then other indicators, such as the ability to engage in policy dialogue, participation, and presentation of key findings in ministry meetings, and perspectives of stakeholders on research findings must also be assessed.

Financial Resources

Globally, investment in research and development remained stable at around 1.7% of gross domestic product (GDP) between 2002 and 2007, but the actual amount of money invested grew by 45%.[31] The "emerging developing countries"—Brazil, India, China, Mexico, and South Africa—are among those increasing research investments, but significant variation across countries persists. In China, accompanying growing investment is a growing number of researchers, placing the country squarely among the "Big Five" (U.S., EU, China, Japan, and Russia) that account for 35% of the world's population but 75% of its researchers. By contrast, all of Africa and Latin America combined contribute 5.7% of the world's researchers. Gross expenditures on research and development in Latin America and the Caribbean constituted just 0.68% of GDP in 2006, and less than 2% of global spending.

Respondents to the WHO mapping study of mental health research identified lack of funding as a key challenge for researchers.[5] A sustainable and diversified funding stream should support every budding research program. A diverse set of funders (e.g., institutional, private, corporate, bilateral, and multilateral donors) and types of grants (e.g., reentry, seed, and travel grants; core funding; competitive fellowships) can provide individuals and institutions a range of options to cover the human, infrastructure, and administrative costs associated with research. Development agencies may be one source of funding for research activities that are integrated into larger efforts to implement mental health services. Two projects supported by the Swedish International Development Cooperation Agency (SIDA) since 2010 examine barriers to mental health care in Rwanda and the right to health care for people with mental illness in South Africa. One particularly important funding strategy is resource concentration; i.e., creation of a critical mass of researchers who have the ability then to carry out research, compete for funds, and train and mentor research students and early career researchers.[15] A resource concentration strategy supports both individual and institutional capacity building.

National funding agencies and multilateral organizations are investing significantly in global health research capacity building. Increasingly, middle-income countries like Brazil are developing robust national research programs that include investment in mental health research. A decade ago, Brazil committed about US$101 million to health research, with US$3.4 million invested in mental health research.[32] The São Paulo State Funding Agency and the Ministry of Education provided the bulk of these resources. From 1998 to 2002, 37 new trainees in areas of mental health received doctoral degrees each year, and a total of 481 theses were published. Mental health investigators published 637 scientific manuscripts in ISI-indexed journals, demonstrating a doubling in publications over previous years, most likely due to a stronger research orientation in postgraduate health programs. Ten years later, Brazil has taken further steps to increase scientific collaboration with international researchers, including in mental health relevant fields such as neuroscience.[33] The Science Without Borders Program sponsored by the National Council for Scientific and Technological Development, under the Ministry of Science and Technology (CNPq/MCT), aims to permit Brazilian scientists access to leading research institutions around the world while simultaneously encouraging young international investigators and well-established researchers to conduct research and training in Brazil. These collaborative research activities within Brazil are meant to generate well-trained scientists at various stages of development (i.e., from undergraduate to postdoctoral).

The U.K. Department for International Development (DFID) Research Programme Consortiums mandate allocation of a specified amount of time and funding towards research capacity building and dissemination activities.[34] The Wellcome Trust's African Institutions Initiative supports research capacity in 50 African institutions from 18 countries partnered in several international pan-African consortia. The WHO Alliance for Health Policy and Systems Research supports LMIC capacity building that focuses on application of research evidence into policy and practice.[35] Both North-South and South-South research partnerships figure greatly in strengthening capacities.[26] The research programs generated through these efforts could potentially serve as platforms for mental health research in the future. The Wellcome Trust and Canada's Global Health Research Initiative also invest in individual investigators from LMICs through scholarships and career phase–appropriate fellowships.

In tandem with opportunities for LMIC investigators, career development funding for HIC investigators interested in global mental health is also on the rise. Over the past two years, NIMH has, in collaboration with the Fogarty International Center at the NIH, worked to identify, convene, and support a cadre of young researchers interested in global mental health through workshops. To the best of our knowledge, in 2010, NIMH convened the first meeting in North America of students and early-career researchers (ranging from undergraduates to junior faculty members) with an interest in global mental health. The group heard the stories of career trajectories, the challenges of collaborations, the importance of mentorship, and opportunities for gaining experience from investigators at the start of their careers as well as those more senior. They interacted with NIMH staff, directors of nascent global mental health training programs in academic centers, and representatives of global health non-governmental organizations conducting mental health research in LMICs. The participants discussed the identified gaps in the established funding mechanisms for research training that created barriers to a sustainable research career focused on global mental health questions. Participants also discussed the need for research experiences in LMICs and the challenges of finding resources to support these opportunities.

In response to these concerns, NIMH took steps to help support a new cadre of global mental health investigators through actions that provided *access to information* about funding through the establishment of an electronic newsletter, "Global Tracks"; *more funding opportunities* for young researchers through collaborative funding with the Fogarty International Center and by supporting new postdoctoral global mental health training programs at U.S. universities; and *opportunities to interact with mentors* by supporting travel to international meetings and networking events, as well as providing early career researchers opportunities to present their research and viewpoints at global mental health workshops sponsored by NIMH. Figures 19.1 and 19.2 show a progression of funding opportunities—beginning with earlier career phases—that can support global mental health research activities for U.S. and non-U.S. investigators, respectively.

Institutional Resources and Capacity

A *sine qua non* for research workforce development is the availability of a functional physical, virtual, and administrative infrastructure. A well-developed infrastructure creates an enabling and supportive environment for the uptake, production, and dissemination of research. Adequate physical infrastructure includes providing and maintaining well-designed and equipped laboratories, clinics, libraries stocked with up-to-date text books and a wide range of journals, and functional classrooms or other spaces for learning. These might include virtual infrastructure that supports reliable Internet access and

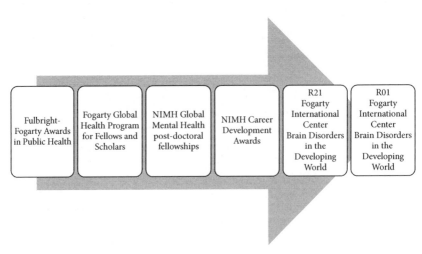

FIGURE 19.1

Selected National Institutes of Health funding mechanisms that support global mental health research training activities for U.S. investigators.

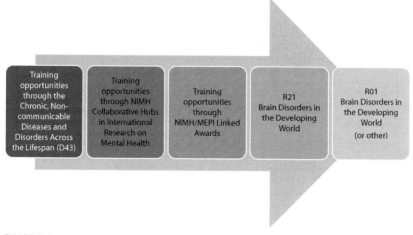

FIGURE 19.2

Selected National Institutes of Health funding mechanisms that support global mental health research training activities for which non-U.S. investigators are also eligible.

facilitates use of Open Access journals, distance learning, and e-mentoring, which also aid in reducing scientific isolation. Administrative infrastructure ideally provides research management such as support for submission of grant applications, accounting, disbursement of funds, and financial reporting. Structures to ensure the ethical conduct of research, such as institutional review boards or research ethics committees, can be maintained through the research administrative infrastructure.

RESEARCH PRIORITIES FOR GLOBAL MENTAL HEALTH

Why Set Priorities?

Priority-setting is one of the central functions of a global health system. Moon and colleagues identify establishing an agenda (through priority-setting) as the first of five elements of a global health system.[36] Others include financing and resource allocation; research and development; implementation and delivery; and monitoring, evaluation, and learning. More than $130 billion is invested globally into health research each year.[37] This figure has been growing, but in spite of this, the need for more research funds far exceeds the money available. Given this disjuncture, priorities must be set using feasible, transparent methodologies that include all stakeholders.

Who Sets Priorities?

Although multilateral organizations and national governments traditionally wielded much of the influence in priority setting, an increasingly broad set of stakeholders participates in most global priority-setting efforts.[36] Stakeholders are a large and highly heterogeneous group, but the extent of their engagement varies across priority-setting exercises. Donor organizations may wish to set priorities, and their reference group may be relatively small and homogenous. On the other hand, the setting of national priorities by governments often involves a larger, heterogeneous group, from policymakers to end users of interventions and treatments. The use of methods that rely on expert consensus is a valuable approach when other evidence is unavailable, which is very frequently the case in low- and middle-income countries.[38]

Methodologies

A number of priority-setting methodologies have been developed in the field of health research in recent years (see Table 19.1 for a summary of the four most commonly used methodologies). Of these methodologies, the Combined Matrix Approach has been applied to schizophrenia;[39] the methods utilized by the Child Health and Nutrition Research Initiative (CHNRI),[40] a modification of this approach,[41] and Delphi approaches[42,*] have been used to set global mental health priorities (see below for an outline of the results from these processes).

Global Priority-Setting Exercises and Outcomes

In recent years, a number of priority-setting exercises have been conducted in the area of mental health. We outline the underlying themes, principles, and top priorities of these priority-setting processes.

The Lancet GMH Research Priority Setting

As part of the first global mental health series the Lancet Global Mental Health Group conducted a priority-setting exercise in order to identify gaps in the evidence base in global mental health for four categories of mental disorders (schizophrenia and other major psychotic disorders, major depressive disorder and other common mental disorders, alcohol abuse and other substance abuse disorders, and the broad class of child and adolescent mental disorders).[17,40] The group employed the methods utilized by CHNRI, and they listed and scored research options.

The highest research priorities that emerged were related to health policy and systems research, and how to deliver cost-effective interventions.[40] The top five research options in this exercise were:

1. Implement health policy and systems research (HPSR) to determine the most effective intersectoral (social, economic, and population based) strategies to reduce consumption in high risk groups (particularly men) thus reducing the burden of alcohol abuse
2. What training, support, and supervision will enable existing maternal and child health workers to recognize, and provide basic treatment for, common maternal, child, and adolescent mental disorders?
3. Study the effectiveness, and cost-effectiveness of school-based interventions, including children with special needs
4. Conduct HPSR to integrate child and adolescent mental-disorders management with other child and adolescent physical-disease management, including nutrition
5. Conduct research into the effectiveness of early detection and simple brief treatment methods that are culturally appropriate, that are implemented by non-specialist health workers in the course of routine primary care, and that can be scaled up

In addition, the highest scoring research options addressed either alcohol and drug abuse or the category of child and adolescent mental disorders. The lowest scoring

* A Delphi process is a structured communication technique for forecasting and goal-setting that makes use of expert opinion, anonymity, and iterative, controlled feedback to arrive at a statistical group response. See Goodman C. M. The Delphi technique: a critique. *Journal of Advanced Nursing*, 1987, 12 (6): 729–734.

Table 19.1 Priority Setting in Global Mental Health: Actors and Approaches

Council on Health Research and Development (COHRED)	• Defines who sets priorities and how to get participants involved; the potential functions, roles, and responsibilities of various stakeholders; information and criteria for setting priorities; strategies for implementation and indicators for evaluation • Specifies broad research avenues
Combined Approach Matrix (CAM)	• Systematic classification, organization, and presentation of large body of information • Incorporates many dimensions • Specifies broad research avenues • CAM can be applied at the level of disease, risk factor, group, or condition, and also at local, national, or international level
Child Health Nutrition Research Initiative (CHNRI)	• Principles of legitimacy and fairness • Detailed listing of specific research questions • Individual questions scored against predefined criteria. Technical experts independently score each research option • Stakeholder input is sought and used to provide relative weight of the criteria
Delphi approach	• Group communication process to achieve convergence • Principle of consensus building • In principle there can be infinite iterations—usually three rounds • Can specify broad research avenues or specific research questions

research options were those that proposed the development of new interventions and technologies such as those targeted at the development of new drugs, vaccines, or pharmacological agents.[17,40] The Lancet exercise emphasized the need for research into the implementation of existing interventions and how to overcome health system constraints in developing countries.[17] This exercise demonstrated that in a context of global mental health, research funding is best placed into health policy and systems research that would fill the critical gaps in knowledge and suggest where and how to deliver the existing cost-effective interventions.

Mental Health Research Priorities in Low- and Middle-Income Countries of Africa, Asia, Latin America, and the Caribbean

Sharan and colleagues (2009) surveyed researchers and stakeholders in 114 countries of Africa, Asia, Latin America and the Caribbean.[43] In this extensive survey, they described broad agreement on research priorities in low- and middle-income countries, including epidemiology, health systems, and social science research. Children, adolescents, women, and people exposed to violence and trauma were prioritized. In terms of disorders, depression/anxiety, substance use, and psychosis were prioritized disorders, while suicide was lower on the list of priorities.

Mental and Neurological Health Research Priorities in LMICs

Khandelwal and colleagues[44] employed a combined matrix approach to conduct a consultation process in six regions across LMICs that aimed to produce regional as well as global research priorities on mental and neurological health in low- and middle-income countries.

The following priorities emerged:

1. Awareness and advocacy—Epidemiology; burden of disease; socio-economic impact; advocacy programs for decision makers in health services development (HSD); awareness programs; advocacy groups.
2. Research capacity—Tools, instruments and mechanisms; international links; network of centers of excellence
3. Training for service delivery—Evaluation of existing programs; identification of obstacles to service delivery; adaptation of training programs.
4. Policy—Guidelines for integrating mental and neurological health programs into broad programs of HSD

Grand Challenges in Global Mental Health

In the most comprehensive study to date on the setting of global mental health research priorities, Collins and colleagues employed a Delphi method to identify priorities in the full range of mental, neurological, and substance-use (MNS) disorders.[42] This initiative was the first to employ the Delphi method, and take a global approach, as well as the first to cover all MNS disorders. The Delphi panel consisted of 422 researchers, advocates, program implementers, and clinicians from 60 countries. Basic researchers comprised just over a third of the panel; a quarter were mental health services researchers; a third were clinical researchers and epidemiologists.

The priority-setting exercise identified 40 leading challenges that included implementation and policy needs, the scaling up of effective interventions, as well as etiological and treatment questions related to MNS disorders. Children were seen as a particularly important priority population in need of prevention and care, which, according to the authors, reflects the developmental nature of many mental disorders. There were four main themes captured by the exercise:

a. Research should adopt a life course approach based on the knowledge that many MNS disorders originate early in life, but also the acknowledgement of the importance of being attentive to risk factors in the elderly;
b. MNS disorders require system-wide approaches in order to address the suffering they cause;
c. Interventions should be evidence-based; and
d. Environmental exposures influence risk and resilience to MNS disorders.

The top five challenges, after ranking by feasibility, immediacy of impact, impact on equity, and disease burden reduction in this exercise were:

1. Integrate screening and core packages of services into routine primary health care
2. Reduce the cost and improve the supply of effective medications
3. Provide effective and affordable community-based care and rehabilitation
4. Improve children's access to evidence-based care by trained health providers in low- and middle-income countries
5. Strengthen the mental-health component in the training of all health-care personnel

Tol and colleagues[41] developed a consensus-based research agenda using an adaptation of the methods applied in the CHNRI aimed at supporting the prevention and treatment of mental disorders and the protection and promotion of psychosocial well-being in humanitarian settings. In this field, key ideological divisions exist between researchers and practitioners regarding issues such as the focus on post-traumatic stress disorder (PTSD) as a central research and intervention subject,[45] the distinction between normal psychological distress and mental disorders in situations of adversity,[46] and whether interventions should target mental disorders or ongoing structural and situational stressors these environments. Given these ideological and knowledge gaps, the Mental Health and Psychosocial Support in Humanitarian Settings—Research Priority SETting (MH-SET) project was initiated to establish a consensus-based research agenda designed to support the prevention and treatment of mental disorders and the protection and promotion of psychosocial well-being in humanitarian aid settings. The MH-SET project aimed to set research priorities based on the perspectives of a range of key stakeholders, including academics, practitioners, and policymakers from a variety of disciplines, ensuring representation from locations where humanitarian crises occur.

The most highly prioritized research questions favored practical initiatives with a strong potential for translation of knowledge into mental health and psychosocial support programming.

The top five research options in this exercise were the following inquiries:

1. What are the stressors faced by populations in humanitarian settings?
2. What are appropriate methods to assess mental health and psychosocial needs of populations in humanitarian settings?
3. How do affected populations themselves describe and perceive mental health and psychosocial problems in humanitarian settings?
4. What are appropriate indicators to use when monitoring and evaluating the results of mental health and psychosocial support in humanitarian settings?
5. How can we best adapt existing mental health and psychosocial interventions to different socio-cultural settings?

The exercise emphasized the importance of including the perspectives of affected people, and highlighted the importance of involving grass roots workers in an attempt to make research as relevant to their concerns as is possible.

Summary

Most research priority-setting exercises result in messages that are acceptable but general. Policymakers have little specific guidance on how to distribute research funds in such cases. One advantage of the methods applied by the CHNRI (and the recent use of the Delphi method in the Grand Challenges in Global Mental Health) is that they provide more specific outcomes and suggestions, with a priority score that can be used to assist policymakers in determining the level of risk associated with a specific research option. It also enables funders to develop a portfolio of research options that minimize risk and respect the values of stakeholders.

Ensuring a fair and inclusive priority-setting process is essential, but it is important to acknowledge that agreeing and acting upon priorities means making tradeoffs. Priority setting results in shifts in political and funding support, better training programs and rapid development of interventions in areas that are prioritized, and job losses and funding shortages in areas that were previously prioritized or are now low on the current list of priorities. In addition, when a particular health concern, such as mental health, forms part of a broader health domain (i.e., non-communicable diseases) it runs the risk of losing out to other priorities within the broad domain when political bargaining elevates one component over another.

Several themes predominate across the five research priority-setting exercises presented here. All of the exercises highlighted the need for research related to health policy and health systems; delivery of effective and cost-effective treatments at scale; the integration of mental health care into primary care; as well as the needs of children, with a particular prioritization of prevention and care; and the development of human resources of for MNS service delivery.

Progress towards ensuring that these priorities are achieved will depend on significant research funding being made available in the next decade. Significant strides have been made in this regard with the establishment of the U.S. NIMH Collaborative Hubs (in Africa, South Asia, and Latin America); the Programme for Improving Mental Health Care (PRIME) funded by the U.K. Department for International Development (DfiD) focusing on Ethiopia, India, Nepal, South Africa, and Uganda; and the multiple mental health projects supported by Grand Challenges Canada in LMICs.

FROM PRIORITIES TO UPTAKE: IMPLEMENTING AND TRANSLATING RESEARCH TO POLICY AND PRACTICE

The values conveyed in several global mental health priority-setting exercises—such as ensuring that interventions have an evidence base and involving grass-roots constituents in identifying priorities—lay the groundwork for increasing the relevance of research to affected communities. Ensuring the conduct of ethical research, engaging communities in research activities and dissemination, and creating demand for research form aspects of research capacity; we discuss each in turn.

Respecting the Research Process: Using Ethical Research Practices in Global Mental Health

As mental health research activities increase in LMICs, adequate ethical oversight will be essential. Cognitive impairment, poor judgement, and poor impulse control are some of the symptoms that make individuals with certain mental illnesses more vulnerable in the context of research. When compounded by poverty, the ethics of conducting research become increasingly complex. Nine factors that need to be considered in the conduct of mental health research include: social value of the research, study design, study population, informed consent, risks and benefits, confidentiality, post-trial obligations, legal versus ethical obligations, and oversight.[47]

The study design determines the kind of data to be generated, and the desired data inform the kind of intervention (and attendant risks) to which participants will be exposed. The issue becomes particularly complex when one design may generate very useful knowledge, but may put participants at greater risk. In international settings, the question of offering the existing standard of care in the context of controlled trials raises ethical issues. If, for example, a proposed randomized controlled trial will assign participants in the control group to receive the standard of care in a low-income country with extremely limited mental health resources, while the participants in the experimental group receive a highly effective medication or psychotherapy, is the clinical duty to provide the best care being forfeited? Ethics committees and institutional review boards, whose standards are typically based on principles of the Nuremberg Code or the Belmont Report (of the U.S. National Commission for the Protection of Human Subjects of Biomedical and Behavioral Research) assist investigators in determining how to respond to such questions and best protect the welfare of research participants.

The Belmont Report requires that potential research participants be treated equally; i.e., they should not be unfairly excluded from research that may benefit them, nor should they be unfairly committed to research that may have a greater chance of harming them. The report also requires that the impact of the research on "social justice" be considered. According to this principle, research should not augment social inequalities; i.e. people that are bad off should not be made worse off by participating in research.[47]

Research frequently exposes participants to some level of risk. Mental health research may present risks (1) due to psychological harm that may occur through participating in a trial (e.g., an experimental medication may have adverse effects); (2) because for participants with existing disorders, participation may require stopping a medication and risking the onset of symptoms or dangerous behavior like suicide; (3) because lack of access to a medication after the trial is complete can also lead to relapse, if the treatment controlled symptoms.[47] An additional risk in poor countries may be lack of access to psychopharmacological agents after the study ends. Another risk occurs in settings where having an identified mental illness increases the patient's social exclusion or discrimination; participation in a study can lead to disclosure of one's status depending on the study design.

Bioethicist Joseph Millum writes, "Research participants with a psychiatric diagnosis often retain the capacity and legal status to give informed consent.[47]" At times, however, for some people with certain disorders, cognitive impairment or impaired judgement as a result of symptoms can limit capacity to consent. Protocols for assessing capacity need to be included in the study design. Millum explains, "If she understands that project and what it implies for her and is capable of articulating her reasoning about it, then…she is capable of consenting to participation, independent of her more general capacities." Proxy consent (i.e., consent given by an appointed decision maker) should only be used if a study poses low risk or stands to benefit the participant. Additionally, standards for medical care should not be confused with standards for research participation. Medical care is meant, by definition, to benefit a person, whereas research is not.

Keeping Research Relevant: Engaging Communities and Respecting Responsibilities

Researchers who implemented projects in response to previous Grand Challenge initiatives identified a set of considerations to ensure that research activities that flow from priority-setting also address the needs of communities and the end users of research.[48] These include community engagement, public engagement, consideration of cultural beliefs, and respect for post-trial obligations.

Community engagement ensures that research occurs in the context of collaborative relationships with the communities where research will be conducted and requires that investigators listen to and address the concerns of community members, support open communication between researchers and community members, and facilitate ownership of the research by the community. Moving beyond the particular populations participating in the research, effective engagement of the broader public can facilitate the translation of research to social action. Public engagement keeps a broad range of stakeholders informed of key policy issues relevant to the research, provides avenues for investigators to receive input from the public, and permits continual assessment of public perception of research activities. Most importantly, successful engagement encourages integration of the public's views into decision-making and action. How can engagement best be carried out? Box 19.3 displays eight actions that can assist in establishing meaningful community collaborations.[49]

Box 19.3 Engaging Communities: Eight Ingredients to Consider

1. Do your homework prior to entering a community.
   - Know the structure of a community.
   - Be aware of attitudes toward mental illness or experiences with mental health research or services.
2. Earn the trust of the community.
   - Be honest when describing the research you will conduct.
   - Take time to get to know community members.
   - Listen to the viewpoints of community members.
3. Spend time in the community.
   - Avoid showing up just for meetings and leaving immediately.
   - Demonstrate your interest in the community and its members.
4. Encourage full participation of community members in research and in opportunities to develop research capacity.
   - Share decision-making with community members.
   - Involve community members in planning.
   - Provide training that increases understanding of research, budgeting, leadership, etc.
5. Recognize/identify the strengths of community members.
6. Be compassionate and listen well.
7. Respect the time of those members with whom you collaborate.
8. Ensure that other organizations you work with will also welcome community participation.

Adapted from Franco et al.[49]

Integral to public and community engagement is an acknowledgement of cultural beliefs that may support or conflict with the successful implementation of health-promoting interventions. Community members and investigators can negotiate the conduct of activities that respect cultural beliefs, and at the same time, acknowledge and address culturally ingrained negative actions (e.g., gender discrimination) that hinder effective public health interventions. Finally, at the end of a study, when the research-supported intervention is complete, post-trial obligations include ensuring that the active and effective intervention (whether a medicine or other therapeutic intervention) remains available to communities. This can also be accomplished by scaling up successful interventions so that they become part of the existing health care system, but a prerequisite for this step is ensuring that research results are actually applicable to real-life settings.

Creating Demand for Research

Conducting research and demonstrating that a mental health intervention works—i.e., establishing the evidence base—does not ensure that the intervention will become a widely adopted practice. Although a range of political, economic, social, scientific, and cultural barriers can contribute to the lack of translation to practice, so can costs related to an intervention, target population characteristics, competing demands for staff members, and organizational culture, limit generalizability of study findings and hence the likelihood of broad uptake[50] (Box 19.4). Researchers must carefully consider the context of their research activities and the differing needs of stakeholders, be they local decision makers (e.g., clinicians, organizations, patients) or policymaking bodies (city, state,

Box 19.4 Assessing Barriers to Translation from Research to Practice: Guiding Questions

1. Intervention:
   - Is it costly?
   - Is a high level of staff expertise needed?
   - Is there no intervention package or manual?
   - Is it highly specific to a particular settings?
2. Target settings:
   - Are there too many competing demands?
   - Is the program imposed from the outside?
   - Are resources limited?
   - Is time limited?
   - How do current practices work against innovation?
3. Research or evaluation design:
   - Can the study sample used lead to findings that can be generalized to a variety of patients, staff, clinical settings?
   - Have the outcomes relevant to decision makers and other end users been evaluated (e.g., intervention costs, cost-effectiveness, adoption of the intervention in the setting, implementation, maintenance, and sustainability of the intervention)?
4. Interactions among these three:
   - Barriers to participation lead to poor program reach or participation.
   - Interventions are not flexible.
   - Interventions are not appropriate for the target audience.
   - Staffing patterns do not match the intervention needs.
   - Organization and intervention philosophies are not aligned.
   - Organization is unable to implement the intervention adequately.

Adapted from Glasgow & Emmons.[50]

federal governments), as they collect information so that study findings provide information about the external validity of the intervention.

A study among a sample of health care providers working in LMICs reported that they were more likely to adopt evidence-based practices if the research was conducted and published in their own country, not from high-income countries.[51] At the same time, the providers were more likely to believe that research from high-income countries was above average or excellent compared to their assessment of research conducted in their countries. Having access to and using hard copies of clinical guidelines, scientific journals from their own country, viewing research performed in their own country as being above average or excellent, and trusting systematic reviews of randomized controlled trials were all associated with an increased likelihood that research evidence would influence practice.

Quality of research evidence is not the only factor that drives the link between research, policy, and action. Civil society organizations, advocates, private sector providers of health and education, and media play important roles in influencing the use and dissemination of research findings. More interaction with policymakers, and learning to anticipate the needs of policymakers could also inform the directions and subsequent policy relevance of research. Various methods of knowledge transfer between researchers and policymakers have evolved to make this possible. These include researchers serving as consultants who work closely with decision makers to define central issues to address, analyze relevant information, interpret results, and present findings to the decision makers.[52] Through this process, researchers and decision makers determine how best to frame findings and communicate them in ways that may stimulate change. The very act of involving the end users of research in identifying areas where research is needed can fuel the demand for research, and regular engagement by researchers with these broader networks supports that goal.

A critically important element of creating demand for research is strengthening the research culture, so that the production, dissemination, and use of high-quality research is valued as an integral part of the health system.[13] National research capacity reflects national values, beliefs, practices, language, and systems of power. A fundamental cultural belief concerns the origins of knowledge. Where societies believe that knowledge is created or discovered rather than "received" or "revealed," and that it is provisional, always open to change in the face of new evidence, there is likely to be a vibrant research culture. Where social relations reflect hierarchies of prestige and power, it is likely that prevailing beliefs and practices, including health-relevant practices, will be exempt from scrutiny and challenge. When populations believe that knowledge should be publicly owned, widely disseminated and shared, and should be used for public benefit, the research priorities differ from circumstances where people view knowledge as a reliable means of enrichment and control—as something to be closely held. The dominant culture will influence whether high-quality research flourishes and challenges current beliefs and commitments, or whether existing political, economic, religious, and social orthodoxies prevail. The values that are essential for a thriving research culture include: a commitment to *excellence*—ensuring that research is of the highest quality; promotion of *curiosity*—encouragement of questioning and exploration; encouragement of *free inquiry*—removal of impediments to free inquiry; attitude of respectful skepticism in relation to *authority*—open examination and questioning of prevailing views; a commitment to *justice and equity*—ensuring that research contributes to the public good; and a commitment to ethical conduct of *research*—protection and enhancement of the rights and interests of research participants by establishing processes that ensure ethical research practice.[13]

CONCLUSIONS

A dynamic relationship exists among (1) generation of research priorities and the growth of knowledge development in specific areas, (2) translation of research to priority policies and interventions, (3) the demand for research and (4) the necessity for research capacity-building, all of which ultimately aim to improve mental health outcomes in individuals and communities (Figure 19.3).

Although research is central to guiding communities to better health, every community does not benefit equally from the opportunity to design, participate in, or receive the outputs of research. This is particularly true with respect to mental health research. The ability to build capacity and to conduct mental health research globally is marked by very real constraints, most of which are interrelated. Two in particular—availability of health research funding and stated priorities for health research—drive the activities of scientists in a given context. Voices of community members, decision-makers, people suffering from mental illness, and their families and friends become particularly important in the context of low resources—both as advocates for mental health research, but perhaps more importantly, as advocates for research that yields systems of comprehensive and inclusive care for people and their communities. This kind of advocacy will help move governments and donors from overly fragmented and siloed systems of care and funding as well as disjointed approaches to health and healing, which frequently inadequately address the needs of people with mental illness. This is risky business, however, because priority

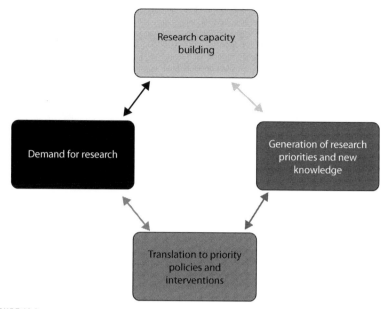

FIGURE 19.3

Research priorities, translation of research into policy and practice, creating demand for research, and research capacity-building.

setting is essential, something will be left out, and funds never equal the needs. Here again, research and global cooperation can play a role: knowledge generated by research offers our best chance to build better *comprehensive* preventive, treatment, and systems interventions that meet the needs of people with mental illness.

REFERENCES

1. Minas H, Diatri H. Pasung: physical restraint and confinement of the mentally ill in the community. *Int J Ment Health Syst.* 2008;2:8.
2. Puteh I, Marthoenis M, Minas H. Aceh free Pasung: releasing the mentally ill from physical restraint. *Int J Ment Health Syst.* 2011;5.
3. O'Shea B. Psychiatric patients with no place to go but jail. *New York Times/Chicago News Cooperative*, Health section, Feb. 19, 2012: A25A.
4. Szlezák NA, Bloom BR, Jamison DT, Keusch GT, Michaud CM, Moon S, et al. The global health system: actors, norms, and expectations in transition. *PLoS Med.* 2010 7(1):e1000183. Epub 2010 January 5.
5. Sharan P, Levav I, S Olifson, A de Francisco, Saxena S. Research capacity for mental health in low- and middle-income countries: results of a mapping project. 2007. Available from: http://www.who.int/mental_health/MHRC_FullText.pdf.
6. Saxena S, Paraje G, Sharan P, Karam G, Sadana R. The 10/90 divide in mental health research: trends over a 10-year period. *Br J Psychiatry.* 2006;188:81–2. Epub doi:10.1192/bjp.bp.105.011221.
7. Kieling C, Herrman H, Patel V, de Jesus Mari J. Indexation of psychiatric journals from low- and middle-income countries: a survey and a case study. *World Psychiatry.* 2009;8:40–4.
8. Razzouk D, Sharan P, Gallo C, Gureje O, Lamberte E, de Jesus Mari J, et al. Scarcity and inequity of mental health research resources in low-and-middle income countries: a global survey. *Health Policy.* 2010;94:211–20.
9. Lansang MA, Dennis R. Building capacity in health research in the developing world. *Bull World Health Organ.* 2004;82(10):765–9.
10. Thornicroft G, Cooper S, Bortel TV, Kakuma R, Lund C. Capacity building in global mental health research. *Harv Rev Psychiatry.* 2012;20:13–24.

11. World Health Organization. *Mental Health Atlas 2005.* Geneva: World Health Organization; 2005.

12. Whitworth JA, Kokwaro G, Kinyanjui S, Snewin A, Tanner A, Walport M, et al. Strengthening capacity for health research in Africa. *Lancet.* 2008;372(9649):1590–3.

13. Minas H. International observatory on mental health systems: structure and operation. *Int J Ment Health Syst.* 2009;3(1):8.

14. Minas H. The Centre for International Mental Health approach to mental health system development. *Harv Rev Psychiatry.* 2012;20(1):37–46.

15. Minas H, Mahoney J, Kakuma R. *Health for the South community mental health project.* Melbourne: Centre for International Mental Health, 2011.

16. IDRAAC. *Institute for Development, Research, Advocacy and Applied Care.* 2006 [September 24, 2012]; available from: http://www.idrac.org.lb.

17. Chisholm D, Lund C, Saxena S. Cost of scaling up mental healthcare in low- and middle-income countries. *Br J Psychiatry.* 2007;191:528–35.

18. Lund C. Mental health in Africa: findings from the Mental Health and Poverty Project. *Int Rev Psychiatry.* 2010;22:547–9.

19. Lund C, Breen A, Flisher A, Kakuma R, Corrigall J, Joska J, et al. Poverty and common mental disorders in low-and middle-income countries: a systematic review. *Soc Sci Med.* 2010;71:517–28.

20. Petersen I, Bhana A, Campbell-Hall V, Mjadu S, Lund C, Kleintjies S, et al. Planning for district mental health services in South Africa: a situational analysis of a rural district site. *Health Policy Plan.* 2009;24:140–50.

21. Sikwese A, Mwape L, Mwanza J, Kapungwe A, Kakuma R, Imasiku M, et al. Human resource challenges facing Zambia's mental health care system and possible solutions: results from a combined quantitative and qualitative study. *Int Rev Psychiatry.* 2010;22:550–7.

22. Ruffin J, Flagg-Newton JL. Building capacity for health disparity research at minority institutions. *Am J Med Sci.* 2001;322(5):253–8.

23. Manson S. Personal journeys, professional paths: persistence in navigating the crossroads of a research career. *Am J Public Health.* 2009;99(1):20–5.

24. Nakanjako D, Byakika-Kibwika P, Kintu K, Aizire J, Nakwagala F, Luzige S, et al. Mentorship needs at academic institutions in resource-limited settings: a survey at Makerere University College of Health Sciences. *BioMed Central Med Educ.* 2011;15(23).

25. Kahn JS, Greenblatt RM. Mentoring early-career scientists for HIV research careers. *Am J Public Health.* 2009;99 (Suppl 1):S37–42.

26. The Royal Society. *Knowledge, networks and nations: Global scientific collaboration in the 21st century.* London: The Royal Society; 2011 [cited 2012 May 31]; available from: http://royalsociety.org/uploadedfiles/royal_society_content/influencing_policy/reports/2011-03-28-knowledge-networks-nations.pdf.

27. Jones C. *An environmental scan of practice based research networks in Canada.* Kingston, Ontario: Centre for Studies in Primary Care; 2006 [cited 2012 16 February]; Available from: http://www.cfpc.ca/uploadedFiles/Research/An_Env_Sca_of_PBRN_PCNs.pdf.

28. The Working Group on Priority Setting. Priority setting for health research: lessons from developing countries. *Health Policy Plan.* 2000;15(2):130–6.

29. ESSENCE on Health Research. *Planning, monitoring and evaluation: Framework for capacity strengthening in health research.* Geneva: WHO; 2011.

30. Panel on Return on Investment in Health Research. *Making an impact: A preferred framework and indicators to measure returns on investment in health research.* Ottawa: Canadian Academy of Health Sciences; 2009.

31. UNESCO. *UNESCO Science Report 2010.* Paris: UNESCO; 2010.

32. de Jesus Mari J, Bressan RA, Almeida-Filho N, Gerolin J, Sharan P, Saxena S. Mental health research in Brazil: policies, infrastructure, financing and human resources. *Revista Saude Publica.* 2006;40(1):161–9.

33. CNPq/MCT. *Science without borders: The Brazilian scientific mobility program at CNPq/MCT.* 2011 [September 25, 2012]; available from: http://www.access4.eu/_media/2011_science_without_borders.pdf.

34. Flisher AJ, Lund C, Funk M, Banda M, Bhana A, Doku V, et al. Mental health policy development and implementation in four African countries. *J Health Psychol.* 2007;12(3):505–16.

35. Alliance for Health Policy and Systems Research. *Innovative strategies to enhance capacity to apply health policy and systems research evidence in policy making*. 2012 [cited 2012 June 5, 2012]; available from: http://www.who.int/alliance-hpsr/projects/strategies_capacity/en/index.html

36. Moon S, Szlezák NA, Michaud CM, Jamison DT, Keusch GT, Clark WC, et al. The global health system: lessons for a stronger institutional framework. *PLoS Med.* 2010;7(1): e1000193. doi:10.1371/journal.pmed.1000193.

37. Rudan I, Chopra M, Kapiriri L, Gibson J, Lansang MA, Carneiro I, et al. Setting priorities in global health research investments: universal challenges and conceptual framework. *Croatian Med J.* 2008;49:307–17.

38. Minas H, Jorm A. Where there is no evidence: use of expert consensus methods to fill the evidence gap in low-income countries and cultural minorities. *Int J Ment Health Syst.* 2010;4:33.

39. Ghaffar A, Francisco Ad, Matlin S, editors. *The combined approach matrix: A priority-setting tool for health research*. Geneva: Global Forum for Health Research; 2004.

40. Tomlinson M, Rudan I, Saxena S, Swartz L, Tsai A, Patel V. Setting priorities for global mental health research *Bull World Health Organ*. 2009;87:438–46.

41. Tol W, Patel V, Tomlinson M, F FB, Galappatti A, Panter-Brick C, et al. Research priorities for mental health and psychosocial support in humanitarian settings. *PLoS Med.* 2011;8:9.

42. Collins PY, Patel V, Joestl SS, March D, Insel TR, Daar AS. Grand challenges in global mental health. *Nature.* 2011;475:27–30.

43. Sharan P, Gallo C, Gureje O, Lamberte E, Mari J, Mazzotti G, et al. Mental health research priorities in low- and middle-income countries of Africa, Asia, Latin America and the Caribbean. *Br J Psychiatry.* 2009;195:354–63.

44. Khandelwal S, Avode G, Baingana F, Conde B, Cruz M, Deva P, et al. Mental and neurological health research priorities setting in developing countries. *Soc Psychiatry Psychiatr Epidemiol.* 2010;45:487–95.

45. van Ommeren M, Saxena S, Saraceno B. Mental and social health during and after acute emergencies: emerging consensus? *Bull World Health Organ.* 2005;83:71–5.

46. Horwitz AV. Transforming normality into pathology: the DSM and the outcomes of stressful social arrangements. *J Health & Soc Behav.* 2007;48:211–22.

47. Millum J. Introduction: Case studies in the ethics of mental health research. *J Nerv Ment Dis.* 2012;200:230–5.

48. Berndtson K, Daid T, Tracy CS, Bhan A, Cohen ERM, Upshur REG, et al. Grand challenges in global health: ethical, social, and cultural issues based on key informant perspectives. *PLoS Med.* 2007;4(9). Epub doi:10.1371/journal.pmed.0040268.

49. Franco LM, McKay MM, Miranda A, Chambers N, Paulino A, Lawrence R. Voices from the community: key ingredients for community collaboration. In: McKay MM, Paikoff RL, editors. *Community collaborative partnerships: The foundation for HIV prevention research efforts.* Binghamton, NY: The Haworth Press; 2007: 313–32.

50. Glasgow RE, Emmons KM. Evaluating the relevance, generalization, and applicability of research: issues in external validation and translation methodology. *Annu Rev Public Health.* 2007;28:413–33. Epub DOI:10.1146/annurev.publhealth.28.021406.144145.

51. Guindon GE, Lavis JN, Becerra-Posada F, Malek-Afzali H, Shi G, Yesudian CK, et al. Bridging the gaps between research, policy and practice in low- and middle-income countries: a survey of health care providers. *CMAJ.* 2010;182(9):E362–E372.

52. Jacobson N, Butterill D, Goering P. Consulting as a strategy for knowledge transfer. *Milbank Q.* 2005;83(2):299–321.

20 Generating Political Commitment for Mental Health System Development

José Miguel Caldas de Almeida,
Harry Minas, and Claudina Cayetano

POLITICAL COMMITMENT

The concept of *political commitment*, as it is used in this chapter, encompasses other terms that are frequently used and that have overlapping meanings, such as *political will*[1,2] and *political priority*.[3,4] All of these constructs are also related to the concept of *agenda setting*.[2,5,6] By "political commitment for mental health system development" we mean the organized intentions and actions of key decision-makers in a society, especially political leaders, to respond effectively to the mental health needs of the population. This is the public—including political—will to marshal intellectual, social, and economic resources to achieve valued population mental health objectives,[7] which will generally include reform of legal, policy, and regulatory frameworks; increasing investment in mental health; modification or reform of existing programs, and establishment where necessary of new programs; strengthening of human resources for mental health; and generation and systematic use of evidence to inform decision-making.

PROGRESS IN GLOBAL MENTAL HEALTH

In the last 20 years, efforts have been made all over the world to encourage national and international political leaders to give more attention to mental health, and to provide financial and human resources commensurate with the magnitude and impact of mental health problems.

These efforts grew from the recognition of two different facts. First, despite the significant advances in the development of effective interventions for the treatment of mental disorders in recent decades, a large proportion of people suffering from these disorders across the world continue to have limited access to the effective treatments and interventions that are currently available. Second, it is not possible to significantly change this situation if, at the national level, mental health policies and plans are not developed and implemented, and if, at the international level, mental health initiatives are not developed to support countries with limited resources.

Mental health system reform is a complex process,[8] requiring the closure or downsizing of traditional institutional services; the development of new services, programs, and interventions; and the integration of mental health in primary care. This reform cannot be achieved without a complex reallocation of resources, and in many cases without additional resources in the transitional period. Usually it requires the training of human resources in the use of new models of intervention, as well as the establishment of close collaboration with other sectors. In such a complex process, resistance to change, together with difficulties in ensuring the needed resources and collaborations, is common, and the strong commitment of policy makers is vital for the development of the policies that are indispensable to overcoming all these barriers.

In many countries, generating the commitment of donors is no less important. Most low-income countries have a very limited proportion of their already limited health budgets allocated to mental health[9] and are significantly dependent on external support to initiate a mental health reform process and to fund the costs of the transition phase.

Until recent times, mental health was one of the last priorities in the public health agenda everywhere. Significant efforts have been developed in the last two decades to give mental health the attention it deserves.[10]

All these efforts have had an appreciable impact. Comparing the way mental health is currently seen in most sectors with how it was seen twenty years ago, we have to conclude that important advances have been achieved. Looking at developments that have occurred at the policy and services levels in many countries, we arrive at the same conclusion.

However, much still remains to be done. The level of implementation of the political, legal, and technical principles that are fundamental to development of effective responses to the basic mental health needs of populations has been, so far, very limited. Despite the work done by the mental health advocacy movement, we are still far from a general recognition of the real importance of mental health by policy makers, donors, and public opinion.

Several factors continue to be obstacles to progress. Stigma is, undoubtedly, one of the most important. Myths, taboos, and misconceptions associated with mental ill-health, continue to be common among general populations, professionals, and policy makers all over the world, and are an impediment to development and implementation of necessary mental health policies, plans, and programs.

The specific obstacles and difficulties associated with the restructuring of mental health systems represent another important group of barriers. Mental health system reform is complex and technically difficult, requiring strong political support, good leadership, technical capacity, and adequate resources. Without these ingredients it is very difficult to achieve the changes that are needed, to develop the new attitudes and interventions that must be introduced, and to overcome the resistances that are common in this process.

The financial constraints currently found in most countries, with a particular impact on the funding of health care systems, is a particularly important barrier. All countries, with no exception, have been struggling with the increasing costs of health care. After the financial and economic crisis that started in 2007, many countries are adopting tough measures to reduce government expenditures, often with substantial reductions of health budgets.

In this context, increasing competition for funds among the different areas of health is inevitable, and mental health has some competitive disadvantages: first, because of the stigma associated with mental disorders; second, because, despite the advances made in mental health services research, we still need more solid evidence for the proposition that investment in mental health produces health, social, and economic returns that justify allocating high priority to such investment.

In May 2012, the 65th World Health Assembly passed Resolution 65.4, "The global burden of mental disorders and the need for a comprehensive, coordinated response from health and social sectors at the country level."[11] The resolution urges member states to "to develop and strengthen comprehensive policies and strategies that address the promotion of mental health, prevention of mental disorders, and early identification, care, support, treatment and recovery of persons with mental disorders" and requests the director-general of WHO "to strengthen advocacy, and develop a comprehensive mental health action plan with measurable outcomes." The draft Global Mental Health Action Plan 2012–2020,[11] developed by WHO and released for consultation, identifies commitment by governments as one of the key issues in developing effective policies and plans, and commitment of resources towards implementation as required for decisive action.

Although there has been rapid development of an evidence base for mental health development,[6,12-22] technical guidance concerning packages of care,[23-29] and development of mental health legislation, policies, and services,[30] there is little guidance in how to generate and strengthen political commitment to mental health development. In this chapter, we review the factors that play a significant role in generating political commitment and discuss how to develop a plan of action to strengthen such commitment.

POLITICAL COMMITMENT: WHAT IS IT?

Although the central need for political commitment is often asserted in the public health literature, what it is and how it is to be generated have received surprisingly little research attention.[31] The issue has been most extensively explored in relation to HIV[32,33] and safe motherhood,[2-4] and more broadly in relation to public health.[34]

A review of the literature on political commitment in relation to HIV[31] identifies three main components:

1. Expressed commitment: The extent to which decision-makers publicly make statements of support about the issue in question.
2. Institutional commitment: Whether institutional arrangements are put in place to implement the stated intent. This may include legal and policy frameworks, management arrangements, program and service delivery structures, and monitoring and evaluation strategies.
3. Budgetary commitment. Allocation of the necessary funds to give effect to the expressed intent.

Goldberg and colleagues[31] have highlighted the complexity of political will.

[G]overnments may verbally commit to HIV, making public pronouncements for instrumental reasons (e.g., to attract donor funds), but fail to translate this rhetoric into action in the form of laws or investments in actual programmes. Conversely, governments may remain silent, but have all of the institutional infrastructure in place and invest resources towards HIV. It is also possible for governments to commit institutionally, but to underfund programmes, leading to incomplete policy implementation. Governments may invest in programmes but undermine them through public discourse or lack the institutional capacity to make use of funds. Judgements on the level of political commitment should therefore take simultaneous account of different components of commitment.[31]

In addition, the authors identify two factors that cut across the three dimensions above—the extent to which ethics and human rights underpin the commitment, and the extent to which the political response is informed by scientific evidence.[31]

THE KEY DETERMINANTS OF POLITICAL COMMITMENT

To improve our capacity to generate political commitment in mental health, we must understand the factors that influence the degree to which international and national political leaders actively give attention to a health issue.

We know that some areas of health have been much more successful than others in being recognized as political priorities and mobilizing significant resources at the global level. Vaccines, HIV/AIDS, malaria, and maternal and child health are good examples. Which are the factors that explain this success? Researchers in the area of health advocacy have identified four different kinds of determinants of success in global health initiatives: the power of the actors involved, the power of ideas and facts, the political context, and characteristics of the issue itself.[4] Using this framework in the analysis of global mental health advocacy initiatives specifically developed to generate political commitment, we can reach some conclusions that may be helpful to increase the success of future initiatives in the field.

The Power of Actors Involved

Global mental health initiatives can involve a large range of actors: consumers, families, professionals, non-governmental organizations, government officials, international organizations, academics and researchers, scientific organizations, and human rights organizations. The success of each initiative depends on the strength and representativeness of the actors involved, the relationships they have established between them, the leadership and cooperation models adopted, and the capacity they have to confront the obstacles they will have to face.[4]

The global mental health policy community—government officials, leaders of non-governmental organizations, bilateral donors, members of WHO and other international organizations, and academics—that has been operating globally in defense of mental health, has made significant advances, due in great part to its capacity to focus on common goals (e.g., decreasing the burden of mental disorders) and to agree on the same solutions (e.g., development of community-based services). These actors have a decisive role in influencing policy makers, at the international and national level, as they are recognized as the main authorities in the field. It is crucial to preserve the consensus that has been reached among them and to use their authority in the presentation of clear proposals regarding policy and service development.

The participation of consumers and families in this process is especially important. For a long time neglected, their participation has proved to be key in activities calling attention to the importance of improving access to mental health care of good quality and the need to protect the human rights of people with mental health problems, and is now considered obligatory.

Grassroots organizations in civil society have also proven to be absolutely indispensable for the success of global mental health initiatives. The capacity of WHO to mobilize these organizations in 2001 was crucial for the success of the 2001 World Mental Health initiatives. The World Mental Health Day celebrated every year on October 10th, under the leadership of World Federation for Mental Health (WFMH),[35] became a significant component of the mental health advocacy movement, offering a unique opportunity to raise awareness of mental health, thanks to the involvement of thousands of grassroots organizations across the world. Other global initiatives, especially on human rights and mental health, have been possible because of their capacity to involve consumers and family organizations.

It is also important to ensure the participation of all groups of professionals involved in mental health care. Some of them, psychiatrists, general practitioners, psychologists, and nurses for instance, are very powerful in many places, and their support proved to be essential to the success of advocacy initiatives.

Personal and institutional leadership is crucial. Looking to the most successful mental health initiatives to generate political commitment, both at the national and international level, we always find behind them respected leaders that provide guidance and have the authority that is needed to strengthen partnerships and convince policy makers.

The same can be said of the institutions that have led global mental health initiatives. WHO, the preeminent institutional leader in global mental health, has proven to be particularly effective in the leadership of initiatives that encourage and support policy makers to improve mental health services, ensure access to and equity in care, and promote the human rights of people with mental health problems. Other organizations, such as the World Federation for Mental Health and the Movement for Global Mental Health, play a leadership role in important global initiatives. All these organizations have been able to establish active links and strong partnerships between them, which certainly should be further strengthened in the future.

The Power of Ideas and Facts

The way a health issue is understood and portrayed publicly is a decisive factor in the process of generating political commitment to actions in favor of that issue. Policy makers are pressured to support many different health issues; they will prioritize the areas that are seen as serious health problems, with a severe impact for society, and to which there are effective solutions. If the available solutions are easily affordable, this will certainly help, but the crucial point is that there be a solution and that there be strong and consensual evidence supporting its effectiveness.[4]

One of the main weaknesses of mental health initiatives to generate political priority was, for a long time, the way mental health was traditionally portrayed in the past: as an area of health having as its object disorders resulting from causes that were unknown or controversial, with prevalences and impacts that could not be rigorously measured, for which there were no really effective treatments, and that was associated with images of old psychiatric institutions separated from the general health system.

Although psychiatric institutions with terrible living conditions continue to exist in many places, a large number of people with mental disorders continue to have no access to treatment, and the scientific quality of many services is poor, the situation today is completely different. As considered in depth in other chapters of this book, now we have reliable data on the prevalence and burden of mental disorders in a large number of countries; we know that mental health services can be community-based, of good quality, and respectful of human rights; for most mental disorders, effective treatments are available; and important scientific advances are being made every day.

The new knowledge developed in the last twenty years on the burden of mental disorders and the treatment gap proved to be a strong and compelling argument in favor of the importance of mental health and the need to include mental health in the public health agenda. Thanks to the epidemiological studies and the burden of diseases studies, we have facts, and the facts are impressive. Mental disorders are not only highly prevalent—they have also a huge impact on individuals, families, and societies. Millions of people suffer from mental disorders across the world. All people can be affected, independent of age, gender, and social factors. Mental disorders interfere with the lives of children and adults, men, and women from all regions of the world, causing enormous suffering and disability.[36]

Positive mental health, though more difficult to measure, has also a profound impact in many aspects of the life of individuals and groups.[37] Being an inseparable part of health, it forms the basis of an individual's well-being and effective functioning, playing a fundamental role in interpersonal relations, family life, social inclusion, and the full participation of citizens at the social and economic levels.

In the last 20 years, significant advances have taken place at both the molecular and the more integrative aspects of neuroscience. These scientific accomplishments, together with advances in psychosocial research, have made possible enormous progress in the development of new and more effective treatments. A wide range of interventions and services has proven to be effective in the treatment and rehabilitation of most mental disorders. Advances in the development of effective interventions to prevent mental disorders and promote mental health have occurred more slowly. Nevertheless, there is already a significant array of available interventions[28] in these areas; for instance, evidence-based packages of care for depression,[27] schizophrenia,[24] ADHD,[25] alcohol use disorders,[23] epilepsy,[26] and dementia.[29]

Finally, new models of mental health care, more centered in the community, have been developed and evaluated in many countries. Most studies support the idea that the new models of care are more effective and preferred by patients and their families, and that integration of mental health into primary care is a strategy that contributes to the improvement of access to mental health care.[38]

All this knowledge has contributed to changing the old ideas about the effectiveness of mental health interventions, and to supporting the calls for action to invest in the development of mental health policies and services.

The Political Contexts

Political contexts can have a significant influence on the support given by policy makers to mental health policy and services development. In general, we can say that periods of political and social innovation are favorable to generating more interest in the improvement of mental health care. The support given to mental health reform in Latin American countries (e.g., Brazil and Chile), after democratic governments replaced dictatorships, is a good example of this principle.[39]

Political contexts in which the defense of values such as equity and social inclusion are prioritized can also enhance the probability of mental health being given special attention. Human rights initiatives, in particular, have proven to be instrumental in calling the attention of policy makers to the problems of exclusion and abuse experienced by people with mental disorders.

Some special contexts can represent policy windows in which mental health advocates find especially favorable opportunities to get the commitment of political leaders. This happened in the period after the WHO global mental health initiatives in 2001, when the momentum created by those initiatives facilitated the success of many national and international mental health projects.

Disasters and emergencies can also present unique opportunities to raise awareness of the importance of mental health and to improve nationwide mental health services. The mobilization of resources for mental health care in the aftermath of the September 11, 2001, attacks and the Indonesian tsunami in 2005 provide excellent examples of the opportunities created by emergencies, but many other situations of earthquakes and other disasters have had the same effect of creating new opportunities for mental health initiatives.[40]

Some great global health initiatives and projects not specifically dedicated to mental health, but addressing themes involving mental health aspects, can also be good policy windows. This could have been certainly the case with the UN Millennium Development Goals,[41] but unfortunately it was a missed opportunity, because mental health was not explicitly included in the selected goals. Despite the absence of specific inclusion of mental health goals, the achievement of the other development goals included in the MDGs will produce substantial mental health benefits for populations.[42] The 2011 United Nations Summit on Non-Communicable Diseases[43] was also a great opportunity to bring attention to the importance of mental health among the non-communicable diseases (NCD). Thanks to the efforts led by WFMH, several organizations have come together to promote the inclusion of mental health in the NCD agenda at the United Nations General Assembly High-Level Meeting on Non-Communicable Diseases in 2011 and in the global health and development agenda in the future.

The adoption by WHO executive board, in the beginning of 2012, of a draft resolution[44] moved by India, focusing on the global burden of mental disorders and the need for a comprehensive, coordinated response from health and social sectors at the country level, represents very important progress in the creation of a framework for action supporting political commitment from governments and international organizations in mental health. It is an excellent example of a successful strategy involving many actors at the international level, which created a new context facilitating the commitment of policy makers to action in favor of mental health.

GENERATING POLITICAL COMMITMENT: THE MAIN STEPS

Generating political commitment to support mental health requires a process that usually involves several important steps.[45] The first step consists in gathering the information that is available on the mental health problems we want to address. Building the networks that are fundamental to implement a successful advocacy initiative is the second step. Once we have this collaborative network, we can move to the third step and start working with our partners in the elaboration of a plan of action, including the specific objectives we want to achieve, the strategies and the activities that will be developed to attain these objectives, as well as the monitoring and evaluation procedures. The fourth step—implementation of the plan—should always include several components: development of ideas and messages; creation of messages for the specific audiences we want to reach, integration of champions and a specific strategy of work with the media.[45]

Gathering Information

Before starting advocacy initiatives to generate political commitment it is essential to collect all information that is available in the areas that are most relevant for our purpose. It is indispensable, in the first place, to collect the evidence that is required to prove to policy makers why they should make a commitment for action. This includes data on the magnitude and impact of the mental health problem we want to address, as well as evidence on the effectiveness of the actions that are proposed.

On the other hand, it is necessary to map the decision makers who may have a significant role in the process of change we want to promote: Who makes the important decisions? Who influences policy? Who may be interested in financing mental health projects? Finally, we should try to have all the available information about previous initiatives in the field and the organizations that should be approached and invited to become partners.

Building Networks

Establishing alliances with other partners who share common goals and are also interested in changing the situation in mental health is usually an obligatory component of initiatives calling for more support from policy makers in the development of mental health projects. Working together with others has several advantages. It can increase our knowledge, resources and skills. It can allow sharing of experience in relevant areas of mental health work. It can bring added value in terms of visibility and credibility. It can also facilitate access to important decision makers.[45]

In a field with so many different stakeholders, a significant effort should always be made to involve representatives of all relevant actors and sectors (professionals, users, and families; health sector and other sectors; governments and civil society, among others). By doing this, it is possible to prevent possible barriers, increase the capacity to influence others, and strengthen the ability to promote actions leading to better mental health, at both the national and international levels.

Building a network requires persistent work. It is necessary to identify the individuals and organizations that should be included in the network. It is also necessary to approach all possible partners, giving them good reasons to join the project and negotiating with them the rules that will be followed in the collaborative work to be developed.

The success of the partnerships depends in large measure on trust and reciprocity. From the beginning, all partners have to be sure that relevant information will be shared, and that clear rules exist about leadership, internal communication, distribution of tasks, and use of resources. It is also important to agree on the mechanisms that will be used to maintain group cohesion and resolve possible conflicts.

Defining the Plan of Action

The definition of a plan of action, with the collaboration of all partners, is essential for the success of any project. It should include defining the objectives, strategies and activities chosen for each objective, the indicators, as well as the methods that will be used in the monitoring and evaluation of the project.

A clear and precise definition of the objectives we want to achieve is the most important part of any initiative aiming at generating political commitment for action to support mental health. Our goal is to persuade policy makers that there is a mental health issue that should be addressed, and that their support can be a very important contribution to tackling this problem.

Therefore, we have to be able to explain in a very simple and clear way what problem we want to address, why this problem is important, and what are the actions that can change the existing situation and overcome the problem. All efforts we can make to describe the specific expected outcomes we want to achieve, and to define the concrete and realistic actions that may change the situation, are never too much.

Political commitment can be sought for a wide range of objectives in mental health: from very specific objectives related to interventions and services, to broader objectives related to legislation and policies. In all cases, it is necessary to define the objectives in such a way that someone who is not a mental health expert can easily understand what really needs to be changed and which are the concrete actions that should be developed to ensure that the change will take place.

Building Capacity

Development of the capacity of mental health leaders and different stakeholders involved in mental health policy implementation is a key component of advocacy initiatives aiming at generating political commitment. Building capacity in this area has been successfully developed through teaching programs of different sorts, ongoing support and supervision, and through the development of regional networks for mental health policy.[46]

Developing a Communication Strategy

A communication strategy is a key component of all advocacy initiatives to generate political commitment for mental health policy. It must include a set of messages specifically developed to persuade particular audiences to take action or provide support, as well as a selection of methods that will be used to deliver the messages. Some messages should contribute to making people aware of the importance of mental health problems and to sensitizing the audiences about the need to develop policies that may decrease the burden of mental disorders and diminish the treatment gap in mental health. Other messages must focus on the available solutions, calling attention to the effectiveness of mental health policies, and proposing concrete actions to be taken by the target audience in order to change the situation. Messages should be tailored for each audience, must be based on available evidence, and should be as brief and simple as possible.

The dissemination of the messages should start with the identification of databases of different audiences that may be involved in the process: policy makers and health authorities, scientific associations related with mental health, professional associations from mental health–related fields, representatives of patients and families, NGOs, and key agents in the community, among others. Specific actions, conceived to maximize the impact in accordance with the characteristics of the target group, can include the development of fact sheets for distribution among the media, the organization of workshops or high-level meetings, the publication of papers in scientific journals, or the presentation of the messages to the national and international agencies related to mental health policy development. If it is necessary to ensure dissemination of all relevant information to the different target groups, including the general population, the development of a website should be contemplated.

Integrating Champions

The integration of champions can significantly contribute to the success of a project. Champions—persons with high visibility who take an active role in the public promotion of a cause—can increase the credibility and visibility of the project. They can help in calling the attention of the media, general public, and policy makers to the importance of mental health issues. They can also facilitate the creation of partnerships and building of networks. Several mental health initiatives in the past were effectively supported by different kinds of champions: first ladies, members of governments and parliaments, well-known writers and artists, among others. In some cases, the fact that they had suffered from a mental disorder, or had a close relative with a mental disorder, was a significant factor in their involvement and made them especially effective in reaching the general public.

Monitoring and Evaluation

Monitoring and evaluation are fundamental to obtaining the information needed to take decisions related to the management and improvement of the plan of action, and to generating data to satisfy accountability requirements.

To evaluate the success of our plan of action, effective political commitment is the best outcome indicator we can use. A framework for measuring political commitment is offered by Fox and colleagues.[31,32] We should also use other important outcomes, such as strengthening the networks that were involved, the alliances established, and the organizations created.

Case study Belize—Generating Political and Donor Commitment for Mental Health Reform Implementation

Belize, the only English-speaking country in Central America, is an upper-middle-income country (according to World Bank classification in 2010) with a total area of 22,700 square kilometers and a population of 291,800 inhabitants. Approximately 33.5% of the population lives in poverty, and 13.4% lives in extreme poverty.

The first service specifically dedicated to the treatment of mental disorders, the Seaview Hospital, was created in Belize City in 1912. Like most of the psychiatric institutions created at that time in the region, the Seaview Hospital was for many years an asylum offering custodial care to patients with long-term mental disorders. It displayed the low quality of care and the violations of human rights that usually characterized this kind of institution.

With the arrival of the first staff psychiatrist in the 1960s, several measures were taken to change this situation and to introduce a medical approach in the hospital. New treatment regimens were established, including the use of the new drugs developed at the time, nurses and attendants were trained, and occupational therapy activities were developed.

However, in 1979, the Belize government decided to transfer psychiatric care to the facilities of a former minimum-security prison in the village of Rockville. This move created significant difficulties for the previous efforts to improve mental health care, and represented a serious setback in the modernization of mental health services. Rockview Hospital was a collection of dilapidated buildings located 22 miles from Belize City, without any conditions to function as a hospital. The remote location of the new facility posed significant challenges for the transportation of staff and the delivery of service utilities, and contributed to making all interactions with the community even more difficult than before.

In the late 1980s, several initiatives, such as the collaboration with the Memorial University of Newfoundland in Canada and the Pan American Health Organization, led to visits of staff to the mental health services in Canada at the Homewood Health Center and the organization of workshops in collaboration with the University of Louisville (Kentucky) and the University of Mount Sinai in New York. These initiatives created important opportunities to increase the knowledge of professionals about new models of intervention, and facilitated the establishment of collaborations with other countries.

At the time, the immediate impact of these initiatives on the functioning of the services was practically nonexistent. Barriers to change resulting from the custodial model of Rockview were too strong, and mental health was not yet a priority for the government.

However, the contact of Belizean professionals with the experience of other countries was instrumental in developing an increasing awareness by Belizean professionals of the need to improve mental health care in their country. It also helped create a pressure group that later would come to play a key role in generating the commitment of policy makers, which in turn was crucial for the launching of a mental health reform in Belize in the early 1990s.

The reform of the mental health system in Belize, one of the most innovative in the Americas, proved that it is possible to successfully and significantly improve mental health care in a country with very limited resources. It is also a good example of the fundamental role played by strategies to generate political commitment in a process of mental health reform.

(continued)

The reform, initiated in the beginning of the 1990s, has developed through different phases, which we describe below.

First Phase (1992–2004)

In the beginning of the 1990s, mental health care in Belize continued to be almost exclusively provided by Rockview Hospital. There were neither community mental health services nor any psychiatric units at general hospitals. Mental health care was not integrated in primary care services. Mental health legislation was still based on the antiquated laws established during British rule, ignoring all the advances made in the last decades in the protection of the rights of people with mental disorders.

The change that occurred at that time, and it was really a significant change in relation to the past, consisted in the government recognizing that some action was urgently needed to improve mental health care. There were three main reasons for the government's changed attitude in relation to mental health care. First, the contact of professionals with new models of care developed in countries like Canada and Jamaica, where mental health care had been decentralized, had encouraged an increasing number of people in Belize to advocate for changes in the country's mental health services. Second, after the Caracas Declaration (which was issued at the Regional Conference for the Restructuring of Psychiatric Care in Latin America, held in Caracas, Venezuela, in 1990), projects of reorganizing mental health services had been undertaken in several Central American countries, and the effects of these developments in neighboring countries could not fail to be felt in Belize. Finally, through the technical cooperation provided by the Pan American Health Organization (PAHO) and other international organizations, several activities had been developed that contributed to increasing the knowledge in Belize about the importance of mental health problems and the best ways to manage these problems.

Confronted with the need to improve mental health care, the Ministry of Health did not have many options. The existing psychiatric hospital was so deteriorated that it was not justifiable to invest in its recovery. With just one, and at intervals two, psychiatrists and very few nurses with psychiatric training, and with a large part of the population living very far from the capital city, the only possible way to facilitate access to mental health care passed through the training of non-medical professionals and through assigning them the responsibility for a significant part of mental health care.

It was in this context that the Ministry of Health decided to embark on a program to train nurses in psychiatric care in order to develop community-based mental health care, which would be provided by Psychiatric Nurse Practitioners (PNPs) with supervision from psychiatrists. The program was developed through financial support from the Canadian International Development Agency (CIDA). The curriculum, developed by the faculty from Memorial University in Newfoundland, Canada, aimed at giving the nurses the skills they would need to treat people with mental disorders in the community. In 1992, 16 PNPs completed a ten-month training program and started working in different locations throughout the country. Their work consisted of providing mental health care in outpatient clinics, conducting home visits, and providing mental health education in schools and in the community.[47] The psychiatrist regularly visited the PNP teams to provide clinical supervision, work that would later be supported by a tele-psychiatry program.

Three years later, an evaluation of the PNP program showed a high level of satisfaction felt by patients treated by the PNPs, and revealed that the PNPs felt they had been well prepared by the program for the tasks for which they were responsible.[47] The success of the program contributed to creating a momentum that was crucial for the generation of additional support for mental health reform in Belize, both at the national and the international level. Internally, this success was fundamental to strengthening the individuals and the groups previously engaged in promoting change, and encouraged them to propose further steps in the process of reform. At the international level, it helped attract the interest of several organizations in supporting an experience of community-based care undertaken with very few resources, which seemed to have the potential to be replicated in other countries with similar characteristics.

The involvement of Mrs. Kathy Esquivel, the First Lady, in the advocacy movement had a particularly important role, confirming the effectiveness of the integration of champions in the generation of political commitment. Her participation in a mental health conference promoted by Mrs. Rosalynn Carter, and specially the impressive way she presented the Belize experience at this conference, helped give more visibility to this experience at the international level, as well as to mobilize new technical and financial support for mental health reform in Belize.

On the other hand, the fact that the First Lady of Belize assumed the leadership of the Mental Health Advisory Board (MHAB) in 1997 was instrumental in making this body an important instrument of advocacy. The mission of the MHAB was to advise the Ministry of Health on mental health care issues and to develop advocacy activities. It included representatives from different ministries and mental health professionals and organizations. In 1998, it successfully lobbied for the decriminalization of attempted suicide. After being transformed into the national Mental Health Association, a nonprofit organization, in following a change of government, it had a key role in raising funds from the Japanese Small-Scale Grant Assistance Program. This made possible, in 2001, the development of the first acute psychiatric unit within a Belizean general hospital, in Belmopan. It had also an important role in the promotion of campaigns against depression and the development of initiatives to generate the commitment of policy makers in the implementation of mental health reform.

In 1997, a project to strengthen community-based mental health care in Belize was officially integrated into the WHO Nations for Mental Health Program.[48] The project, which included technical cooperation and financial support, was implemented by the Ministry of Health and the Pan American Health Organization/WHO. In 2002 it had contributed to several important achievements:

- A mental health advisory board with its own terms of reference was established.
- Community mental health training workshops were implemented.
- Mobile psychiatric units were set up in the villages most in need.
- A community education committee for mental health was established.
- A media strategy for mental health was implemented.
- The referral system for mental health problems was reorganized.
- Forms for reporting mental health problems and for admission and discharge to and from hospitals were updated.
- A plan was developed to reorganize the psychiatric and mental health services with an emphasis on deinstitutionalization.

This partnership with PAHO/ WHO played a key role in the first phase of the mental health reform in Belize. However, other partnerships were also established in this phase. As mentioned above, partnerships with Japanese resulted in infrastructure improvements, and partnerships with American and Canadian institutions resulted

(continued)

in personnel development. The relationship with the Homewood Foundation, a Canadian NGO, was particularly fruitful, having contributed to training opportunities of professionals in Canada, development of training materials, and the launching of a tele-psychiatry project.

Second Phase (2004–2008)

In the beginning of the new millennium, despite the advances registered in the development of community-based care, Belize still faced three major problems in mental health care. First, to ensure the sustainability of the community care provided by the PNP program: Some of the nurses trained in 1992 had left; it was necessary to create mechanisms guaranteeing the regular training of new professionals. On the other hand, the experience of the previous years had showed that it was indispensable to strengthen the teams led by the PNPs in order to improve the integration of these teams in primary care, and it was necessary to consolidate the supervision of clinical activities.

Second, the structural deficiencies of Rockview Hospital were so pronounced, and its facilities had reached such a high level of deterioration, that it was obvious the solution to Rockview's problems involved the closure of the hospital and its replacement by other facilities, preferably in the community.

Finally, there remained the problem of the lack of adequate legislation protecting the human rights of people with mental disorders. Thanks to the efforts by the groups advocating the consolidation of the mental health reform, the Ministry of Health, in collaboration with the University of Belize, promoted, in 2004, a new training program to integrate more PNPs in the mental health system. With this program, 13 new PNPs graduated and were integrated into the network of community mental health services.

By the end of the 1990s, the government had already recognized that the conditions at Rockview Hospital were clearly unacceptable, recognizing the need to close down the hospital and to replace it with an acute psychiatric unit within a general hospital, a day hospital in Belize City, and sheltered housing for the chronically ill patients nearer to or within Belize City.

The creation in 2001 of an acute psychiatric unit in Belmopan General Hospital had represented a first step in the creation of alternatives for the inpatient treatment of acute patients. However, a lot of work remained to be done in the creation of better alternatives for Rockview, and views on how to ensure the creation of these alternatives differed significantly.

These differences reached a critical point when the government announced its intention of building a new psychiatric hospital near Belmopan, using funds available in the framework of a project intended for the development of new structures in the country. The representatives of professionals, users, and families opposed this project, arguing that concentrating the inpatient treatment of all psychiatric patients once again in a single institution, separated from the general health system, and in a location away from the community, ran a huge risk of reproducing once more the custodial model of Rockview.

Confronted with the pressure from the advocacy groups, the government decided to request an external evaluation of the mental health situation in Belize and to organize a national debate on the best ways to continue mental health reform.

In the end of 2004, with the support from PAHO, an international expert carried out an evaluation of the mental health situation, and, in February 2005, two workshops, one on human rights and mental health legislation and another on mental health policy and services, took place in Belize City. The workshops counted with the participation of Ministry of Health personnel, personnel from Rockview Hospital, the Association of Consumers and Families, as well as other relevant NGO's (disability, human rights, mental health, etc.), and staff from PAHO. The workshops led to the following recommendations:

- Formulation of a national mental health policy and plan, and updating of the mental health legislation
- Creation of the National Mental Health Committee
- Implementation of the National Mental Health Plan
- Reorganization of services, with five main objectives: closing Rockview Hospital, strengthening of the CMHC, creating a psychiatric unit at Karl Heusner Memorial Hospital, creating residential facilities for patients discharged from Rockview Hospital and for new chronic patients, and developing day centers in the different sectors of the country.
- Program against stigma

The developments that took place in the following years proved that the external evaluation and the national debate carried out through the workshops proved to be effective strategies for reaching a general consensus on the objectives that should be prioritized and for ensuring a strong commitment on the part of the government.

In May of 2007, the National Mental Health Committee had drafted its Mental Health Policy. In that same year, important steps were taken in the collection of data essential for the planning, evaluation, and monitoring of mental health services. On one hand, relevant information on the country's mental health system was gathered through the WHO–AIMS project (WHO and Ministry of Health Belize, 2009). On the other hand, mental health information was integrated in the computerized health information system.

In 2008, with the establishment of a day hospital within the premises of the Port Loyola Centre, another important objective of the reorganization of services was attained. Thanks to this new service, provided by a team including PNPs, a social worker, and an occupational therapist, it became possible to offer rehabilitation programs in Belize City. On October 18, 2008, with the transfer of the last 38 patients in Rockview Hospital to a sheltered housing facility in Belmopan, the Palm Center, the Rockview Hospital, symbol of the old custodial mental health care, was finally closed.

Third Phase (2008–2012)

After the closure of the mental hospital, a new program started in Belize City, designated the Community Treatment Program (CTP). This program was introduced to address the needs of individuals who are discharged from the mental hospital, have persistent mental illness, and are living in the community.

The CTP staff were originally working at the mental hospital. When it was closed down, they were retrained to work in the community. The program's objective is to provide practical assistance at home, on the streets, or anywhere in the community, including such aspects as medication management, self-care, recreation, leisure, and medical support, among others. The program handles around 80 patients, female and male.

It is also worth noting that during this phase the Ministry of Health established a dedicated budget for the Mental Health Program and created an Operational structure

(continued)

for program implementation within the Ministry. The other objectives of the third and current phase are the updating of the mental health legislation, the strengthening of community-based services, the establishment of emergency psychiatric services in all district hospitals, and the development of a mental health disasters plan.

Why it worked in Belize

In little more than twenty years, Belize radically transformed its mental health services, improving in a significant way the access to and the quality of mental health services. To implement the changes that made this progress possible, it was necessary to generate the commitment of policy makers and international donors at several stages of the process.

Different factors can be invoked to explain the success in generating political and donor commitment in this process. The existence of clear leadership in the implementation of the reform was certainly a major factor in its success. It facilitated the definition of priorities and made possible the creation of consensus between the different stakeholders.

The capacity to establish alliances and partnerships, both at the national and the international level, was also of utmost importance. It was this capacity that allowed the building of a strong network to defend the reform, including professionals, users, families, and NGOs, and contributed to attracting the interest of so many international organizations. The power of the people involved was, therefore, the key factor in this process, confirming the lessons taken from similar processes.

The power of facts was also confirmed in Belize. Identifying the problems existing in the Belizean mental health system and presenting evidence of effective strategies to overcome those problems proved to be a good strategy to persuade policy makers and donors to support the reform. In this respect, proving that it had been possible to significantly improve mental health care through the PNP program was particularly effective, because it showed to policy makers and donors that it is worth investing in mental health in Belize.

Finally, the use of opportunities offered by the health sector reform, that took place in Belize in the 1990s, proved also to be an effective strategy for generating political commitment to the implementation of the mental health reform.

Synopsis

First Phase

1992	Establishment of Psychiatric Nurse Practioners (PNP) Community Mental Health Program.
1995	Evaluation of the PNP program revealed high level of satisfaction of patients receiving care provided by the program.
1997	First Lady, Mrs. Kathy Esquivel, presents the Belize reform at a Mental Health Conference invited by Mrs. Rosalynn Carter and subsequently leads the formation of the National Mental Health Advisory Board.
	WHO Nations for Mental Health integrates a demonstration project in Belize aiming at the strengthening of community mental health care.
1998	Mental Health Advisory Board is reorganized into a nonprofit organization, the Mental Health Association.

Thanks to lobbying from Mental Health Association, attempted suicide is decriminalized.

2001 Launching of the first Community Mental Health Project funded by PAHO/WHO.

First acute psychiatric unit within a general hospitals created in Belmopan, with funds from Japan raised by the Mental Health Association.

Second Phase

2004 Second training program for PNP conducted to integrate a greater number of PNPs in the mental health services: 13 new PNPs graduate.

First workshop on human rights is conducted with support from PAHO.

Government asks for an assessment of the mental health program. With PAHO collaboration, an international consultant makes a comprehensive evaluation of the program and presents recommendations for the future.

2005 Workshop on mental health policy and services is organized by the Ministry of Health with participation of professionals, users, and families and support from PAHO. Main recommendations include the development of a mental health policy and the replacement of Rockview Hospital by community service.

Second workshop on mental health legislation and human rights. Recommendations include the updating of the mental health legislation.

2007 Belize's Mental Health Policy approved by the Ministry of Health.

Mental health information integrated in the computerized health information system.

Baseline information on mental health system in Belize gathered with the WHO–AIMS.

Development of the Mental Health Training Manual for Police Officers.

2008 Rockview Psychiatric Hospital is closed down.

The last 38 patients from the Psychiatric Hospital are transferred to Palm Center, a sheltered housing facility located in Belmopan.

Day Hospital is established at the Port Loyola health center.

Establishment of the Community Treatment Program (CTP) in Belize, to address the needs of persons with long-term mental disorders living in the community.

Third Phase

2011 Training of 170 Community Health Nurses in collaboration with PAHO, the University of West Indies, and the Mental Health Reform Research Trust of the Royal Free Hospital in London.

Integrating Mental Health into Primary Health Care in the Caribbean: A demonstration project in Belize and in Dominica.

Annual mental health consumer workshops.

2013 Passing of new mental health legislation.

CONCLUSIONS

Important advances have occurred in mental health advocacy at the global level in recent years. These advances were possible because scientific progress contributed to changing the perception we have today of mental health issues, and because strong networks were created with the participation of professional and scientific associations, users and families, NGOs, universities, governments, and international organizations.

The contribution of the human rights movement has been key in this process. It helped focus the objectives of the global health movement on some key rights, such as the right to the highest attainable standard of physical and mental health (including access to appropriate and professional services, the right to individualized treatment, the right to rehabilitation and treatment that enhances autonomy, the right to community-based services, the right to the least-restrictive services), the right to liberty and security, freedom from discrimination, and freedom from inhuman and degrading treatment.

These values, together with the available evidence on the impact of mental disorders, the treatment gap and the human rights violations that continue to exist across the world, created the basis of compelling arguments that have been successfully used in favor of a new attention to mental health.

Our understanding of the factors that influence the capacity to generate political commitment for action in the area of mental health has also significantly increased. Therefore, we are now in a better situation than we were twenty years ago: we have strong values, sound scientific evidence, and experience with developing a process to generate political commitment.

However, the problems that we will have to face in the near future are huge. New policy and clinical responses are needed to address the increasing frequency of psychiatric morbidity and psychosocial problems among vulnerable populations, and the competition for resources with other sectors is expected to become more difficult in the future.

In this context, generating political commitment is one of the most important challenges for global mental health. To address this challenge, we need to develop capacity, share best experiences, and find new and more effective ways of developing international cooperation in this field.

REFERENCES

1. Catford J. Creating political will: moving from the science to the art of health promotion. *Health Promot Int.* 2006;**21**(1):1–4. Epub 2006/02/03.
2. Shiffman J. Generating political will for safe motherhood in Indonesia. *Soc Sci Med.* 2003;**56**(6):1197–207. Epub 2003/02/26.
3. Shiffman J. Generating political priority for maternal mortality reduction in 5 developing countries. *Am J Public Health.* 2007;**97**(5):796–803. Epub 2007/03/31.
4. Shiffman J, Smith S. Generation of political priority for global health initiatives: a framework and case study of maternal mortality. *Lancet.* 2007;**370**(9595):1370–9. Epub 2007/10/16.
5. Williams R. Setting the agenda—The interaction between research and the strategic leadership of child and adolescent mental health services. *Curr Opin Psychiatr.* 1997;**10**(4):265–7.
6. Patel V, Boyce N, Collins PY, Saxena S, Horton R. A renewed agenda for global mental health. *Lancet.* 2011;**378**(9801):1441–2. Epub 2011/10/20.
7. Lezine DA, Reed GA. Political will: a bridge between public health knowledge and action. *Am J Public Health.* 2007;**97**(11):2010–3. Epub 2007/09/29.
8. Lund C. Mental health policy development. In: Patel V, Minas H, Cohen A, Prince M, editors. *Global mental health: Principles and practice.* Oxford: Oxford University Press; 2014.
9. World Health Organization. *Mental Health Atlas 2011.* Geneva: World Health Organization; 2011.
10. Cohen A. A brief history of global mental health. In: Patel V, Minas H, Cohen A, Prince M, editors. *Global mental health: Principles and practice.* Oxford: Oxford University Press; 2014.

11. World Health Assembly. *The global burden of mental disorders and the need for a comprehensive, coordinated response from health and social sectors at the country level. WHA A65/R4.* Geneva: World Health Organization; 2012.

12. Jacob KS, Sharan P, Mirza I, Garrido-Cumbrera M, Seedat S, Mari JJ, et al. Mental health systems in countries: where are we now? *Lancet.* 2007;**370**(9592):1061–77.

13. Patel V, Araya R, Chatterjee S, Chisholm D, Cohen A, De Silva M, et al. Treatment and prevention of mental disorders in low-income and middle-income countries. *Lancet.* 2007;**370**(9591): 991–1005.

14. Prince M, Patel V, Saxena S, Maj M, Maselko J, Phillips MR, et al. No health without mental health. *Lancet.* 2007;**370**(9590):859–77.

15. Saraceno B, van Ommeren M, Batniji R, Cohen A, Gureje O, Mahoney J, et al. Barriers to improvement of mental health services in low-income and middle-income countries. *Lancet.* 2007;**370**(9593):1164–74.

16. Saxena S, Thornicroft G, Knapp M, Whiteford H. Resources for mental health: scarcity, inequity, and inefficiency. *Lancet.* 2007;**370**(9590):878–89.

17. Lancet Global Mental Health Group. Scale up services for mental disorders: a call for action. *Lancet.* 2007;**370**(9594):1241–52.

18. Eaton J, McCay L, Semrau M, Chatterjee S, Baingana F, Araya R, et al. Scale up of services for mental health in low-income and middle-income countries. *Lancet.* 2011;**378**(9802):1592–603. Epub 2011/10/20.

19. Kakuma R, Minas H, van Ginneken N, Dal Poz MR, Desiraju K, Morris JE, et al. Human resources for mental health care: current situation and strategies for action. *Lancet.* 2011;**378**(9803):1654–63. Epub 2011/10/20.

20. Drew N, Funk M, Tang S, Lamichhane J, Chavez E, Katontoka S, et al. Human rights violations of people with mental and psychosocial disabilities: an unresolved global crisis. *Lancet.* 2011;**378**(9803):1664–75. Epub 2011/10/20.

21. Tol WA, Barbui C, Galappatti A, Silove D, Betancourt TS, Souza R, et al. Mental health and psychosocial support in humanitarian settings: linking practice and research. *Lancet.* 2011;**378**(9802):1581–91. Epub 2011/10/20.

22. Kieling C, Baker-Henningham H, Belfer M, Conti G, Ertem I, Omigbodun O, et al. Child and adolescent mental health worldwide: evidence for action. *Lancet.* 2011;**378**(9801):1515–25. Epub 2011/10/20.

23. Benegal V, Chand PK, Obot IS. Packages of care for alcohol use disorders in low- and middle-income countries. *PLoS Med.* 2009;**6**(10):e1000170. Epub 2009/10/28.

24. de Jesus MJ, Razzouk D, Thara R, Eaton J, Thornicroft G. Packages of care for schizophrenia in low- and middle-income countries. *PLoS Med.* 2009;**6**(10):e1000165. Epub 2009/10/21.

25. Flisher AJ, Sorsdahl K, Hatherill S, Chehil S. Packages of care for attention-deficit hyperactivity disorder in low- and middle-income countries. *PLoS Med.* 2010;**7**(2):e1000235. Epub 2010/02/27.

26. Mbuba CK, Newton CR. Packages of care for epilepsy in low- and middle-income countries. *PLoS Med.* 2009;**6**(10):e1000162. Epub 2009/10/14.

27. Patel V, Simon G, Chowdhary N, Kaaya S, Araya R. Packages of care for depression in low- and middle-income countries. *PLoS Med.* 2009;**6**(10):e1000159. Epub 2009/10/07.

28. Patel V, Thornicroft G. Packages of care for mental, neurological, and substance use disorders in low- and middle-income countries: PLoS Medicine Series. *PLoS Med.* 2009;**6**(10):e1000160. Epub 2009/10/07.

29. Prince MJ, Acosta D, Castro-Costa E, Jackson J, Shaji KS. Packages of care for dementia in low-and middle-income countries. *PLoS Med.* 2009;**6**(11):e1000176. Epub 2009/11/06.

30. World Health Organization. The WHO mental health policy and service guidance package. Available from: http://www.who.int/mental_health/policy/essentialpackage1/en/index.html.

31. Fox AM, Goldberg AB, Gore RJ, Barnighausen T. Conceptual and methodological challenges to measuring political commitment to respond to HIV. *J Int AIDS Soc.* 2011;**14** Suppl 2:S5. Epub 2011/10/14.

32. Goldberg AB, Fox AM, Gore RJ, Barnighausen T. Indicators of political commitment to respond to HIV. *Sex Transm Infect.* 2012;**88**(2):e1. Epub 2012/02/22.

33. Patterson D. Political commitment, governance, and HIV/AIDS. *Can HIV AIDS Policy Law Rev.* 2001;**6**(1-2):39–45.

34. Chemtob D, Kaluski DN. Political commitment and public health prioritization. *IMAJ.* 2002;**4**(3):234. Epub 2002/03/23.

35. World Mental Health Day. Available from: http://www.wfmh.org/00WorldMentalHealthDay. htm.

36. Kessler R, Aguilar-Gaxiola S, Alonso J, Chatterji S, Lee S, Ormel J, et al. The global burden of mental disorders: an update from the WHO World Mental Health (WMH) surveys. *Epidemiol Psichiatr Soc.* 2009;**18**(1):23–33.

37. Herrman H, Saxena S, Moodie R, editors. *Promoting mental health: concepts, emerging evidence, practice: A report of the World Health Organization, Department of Mental Health and Substance Abuse in collaboration with the Victorian Health Promotion Foundation and the University of Melbourne.* Geneva: World Health Organization; 2005.

38. World Health Organization. *The World Health Report 2001—Mental health: New understanding, new hope.* Geneva: World Health Organization; 2001.

39. Caldas de Almeida J, Horvitz-Lennon M. Mental health care reforms in Latin America: an overview of mental health care reforms in Latin America and the Caribbean. *Psychiatr Serv.* 2010;**61**(3):218–21.

40. Caldas de Almeida J. Mental health services for victims of disasters in developing countries: a challenge and an opportunity. *World Psychiatry* 2003;**2**(3):155–7.

41. United Nations. *The Millennium Development Goals report 2012.* New York: United Nations; 2012.

42. Minas H. Human security, complexity and mental health system development. In: Patel V, Prince M, Cohen A, Minas H, editors. *Global mental health: Principles and practice.* Oxford: Oxford University Press; 2014.

43. President of the General Assembly. *Political declaration of the High-Level Meeting of the General Assembly on the prevention and control of non-communicable diseases. A/66/L.1.* New York: United Nations General Assembly; 2011.

44. World Health Organization. *Global burden of mental disorders and the need for a comprehensive, coordinated response from health and social sectors at the country level. A/65/10.* Geneva: World Health Organization; 2012.

45. International Planned Parenthood Federation. *Generating political change: Using advocacy to create political commitment.* London: International Planned Parenthood Federation; 2009.

46. Collins PY. Research priorities, capacity and networks in global mental health In: Patel V, Minas H, Cohen A, Prince M, editors. *Global mental health: principles and practice.* Oxford: Oxford University Press; 2014.

47. Government of Belize. *Identification of best practices in primary care.* Belmopan, Belize: Mental Health Program, Ministry of Health; 2007.

48. World Health Organization. *Nations for mental health. Final report.* Geneva: World Health Organization; 2002.

Index

Made in the USA
Middletown, DE
03 January 2025

68738578R00285